Medical Association

HAMILTON

Physical Signs

Demonstrations of Physical Signs in Clinical Surgery

D1342540

HAMILTON BAILEY'S

Physical Signs

Demonstrations of Physical Signs in Clinical Surgery

18th Edition

Professor John S P Lumley MS FRCS

Professor of Surgery
St Bartholomew's Hospital
London

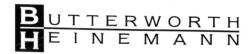
BUTTERWORTH
HEINEMANN

Butterworth–Heinemann
Linacre House, Jordan Hill, Oxford OX2 8DP
A division of Reed Educational and Professional Publishing Ltd

A member of the Reed Elsevier plc group

OXFORD • BOSTON • JOHANNESBURG • MELBOURNE • NEW DELHI • SINGAPORE

First published 1927
Second edition 1930
Third edition 1931
Fourth edition 1933
Fifth edition 1935
Sixth edition 1937
Seventh edition 1940
Eighth edition 1942
Ninth edition 1944
Tenth edition 1946
Eleventh edition 1949
Twelfth edition 1954
Thirteenth edition 1960
Fourteenth edition 1967
Fifteenth edition 1973
Reprinted 1976, 1978
Sixteenth edition 1980
Reprinted 1984
Seventeenth edition 1986
Reprinted 1992
Eighteenth edition 1997

British Library Cataloguing in Publication Data
A catalogue record for this book is available from the British Library

Library of Congress Cataloguing in Publication Data
A catalogue record for this book is available from the Library of Congress

ISBN 0 7506 1621 0

Text Management: John Ormiston
Design and Illustration: edi The EDI Partnership
Layout artist: Jenni Miller

Printed and bound in Italy by Vincenzo Bona

Contents

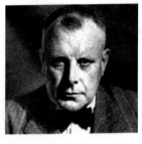

Hamilton Bailey 1894–1961

Born in Bishopstoke, Hampshire, where his father was a general practitioner, Henry Hamilton Bailey grew up in Southport, Eastbourne, and Brighton, England, where his father was successfully in practice. His mother was a nurse, so not surprisingly he became a medical student at the London Hospital at the early age of sixteen years, after schooling at St. Lawrence College, Ramsgate.

At the outbreak of the First World War he was a fourth-year medical student, and volunteered for the Red Cross, being dispatched with the British Expeditionary Force to Belgium. Almost inevitably he was taken prisoner-of-war and set to work on the German railways. A troop train was wrecked and Bailey, with two Frenchmen, was held on suspicion of sabotage. One of the latter was actually executed but Bailey was reprieved (apparently by the good offices of the American Ambassador in Berlin) and repatriated via Denmark, where he continued his medical studies temporarily.

In 1916 he joined the Royal Navy as a Surgeon-Probationer, serving in HMS Iron Duke at the Battle of Jutland. During the battle he helped with casualties in near darkness, the electricity supply being damaged for most of the action. While in the Navy he qualified, and later returned to the London Hospital, where he gained the FRCS (Eng) in 1920. During his period as surgical registrar at the London Hospital he pricked his left index finger, and tendon-sheath infection, a common sequel in those days, ensued. The end result was an amputation of the stiff finger, but he soon overcame the disability.

Appointments as Assistant Surgeon at Liverpool Royal Infirmary, Surgeon to Dudley Road Hospital, Birmingham (1925), and finally as Surgeon to the Royal Northern Hospital, London (1931) followed.

In a quarter of a century Bailey produced this work, his *Emergency Surgery*, and *Short Practice of Surgery* [jointly with R.J. McNeill Love (1891–1974), contemporary as a surgical registrar at the London Hospital and as a Surgeon at the Royal Northern Hospital], edited *Surgery of Modern Warfare* during the Second World War, and revitalized *Pye's Surgical Handicraft*. These were his most successful works; all rapidly attained a wide circulation with many editions, and it has been said '... it will readily be conceded that the present excellence of illustrations in medical textbooks owes much to his inspiration and striving for perfection'. In addition to these major contributions, he wrote over 130 original papers and nine other books.

All this, together with a busy practice, particularly in surgical emergencies, was too much even for Hamilton Bailey's massive frame, and in 1948 he suffered a breakdown in health, aggravated, no doubt, by the death of his only child, a son, in a railway accident in 1943. He retired to Deal, Kent, and later to Malaga, Spain, but continued his literary work. He died of carcinoma of the colon, and is buried in the peaceful little English cemetery in Malaga. His missionary zeal for teaching medical students has been perpetuated by the use of the royalties from his books to expand medical libraries in developing countries.

Contributors

Dominic Corry, BSc FRCS
Specialist Registrar, General Surgery, Royal London Hospital
Chapters 18, 21–26

Athanasios D Giannoukas, MSc MD
Consultant Vascular Surgeon, University of Crete Medical School
Chapters 28, 29

Fares S Haddad, BSc FRCS FRCS(Ed)
Senior Orthopaedic Registrar, Royal National Orthopaedic Hospital, London
Chapter 30

Simon A V Holmes, MS FRCS(Urol)
Consultant Urological Surgeon, St Mary's Hospital, Portsmouth
Chapter 27

Philip Hornick, BSc MB BChir FRCS(Eng)
Department of Cardiothoracic Surgery, Royal Postgraduate Medical School,
Hammersmith Hospital, London
Chapters 19, 20

Eleanor A Ivory, MA FRCS(Ed)
Specialist Registrar, Accident and Emergency, Princess Margaret Hospital, Swindon
Chapter 7

John P Ivory, MA FRCS(Orth)
Consultant Orthopaedic Surgeon, Princess Margaret Hospital, Swindon
Chapters 31–40

John S P Lumley, MS FRCS
Professor of Surgery, St Bartholomew's Hospital, London
Chapters 1–4, 6–8, 19, 28, 31

Peter J Lunniss, BSc MS FRCS
Senior Lecturer, St Bartholomew's and the Royal London School of Medicine and Dentistry
Chapters 21–26

M H H Nordeen, MA BM MCh(Orth) FRCS(Orth)
Consultant Orthopaedic and Spinal Surgeon, Royal National Orthopaedic Hospital and Great Ormond
Street Hospital for Children, London; Hon Senior Lecturer, University College, London
Chapter 30

Saeed M Rakha
Research Assistant, Surgical Unit, St Bartholomew's Hospital, London
Chapter 6

Lynn Riddell, BSc MBChB MRCP(London)
Research Registrar, Immunology Department, St Bartholomew's Hospital, London
Chapter 5

Sandip Sarkar, FRCS
Specialist Registrar, Royal National Orthopaedic Hospital, London
Chapters 31–40

Paul D Srodon, FRCS
Lecturer in Surgery, St Bartholomew's Hospital, London
Chapters 9–17

Preface to the Eighteenth Edition

Hamilton Bailey was a great teacher and the most prolific medical author of his generation; at the height of his output he had six full-time secretaries working on his books. Although he died more than 30 years ago, Vita Bailey, his wife and partner in the illustrative material in his books, died only recently (since the seventeenth edition of this text was published). One of the great innovations of the Hamilton Bailey books was the use of photography and added colouring: this was, to a large extent, Vita's personal contribution. After Hamilton Bailey's death, Vita maintained a close watch on his books and directed their royalties into ongoing medical charities. As the first recipient of the Hamilton Bailey Travelling Fellowship of The International College of Surgeons, and having had the great delight of listening to many of Vita Bailey's reminiscences, it will come as no surprise to the reader that I dedicate the present edition to her memory.

This 18th edition is the most radical revision of Hamilton Bailey's *Physical Signs* since its first publication in 1927. The aim of the book is still the demonstration and discussion of abnormal physical signs. In keeping with previous editions, little attempt has been made to cover the investigation and treatment of disease. Standard examination techniques are summarized at the beginning of each section. More details of the examination of each system can be obtained in the companion volume *Clinical Examination of the Patient* (Lumley and Bouloux, Butterworth–Heinemann), together with sections on psychiatric assessment, normal laboratory values, and a glossary of medical terms. A number of figures have been duplicated from this text.

The desire to streamline the book, while retaining all factual material, necessitated four changes of policy. It was not possible to cover exhaustively every abnormal physical sign; the annotated derivation of every sign has been removed; some rare diseases have not been included; and all black and white illustrations from the original edition have been removed.

The purist will mourn the loss of footnotes and it is sad to see the disappearance of some of the most memorable illustrations, such as the smiling psychiatric patient with a pin-filled left arm, debauched noses and the inflammatory lesions touched-up by Vita's artwork. However, these illustrations had become very out-dated and the Baileys would have been delighted to use the full colour potential of modern publishing software and printing techniques.

The ease of world-wide travel has meant that all clinicians must be aware of the features of tropical and other regional diseases. Tropical conditions have therefore been included as a separate chapter and grouped by their common presenting symptoms. The chapter on multiple injuries is also new. This chapter differs from the rest of the text in that it includes therapeutic measures, since the clinical status of the severely injured patient is in continuous change, and urgent treatment has to begin alongside clinical assessment. The chapter incorporates the basic principles enumerated in the Advance Trauma Life Support (ATLS) system.

The inclusion of a chapter on HIV and AIDS reflects the world-wide increased incidence and the importance of this condition. We are grateful for the help of Mark Holbert and Catriona Good with this section, and for the slides contributed by other experts. In particular, we pay our tribute to the great surgical contribution made by the late Adrian Tanner. His premature death has deprived both patients and doctors of his skills and dedication to this field.

The bulk of the illustrative material has come from the slide collection at St Bartholomew's Hospital, and we are grateful to the clinicians and photographers who have contributed to this collection over the last half century. As the prime function of this text is the demonstration of abnormal physical signs, pathological and radiological illustrations have been kept to a minimum. The exception is the radiological demonstration of bony and lung abnormalities, since these appearances are usually diagnostic.

Seven orthopaedic illustrations have been reproduced from Apley and Solomon's text, *Physical Examination in Orthopaedics*, and we are grateful to authors and publishers for this material. The recent death of Allan Apley was a sad loss to the surgical community. He, like Hamilton Bailey, was renowned for his clinical teaching and his textbooks. *Figure 30.12* shows Apley, as he was known to so many, enthusiastically demonstrating physical signs.

The evolution of radiological imaging in recent years has provided the clinician with a wide range of diagnostic tools. The efficient use of these techniques, however, is dependent on a reliable initial clinical assessment. The skills of history taking and eliciting abnormal physical signs are thus as important today as in Hamilton Bailey's time. Developing clinical skills is largely dependent on clinical experience, but the identification of abnormalities requires a well-tried system, a keen eye, and a delicate touch.

This text is intended to direct and facilitate the acquisition of these skills. It introduces the reader to all common physical signs, so that they can subsequently be recognized in the clinical setting. The book is intended for medical students and surgeons in training world-wide.

John S P Lumley

1 History taking and general examination

History taking

A patient usually comes to see a doctor with a specific problem (symptom) and the doctor's aim is to make the patient better. To do this, the doctor tries to work out what is causing the problem (diagnosis), determine its severity (assessment) and then institute appropriate treatment. The total process of assessment and treatment is termed management.

Disease may be due to social and psychological as well as physical abnormalities – the surgeon must be aware of, and sensitive to, all of these factors. To diagnose and assess a patient's problems the doctor can obtain information from three sources:

- Take a history.
- Carry out a physical examination.
- Request appropriate investigations.

The history is the single most important factor in making a diagnosis. Although this text is primarily concerned with eliciting abnormal physical signs, these are not always present at the time a patient presents. The history directs the clinician to search for the physical abnormalities and find them at the earliest possible stage of the disease, thus facilitating further management.

The skilled clinician becomes an expert on the pattern of diseases but the greatest skill is to listen to what the patient volunteers. This is the key to the diagnosis and the clinician must not shape, elaborate, flavour or direct a history into a particular category just so that it fits a classical package. Such prompting may result in misdiagnosis.

Sometimes it is not possible to make a diagnosis. However, the process of assessment serves to exclude serious abnormalities, allowing the clinician to reassure the patient and advise symptomatic treatment. This strategy is based on the nature and duration of the symptoms and on the type of patient. It allays the patients' fears and avoids over-investigation of trivial and self-limiting disease.

A decision must be made, however, as to whether the patient needs to be seen again, and whether they are likely to default from attending. Explanations to the patient markedly depend on the outcome of any previous encounters and on their intelligence, education, background and personality. Occasionally management may have to be initiated before a definitive diagnosis is made, such as in the control of severe pain or haemorrhage.

The following scheme for history taking is intended as an introduction to the subject and outlines the prime headings that need to be considered when interviewing each patient.

Scheme for history taking

First record the **date** of the examination. Note the patient's **name**, **age**, **sex**, **occupation** (past and present) and **marital status** (including any children). The history emerges from the patient's description of the problem, directed by your planned questioning. It is conveniently recorded under the following six headings.

Present illness
Presenting complaint(s)
What brought you to hospital? This must be put in a short statement preferably in the patient's own words, for example c/o (complaining of) abdominal pain and vomiting for the last 24 hours; increasing breathlessness for 2 weeks. If there is more than one complaint, these are listed and then taken in turn through the following two sections.

History of present complaint(s)
This should record details of each problem, using mainly the patient's own words. Record as accurately as possible how long the complaint has been present and include the sequence of events in chronological order with dates (e.g. 1 year ago; 1 month ago; yesterday). Let the patient begin by telling the story in their own words without interrupting. Afterwards, ask specific questions, using terms readily understood by the patient, either enlarging upon or clarifying their symptoms.

The presenting disorder is usually related to one system and questions referable to this – and any other system involved in the presenting complaint – are delivered at this stage. Pain is one of the most common symptoms; appropriate questions are given below. Many of these questions can also be applied to other symptoms.

If the patient is a poor historian, unable to give a history, or you suspect is giving unreliable information, it may be helpful to talk to relatives or witnesses. Record the source of this and all aspects of the history that are not directly from the patient.

Previous history of present complaint(s)

If the patient has had similar symptoms in the past, obtain detailed information in chronological order, including any treatment received and the results of any investigations (if known). Report any past event with a clear bearing on the present condition, such as operations, trauma, weight loss, medication, contact with others with disease or any recent travel abroad.

Past medical history

Note all other previous non-trivial illnesses, operations, accidents and periods of admission to hospital for non-related illnesses, together with their dates. In children, note illnesses, investigations, and immunizations. In adults, note relevant childhood problems, for example chronic respiratory disease, cardiac problems and rheumatic fever.

Drugs and allergies

Note all drugs being taken, their doses and for how long they have been taken. Enquire what drugs have been taken in the past and for what conditions. Record drug allergies and any allergic symptoms. Ask what is meant by any admitted allergy.

Social and personal history

Note any current smoking habit, the number of years smoked and changes over this time. Note the usual alcohol consumption in units per day or per week and what is drunk. Question whether the subject has ever been a heavy drinker. Ask whether any recreational drugs are used.

Record details of work and, where relevant, any difficulties with job, family or finances. Note any recent mental stress or problems with sleeping pattern. Does the patient live alone? Which floor? Are there lifts? Is the lavatory on a different floor? Are friends and/or relatives nearby? Do they receive or need home help or meals on wheels? Will the patient be able to return to previous residence and/or employment?

Family history

Enquire of the state of health or cause of death of the patient's parents, siblings, other close relatives and spouse. Question whether any members of the family are suffering, or have suffered from the presenting condition(s). It often helps to draw a family tree.

Review of systems

The history of the present complaint encompasses a detailed enquiry of at least one of the systems of the body; this part of the history reviews the remaining systems for unsuspected abnormalities. It is carried out by the use of specific questioning pertinent to each system; these are considered with the examination of each system. Non-specific symptoms may also be present, such as fever, lassitude, malaise and weight change.

Pain

Pain is an indicator of disease and is frequently the presenting symptom in every body system. It varies with the disease process and the tissue involved, and may be characteristic and diagnostic. Pain may be present at the time of interview but – although this allows firsthand experience of the patient's problem – it can also interfere with the assessment.

Pain is very subjective and can be influenced by what the patient thinks or suspects its cause to be and its implications. They may have worries of the seriousness of a certain condition and because relatives or friends have been disabled or died from similar problems. They may want to impress or convince the doctor, or may underplay the symptom in order not to interfere with their own plans and needs. Responses to pain also vary with age, sex, ethnic origin, education and personality. A doctor should guard against categorizing and interpreting a pain to suit a chosen diagnosis and – even if leading questions are needed – there must be a free choice of answers.

Although friends and relatives can provide a good indication of how pain interferes with a patient's every day activities, they cannot describe features of the pain. In this respect use of interpreters can be difficult, since words used to describe the nature and severity of pain may have different meanings in different languages – the interpreter may be giving their own opinion rather than that of the patient. Also, patients may be unwilling to admit fears or disclose precipitating causes of a pain through an interpreter.

Each doctor must therefore develop an efficient and reliable method of questioning a patient about their pain, using clear, understandable language. The following section outlines the areas that need to be covered. It is worth studying these questions and reshuffling them into a form which you can easily remember, perhaps converting them into an acronym or an anagram.

Site

The site of the pain is a good indicator of its origin. Ask the patient where the pain is and to point to the area of maximum intensity. This may be **focal** and indicated with one finger, such as an infected maxillary air sinus or a fractured lateral malleolus. Injuries, in particular, can usually be localized by the site of the pain and tenderness (pain is what is experienced by the patient while tenderness is elicited by the examining doctor).

Pain arising from the skin and subcutaneous tissues is better localized than that from the deeper structures, as pain in the latter may be **diffuse**. Headache from an intracranial lesion may be indicated by the whole hand placed over the side or the top of the head. Similarly, cardiac pain may be demonstrated by a hand over the central chest wall, and abdominal pain over a quadrant of the abdomen. Severe limb ischaemia is another example of diffuse pain, the rest pain involving the forefoot or sometimes the whole foot and lower leg.

Pain may **radiate** from the site of origin to another region of the body, for example protrusion of an intervertebral disc may trap a nerve, giving local back pain, but also produce pain down the back of the thigh and possibly into the calf or foot. Pain from posterior abdominal wall structures – such as the pancreas and abdominal aorta – may radiate through to the back. Renal colic may radiate from the loin around to the iliac fossa and on to the groin. Gall bladder pain may be felt between the shoulder blades; the pain of myocardial infarction may radiate from the chest into the neck and down the left arm. The radiated pain may have different features from the local pain and it may occur independently.

Referred pain implies pain occurring at a site far removed from the originating disease. It is due to visceral nerve impulses stimulating the somatic afferent pathways of the same dermatome. A classic example is pain over the tip of the shoulder from disease under the diaphragm, the visceral nerve being the phrenic, and the somatic dermatome the fourth cervical.

Timing

When questioning the timing of a pain, include its onset, progress and offset. The **onset** may be sudden or gradual. Sudden pain is typical of that associated with injury, with blocking or rupture of an artery (as in myocardial infarction or ruptured abdominal aorta) and rupture of a viscus (such as a spontaneous pneumothorax or a perforated peptic ulcer). Most patients are be able to describe the precise time of onset in these examples.

Gradual onset times vary greatly. Acute inflammatory lesions may progress during a day or overnight, while claudication from degenerative arterial disease or the pain of osteoarthritic knees may take many years before the patient realizes that a vague ache is a specific problem and seeks medical advice. Gradual in these examples implies a gradual awareness of pain; it also indicates a gradual increase in the severity of pain.

Note the **progress** of the current attack, if it is changing and if there is any **pattern** to the pain. Pain may gradually increase or decrease, or become continuous or persistent. It may also fluctuate. There may be total relief between bouts. The latter is characteristic of **colic,** which is due to waves of contraction down an obstructed hollow viscus, such as with adhesions obstructing the small bowel, a cancer obstructing the large bowel or a stone blocking the ureter. Note how often these attacks occur and their duration. The pain may be continuous with exacerbations producing peaks of pain. Factors exacerbating or precipitating the pain are considered below (see Modification).

Enquire carefully about **previous** bouts of pain or anything similar in the past. Record the patterns of previous attacks, their frequency, how many in all and their duration. Note if they are changing in character. The terms exacerbation and recurrence are used to denote changes in disease as well as its symptoms.

Like the onset, the **offset** of pain may be gradual or sudden and this may be characteristic of the condition. Relief of pain usually indicates improvement of the disease or removal of the precipitating cause. Improvement may be obtained by treating with analgesics, surgically or with other therapies. Very occasionally, reduction of pain is a bad sign, e.g. the rupture of a tense abscess into the cerebral ventricles or the peritoneal cavity. The previous history and knowledge of any underlying disease can provide guidelines on the likelihood of further recurrence of the pain.

Severity

The quantity of pain is generally related to the severity of the underlying disease. However, individuals vary extensively in their pain tolerance and this is further influenced by anxiety and a fear of the possible implications of the pain. Sometimes there may be a desire to impress the doctor on the extent of the problem or conversely to play down the symptoms for some personal reason.

A useful indicator is the influence of the pain on the patient's lifestyle. Enquire whether they have had to stop work or go to bed, and whether they are losing sleep through the pain. If they have pain at the time of the interview, their response to it can be directly assessed. However, by this time they may have already had some appropriate analgesia.

A rough quantitative measure can be obtained from a pain scale of 1 to 10. The patient is asked to grade their pain on this scale, when 0 is no pain at all and 10 the worst possible pain imaginable. Although this is still very subjective, and dependent on the individual's response, it can be of value in assessing change within the individual.

Quality

The quality or nature of the pain is another subjective assessment, it may have specific characteristics but these are difficult to categorize. The terms used can be linked to previous experiences – common terms are sharp, stabbing or knife-like. Such terms are associated with most wounds.

Inflammation and pain from deeper organs are often described in less precise terms, such as aching, bruising, burning, gripping, crushing, twisting and breaking. Colic has already been referred to in gut obstruction when the patient may also complain of a distended or bloated feeling; this may also occur in childbirth and urinary retention.

A throbbing pain implies a tense, sensitive area with an increase of tension with each heart beat. Such situations can occur in vascular tumours, acute inflammation with or without an abscess, with raised intracranial pressure and vascular lesions, such as an expanding aneurysm or a complicated arteriovenous malformation or fistula.

Modification

Some of the factors precipitating and influencing a pain may have already been elicited by this stage in the history. Now ask the patient specifically what makes the pain worse or better, and what they do in an attack.

Aggravating factors include eating spicy foods (in peptic ulcers) and fatty foods (in biliary disease), movement such as coughing (in pleuritic pain and that due to peritonitis) or walking (in lower limb injuries or ischaemia), certain postures such as sitting and standing (with lumbar disc protrusions) and raising the leg (in severe foot ischaemia or sacral nerve root compression).

Relieving factors include analgesics and specific medication such as antacids. Eating may relieve the pain of duodenal ulcers, and resting a limb may ease inflammatory pain and that of injuries. The severe pain of lower limb ischaemia may be helped by hanging the leg out of bed.

The application of heat from a hot flannel, a fire or a hot water bottle is often used, and specific aids such as transcutaneous electrical nerve stimulation (TENS) can help. The repeated use of heat, such as a fire to the shins or a hot water bottle on the abdomen, may produce a characteristic mottled brown skin pigmentation (erythema ab igne), providing an important physical sign.

Remember that denervation may render an area insensitive and therefore subject to repeated trauma and inflammatory changes, without the protective benefit of pain sensation. Such examples are seen in a diabetic neuropathy where perforating ulcers are commonly seen over the pressure areas of the sole. Extreme examples are seen in leprosy where there can be progressive loss of digits and limbs.

Associated symptoms

Systemic effects of pain may be primary or secondary. Primary are specific events, such as the vomiting with peptic ulcers and the diarrhoea in inflammatory bowel disease. However, these same symptoms can be seen as non-specific effects in severe pain originating outside the alimentary tract. Similarly, nausea, malaise, sweating, loss of sleep and restricted fluid and food intake are frequently encountered.

Cause of pain

It is important to ask the patient's opinion on the cause of their pain. They may know or think they know what this is. They may be afraid or unwilling to tell you the cause as there may be a guilt complex, such as in current or previous self-abuse, but there may still be some hints as to the underlying cause of pain. Such clues must be carefully noted. The patient may well have given a lot of thought as to the potential causes of their pain and it is important to identify areas of anxiety which can often be treated by immediate reassurance.

General physical examination

When undertaking a physical examination, aim to keep a patient comfortable, relaxed and reassured. Talk through what is going to happen – if this is not obvious – and ensure minimal discomfort and inconvenience. A warm environment is essential and, similarly, the examiner's hands must be at a warm temperature. The privacy of a small room or a curtained area is desirable, with optimal – preferably natural – lighting.

The patient undresses down to underclothes and puts on a dressing gown. They then lie supine on a couch, with an adjustable back to provide head support, covered with a sheet or blanket. Each area must be adequately exposed as required without embarrassment to the patient. A cardinal principle is to expose both sides when examining paired structures in order to compare the diseased with the normal, e.g. a limb or breast. A chaperon may be appropriate when examining members of the opposite sex. Relatives are usually best excluded except when examining children.

The examiner stands on the right side of the patient. The order of examination is **regional** rather than by system, although the central nervous system is often examined as an entity, together with various parts of the locomotor system, at the end of the procedure.

It is usual to commence the examination with the hands and then to proceed methodically from head to toe, surveying all systems and later integrating these findings, as subsequent verbal presentations and recording in the notes are usually by system. Thoroughness is important – efficiency and speed develop with practice. The examination time should not be prolonged in ill or frail patients and, in emergencies, it may be appropriate to concentrate on diseased areas, completing a routine examination at a later time.

General impression

Throughout history taking the clinician is gaining an impression of the physical and mental status of the patient and the severity of his disability, as well as attempting to make a diagnosis. Physical examination continues these observations giving information on the patient's general state of health, his or her shape, posture, state of hygiene and mental and physical activity. The patient must be considered as a whole but initially the doctor should observe the exposed parts, particularly the hands, skin, head and neck.

The patient may be fit and well but problems with diet and disease can lead to alteration of nutrition and hydration such as obesity, weight loss, cachexia, loss of skin turgor and skin laxity. In the clinic it is important to weigh the patient; other factors that should be charted routinely are pulse rate, blood pressure and urine testing. A subject can usually state their height but accurate assessment may be important when considering endocrine abnormalities, together with measurements of segments and spans. Admission to hospital usually indicates more severe disease states and additional monitoring includes temperature, respiratory rates, bowel habit and the examination of sputum and faeces.

Mental status

A patient's behaviour may be influenced by the unaccustomed situation of being a patient or by the effect of his disease, particularly if there is pain. This may be manifest by facial expression, the degree of eye contact, restlessness, sweating, anxiety, apathy, depression, lack of co-operation or aggression. Stress may be indicated by rapid respiration, rapid pulse rate and sweating. Note whether the patient's intelligence and personality equate to what one would expect from the history or whether this could have changed in relation to the disease.

Drugs, head injuries and other diseases of the central nervous system can affect the level of consciousness, varying through alert, slow and confused, lacking concentration and reduced level of response to spoken and physical stimuli. The patient's orientation in time, place and person should be noted: the Glasgow coma scale (p. 157, *Table 9.1*) is a valuable way of documenting the level of consciousness for serial measurement. A patient's speech may be impaired by diseases of the central nervous system, producing dysphasia or dysarthria and there may be voice changes such as hoarseness in laryngeal infection or myxoedema. Impairment of motor function can produce weakness or spasticity and these may affect the speech.

The posture and gait should be noted and other activities, such as undressing. There may be added movements, such as the fine tremors of age, thyrotoxicosis, parkinsonism and alcoholism, the flapping tremors of hepatic, respiratory, renal and cardiac failure, or more specific neurological abnormalities producing lack of co-ordination and involuntary movements.

Psychiatric assessment is not usually part of a surgical examination but if abnormalities are present or suspected, note the general behaviour, disturbances of consciousness and orientation. Record the emotional state, the insight, thought processes and content, hallucinations, delusions and compulsive phenomena, and include an assessment of cognitive and intellectual function.

Abnormal facies and body configuration

A number of congenital and endocrine diseases have characteristic general features amenable to spot diagnosis. However, one needs experience to differentiate between minor changes and the extremes of normality, thus be aware of the danger of jumping to false conclusions. Congenital examples are Down's, Turner's and Marfan's syndromes, achondroplasia and hereditary telangiectasia. Endocrine abnormalities include acromegaly, Cushing's disease, myxoedema and thyrotoxicosis. Other spot diagnoses included Paget's disease, parkinsonism and myopathies (see *Chapter 2*). Some general disease states are added to the end of this chapter and include weight loss, dehydration, oedema and pyrexia of unknown origin, as well as examples from the above list. Other examples included elsewhere are the features of hepatic and renal failure.

The hands

The general examination starts with the hands: sweating or abnormal soft tissue may have been noted during the introductory hand shake. The hand may be unusually large as in acromegaly (*Figure 1.1*) or small or deformed, perhaps relating to a previous injury or to systemic disease. Skin abnormalities of the palm and dorsum of the hand are usually easier to see in a white-skinned individual but are usually visible in all races and should be carefully noted. They include pallor, cyanosis, polycythemia, pigmentation (*Figure 1.2*), bruises, rashes (*Figures 1.3 and 1.4*) and nicotine stains (*Figure 1.5*). Many of these features are more easily seen in the head and neck, and are further considered in the next section.

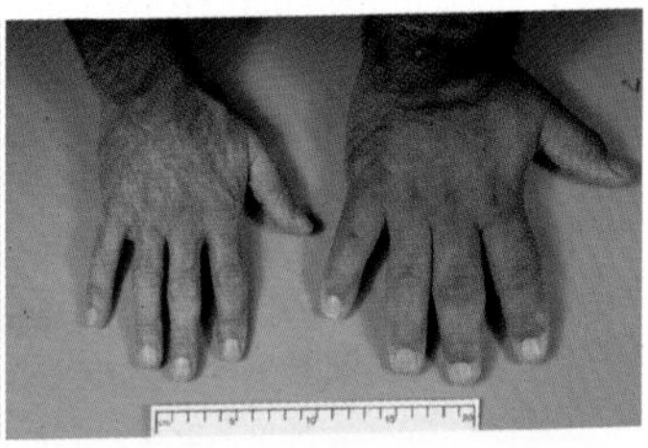

Figure 1.1. The acromegalic hand is large with wide long fingers.

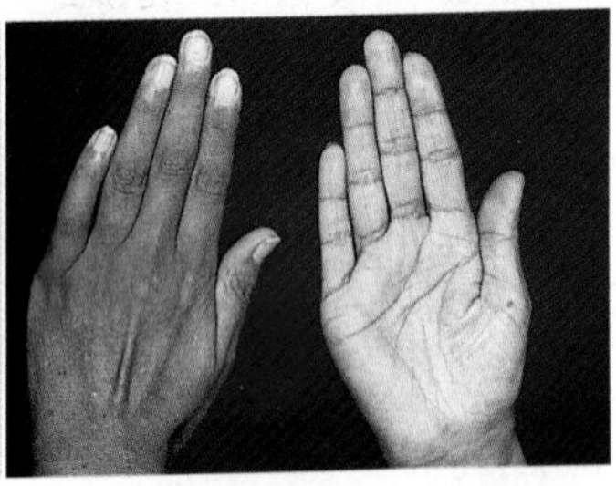

Figure 1.2. Skin pigmentation of the dorsum of the hand in a Caucasian patient with Nelson's syndrome.

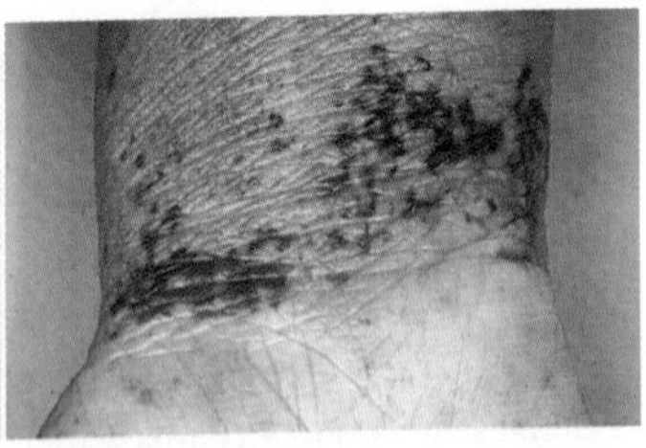

Figure 1.3. Hyperpigmentation of an area of atopic eczema on the wrist of a patient with Addison's disease.

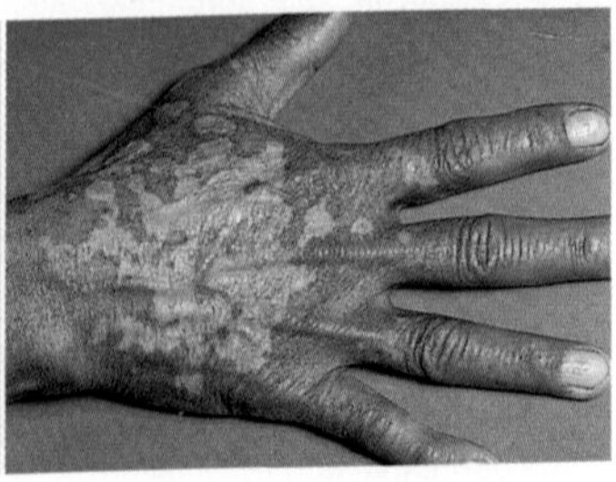

Figure 1.4. The rash on discoid lupus erythematosus of the dorsum of the hand.

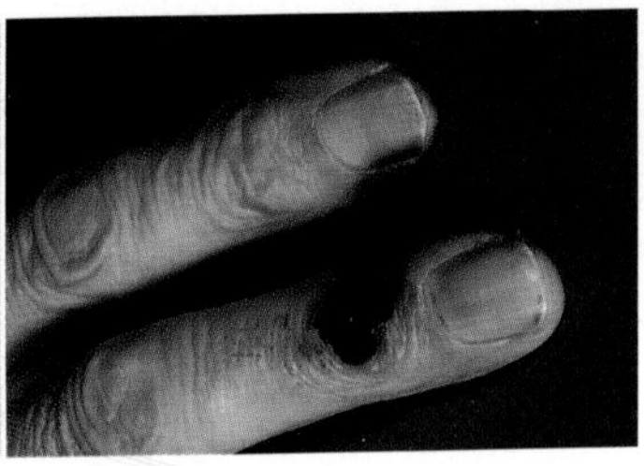

Figure 1.5. Nicotine-stained fingers of a chain smoker.

Nails

Nails can be an indicator of local and systemic disease. There can be stunted growth, and they may be brittle and deformed. Nail biters can be identified from the loss of the projecting nail in all the digits of both hands. Whitish spots (*Figure 1.6*) under the nail (leukonychia punctata) are associated with minor trauma. The pallor of anaemia (*Figure 1.7*) and hypoalbuminaemia, the colour of jaundice and cyanosis (*Figure 1.8*) are usually well shown, and pitting of the nails is common in psoriasis (*Figure 1.9*). Splinter haemorrhages (*Figure 1.10*) are longitudinal brown strips along the length of the middle of

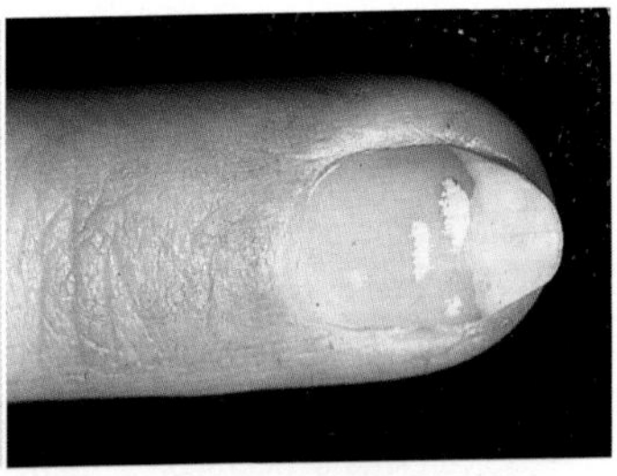

Figure 1.6. White spots within the nails indicating previous trauma.

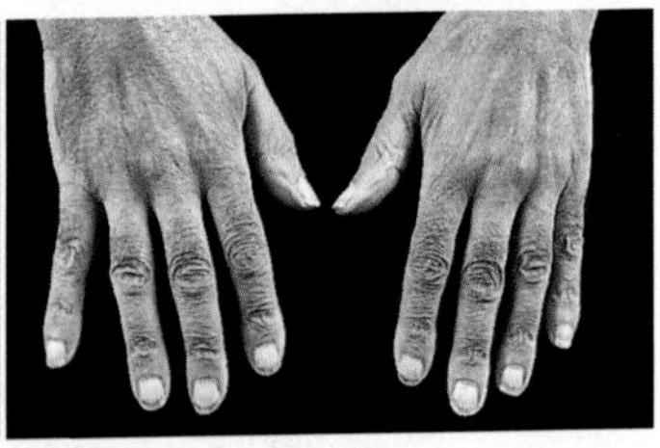

Figure 1.7. The colour of the nails in an anaemic patient.

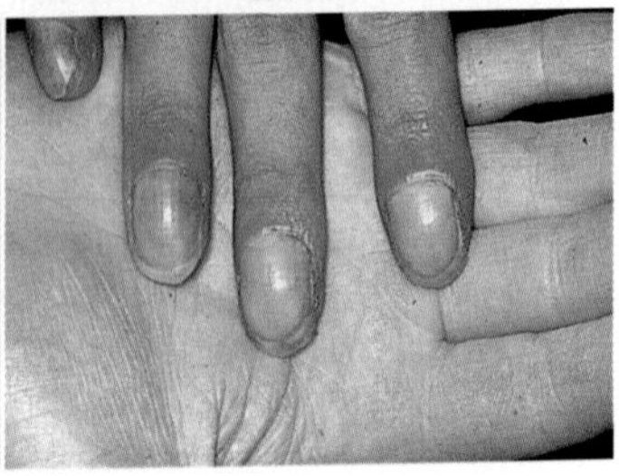

Figure 1.8. Marked cyanosis of the nails in a patient with Fallot's tetralogy.

Figure 1.9.
Pitted nails of psoriasis.

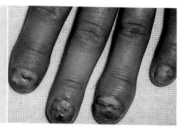

Figure 1.13.
Paronychial infection around the lateral border of the nail.

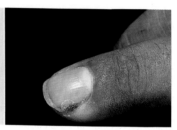

the nail which are seen in subacute bacterial endocarditis and vasculitic disorders. A spoon-shaped depression of the nail is seen in iron deficiency anaemia and is termed koilonychia (*Figure 1.11*).

Transverse grooves at a similar level in a number of nails (Beau's lines, *Figure 1.12*) can denote growth abnormalities related to the onset of a severe systemic disease. The arch over the base of the nail may become brown (Mei's lines) in renal insufficiency, poisoning and some inflammatory disorders. Infections around the nail (paronychia, *Figure 1.13*) are common but always exclude a diabetic aetiology.

Clubbing

In clubbing of the fingers, the tissues at the base of the nail are thickened and the angle between the nail base and the adjacent skin of the finger, which should measure approximately 160°, becomes obliterated. Application of light pressure at the base of the nail is associated with excessive movement of the nailbed. In clubbing, the nail loses its longitudinal ridge and becomes convex from above downwards as well as from side to side. In the later stages there may be associated swelling of the tips of the fingers. Hypertrophic pulmonary osteoarthropathy may be associated with clubbing in bronchial carcinoma (*Figure 1.14*); involvement of the wrist joint can be looked for at this stage.

Clubbing may also involve the feet (*Figure 1.15*), particularly the congenital variety. Common causes of clubbing are carcinoma and purulent conditions of the lung (bronchiectasis; lung abscess; empyema), congenital heart disease and infective endocarditis. Less common conditions are pulmonary fibrosis, fibrosing alveolitis, pulmonary tuberculosis, pleural mesothelioma, cystic fibrosis, coeliac and inflammatory bowel

Figure 1.10.
Splinter haemorrhages associated with bacterial endocarditis.

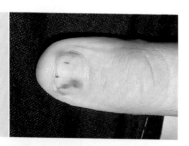

Figure 1.11.
Spoon-shaped depressions of koilonychia.

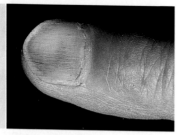

Figure 1.14.
Clubbing associated with bronchial carcinoma.

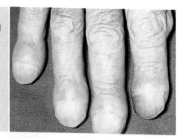

Figure 1.12.
Beau's lines.

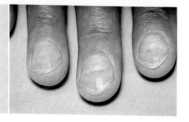

Figure 1.15.
Congenital clubbing of the feet.

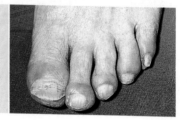

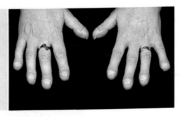

Figure 1.16.
Clubbing associated with hepatic cirrhosis.

spider naevi (*Figure 1.18a, b*). The skin on the back of the hand is a useful site to assess skin turgidity and to look for generalized pigmentation (*Figures 1.19–1.21*) and bruising (*Figure 1.22*). Other cutaneous abnormalities (*Figures 1.23–1.25*) are considered on p. 129. Laxity (*Figure 1.26*) is seen in older subjects but may indicate extensive dehydration at all ages. Similarly, areas of bruising and senile keratosis (*Figure 1.27*) are normal features of ageing but may also indicate disease. Skin nodules and moles are common (p. 143).

disease, cirrhosis (*Figure 1.16*), malabsorption, thyrotoxicosis and bronchial arteriovenous malformations.

Skin

Examination of the skin of the palm of the hand gives some indication of the type of work undertaken. Stretch the skin of the palm to examine the colour of the skin creases – these provide a better indication than the more exposed areas. Erythema of the palmar skin is most marked over the thenar and hypothenar eminences (*Figure 1.17*). It is an important finding in liver disease but may also occur in pregnancy, thyrotoxicosis, polycythemia, leukaemia, chronic febrile illnesses and rheumatoid arthritis. Liver disease may also give rise to

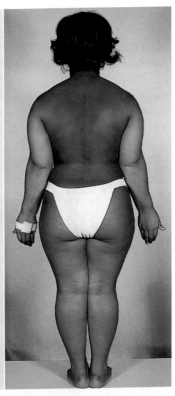

Figure 1.19.
Acanthosis nigricans. Cutaneous pigmentation and thickening associated with an underlying malignancy. It is common in older individuals associated with itching and commonly seen in the groin, hands and face. It may also affect the oral mucosa.

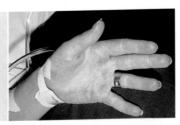

Figure 1.17.
Palmar erythema of a patient with chronic liver failure.

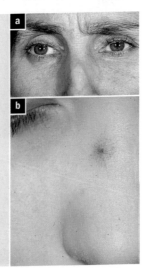

Figure 1.18.
Primary biliary cirrhosis.
a. Yellow discoloration of the conjunctivae from jaundice;
b. Spider naevi. Spider naevi are usually the result of abnormalities of subcutaneous connective tissue, particularly in liver disease, resulting in dilation of small vessels. They may also be congenital in origin.

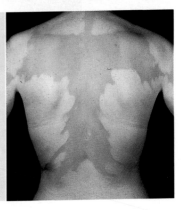

Figure 1.20.
Vitiligo. An autoimmune destruction of melanocytes often associated with other autoimmune diseases. The condition may be familial, lesions occasionally developing with changes in melanoma.

Note the nutrition of the fingertips in scleroderma (*Figure 1.28*), rheumatoid arthritis (*Figure 1.29*), other collagen diseases and ischaemic conditions. There may be loss of pulp and small areas of ulceration around the fingertips. Painful nodules around the fingertips are seen in infective endocarditis (Osler's nodes). Thickening of the palmar fascia – Dupuytren's contracture (*Figure 1.30*) – may be idiopathic, hereditary or associated with cirrhosis and various gut and pulmonary disorders.

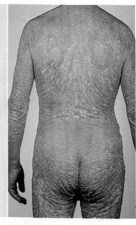

Figure 1.25.
Exfoliate dermatitis. Dermatitis is inflammation of the skin and may be in response to an allergen but the cause is often unknown.

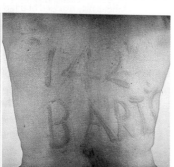

Figure 1.21.
Erythema ab igne. Reticular pigmentation following repeated application of a heat source, in this case a hot water bottle to soothe local pain.

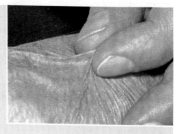

Figure 1.26.
Laxity. With ageing, skin becomes thinner and loses its elasticity as demonstrated by laxity.

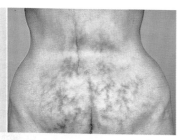

Figure 1.22.
Bruising. Individuals vary in their ease of bruising but spontaneous or major bruising requires investigation.

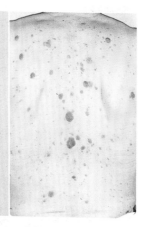

Figure 1.27.
Senile keratosis. Aged skin is also subject to weathering, bruising and pigmentation and occasionally as pigmented hyperkeratosis particularly in areas subject to continuous rubbing or exposure to the elements.

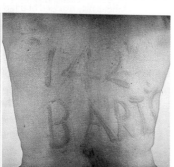

Figure 1.23.
Dermography. Urticaria is a transient swelling with or without flushing, produced by physical and chemical agents. The demographia shown is a hypersensitive response to scratching.

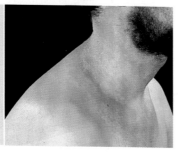

Figure 1.24.
Light-sensitive dermatitis. Sunburn occurs a number of hours after exposure but light sensitivity as demonstrated occurs immediately, particularly over infrequently exposed areas.

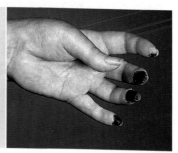

Figure 1.28.
In scleroderma there is connective tissue proliferation and inflammatory cell infiltration. It usually affects the skin layer, also producing necrosis or other tissue abnormalities.

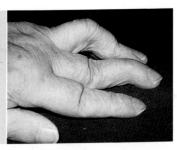

Figure 1.29.
Rheumatoid arthritis. The chronic inflammatory changes in rheumatoid arthritis mostly affect the joints producing deformity and disability.

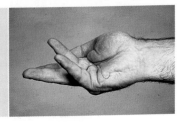

Figure 1.30.
Dupuytren's contracture.

Muscles and joints

The small muscles of the hand provide an early indication of general and muscular wasting as well as peripheral nerve injury. Note particularly the dorsum of the hand, the loss of substance of the interossei of the thumb and index finger (*Figure 1.31*), and the loss of muscle bulk deep to the long extensor tendons. Local causes of muscle wasting include carpal tunnel syndrome, proximal lesions of the median and ulnar nerves and their roots (*Figure 1.32*), motor neurone disease, poliomyelitis, syringomyelia, peripheral neuropathy and rheumatoid arthritis.

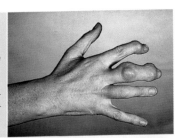

Figure 1.31.
Small muscle wasting. Wasting of the small muscles in the hand may be part of general weight loss or specific abnormalities of muscle innervation.

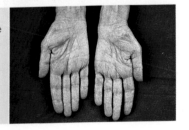

Figure 1.32.
Leprosy. The muscle wasting is due to peripheral nerve damage.

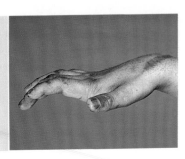

Figure 1.33.
Heberden's nodes. Inflammatory nodules of the skin overlying the joints in osteoarthritis.

The joints of the hands are commonly affected in rheumatoid arthritis (p. 432) and occasionally the terminal interphalangeal joint is involved with osteoarthritic changes. There may be palpable osteophytes in this area, e.g. Heberden's nodes in osteoarthritis (*Figure 1.33*).

Examination of the pulse is considered in more detail under Vascular system (p363) but at this stage in the general examination it is counted for at least half a minute, and abnormalities of volume, character and rhythm noted. The pulse rate at birth is approximately 135 beats per minute, falling to 100 at 5 years, 80 in the teens and 72 in the adult. This is also a useful point at which to note the blood pressure as it may be inadvertently omitted if not routinely positioned in the examination.

Blood pressure

The upper limb is fully exposed and the patient sits or lies on a couch. An appropriately sized blood pressure cuff must be used: in adults this is 12.5cm. It should not impinge on the axilla or the cubital fossa and should be wrapped closely and evenly around the upper arm. Smaller cuffs are available for children. Too small a cuff can give a falsely high reading, while too large a cuff prevents access to the brachial artery. The manometer should be at the eye level of the observer.

The radial pulse is palpated as the cuff is inflated. The pressure is raised to approximately 30mmHg above the level at which the pulse disappears. A stethoscope is lightly applied over the brachial artery on the medial aspect of the cubital fossa and the cuff pressure lowered 5mmHg at a time. The systolic blood pressure is the level at which the sound is first heard. The diastolic is the point at which the sound becomes suddenly faint or inaudible (Korotkoff sounds: I – appearance; IV – muffling; V – disappearance.)

In cardiovascular disease the blood pressure is taken in both arms and – in patients with treated or untreated hypertension – in lying and standing positions. If a patient is anxious, a falsely high reading may be obtained together with an increased pulse rate. When abnormal readings are obtained the recording should be repeated, the pressure in the cuff being allowed to drop to zero between measurements.

In peripheral vascular disease the blood pressure may also be measured in the lower limbs. A wider cuff is required for thigh compression and a Doppler probe is used to detect the presence or absence of a distal pulse. The systolic blood pressure is the point of reappearance of audible pulsation when letting down the cuff.

The face

Generalized weight loss may be apparent in changing facial and cervical contours. Excess tissue fluid – oedema (*Figure 1.34*) – is subject to the effect of gravity and although mostly observed in the lower limbs towards the end of the day, it may also be obvious within the face, particularly the eyelids, after a night's sleep. Regional oedema of the head, neck and upper limbs is seen in superior vena caval obstruction and the oedema of myxoedema may be particularly obvious in the eyelids, associated with skin and hair changes (*Figures 1.35* and *1.36*).

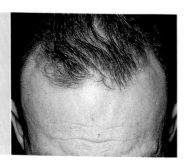

Figure 1.36.
Alopecia. Frontal recession and thinning of scalp hair is age and sex related. Alopecia also occurs in a number of conditions, particularly with the use of cytotoxic drugs.

Whereas pallor and cyanosis of the hands may be due to the cold or local arterial disease, these signs in the warm, central areas of the lips and tongue have a more generalized significance. The pallor of anaemia is most noticeable in the mucous membranes, although the sign lacks specificity. The inner surface of the lower lid is an important area for demonstration, as well as pallor of the mucous membranes and the palmar creases.

Cyanosis is the blue discoloration given to the skin by deoxygenated blood. However, a minimum of 5g/dL is required to produce visible cyanosis; it is thus not detectable in severe anaemia. Cyanosis is best observed in areas with a rich blood supply such as the lips and tongue. It may also be noted in the ear lobes and fingernails but these areas can react to cold by vasoconstriction, producing peripheral cyanosis in the presence of a normal oxygen saturation.

Central cyanosis is usually due to cardiorespiratory abnormalities (*Figures 1.37* and *1.38*) but may also occur at high

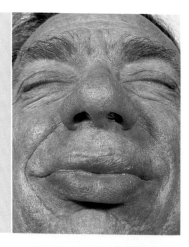

Figure 1.34.
Facial oedema.

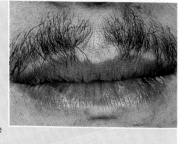

Figure 1.35.
Idiopathic hirsuties. Hirsute usually refers to a male pattern of hair growth in a female patient. Female hair growth varies in different races but is increased in a number of endocrine disorders.

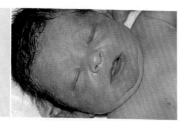

Figure 1.37.
Blue baby with cyanotic heart disease.

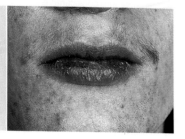

Figure 1.38.
Cyanosis in a child with a single ventricle.

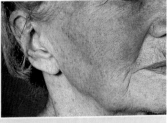

Figure 1.39.
Malar flush. Facial flushing occurs in individuals who are regularly exposed to the elements and is a feature of mitral and pulmonary stenosis. Found in Cushing's and carcinoid syndromes and some collagen diseases.

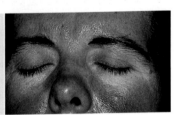

Figure 1.40.
Flushing in a patient with carcinoid syndrome.

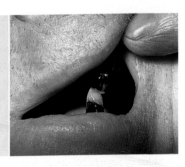

Figure 1.41.
Poor dentition.

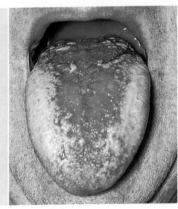

Figure 1.42.
Oral candidiasis.

altitudes, with methaemoglobinaemia and sulphhaemaglobinaemia. Cardiac conditions include a number of congenital abnormalities with a right-to-left shunt, while cyanosis may be related to hypoventilation (head injuries; drug overdosage), chronic obstructive airways disease and mismatched arterial ventilation and perfusion (pulmonary embolism; pulmonary shunts; AV fistulae). Cyanosis is difficult to elicit in dark-skinned people with anaemia. Polycythemia is an excess of circulating red cells and may produce a purple–blue skin discoloration, mimicking cyanosis. However, it is also prominent in the cheeks and the backs of the hands (*Figures 1.39* and *1.40*).

Jaundice is a yellow discoloration due to excess circulating bile pigments. Mild degrees of jaundice are easily picked up by staining of the sclera (*Figure 1.18a*, p. 8. Be careful not to confuse the uniform yellow colour of jaundice with a yellowish peripheral discoloration of the sclera that can be seen in normal individuals. As the jaundice becomes more pronounced there is yellow discoloration of the skin and this may progress to yellow/orange or even dark brown with high levels of plasma pigment. Other generalized changes in skin pigmentation are considered on p. 143.

The mouth

The mouth is a valuable indicator of systemic illness as well as local pathology. The mouth has a complex embryological origin being the site of the junction of ectoderm and endoderm, and receiving contributions from pharyngeal arch mesoderm. The tongue muscles are derived from suboccipital somites that have migrated forwards around the pharynx,

bringing their nerve supply with them. This origin is also reflected in the variety of diseases. These include skin and gut mucosal abnormalities together with other lesions that encompass a number of medical and surgical disciplines.

The breath must be examined for halitosis (offensive or abnormal – foetor oris); this may be an indicator of respiratory, upper alimentary or systemic disease. Purulent oral infection, producing halitosis, most commonly involves the gums in association with poor dentition (*Figure 1.41*). Oral candidiasis (*Figure 1.42*) – a white coating with fungus – may occur in relation to debilitating disease, prolonged antibiotics or steroid therapy, immunological diseases (such as sarcoidosis), immunodeficient disorders (such as HIV infection) and immunosuppressive drugs. Certain drugs – such as paraldehyde – have a specific foetor.

Nasal and sinus infections and degenerative tumours in these areas may give offensive odours, as does the infection of bronchiectasis.

Alimentary odours may be related to gastroenteritis, obstruction of the pylorus and small or large gut, and over-indulgence of food or alcohol. The latter aroma depends on the timing and the quantity imbibed.

Systemic disease producing characteristic odours are diabetic ketosis, and renal and hepatic failure. The sweet smell of ketotic breath may be related to insulin deficiency but also increased metabolic rate – such as with a fever and fasting – particularly in childhood disorders. In renal and hepatic disease there may also be systemic manifestations of the conditions. The amoniacal smell of hepatic coma has been likened to musty old eggs.

Examination of the mouth

Examination of the mouth requires a good light. This may be provided by daylight but usually a torch or lamp is necessary. A spatula allows movement of the lips, cheeks and tongue to observe all areas; this may be aided by a dental mirror. Palpation is with a gloved finger, the second hand being used for bimanual exploration of the floor of the mouth and the cheeks. The tongue may be pulled forward by holding it with a swab to examine its sides and the adjacent structures.

Specific disorders of the tongue – such as congenital abnormalities – and benign and malignant tumours are considered on p. 198, but it is often a good indicator of systemic disease. There is a good deal of variation of ethnic pigmentation and papillary patterns, such as 'geographic tongue'. The pallor of anaemia, central cyanosis and the yellow tingeing of jaundice may be recognized in all races.

Many tongue coatings have no clinical significance or may reflect a recent meal. Roughage in the diet can serve to remove particulate matter and, therefore, coatings do relate to dietary habit. Dietary deficiencies such as vitamins C and D may produce an abnormally smooth tongue. Coating is increased in heavy smokers and mouth breathers. Mouth breathing may also dehydrate the surface of the tongue. However, this, together with the loss of skin turgor and sunken eyes, is a valuable indicator of the general state of dehydration postoperatively, in fevers and with reduced fluid intake. There may be tongue atrophy in the Plumber–Vincent syndrome, associated with angular stomatitis (*Figure 1.43*) and abnormalities of the gastric mucous membrane.

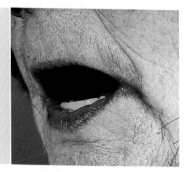

Figure 1.43.
Angular stomatitis with cracking and fissuring of the lips: a feature of vitamin deficiency.

Ulcerated tongue

Ulceration of the tongue is common and is usually due to dental trauma or aphthous ulcers. In the former, there may be sharp teeth or poorly fitting dentures and the gums must be carefully checked for any associated damage. Falls, fits and sports or other injuries may be associated with tongue biting and fish bones may lodge anywhere in the tongue or alimentary tract, producing trauma and infection.

Aphthous ulcers (*Figure 1.44*) may be associated with generalized disease but are usually of unknown aetiology. Ulcers may also be associated with inflammatory changes of the tongue and this glossitis may be due to generalized disease. Examples are drug reactions such as Stevens–Johnson and Magic syndromes. Sexually transmitted diseases causing glossitis and inflammation include HIV, syphilis and gonorrhoea, and may be part of Reiter's syndrome. Autoimmune, connective tissue disorders and occasionally gut abnormalities – such as ulcerative colitis and Crohns (*Figure 1.45*) – may have associated mouth ulceration.

A coating of candida has already been considered in the mouth. White patches also include lichen planus, a disorder of unknown aetiology. It has a number of characteristic patterns, usually involving the edges of the tongue, associated

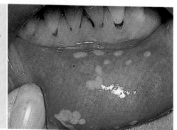

Figure 1.44.
Aphthous ulcers are common and usually of unknown aetiology. Frequent complications of autoimmune deficiency.

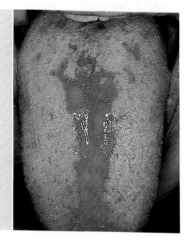

Figure 1.45.
Crohn's disease affecting the oral mucosa.

with mucosal atrophy and erosion. An important differential diagnosis of a white coating is leukoplakia (*Figures 1.46* and *1.47*), a premalignant condition. An important finding is that it cannot be removed by scratching the mucosal surface.

Large tongues are seen in hypothyroidism and acromegaly (*Figure 1.48*), in developmental abnormalities and associated with some congenital syndromes such as Down's syndrome.

The tongue receives bilateral cortical innervation, therefore wasting only occurs with bilateral upper motor neurone lesions (pseudobulbar palsy). However, the 12th nerve nucleus may be affected by motor neurone disease and the nerve damaged in surgical or other trauma. With a lower motor neurone paralysis the tongue deviates towards the side of the lesion. Tongue weakness and difficulty in swallowing may be present in myasthenia gravis and the tremor of Parkinson's. Thus disease can often be well demonstrated by asking the patient to stick their tongue out.

Many of the features described in the examination of the mouth and tongue apply equally to the mucous membrane of the oropharynx.

Systemic examination

After completing the general examination – as outlined above – the examination takes a regional approach, as indicated in subsequent chapters. Some specific clinical syndromes that need to be identified and understood are covered in chapter 2.

The skin of each area provides further information on the state of nutrition and hydration, colour changes and scratch marks. Venous and arterial pulsation can be observed in the neck, and respiratory movements in the chest and abdomen. Abnormal movements such as neurological abnormalities (p. 435) and hiccups may become more obvious, as well as an abnormal posture, in relation to pain and deformity.

On completion of the examination of each region and system, cover the patient and make sure they are comfortable. Examine all excreta available and request the collection of these when appropriate. The excreta include sputum, vomit, faeces, the contents of surgical drainage bottles and any discharges. Discharges may be from ulcers, wounds or other sites and smaller amounts can be observed on dressings also.

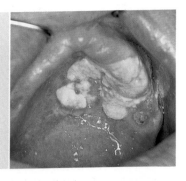

Figure 1.46.
Leukoplakia.

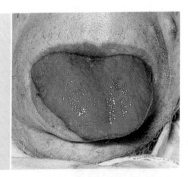

Figure 1.48.
Macroglossia of acromegaly.

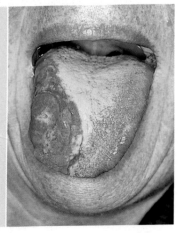

Figure 1.47.
Carcinoma of the tongue.

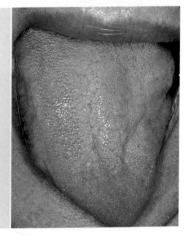

Figure 1.49.
Twelfth nerve palsy (hypoglossal).

Formulating a diagnosis

On completion of the history and examination the clinician has usually come to a working diagnosis. This is supported or not by further investigations and the subsequent progress of the disease.

Sometimes it is difficult to diagnose a patient's problem. This may be linked to inexperience, the condition may already be resolving or difficulty may be encountered in the very early stages of presentation. *Table 1.1* is intended to generate ideas for possible diagnoses and differential diagnoses in these circumstances.

First try to identify the system involved. Backache, for example, may be musculoskeletal but consider neurological causes or referred pain from the cardiovascular system (e.g. ruptured abdominal aortic aneurysm) or alimentary system (e.g. pancreatic or biliary disease). The anatomy of the region of interest should be considered with a pain or a lump. This may be sited superficially in the skin, subcutaneously or more deeply in muscle or viscera. The pathology list – 'diagnostic sieve' – is of particular value when assessing a lump but is equally applicable to any symptom.

The original 'surgical sieve' included the five headings: congenital; infection; traumatic; neoplastic and degenerative. Inflammation is 'the body's response to injury' and is a wider title than infection. The injury not only includes infection from a virus or bacteria but also from other organisms, an antigen and that surrounding a traumatic wound or infiltrating neoplasm. It is a useful heading under which autoimmune diseases can be placed.

Table 1.1. Aids to diagnosis.

System	Anatomy	Pathology
Cardiovascular	Skin	Congenital
Respiratory	Subcutaneous tissues; fat;	Inflammatory
Gastrointestinal	vessels; nerves	Traumatic
Genitourinary	Muscles	Neoplastic
Musculoskeletal	Bones	Degenerative
Neurogenic	Joints	Metabolic
Haemopoietic	Related viscera	Hormonal
		Haematological
		Poisons
		Chemicals
		Psychiatric
		Idiopathic
		Iatrogenic

Neoplasia should be divided into benign and malignant and the latter into primary and secondary lesions. Degenerative disease is a useful heading under which to place atheromatous disease, dementia and other diseases of the aged.

Communication

Taking a detailed history and performing a thorough examination establishes a unique doctor–patient relationship. This privileged relationship must be reinforced by frank explanation of the findings to the patient in terms that they fully understand, together with the proposed course of action. The degree of empathy that a clinician achieves with different patients is dependent on both their personalities. However, with all patients, the clinician must aim to establish mutual respect of the relationship based on sympathy, trust and honesty. In the case of children or mentally disabled patients, these discussions should be with the appropriate guardian.

In the case of a specialist referral, the letter must ensure that the referring clinician is kept fully informed of all actions taken. This is similarly true when a patient is discharged from hospital, when the general practitioner should receive an immediate discharge letter followed, as soon as possible, by a summary of the admission.

Accurate records are essential to document progress and to ensure effective continuity of care; they also have important medicolegal significance.

Surgical examination of the child

Many relatively common surgical conditions occur exclusively during childhood. In addition, each stage of childhood has specific problems. Childhood is characterized by growth which can lead to its own disorders, while other conditions can adversely affect the growth and development of the child. Children also pose difficulties in examination, especially in infancy and early childhood.

This section deals with the approach to the child as a whole during the different stages of growth and development, referring the reader to other parts of the text when disorders are discussed with related adult conditions.

Examination of the neonate
The growth and development of the individual begins at conception and even at this stage disease may become evident. Most genetic disorders and genetically damaged blastocysts

or embryos do not implant or are miscarried before the mother is even aware that she is pregnant. Previous pregnancies or the family histories of the parents may point to the possibility of genetically determined disorders and, in future, genetic population screening will lead to an increased awareness of these problems. *In vitro* fertilization techniques provide a means by which abnormal embryos may be diagnosed and excluded from implantation. Genetic information can also be obtained by taking a sample of the covering membranes of the foetus (chorionic villous sampling) or of cells in the amniotic fluid (amniocentesis). Further assessment of the growth and development of the foetus is by ultrasound examination of the foetus *in utero*. In particular, defects affecting the spine and the neurological and cardiovascular systems may become apparent.

Apart from predetermined genetic disease, the growing and developing foetus is in danger from infective agents that can cross the placenta such as the rubella virus, cytomegalovirus or toxoplasmosis – these organisms can lead to disorders of organ growth and development. Maternal health and adequate nutrition also determine the health of the foetus, as do the mother's ingestion of alcohol and drugs, and the inhalation of tobacco.

The general health of the growing foetus can, to a large extent, be assessed by examination of the mother. The growth (by fundal height), heart rate (by auscultation) and foetal movement are useful markers. The amount of amniotic fluid is a guide to the function of the gastrointestinal tract and urogenital systems. Excess amniotic fluid – polyhydramnios – may be a sign of a high gastrointestinal defect or diabetes mellitus, and reduced volume may be a sign of a problem in renal failure or expulsion of urine, or intra-uterine growth retardation.

Finally the baby may undergo harm or injury during birth. Anoxia during birth may lead to neurological impairment and the baby can suffer serious nerve (in particular brachial plexus) and musculoskeletal injury (including fractures) during obstructed or otherwise complicated deliveries, e.g. shoulder dystocia; these injuries may be iatrogenic, though occasionally unavoidable. Forceps- or suction-assisted deliveries have characteristic injury patterns, and the baby may be injured during Caesarean section. Examination of the newborn infant should, therefore, take into account the health and medical history of the mother and any previous siblings, the health of the mother during pregnancy, the progress of the pregnancy and the mode of delivery.

All parents are keen to know that their newborn child is normal and so a brief but important examination is always carried out immediately. The baby is first inspected for signs of life, such as adequate spontaneous respiration and adequate circulation, leading to a healthy skin coloration and spontaneous activity of all limbs, eyes and head. If these are not present the baby requires immediate resuscitation. These initial physical signs are grouped together and scored to give the 'Apgar' score – this is an index of the immediate physical state of the neonate, usually recorded at 1 and 5 minutes after delivery (*Table 1.2*).

The baby can then be examined more carefully, first by inspection. Particular attention is paid to the head and spine. Meningomyeloceles and anencephaly are usually obvious but other types of spinal dysraphism may not be immediately apparent. They may be evident from a degree of abnormal curvature of the spine or a patch of hair over the spine. The eyes are inspected. Pronounced canthal folds together with a large tongue and the distinctive continuous single 'simian' crease in the palm lead to a suspicion of Down's syndrome. The syndrome is associated with other abnormalities, notably congenital heart defects and duodenal atresia.

The mouth should be inspected – cleaned out if necessary – to exclude cleft lip or palate. The chest wall and abdominal wall are examined to exclude defects such as bladder extrophy; the umbilical cord is examined to ensure it contains the usual configuration of three vessels – abnormalities are suggestive of renal deformities. Failure of the intestine to return to the abdominal cavity *in utero* leads to exomphalos. The anus is examined to exclude a very low obstruction of the intestinal tract. The genitalia having been examined carefully by one and all to determine the sex of the baby, are examined more carefully to ensure that there is no abnormality.

The limbs are examined, confirming the normal configuration and the correct number of digits. Fractures and dislocations caused during difficult labours are usually obvious, and talipes – club foot – from its characteristic equinovarus deformity. The baby's skin is examined for the presence of rashes, discolorations and accessory skin tags. The chest is auscultated to ensure that the lungs have expanded and that there are no cardiac murmurs.

Finally the baby is weighed. Low birth weight may be due to prematurity, intrauterine growth retardation, congenital abnormalities, intrauterine infection and maternal poor health. Large babies – macrosomia – can be due to maternal diabetes and are in danger of birth injury, hypoglycaemia, neonatal jaundice and respiratory distress.

When all is deemed to be well the child is returned to the mother and feeding is started. Failure to feed – in particular cyanosis during attempted feeding – together with the presence of frothy saliva around the mouth in between feeds, leads to the suspicion of oesophageal atresia and a tracheo-oesophageal fistula.

Vomiting soon after feeding may be due to a more distal obstruction. If bile is present, this is likely to be distal to the second part of the duodenum. Intestinal obstruction may be due to atresia, obstructing bands, intestinal organs compressing the intestine – notably an annular pancreas – or from inspissated meconium. The latter suggests a diagnosis of cystic fibrosis.

Failure to pass urine may suggest urethral obstruction or problems of renal function. Failure to pass stool can be due to obstruction of the distal colon, rectum or anus by agenesis, the presence of bands or the absence of a functioning myenteric plexus – Hirschsprung's disease.

The baby is re-examined carefully and methodically at 48 hours, care being taken to exclude congenital dislocation of the hips and, in boys, absent testes. A more detailed examination of the cardiovascular system is carried out to exclude murmurs and to assess the presence or absence of the femoral arteries. The character of the peripheral pulses may also be significant – if full it may signify a patent ductus arteriosus, if weak, a major defect compromising cardiac output.

A number of abnormalities are commonly found that are benign and either resolve independently or require minor treatment for removal. These include:

- Mongolian blue spots – areas of blue- or black-pigmented areas usually found on the buttocks or the base of the spine, commoner in dark-skinned babies; they usually resolve spontaneously.
- Capillary or macular haemangioma – very common; usually found around the eyes or the neck at the nape. They usually disappear, especially those around the eyes.
- Breast enlargement – common in both boys and girls due to the presence of maternal hormones. Milk – 'witch's milk' – can also be secreted for a short period of time. Both resolve spontaneously.
- Milia – white spots caused by blocked sebaceous glands usually on the nose and cheeks; they clear spontaneously.

Table 1.2. Apgar score chart.

	Apgar score		
	0.00	1.00	2.00
Response to stimulation	None	Facial grimace	Cry
Respiration	Absent	Gasping	Regular
Heart rate	0.00	<100	100+
Colour of trunk	White	Blue	Pink
Muscle tone	Flaccid	Some flexion	Normal with movement

- Mouth cysts – can occur in the midline of the palate (Epstein's pearls), on the gums (epulis) and on the floor of the mouth; most of these cysts disappear spontaneously.
- Accessory skin tags – common on the face and around the ears.
- Dimples – may occur over the sacrum and should be gently palpated to exclude underlying cysts.

Examination of the infant and child

This varies little from the examination of the adult but one has to be flexible, as often each part of the examination has to be carried out when a suitable opportunity arises. The clinician must be sympathetic to the needs of the child and to recognize that he or she may be frightened, especially if in pain.

A number of gambits exist to calm the anxious child, including the use of dolls or parents to show what will be done, and that nothing harmful is to be undergone. The child's hand can be guided over its abdomen for instance, where tenderness is suspected. Each individual finds the best techniques to suit not only themselves but the individual child in terms of its mental and social development. During these examinations always bear in mind the relative growth and development of a child and, if necessary, chart these over time.

2 Distinctive clinical syndromes

Introduction

Many diseases have characteristic and diagnostic physical signs. This text aims to include all those of surgical relevance. The current chapter brings together a number of clinical states in which a disease presents with multiple – often unique – signs. They are important to recognize, as methods of treatment and problems of management are well documented.

Some of the conditions require operative procedures to treat or prevent complications, while others have abnormalities that may produce anaesthetic difficulties and require skilled post-operative care. Once diagnosed, the patients can benefit from previous experience and their prognosis can be clearly defined.

The importance of these conditions to the examination candidate is disproportionately high. The patients have chronic diseases and are frequently available for clinical examinations. The examiners also expect candidates to recognize the signs and know many details of the diseases and their management.

The clinical states included are of mixed aetiology. The reason for inclusion at this point is the generalized nature of the conditions, affecting more than one region of the body and involving more than one system. They include shock, bleeding disorders, anaemia, pyrexia of unknown origin, weight disturbances, endocrine abnormalities and some inherited disorders. Other conditions – such as hepatic and renal failure – and skeletal abnormalities, although producing widespread signs, have fitted more appropriately into the relevant section in the subsequent text.

Abnormalities of fluid balance

Water makes up approximately 55% of body-weight in males but less in the female, because of their higher fat content. About two-thirds of this fluid is intracellular, where potassium is the main ion contributing to the osmolality; 98% of the body's potassium resides within the cells. Sodium is the main extracellular ion, Na/K ATPase is the source of energy required to keep sodium and potassium in the extra- and intracellular compartments, respectively. This ionic balance is influenced by pH, aldosterone, insulin and the adrenogenic nervous system.

The volume of the extracellular fluid is regulated mainly by the kidney, through a number of mechanisms, the most important of which is ADH (antidiuretic hormone – vasopressin). Lowered sodium and reduced blood volume stimulate hypothalamic receptors with the release of ADH; they also stimulate thirst. There are similar osmoreceptors in the aortic arch and probably in the gut and portal circulation. ADH affects permeability in the terminal distal tubule and collecting ducts of the kidney. Other factors influencing renal tubular function include the renin–angiotensin–aldosterone axis, neurogenic reflexes – such as from the baroreceptors – prostaglandins and natriuretic factor. The latter is a peptide stored in granules in the walls of the atria and released in response to excess atrial filling. It increases renal perfusion and salt excretion.

Plasma comprises about one-quarter of the extracellular fluid. A delicate balance is maintained between the colloid osmotic – oncotic – pressure of the plasma and the capillary hydrostatic pressure, forcing fluid through the capillary wall. These are influenced by the arteriolar and venous pressures, the permeability of the capillary membrane and the lymphatic drainage of the interstitial fluid.

The normal fluid intake is approximately 2.5 L per day, drink providing 1.8 L, and food the remainder. Equivalent loss is mainly from urine at 1.5 L. Exhaled gases and insensible loss make up 0.9 L and faeces 0.1 L.

Oedema

Increased fluid intake is usually compensated for by an increase in urine output. The kidney is capable of increasing this to 750 mL/h and fluid overload is well compensated for in the healthy individual. Some generalized or focal diseases can give rise to an excess of interstitial fluid. When this excess is clinically detectable by pitting on digital pressure, it is termed oedema. Common causes of oedema are listed in *Table 2.1*. Generalized causes include cardiac, renal and liver failure, and hypoproteinaemia.

Although it is tempting to think of cardiac oedema as due to an increase in venous pressure due to poor emptying of the right atrium, the capillary hydrostatic pressure in this condition is not markedly raised, the prime cause being a reduced renal perfusion and reduced sodium excretion, with resultant rise in blood volume and pressure in the interstitial fluid. The oedema of renal failure can be due to a failure of salt and water excretion or secondary to hypoproteinaemia, as in the nephrotic syndrome. Liver failure oedema relates to a low plasma albumin but also to interference with the metabolism of enzymes such as aldosterone. Hypoproteinaemia reduces plasma oncotic pressure, altering the balance between plasma and interstitial fluid pressure measurements. The majority of causes of hypoproteinaemia are gut in origin. They include starvation, malnutrition and malabsorption, together with protein-losing enteropathies; vomiting, diarrhoea, and intestinal fistulae are other causes.

Fluid retention occurs pre-menstrually and in pregnancy, and ADH hormone-secreting tumours reduce water and sodium excretion. Inappropriate ADH secretion may also be present in some malignancies. Certain drugs – particularly steroids – promote sodium retention, and similar problems are encountered with excessive sodium intake. This can be a problem in infants if sodium is added to a milk diet. Fluid retention in myxoedema is partly in the interstitial fluid and may pit. Idiopathic oedema of females is an unusual condition, usually diagnosed by exclusion.

Excessive intravenous hypotonic solutions, such as 5% dextrose and the use of water for bladder or peritoneal washouts may give rise to water retention. Similar effects may be obtained if careful fluid balance is not maintained during haemo- and peritoneal dialysis.

Increased capillary permeability can present as an acute, even fatal, event. There is leakage of proteins, markedly influencing the plasma–intercellular pressure gradient; fibrinogen is one of the plasma proteins that readily leaks under these circumstances and can produce additional problems from fibrin deposition blocking lymphatic drainage. Such allergic reactions (*Figure 2.1*) can occur with certain foodstuffs – particularly shellfish – and drugs and chemicals. A snake bite or bee sting can have rapid and serious consequences through this mechanism.

Focal oedema may be related to inflammation associated with infection, collagen diseases or around traumatized tissue and neoplasms. Venous and lymphatic oedema are considered on p. 381.

History and examination in oedema

The history and examination of the patient with oedema is directed at establishing its cause. In cardiorespiratory causes there may be a history of valvular heart disease, myocardial infarction or angina. Dyspnoea is common, and in more severe cardiac and respiratory problems there is orthopnoea, paroxysmal nocturnal dyspnoea and a chronic history of cough and sputum. Signs may include cardiomegaly, heart murmurs and added respiratory sounds. The signs of congestive cardiac failure include raised jugular venous pressure (*Figure 2.2*), ascites, pleural effusion, hepatomegaly, basal creps and central (*Figure 2.3*) and peripheral oedema.

In renal disease, symptoms and signs may be few. There is anaemia with malaise, pallor, renal angle tenderness; palpable renal and pelvic masses should be excluded. Hepatic

Table 2.1. Causes of oedema.

Condition	Cause
Systemic disease	Cardiac failure Renal failure Hepatic failure Hypoproteinaemia (nephrotic syndrome; liver failure; malnutrition; malabsorption; protein-losing enteropathy)
Fluid retention	Pre-menstrual Pregnancy ADH tumours Inappropriate ADH secretion Sodium-retaining drugs/steroids Added salt (infants) Myxoedema Idiopathic oedema (in females)
Water intoxication	Excess intravenous hypotonic solution Bladder/peritoneal wash-out with water or hypotonic solutions Overload during haemo/peritoneal dialysis
Abnormal capillary permeability	Angioneurotic oedema Allergy (food; drugs; chemical; toxins) Snake bites Bee stings
Local oedema	Inflammation Venous hypertension Impaired lymphatic drainage Prolonged dependency Tight bandaging Fictitious

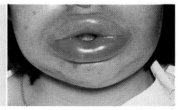

Figure 2.1.
Angio-oedema.

Figure 2.2.
Raised jugular
venous pressure.

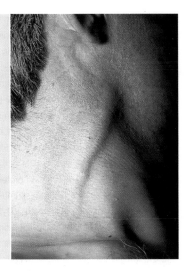

Figure 2.3.
Eyelid oedema.

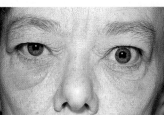

Figure 2.4.
Jaundiced
conjunctiva.

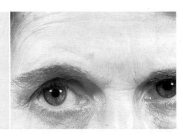

Figure 2.5.
Hepatomegaly.

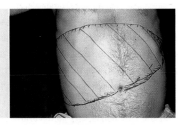

Figure 2.6.
Palmar flush.

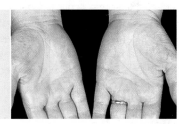

Figure 2.7.
Spider naevi.

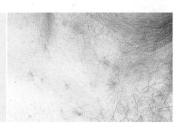

Figure 2.8.
Ascitic liver disease.

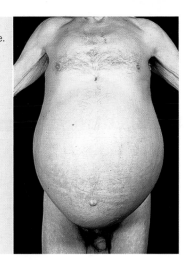

failure is usually obvious, with jaundice (*Figure 2.4*) and
malaise. There may be – at least initially – hepatomegaly
(*Figure 2.5*) and the signs of liver flap, palmar flushing (*Figure
2.6*), cutaneous telangiectasia (*Figure 2.7*) and purpura.

In the alimentary system, note weight loss in the history
and examination and enquire of dietary habits, indigestion,
abdominal pain and the bowel habit, particularly noting
changes and the number, form and colour of the stools.
Examine the hands, mucous membranes, mouth and the
root of the neck for nodes. In the abdomen and pelvis look
for tenderness, enlarged organs, abdominal masses and
ascites (*Figure 2.8*).

In questioning for the miscellaneous other groups causing oedema, discuss all current symptoms and previous illnesses, particularly rashes or vague symptoms following
any particular food and any recent, unusual diets, such as
shellfish. Check the salt and fluid intake, drug history –
whether through prescription or across the counter and any
recreational drugs – and exposure to toxins or chemicals at
work or other environments. In all forms of oedema note
weight changes and keep careful records of weight, and
fluid intake and output.

Reduced body water

Inadequate body fluids may be due to reduced intake, increased needs or increased loss. It is usually accompanied by low body sodium. Common causes of reduced body water content are listed in *Table 2.2*.

Reduced intake may be due to lack of available water or lack of the desire to drink. There may be inability to drink, such as with oral pathology, dysphagia or coma. Increased needs include fever, where every degree of rise in body temperature equates to an increased fluid requirement of 10%. An increased basal metabolic rate – such as in thyrotoxicosis – carries with it an increased water requirement. In raised external temperatures – especially with low humidity – an additional 250 mL of fluid is required for every degree above 29°C.

Fluid loss is commonly related to diseases of the alimentary tract. This loss may be externally – through diarrhoea, vomiting or fistulae – or due to sequestration of fluids within the gut (such as in paralytic ileus) or within the peritoneal cavity (e.g. acute pancreatitis and ascites), particularly if the latter is being continually drained. Fluid loss may be through the skin, such as in widespread burns or extensive weeping eczema. The loss may be through haemorrhage, such as in major trauma or a ruptured aortic aneurysm.

Increased loss through the lungs may be through lack of humidification of a recently fashioned tracheostomy or through hyperventilation. Renal loss can be in the diuretic phase of recovery from renal failure, the over-use of diuretic drugs and in diabetes insipidus.

The clinical features of an abnormally low body water content usually relate to the underlying disease. There is also, at first, lethargy, malaise, drowsiness and muscle twitching, leading eventually to coma. With a few exceptions – e.g. diabetes insipidus – there is oliguria, together with the signs of dehydration, including tachycardia and hypotension. The skin is dry, with loss of elasticity, noted when picking it up between the thumb and finger. The eyes are sunken, the mouth is dry and the tongue usually furred.

Shock

In the extreme cases of fluid depletion – when the circulating volume does not match the circulating capacity – there is an accompanying failure of tissue perfusion. This failure of perfusion to meet the metabolic requirements of the tissues is termed 'shock'. The syndrome incorporates a number of entities such as extremes of cardiac failure and abnormal capillary permeability. The conditions grouped within the syndrome of shock are listed in *Table 2.3*.

The low tissue perfusion produces a profound lactic acidosis, a low pH gives rise to dyspnoea. Initial vasoconstriction is present, although dilatation may occur as a terminal event. There is low cerebral perfusion, producing confusion, agitation and finally coma. Low renal perfusion gives rise to renal failure and, possibly, acute tubular necrosis, while lowered gut perfusion can allow absorption of bacterial vasodilator toxins, accentuating the existing hypotension.

As has already been emphasized, shock is a syndrome encompassing a number of different causes of altered tissue perfusion. The presenting signs and symptoms differ and it is

Table 2.2. Reduced body fluid.

Reason	Cause
Reduced intake	Debilitation Oral pathology Dysphagia Coma (trauma; metabolic; intracranial lesions/surgery)
Fluid loss	Fever Exercise Hot, dry climates Vomiting Gut fistulae Diarrhoea Intestinal obstruction Paralytic ileus Small bowel infarction Peritonitis Acute pancreatitis Drained ascites Severe haemorrhage (multiple trauma; ruptured abdominal aortic aneurysm) Burns Extensive weeping eczema Increased metabolism Respiratory loss (hyperventilation; unhumidified tracheostomy; metabolic acidosis) Diabetes insipidus (hypothalamic disease; idiopathic) Renal diuresis Diuretic drugs

Table 2.3. Causes of shock.

Condition	Type of shock
With high systemic vascular resistance	Cardiogenic Pulmonary embolism Cardiac tamponade Hypovolaemic (fluid loss; haemorrhage)
With low systemic vascular resistance	Septic Anaphylactic Amniotic embolism

important to identify the cause, since treatment is specific and appropriate treatment for one group may be harmful for another. Two main varieties of shock exist: those accompanied by **high** and those with **low systemic vascular resistance.**

High systemic vascular resistance is seen in cardiogenic shock, pulmonary embolism, cardiac tamponade and hypovolaemic shock. In **cardiogenic shock** the heart failure is accompanied by low blood pressure and a tachycardia with a low volume pulse. There may be a gallop rhythm and audible third or fourth heart sounds. Failure of the left ventricle gives rise to acute pulmonary oedema and of the right, raised jugular venous pressure. These features – and the high peripheral resistance – produce a cold, clammy periphery and marked dyspnoea. There may be slight cyanosis with added chest sounds and, possibly, a pleural effusion.

In massive **pulmonary embolism** the signs are similar to those of cardiogenic shock but the symptoms are of very sudden onset, usually 2 to 10 days after an operative procedure. There is acute chest pain and breathlessness, and a vagal reflex may produce a desire to defecate. The ECG may show the typical picture of S1 Q3 T3 (S-wave in lead I, and a Q-wave and an inverted T-wave in lead III). **Cardiac tamponade** – due to fluid within the pericardial cavity compressing the heart – is seen in aortic dissection, after cardiac surgery, acute pericarditis and thoracic malignancy. There is decreased ventricular filling, producing signs similar to those of cardiogenic shock but there may also be pulsus paradoxus, the pulse volume falling with inspiration rather than the usual rise and, similarly, the JVP rising rather than falling in inspiration (Kussmaul's sign).

Hypovolaemic shock is due to a marked loss of tissue fluid. Of particular note are acute pancreatitis, severe burns and acute massive haemorrhage. Hypovolaemia leads to reduced cardiac output and a low blood pressure; there is a tachycardia and the intense peripheral vascular constriction is due to reflex sympathetic stimulation. The patient is cold and clammy with dyspnoea and cyanosis. This pattern is similar to cardiogenic shock but does not show a raised JVP, pulmonary oedema or added heart sounds.

In **septic shock** the septicaemia is usually due to Gramnegative organisms originating from infection in the gastrointestinal or genitourinary systems. Other important sources are infected intravenous lines and large burns. Occasionally, trivial infections of the nasopharynx or skin provide the source, and at times almost every bacterium has been implicated. There is an increased incidence in the aged, malnourished, alcoholics and drug abusers. The toxins produced from the infection give rise to massive arteriolar and peripheral venous dilatation, accompanied by hypotension and a low central venous pressure. The clinical picture differs markedly from the cold, clammy state of cardiogenic and hypovolaemic shock. The sympathetic drive produces a positive inotropic action, there is a full, bounding pulse with a tachycardia, warm extremities and no rise in JVP. However, the gut and kidney are shut down and the poor gut perfusion gives rise to the absorption of further toxins, and there is early acute renal failure. Symptomatically, there is fever, rigor, headache, lethargy and decreasing mental function.

In **anaphylactic shock** the allergic reaction produces a massive histamine response, altering capillary permeability and producing peripheral vascular dilatation. There is increased cardiac output and tachycardia, producing a warm periphery, as with septic shock, but in addition, there is marked pulmonary oedema with bronchospasm and mucosal airway obstruction, giving rise to marked dyspnoea.

Amniotic fluid embolism is due to amniotic fluid – or other material of foetal origin – entering the maternal circulation. There is resulting deposition of fibrin and platelets giving rise to disseminated intravascular coagulation. The circulatory response is rapid and profound, with hypotension and a cold, clammy periphery and cyanosis. If the patient survives the initial reaction they are subject to adult respiratory distress syndrome.

Bleeding disorders

Homeostasis is dependent on free-flowing blood within vessels and effective mechanisms for haemostasis, should a vessel wall be damaged. Failure of this delicate balance can result in death from intravascular thrombosis or from haemorrhage. Control of the system is, therefore, complex, incorporating many inhibitors and feedback loops. The degree of control can be appreciated when one considers that there is enough thrombin in 10 mL of blood to clot the whole of the vascular system if left unopposed. Bleeding abnormalities may give rise to increased natural loss (e.g. as in menorrhagia), spontaneous haemorrhage (e.g. purpura), haemarthrosis and bleeding from the nose and alimentary tract. It is of particular relevance to the surgeon in managing trauma and surgical wounds. **Haemostasis** is achieved by three mechanisms:

- Coagulation of the blood.
- Platelet adhesion and aggregation.
- Vessel wall contraction.

Abnormalities of coagulation, platelets and the vessel wall – although uncommon – encompass a large number of congenital and acquired defects. The more important of these are listed in *Tables 2.4–2.6*. Those of surgical relevance are considered below, after a general discussion of the history and examination of patients with bleeding disorders.

History

The history and examination aim to determine whether there is a potential bleeding problem, which of the three mechanisms

Table 2.4. Disorders of coagulation.

Congenital/acquired	Disorder
Congenital	Haemophilia A and B Von Willebrand's disease Abnormalities of other clotting factors
Acquired	Vitamin K deficiency Acquired anticoagulants Disseminated intravascular coagulation Haemolytic–uraemic syndrome Thrombotic thrombocytopenic purpura Anti-coagulant medication Snake bites

Table 2.5. Platelet abnormalities.

Congenital/acquired	Disorder
Congenital	Hereditary thrombocytopenic purpura Bernard–Soulier syndrome Fanconi syndrome Storage pool failure
Acquired	Reduced platelet production (marrow and megakaryocyte abnormalities) Increased destruction (idiopathic thrombocytopenia; drug induced; infections; autoimmune) Abnormal consumption (disseminated intravascular coagulation; thrombotic thrombocytopenic purpura; infection; haemangioma: Kassabach–Merritt syndrome; pump oxygenation) Splenic sequestration

Table 2.6. Vessel wall abnormalities.

Congenital/acquired	Disorder
Congenital	Hereditary haemorrhagic telangiectasia Connective tissue disorders
Acquired	Endothelial damage (anoxia; chemical; immunological) Abnormal vessel wall (senile purpura; protein abnormalities; scurvy; steroids; amyloid)

it involves, whether it is a congenital or an acquired abnormality and, if the latter, the underlying cause.

A previous history of serious or prolonged bleeding is the most likely way that a bleeding problem comes to light. Enquire about bleeding after dental extraction, trauma, venepuncture and any surgical operation. Spontaneous bleeding commonly comes from the nose, tooth-brushing and from the gastrointestinal tract, although the latter may go unnoticed. There may be a tendency to bruise easily, and purpuric patches may be present. Haemarthroses cause severe pain and must be differentiated from a septic arthritis. Bleeding into the psoas is a common muscular complication and may produce a flank mass and paralysis of the femoral nerve. Bleeding into the central nervous system is the commonest cause of death in bleeding abnormalities.

Congenital problems often first present at 2.5 to 3 years, when a child starts to run and sustain heavier falls. A family history may be present but many congenital lesions occur spontaneously. It is important to determine the mode of transmission – congenital lesions are usually of recessive character, haemophilia being sex linked. A history of previous infection may be present, such as a febrile illness 2 or 3 weeks previously. A full drug history is essential, as drugs influence all three haemostatic mechanisms, and around 100 preparations contain aspirin. Most of these problems resolve within a few weeks of stopping the drug but some preparations – e.g. gold – are bound to the tissues and so take longer to return to normal.

In adults, a large number of diseases give rise to bleeding problems and should be sought for in the history. They include malabsorption, collagen diseases, liver and renal failure, and malignancy, particularly of haematological origin or with bony secondaries.

Examination

Examination must be full, in view of the large number of potentially related diseases. The whole body must be examined for subcutaneous haemorrhage. Small bleeding points are termed petechiae (*Figure 2.9*); they differ from telangiectasia (*Figure 2.10*) in that they do not blanch under pressure. They can occur along scratch lines and at pressure points, such as where clothes rub, and may occur around the lower legs and ankles due to increased hydrostatic pressure.

Blowing up an arm cuff to 80 mmHg can produce underlying and distal petechiae. In the Hesse test, a positive result in this manoeuvre is present if more than 15 petechiae are produced within a 5 cm cutaneous circle. Larger bruises are termed ecchymoses. Purpura is a spontaneous subcutaneous haemorrhage that can be produced by coagulation, platelet

Figure 2.9.
Petechial rash.

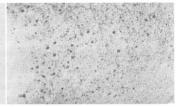

Figure 2.10.
Hereditary
telangiectasia.

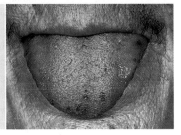

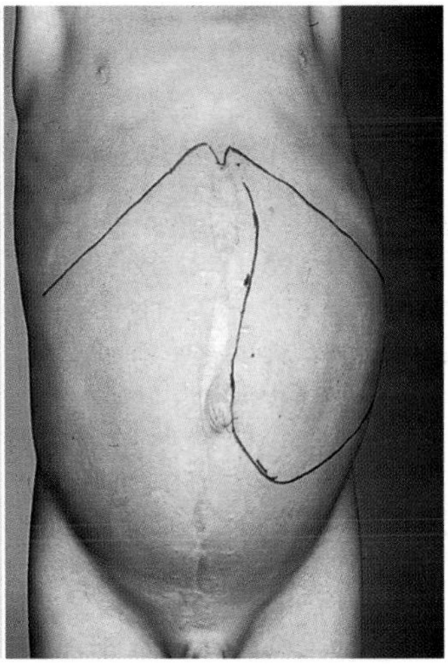

Figure 2.11.
Splenomegaly.

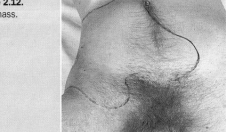

and vessel wall abnormalities. The site of purpuric patches may provide some indication of the underlying disease. Senile purpura and that due to excess steroids are usually over the backs of the hands and arms, Henoch–Schönlein purpura is over the buttocks and thighs, and secondary thrombocytopenic purpura commonly occurs around the ankles, secondary to hydrostatic pressure. Fictitious purpura – and that seen in psychiatric patients – are commonly found over the front and sides of the thighs and legs, sparing the back of the legs and trunk. In general, purpura is the hallmark of platelet abnormalities and haematomas of clotting defects.

Examination of the mouth may show ulceration and haemorrhagic gums in cases of neutropenia, leukaemia and thrombocytic purpura, while congenital haemorrhagic telangiectasia can produce numerous buccal lesions. The joints of haemophiliac patients often undergo progressive degeneration and ankylosis due to recurrent haemarthrosis, whereas they are hyperextensible in patients with Ehlers–Danlos syndrome or pseudoxanthoma elasticum. There may be widespread general features of collagen disease, and of liver and renal failure (pp. 285 and 338); splenomegaly (*Figure 2.11*) may be present. Examine the retina for fundal haemorrhages – they suggest severe thrombocytopenia.

In general, platelet abnormalities produce prolonged bleeding time, whereas coagulation defects prolong clotting time. Routine blood tests include prothrombin time (PT) as an assessment of the extrinsic pathway and activated partial thromboplastin time (APPT) as a measure of the intrinsic pathway. More detailed studies include those of platelet morphology and assaying individual clotting factors.

Disorders of coagulation

Congenital abnormalities of coagulation include haemophilia A (factor VIII deficiency), haemophilia B (factor IX deficiency – Christmas disease) and von Willebrand's disease. Haemophilia occurs in 30–120 cases per million population, affects all races and is widely distributed geographically. It is a sex-linked, recessive transmission but occurs sporadically in one-third of cases. It produces a drastic slowing of thrombin generation via the intrinsic pathway. Haemarthroses are common; in the late stage, fibrosis and ankylosis develop. Spontaneous muscle haemorrhage particularly involves the psoas with associated femoral nerve palsy and a loin mass (*Figure 2.12*). Haematuria and gastrointestinal haemorrhage are common, as is continuous bleeding after dental extraction. Serious consequences include bleeding into the central nervous system and around the sublingual or pharyngeal regions, giving rise to suffocation.

Von Willebrand's disease exhibits autosomal dominant transmission. It is a deficiency of von Willebrand factor, a

Figure 2.12.
Loin mass.

25

protein that promotes platelet adhesion and protects factor VIII against premature destruction. Other deficiencies occasionally encountered include those of factors II, VII, XI and XII, afibrinogenaemia and abnormalities of fibrinogen.

Acquired coagulation defects include vitamin K deficiency. They interfere with hepatic prothrombin metabolism. They may be due to reduced intake – as in starvation (*Figure 2.13*) – or poor dietary habits, malabsorption and primary liver disease. Circulating anticoagulants are probably autoimmune in nature and can occur in collagen diseases, drug reactions and postpartum.

Disseminated intravascular coagulation (DIC) interferes with both coagulation and platelet function. The condition is one of a consumptive coagulopathy, laying down fibrin throughout the microcirculation. Resultant necrosis can lead to damage of essential organs such as the brain, liver and heart. In fulminating cases this is followed by fibrinolysis, depletion of clotting factor and complete thrombocytopenia, the patient paradoxically presenting with widespread haemorrhage. DIC is associated with a number of clinical conditions including malignancy – adenocarcinoma of the gut, prostate, ovary: promyelocytic leukaemia – Gram-negative septicaemia (*Figure 2.14*), fat embolism and severe injuries.

Figure 2.13.
Purpura of scurvy.

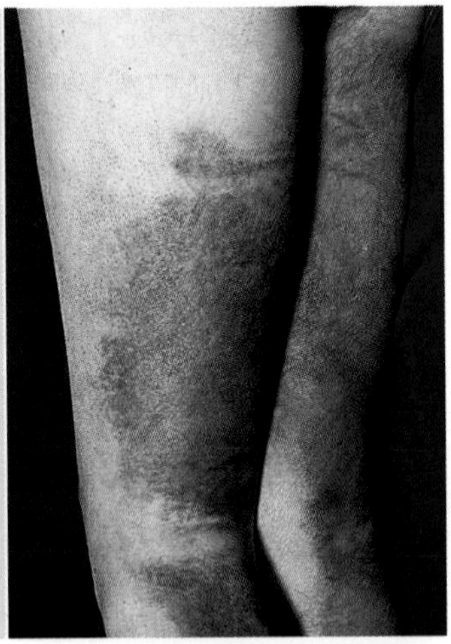

Figure 2.14.
Septic coagulopathy.

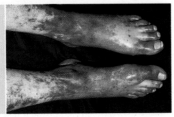

It occurs in obstetric practice in ante-partum haemorrhage, amniotic fluid embolism and – in the more chronic state – a retained dead foetus and pre-eclampsia.

Haemolytic–uraemic syndrome (HUS) and thrombotic thrombocytopenic purpura (TTP), like DIC, have widespread microvascular coagulation but the clotting mechanism is different. They usually follow infection of the respiratory and gastrointestinal tracts. The former predominantly affects the renal vasculature and usually presents in childhood. The latter is commonest in young females.

A detailed anticoagulant history is important as the patient may not have mentioned treatment for prosthetic valves, atrial fibrillation or previous thrombotic episodes. Snake bites need the appropriate anti-venom; if the snake has not been identified an informed guess is based on the locality.

Platelet abnormalities

Platelets contribute to haemostasis in that they adhere to damaged endothelium. They aggregate in response to thrombin, ADP, serotonin and other clotting factors and their presence can accelerate thrombin generation by as much as 1000 times. Congenital disorders of platelet function are rare. They can be reduced in number, such as in hereditary thrombocytopenic purpura and Fanconi's anaemia. There may be reduced platelet adhesion, as in Bernard–Soulier syndrome and there may be failure of platelets to release ADP – with abnormal platelet aggregation – as in storage pool diseases.

There are a large number of acquired disorders of platelet activity, including reduced production, increased destruction, consumptive loss and sequestration. Reduced production occurs in marrow disease – such as bone marrow infiltration with metastases, myeloproliferative disorders, leukaemia – and defective thrombopoeisis, as in vitamin B_{12} and folate deficiency, uraemia, alcohol abuse and some drugs, particularly thiazide diuretics.

Increased destruction of platelets by immune mechanisms – such as idiopathic thrombocytopenic purpura (ITP) – occurs in children at 2 or 3 weeks post viral infections (e.g. mumps, infective mononucleosis, rubella, post-immunization). It can occur as a complication of a large number of drugs – of particular note are chloramphenicol, septrin, sulphonamides, quinine, quinidine, anti-tuberculous drugs, phenylbutazone, aspirin, gold, heparin, high-dosage penicillin and non-steroidal anti-inflammatory drugs. Destruction can also accompany a number of diseases, particularly collagen diseases and infective conditions.

The massive consumption of platelets may be seen in DIC, HUS and TTP (see above). It can also occur with prosthetic heart valves, giant haemangiomas, in extra-corporeal circulation and massive blood loss. Abnormal sequestration of platelets can occur in hypersplenism.

Vessel wall abnormalities

Congenital vessel wall abnormalities are seen in hereditary telangiectasia, most commonly in adults, and in connective tissue disorders such as Ehlers–Danlos syndrome and pseudoxanthoma elasticum. Both of the latter have a lax skin and hyperextensible joints; the patients bruise easily. Acquired vessel wall abnormalities may be limited to the endothelium or represent abnormality of the total wall. The former occurs in anoxia, poisons and immunological disorders, such as Henoch–Schönlein purpura.

More extensive wall abnormalities are seen in senile purpura, disproteinaemias, scurvy, steroids (Cushing's and therapeutic) and amyloid. Most of these conditions present with varying degrees of purpura, particularly over pressure areas, easy bruising and bleeding from mucous membranes.

Anaemia

The prime function of red blood cells is to deliver oxygen to the tissues of the body. Anaemia is the reduction of the haemoglobin concentration, of the red cell count or of the packed cell volume below normal levels. This has the effect of reducing the oxygen-carrying capacity of the red cell mass. Anaemia is one of the commonest conditions encountered and affects in the region of 15–20% of the population worldwide. It may be due to abnormalities of erythropoiesis – red blood cell production – or an increased loss of red blood cells. There are a large variety of causes (*Tables 2.7–2.11*).

Erythropoiesis is considered first – to identify where disorders may occur – followed by comments on classification. Subsequent sections discuss the presenting history and examination in the anaemic patient. Consideration is given to the types of anaemias encountered transglobally.

Erythropoiesis is stimulated by the release of the hormone erythropoietin. In the adult this is stored predominantly in the kidneys and released in response to lowered tissue oxygenation. Maturation of the red blood cell in the marrow, from its precursors, takes 7 days. During this time the nucleus shrinks and gradually disappears, and haemoglobin is synthesized within the cell. The cell becomes enucleate by the seventh day but still contains residual RNA and organelles. In this stage of maturation the cell is termed a reticulocyte and red blood cells are released into the circulation in this form. The

Table 2.7. Anaemia due to defective erythropoiesis.

Type of defect	Disorder
Abnormalities of erythropoietin	Renal disease Reduced oxygen requirements (hypopituitarism; hypothyroidism) Reduced oxygen affinity to haemoglobin Erythropoietin autoantibodies
Defective proliferation	Iron deficiency Marrow failure: – aplastic anaemia (primary; secondary: radiotherapy; chemicals; toxins; drugs) – tumour invasion (leukaemia; lymphoma; myelofibrosis; secondary carcinoma) Chronic diseases (infection; collagen disease; malignancy)
Defective maturation	Nuclear abnormalities (vitamin B_{12} and folate deficiencies) Globin abnormalities: – genetic (thalassaemia; sickle cell disease) – acquired (met-, carboxy- and sulphaemoglobinaemia) Sideroblastic anaemia: – genetic – idiopathic – secondary (alcohol abuse; TB drugs; collagen; infection; lead poisoning; malignancy)

Table 2.8. Haemolytic anaemias.

Genetic/acquired abnormailities	Reason
Genetic (intrinsic)	Haemoglobin (thalassaemia; sickle cell disease) Membrane (hereditary spherocytosis) Enzyme (G6PD)
Acquired (extrinsic)	Trauma (burns; heart valves) Drugs (phenacetin) Immune (incompatible blood; newborn) Autoimmune (leukaemia; lymphoma; SLE) Toxins (lead; copper) Hypersplenism Malaria Snake and insect bites Disseminated intravascular necrosis Haemolytic–uraemic syndrome

nuclear remnants are detectable for a further 24 hours. The life cycle of the mature red blood cell is about 120 days. About 1% of the circulating red cell mass is destroyed daily, being replaced by an equivalent number of reticulocytes.

Initial abnormalities of maturation are due to failure of release of erythropoietin due to renal damage, altered sensitivity to oxygen, reduced oxygen requirement – such as in endocrine abnormalities – and autoimmune destruction of ery-thropoietin. Factors affecting maturation within the bone marrow can be divided into those inhibiting cell proliferation and those affecting the development of the mature cell. Some factors can affect both these aspects of red blood cell development.

Table 2.9. Blood loss through acute haemorrhage.

System	Condition
Gastrointestinal	Haemorrhoids
	Salicylate ingestion
	Non-steroidal, anti-inflammatory drugs
	Peptic ulcer
	Hiatus hernia
	Large bowel tumour
	Hookworm
	Telangiectasia
Uterine	Kidney (autoimmune nephritis; carcinoma)
Genitourinary	Bladder (polyps; schistosomiasis; carcinoma)

Table 2.10. Reasons for vitamin B_{12} and folate deficiencies.

Vitamin B_{12}/folate	Source of deficiency
Vitamin B_{12}	Nutritional (vegan; neglect)
	Malabsorption:
	– gastritis
	– gastric atrophy/carcinoma/resection
	– abnormailities of intrinsic factor
	– blind loop syndrome
	– tropical sprue
	– fish tapeworm
	– drugs (PAS; neomycin; colchicine; metformin; anticonvulsants; alcohol)
Folate	Excess requirements (pregnancy; infection; malignancy)

Table 2.11. Anaemia classified by red blood cell morphology.

Morphology	Condition
Microcytic	Iron deficiency
	Thalassaemia
	Sideroblastic
Macrocytic	Vitamin B_{12} and folate deficiency
	Haemolysis
	Alcohol abuse
Normocytic	Primary disease of the bone marrow (aplastic anaemia)
	Renal failure
	Hypopituitary/hypothyroidism
	Chronic diseases (infection; collagen; malignancy; scurvy)
Leukoerythroblastic	Leukaemia
	Myelosclerosis
	Metastatic carcinoma

Iron deficiency is the commonest factor inhibiting red cell proliferation. Similar effects can occur with primary or secondary marrow failure, or the infiltration of the marrow with malignant disease. Chronic debilitating diseases – such as infection, collagen abnormalities and malignancy – also inhibit proliferation.

Vitamin B_{12} and folate deficiencies inhibit early maturation of the precursor cell membrane. Globin abnormalities include genetic variants – especially thalassaemia and sickle cell disease – and the rare acquired abnormalities of methaemoglobin, carboxyhaemoglobin and sulphaemoglobin. Abnormalities of haem maturation are due to altered iron metabolism, giving rise to iron loading of the red cell, a condition termed sideroblastic anaemia; this can present as a mild genetic form. Acquired sideroblastic anaemia may be idiopathic or secondary to a number of causes, including alcohol abuse and drugs used in the treatment of tuberculosis.

The second group of factors giving rise to anaemia are increased red blood cell loss and haemolysis. Blood loss may be due to acute haemorrhage, but it is more commonly due to chronic loss, particularly from the gastrointestinal tract, the uterus and genitourinary tract. The causes of gastrointestinal haemorrhage vary with age and locality. In western civilization, aspirin ingestion makes up approximately 10% of cases and there is also a high incidence in piles, peptic ulceration and hiatus hernia. In developing countries, hookworm is the commonest cause, another potent cause being schistosomiasis.

Haemolysis may be congenital or acquired. It may be due to abnormal haemoglobin (thalassaemia; sickle cell disease), alteration in the cell membrane (hereditary spherocytosis) or abnormalities of the enzyme systems of the red blood cell (glucose-6-phosphate dehydrogenase deficiency – G6PD). A variety of extrinsic factors make up the acquired group. Haemolysis may be an immune abnormality such as with incompatible blood transfusions or haemolytic disease of the new-born. Blood can be damaged by the trauma of an artificial heart valve or in burns, and abnormal destruction of red blood cells occurs in hypersplenism. The commonest form of acquired haemolytic anaemia is due to the malarial parasite.

Classification of anaemia by red cell morphology

Whereas division of anaemias into abnormalities of erythropoiesis and blood loss helps understanding and memorizing the large number of causes, a useful clinical classification is by the microscopic study of a simple blood film. In this way anaemias can be divided into microcytic, macrocytic and normocytic. These divisions have direct clinical relevance to both the diagnosis and the presenting symptoms and signs.

A microcytic anaemia (*Figure 2.15*) is one in which the red blood cells are reduced in size. It is commonly encountered with reduced circulating or stored iron, and this is usually accompanied by hypochromia, i.e. reduced staining with haematoxylin and eosin due to a decreased amount of cellular haemoglobin. The most useful of the indices in this type of anaemia is a reduction of the mean corpuscular volume (MCV). The mean corpuscular haemoglobin (MCH) and the mean corpuscular haemoglobin concentration (MCHC) are also abnormal.

Microcytosis may also occur in thalassaemia, sideroblastic anaemia and occasionally the anaemia of chronic disorders. Further measurements of body iron, include serum iron, total iron-binding capacity, serum ferritin and the iron stores present in the marrow. In the clinical assessment, include questions on menstruation, post-menopausal bleeding and frank bleeding from the gastrointestinal or urinary tracts. Examine the faeces for occult blood, cysts, ova and parasites. As appropriate, undertake endoscopy and barium studies of the oesophagus, stomach, duodenum, and examine the anus, rectum and colon. Undertake urinalysis to exclude haematuria.

Megaloblastic red blood cells in the peripheral circulation or the marrow commonly occur in relation to vitamin B_{12} (*Figure 2.16*) and folate deficiency. There is also an increase in mean corpuscular volume. Megaloblastic circulating red blood cells also occur in myelodysplasia, anaemia related to alcohol abuse and occasionally haemolytic anaemias. A megaloblastic pattern always warrants further investigation.

Normocytic anaemias occur in a wide variety of disorders. They are usually normochromic and have normal red blood cell indices. They include primary diseases of bone marrow and aplastic anaemias. White blood and red blood cell precursors (*Figure 2.17*) may be present in the peripheral field, including enucleate red cells, myelocytes and metamyelocytes. There may be hypoplasia of all cell groups and also dysplasia. Examination of the marrow may show the underlying cause of disease. The majority of anaemias encountered in chronic disease fall into this category. They include anaemias of renal failure, hypopituitarism, hypothyroidism, inflammation, collagen diseases and malignancy.

Examination of a peripheral blood film may show associated abnormalities of red and white blood cells; such anaemias are termed leukoerythroblastic. They include the anaemias of leukaemia, myelosclerosis and metastatic marrow carcinoma. The film may show the primitive blast cells of leukaemia. White blood cell abnormalities are also seen with iron deficiency anaemia (parasites, especially hookworm; allergic conditions; enteritides and Hodgkin's disease). In vitamin B_{12} and folate deficiency there may be hypersegmented polymorphs and platelet abnormalities, producing a bleeding diathesis (p. 23).

Examination of the peripheral blood film may identify other classical red and white cell abnormalities that may be of diagnostic importance:

- Anisocytes and poikilocytes are abnormally shaped red blood cells that are useful cell markers of iron deficiency anaemia.
- Increased circulating reticulocytes are characteristic of haemolytic anaemia and chronic blood loss. Fragmented cells can be seen in cases of haemolysis and microangiopathies.
- Spherocytes are abnormal, spherically shaped red blood cells encountered in hereditary spherocytosis and malaria.
- Target cells have a characteristic darker centre, providing the multiple ringed appearance. They occur in thalassaemia, liver disease and after splenectomy.
- Punctate basophilia of red blood cells is an abnormality of erythropoiesis seen in lead poisoning.
- Heinz bodies are abnormal sub-units of globin or precipitated haemoglobin, particularly seen in G6PD deficiency.
- Howell–Jolly bodies are nuclear fragments, particularly seen post splenectomy. Sideroblasts are red blood cells with iron granular inclusions, seen in sideroblastic anaemias and post splenectomy.
- Rouleaux formation – i.e. the stacking of red blood cells in columns – occurs in multiple myelomatosis and dysproteinaemia.

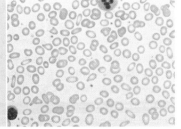

Figure 2.15. Blood film from a patient with microcytic anaemia. Note the hypochromic small red blood cells (also lymphocyte, polymorph, and platelets.

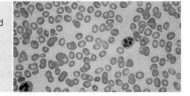

Figure 2.16. Megaloblastic blood film.

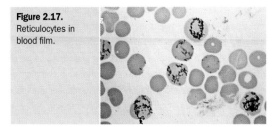

Figure 2.17.
Reticulocytes in blood film.

Haemoglobin abnormalities – such as those of thalassaemia and sickle cell disease – are identified by electrophoresis. More sophisticated tests are becoming available and are used to study milder and rarer forms of haemoglobin abnormality and their mode of inheritance. Different forms of anaemia may coexist, such as iron deficiency in thalassaemia.

Clinical assessment of the anaemic patient

History

The anaemic patient may present with the symptoms of anaemia or its underlying cause. Occasionally, a blood test undertaken for a routine health screen or prior to an operative procedure brings the anaemia to light. The symptoms depend on the rate of onset and severity, for example in chronic, unrecognized bleeding from the stomach, bowel, kidneys or bladder, the haemoglobin can fall to less than 5 g/dL without noticeable symptoms. Similarly, with chronic menorrhagia or hookworm infestation, a haemoglobin of 10 g/dL may well be the norm.

The lowered oxygen tension defining anaemia has widespread effects on all tissues; symptoms are often diffuse. The aim of the history and examination should be to identify the existence of anaemia and to search for any underlying cause. Subsequent investigations help to define the particular type and severity of the anaemia and provide further diagnostic clues, as discussed earlier.

The general symptoms of chronic anaemia are tiredness, weakness and lassitude. There may be a reduced appetite and weight loss. Mental changes of headache and dizziness are common, and to these can be added confusion, particularly in the elderly. Exertional dyspnoea is an early symptom.

More severe symptoms of anaemia usually relate to the effects on cardiac function since the cardiac output has to be increased to deliver adequate tissue oxygen in the presence of an inadequate transport medium. If the disease progresses,

a high-output cardiac failure occurs. Tachycardia and high output give rise to palpitations, increased headache and dizziness. Breathlessness becomes more severe, with orthopnoea and paroxysmal nocturnal dyspnoea. Anaemia accentuates angina and claudication from underlying coronary and lower limb arterial disease. Cardiac failure is accompanied by ankle and sacral oedema and a cough with frothy white sputum.

Having suspected anaemia, explore possible causes, particularly in the gastrointestinal, urological and menstrual history. Fresh alimentary bleeding may be noted from the gums and piles. A painful mouth and tongue may be related to the anaemia and produce eating difficulties. Note low dietary intake due to neglect or starvation, and dietary habits, food fads and psychiatric disorders. A total absence of meat and dairy products can give rise to vitamin B_{12} deficiency. Note dysphagia, indigestion, abdominal pain and distension, and changes in bowel habit. The symptoms may suggest malignancy, other gut disease or sickle cell crises. The locality or overseas trips may suggest specific parasitic problems of the gut or elsewhere, such as hookworm and malaria. Pruritus can occur in iron deficiency anaemia.

In the menstrual history, assess the degree of loss, such as the number of pads used and recent change. Bleeding problems may become apparent through easy bruising after minor trauma, spontaneous purpura or bleeding after tooth extraction, cuts and surgery. Associated diseases may be obvious, such as acute haemorrhage and the symptoms of shock and collapse, severe infections and widespread malignancy. Bone pain may indicate local pathology.

A detailed drug history is essential as the ingestion of nonsteroidal, anti-inflammatory agents is common and patients may be on anticoagulants. Drug reactions are diverse and – once the list is complete – may require reference to the appropriate literature.

Alcohol abuse can produce a number of haematological effects through liver disease as well as specific haemolysis and its effects on bone marrow. Adhesives, lead and some other chemicals linked with occupations or hobbies must be identified. The racial origin of the subject may suggest the possibility of thalassaemia or sickle cell disease, and a detailed family history of bleeding problems should be questioned and a family tree constructed.

Examination

Anaemia is characterized by pallor, though clinical assessment of the degree of pallor is unreliable. It is most easily observed in the mucous membranes of the mouth or the conjunctiva, and peripherally in the nail beds and palmar creases.

Examination of the skin and subcutaneous tissues may reveal bruising, purpura or other manifestations of bleeding diatheses, such as petechiae and telangiectasia. There may be extensive bruising around any venepuncture sites. There may also be fundal haemorrhages noted on retinoscopy.

Cardiac signs include tachycardia, a large pulse volume and a hyperdynamic flow murmur. The hyperdynamic state might give rise to cardiac failure, the signs including peripheral oedema, a raised jugular venous pressure, basal crepitations, hepatomegaly, and fluid collections in the pleural and peritoneal cavities.

In patients with iron deficiency anaemia, there may be weight loss due to deficient intake, from neglect, starvation, food fads and psychiatric problems, or malabsorption and losses through fistulae. The tongue is smooth and shiny (*Figure 2.18*) and there may be angular stomatitis. The nails characteristically show koilonychia, i.e. spooning and widening of the nails, which are brittle and fragile (as shown in *Figure 1.11*).

Patients with vitamin B_{12} and folate deficiencies often have a pronounced pallor but also a lemon-yellow tinge to their skin. They may have angular stomatitis and glossitis, together with mouth ulceration. A specific feature of pernicious anaemia is the presence of subacute combined degeneration of the spinal cord. In this condition the peripheral neuropathy is more pronounced in the lower limbs, especially involving the lateral columns, affecting vibration and position sense, knee jerks are lost, and there may be an extensor plantar response, a positive Rhomberg sign and optic atrophy. Megaloblastic changes may be accompanied by thrombocytopenia, with splenomegaly, hepatomegaly and purpura. Other signs may be related to an underlying carcinoma of the stomach, with weight loss, an abdominal mass, hepatomegaly and supraclavicular nodes.

In haemolytic anaemia there may be a mild jaundice and – if a haemoglobinopathy is present – there may be gall stones, secondary splenomegaly and chronic leg ulceration. Areas of bone necrosis may occur in sickle cell disease. Autoimmune anaemias may occur in chronic lymphatic leukaemia, lymphoma and systemic lupus erythematosis; there may be signs of these diseases and associated splenomegaly.

Malignancy can give rise to other abnormal physical signs. These include an abdominal mass, liver secondaries, hepatosplenomegaly and widespread lymphadenopathy; the latter may be primary or secondary malignant involvement. Endocrine anaemias may be accompanied by pituitary, adrenal or thyroid insufficiency.

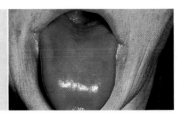

Figure 2.18.
Plummer–Vinson's syndrome: smooth tongue.

Geographic distribution of anaemias

The prominence of anaemia as a world-wide problem has already been emphasized. However, this high incidence has a marked geographical variation. Of particular note is the frequency of anaemia in parts of Africa, Asia and China. The large populations of these areas are dependent on local agriculture and this in turn is subject to many natural and man-made disasters. Of particular note are the effects of drought, flood, earthquake and war.

The ultimate effect is starvation, mass migration and refugee problems. The associated poverty diminishes the potential of alternative food and fresh water supplies. These conditions give rise to deficiency anaemias and anaemias due to infection. The third problem is the genetic haemoglobin abnormalities that already exist in some of these areas.

Starvation gives rise to anaemia through iron, vitamin B_{12}, folate, vitamin C and protein deficiencies. Dietary habits in different continents influence the pattern of endemic anaemias. Common diets are based on rice, wheat and maize, all of which are low in vitamin B_{12}, and this can become a problem if the diet is also low in meat and devoid of dairy products. World-wide, however, folate deficiency is commoner. Folates are destroyed by the prolonged boiling of vegetables and, in this respect, folate deficiency is less seen in China, where vegetables are lightly boiled, than in India, where spicy foods are heated for longer periods. Pregnant women and children are particularly prone to folate deficiency because of their high physiological requirement. Fresh fruit is a valuable source of folate.

Acute infections commonly follow disasters, and the establishment of a clean water supply and adequate sanitation are of prime concern in the management of these events. Many infections, however, are endemic and give rise to widespread, chronic anaemias. Hookworm is a prime offender, it being estimated that 450 million people harbour this parasite, which not only sucks blood through the mucous membrane of the alimentary tract but also secretes an anticoagulant. Although the body is very effective in using ingested iron, it cannot necessarily keep up with the loss produced by such parasites.

There is also an increased requirement in children, and in adolescence, menstruation and pregnancy. Schistosomiasis is another serious cause of anaemia and affects 50 million people world-wide.

In tropical zones it is estimated that 500 million people are exposed to the malarial parasite and probably 100 million are infected at any one time. Such infections can produce mild chronic haemolysis but in other cases this may be profound and lethal. The infant mortality related to malaria is in the region of 250 per 1000 population in some parts of Africa, with a further 150 deaths per 1000 before the age of four.

In malarial regions a number of varieties of haemoglobin have developed that provide partial protection against the haemolytic effects of the parasite. Well over 100 genetic varieties have so far been identified. Many are produced by changes of a single amino acid in the haemoglobin chain, and the majority have no clinical relevance. However, a few, such as those that cause thalassaemia and sickle cell disease, have serious haematological consequences.

Thalassaemia is the commonest inherited haematological abnormality and is probably the commonest genetic disorder in the world. Approximately 240 million people have a heterozygous trait of one of these haemoglobinopathies, and 200 000 have a homozygous pattern, these being approximately equally divided between thalassaemia and sickle cell disease. With the improvement of health care in endemic areas, this figure will probably be doubled by the year 2000.

The thalassaemias are widely encountered, predominantly in Asia but also in the southern Mediterranean and North Africa. Thalassaemia in its severest form gives rise to foetal deaths, therefore it is less commonly encountered in adults. Typical clinical features of α and β, and other varieties of thalassaemia, include failure to thrive, fever, poor feeding and reduced resistance to infection; there is splenomegaly. Late problems include iron overload from repeated transfusion, folate deficiency, weight loss and terminal infections.

Patients with sickle cell disease originate predominantly from North Africa. They have a mild icterus, splenomegaly and a high incidence of leg ulcers. They are also prone to systemic infections. Major problems arise if there are bouts of anoxia, such as with respiratory infections or anaesthesia. These produce acute haemolysis, giving rise to vascular occlusion and focal infarction, presenting with areas of aseptic bone necrosis, and gut and cerebral infarction.

G6PD is a red cell enzyme deficiency widely distributed through Africa, and the Middle and Far East. There are more than 100 variants and it has been estimated that 100 million people are affected. It usually produces mild chronic haemolysis, but acute haemolysis may be precipitated by intercurrent illnesses and exposure to oxidant drugs, including antimalarials.

Urgent treatment is often required for severe anaemia. This may include blood transfusion. However, it is important to take blood for all the appropriate tests prior to the commencement of any therapy as the latter may alter the haematological picture and obscure accurate diagnosis.

Pyrexia

The body temperature can be raised after exercise and is subject to physiological variation, for example at the time of ovulation. The temperature is also raised in response to disease, the condition being known as pyrexia or fever. The mechanism is uncertain but is probably related to the release of endogenous pyrogens from damaged tissue. The highest and most constant fevers occur in infectious diseases but are also associated with collagen disease and some neoplasms, thrombosis, ischaemia and drug reactions.

The cause of a pyrexia is usually obvious. Most acute infections have run their course within 3 weeks and the fever commonly has a characteristic pattern of onset, duration and lysis (p. 106). A few viruses – such as infective mononucleosis, hepatitis and cytomegalovirus – may have a prolonged course, as do chronic granuloma-producing organisms such as tuberculosis, actinomycosis, toxoplasmosis, histoplasmosis and candidiasis. A number of endemic infectious diseases must be considered in their chosen habitat and in visitors from these areas, e.g. malaria, schistosomiasis, amoebiasis and trypanosomiasis (Chapter 6).

The inflammatory response produces pyrexia in non-infective disorders, particularly immunological conditions including the collagen diseases, rheumatoid arthritis, systemic lupus erythematosis, polyarteritis nodosa, temporal arteritis and polymyalgia. Some tumours characteristically have a fever, including hypernephroma, leukaemia, lymphoma and, occasionally, pancreatic carcinoma, liver metastases and sarcomas. Other less common causes include venous thrombosis, pulmonary embolism, cirrhosis and sarcoidosis.

Intracranial disease and associated surgery can interfere with hypothalamic control of temperature, producing marked pyrexia, which may be difficult to control. Almost any drug can produce a febrile reaction but of note are those linked with sulphonamides, penicillin and barbiturates.

A fictitious pyrexia is occasionally encountered, the patient placing a thermometer in a cup of tea or exchanging thermometers. Watching the patient during a sublingual measurement provides an accurate result. Suspicion is raised if the pyrexia is not accompanied by an equivalent rise in pulse rate.

Pyrexia of unknown origin

Patients may present with a pyrexia with no obvious cause. The title of pyrexia of unknown or uncertain origin (PUO) is usually applied when this pyrexia persists for more than 3 weeks or if the diagnosis is not made after 1 week in-patient investigation. A limit of 38.4 °C can be added to provide uniformity for comparative studies. In view of the serious nature of many underlying causes, the patient should be fully investigated. A diagnosis is eventually made in 90% of these cases through careful and repeated history, examination and investigation. About 40% of patients turn out to have an infective source, 20% collagen disease and 20% neoplasia. The diagnosis is usually one of a common condition presenting in an unusual fashion, rather than a rare disease.

History

A patient with a PUO will already have had their history taken on a number of occasions. This means that each subsequent history must be taken in even more detail, although new symptoms may have appeared. Great skill is required and it provides a great diagnostic challenge. Every system must be questioned in detail and even trivial symptoms or slight nuances in the history must be fully assessed. A PUO may be accompanied by anorexia, malaise, lassitude, weight loss and non-specific symptoms of associated anaemia. Skin abnormalities include rashes, eruptions and irritation. Enquire whether the patient has had previous illnesses, accidents, transfusions or surgery. In the alimentary tract question for changes in appetite, dental problems, dysphagia, abdominal discomfort or distension, changes in bowel habit, the presence of mild diarrhoea, changes in stool colour, perianal pain, pruritus or discharge. Enquire of dyspareunia and urethral or vaginal discharge.

In the head, neck and respiratory system, enquire of eye discomfort, redness or discharge, ear-ache or discharge, nasal discharge, pain or tenderness over sinuses, sore throats, cough or dyspnoea. There may be aches or swelling of muscle, bones and joints, or abnormal sensation or motor function. Question for contacts with sick individuals, whether these are in the family, friends or at work. Animal contacts produce a large number of potential pyrexial diseases.

Foreign travel is of prime importance. Visits to malarial zones without appropriate prophylaxis raises the question of malarial infection. Other potential infective diseases from tropical and other zones world-wide include typhoid, paratyphoid, hepatitis, amoebiasis, brucellosis, schistosomiasis, trypanosomiasis, filariasis, *kala azar*, Rocky Mountain spotted fever, typhus, Lassa fever and rabies. Incubation periods vary in these diseases and require reference to appropriate texts (see also Chapter 6).

In the drug history, consider prescribed medications and non-prescriptive drugs, which may have been bought across the counter for minor ailments; also recreational drugs and any injections.

The family history may identify chronic infective diseases such as tuberculosis, collagen diseases or unusual anaemias.

Examination

In the examination, note the pulse, blood pressure and respiratory rate. Check the temperature, watching that the patient is not interfering with the reading. A temperature chart indicates the level and characteristics of the fever. A swinging record implies the presence of pus, while night fever may be associated with tuberculosis.

The general appearance of the patient indicates whether they look unwell and are pyrexial, whether they are pale, jaundiced and whether there is obvious weight loss; also measure the patient's weight. The hands may show clubbing, suggesting respiratory or gut disorders, or splinter haemorrhages of endocarditis. Examine the skin over the whole body for infective lesions, rashes, scratch marks, petechiae, purpura, ulceration and staining, such as in the flanks from pancreatitis, over hernia due to dead bowel and over superficial venous thromboses.

In the head and neck examine for eye abnormalities and tenderness over the mastoid air cells, nasal sinuses, teeth and temporal arteries. Examine the mouth for bad teeth and an inflamed throat. Generalized lymphadenopathy often presents in the neck. Examine all groups, particularly unusually palpable nodes such as the occipital and external and anterior jugular. Examination behind a lax sternomastoid muscle may reveal a palpable scalene node. Examine axillae and groins, as well as the epitrochlear nodes.

The heart valves may be the site of infective carditis. Listen for soft murmurs or established valvular abnormalities, also for pericardial and pleural rubs and focal lung disease. Percuss the lung bases to establish whether the diaphragm is moving or could be splinted by sub-diaphragmatic disease. This is a common site, as evidenced by the aphorism 'pus somewhere, pus nowhere, pus under the diaphragm'.

Hidden and unsuspected causes of PUO are commonly found in the abdomen. Examine for superficial, deep and rebound tenderness and for tenderness in the renal angles. Palpate for masses and viscera, especially hepatosplenomegaly and perinephric masses. Abnormalities along the large bowel – such as malignancy or pericolic abscesses – may be palpable. Check hernial orifices to ensure they do not contain ischaemic bowel or omentum. Listen for peritoneal rubs and hepatic bruits. Pelvic examination is a very important assessment, including rectal and gynaecological digital and instrumental examination. Pus or tumour may be present in the pouch of Douglas and tubovarian disease may be detected.

In the remainder of the examination, note tenderness and swelling of the muscles, bones and joints; look for pain on movement of joints and of the back, and for any neck stiffness. There may be deep tenderness over areas of venous thrombosis.

In a seriously ill patient with a non-specific abnormal white blood count or raised ESR, there is occasionally an indication for laparoscopy or even laparotomy. Also, if certain illnesses are suspected, there may be an indication for prescribing antibiotics, steroids, anti-inflammatory and anti-tuberculous or anti-malarial therapy.

Weight loss

Weight loss in the absence of dieting is usually a symptom of underlying disease and a greater than 5% weight reduction must be fully investigated. Very sudden loss of weight is usually due to fluid loss, from dehydration or operative removal of fluid, correction of fluid overload in renal, cardiac and liver disease, post partum and, to a lesser extent, postmenstrual and after catheterization.

If a patient presents with increased appetite and loss of weight, it is important to exclude thyrotoxicosis, diabetes mellitus and malabsorption. This group of patients may also include unrecognized psychiatric problems (see below), or an early malignancy with a high metabolic rate.

Weight loss is usually due to a decreased intake of food and fluid (dieting; anorexia due to systemic or psychiatric disease), increased loss (diarrhoea, vomiting, fistulae) or increased metabolism (fever, malignancy). In the assessment it is important to establish a patient's normal weight, the usual pattern of intake and output, and to document changes in these patterns.

Weight loss may be evident in any alteration of features or form, and lax skin folds over the arms, trunk and buttocks. The patient's clothes may be too large. Weight reduction can be due to fluid loss, as well as tissue reduction. Signs of dehydration include dry, inelastic skin, sunken eyes and dry mucous membranes.

Table 2.12 indicates the large number of causes of weight loss. General examination must include assessment of the hands and skin for pallor, pigmentation, rashes, clubbing, splinter haemorrhages and spider naevi. Examine for a goitre, eye changes, skin, tremor, sweating and tachycardia to identify thyrotoxicosis. In the abdomen, pelvis, breasts and lymph nodes look for occult malignancy and identify fluid collections in the pleural and peritoneal cavities. Measure the patient's temperature and undertake urinalysis for evidence of glycosuria and proteinuria. After establishing base lines, it is necessary to follow-up with precise measurements of intake and output, weight and skin thickness.

Starvation affects all ages but weight loss at other times is markedly influenced by the patient's age. In children, severe gastroenteritis and malabsorption are frequent causes; the latter may also present in later life. In young adults, common causes are tuberculosis, reticuloses and psychiatric problems. In middle-aged patients consider endocrine disease and malignancy. In older age groups, the cause is usually related to more than one factor. The tissues of old people tend to shrink, and there is a loss of stature. Although this may be associated with reduction of appetite it is important to exclude other causes, particularly neglect and senility. Cancer is common, and cardio-respiratory as well as alimentary diseases are accompanied by weight loss.

Anorexia nervosa is a psychiatric disorder occurring in young adults, particularly women. There is a total preoccupation with the weight in the patient's thought and deed; it overrides any hunger or rational discussion of the problem,

Table 2.12. Causes of weight loss.

Malabsorption	Low intake	Systemic disorders
Chronic diarrhoea	Starvation	Subacute and chronic infection
Laxative abuse	Dieting	
Coeliac disease	Senility	Malignancy
Colitides	Neglect/disability	Cardiorespiratory disease
Crohn's disease	Oral pathology	
Acute/chronic gut infection	Dysphagia	Uraemia
	Obstruction of the upper alimentary tract	Collagen disease
Abnormal gut flora		Alcohol abuse
Liver/biliary/pancreatic disease	Vomiting	Recreational drugs
Gut resection	Anorexia nervosa	Poisons
Endocrine (diabetes mellitus; thyrotoxicosis; panhypopituitarism; hypoadrenalism)	Food fads	
	Psychoses	

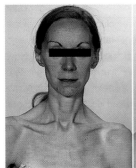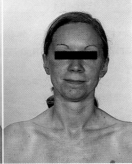

Figure 2.19.
Anorexic twin.

and weight reduction targets are constantly being set. There is rigorous dieting and vigorous exercise programmes – weight loss can be considerable (*Figure 2.19*). Associated endocrine abnormalities include depression of the pituitary–gonadal axis and hypothyroidism, with accompanying loss of libido and potency, and amenorrhoea. In extreme cases of emaciation there may be bradycardia and hypothermia. The condition carries a 5% mortality, usually from a cardiomyopathy induced by nutritional changes in the heart.

Bulimia nervosa is also a psychiatric problem noted in young adults. The preoccupation in this case is with food but there is also a dread of becoming fat. The patient develops a cycle of excessive eating followed by vomiting, these habits taking up much of the day. There may be associated laxative abuse. The weight loss does not equate to that of anorexia nervosa patients, the patients usually maintaining their weight near normal, despite voluminous intake.

Overweight

In the adult, the quantity of most tissues is fixed, however, the amount of fat can vary dramatically. Fat is contained both in the superficial adipose layer and in other tissues such as liver, muscle and bone. In normal adult males fat makes up 12% of the body weight and 26% in females. An individual is termed 'fat' when there is a 20% increase in body weight, and 'obese' after 30%. Obesity is the commonest nutritional disorder in the developed world. Average values are based on height–weight tables and follow-up studies use weight change and measurement of skin fold thickness.

Obesity may also be classified in relation to the body mass index (BMI). This is calculated by dividing the weight in kg by the height in m squared. A BMI greater than 28 is classified as obesity, morbid obesity being greater than 35. An ideal body weight in kg is height in cm –100 in men and –105 in women.

Obesity is usually due to overeating and too little exercise, but it is important to identify weight increase due to focal or generalized fluid retention and that due to pregnancy. Focal fluid collections include ascites and ovarian cysts. Generalized fluid retention may be secondary to cardiac, renal and liver failure.

Obese people eat more but the basis of the hyperphagia can be metabolic or hypothalamic in origin, an example of the latter is a hypothalamic tumour. Genetic causes are usually due to hypogonadism; hormonal causes include hypothyroidism, Cushing's syndrome and abnormal sex hormone metabolism. Drugs include the contraceptive pill and some psychotherapeutic medications.

Eating is influenced by cultural and environmental factors, the variety of food available and its nutritional value; some individuals are habitual or compulsive overeaters.

The distribution of fat is particularly noticeable around the face, abdomen and buttocks, but it may be more focally sited, such as the 'buffalo hump' of Cushing's syndrome. Rapid weight gain may be accompanied by skin stretching, with paper thin striae.

A number of diseases are closely linked with obesity, and these include atherosclerosis, hypertension, hiatus hernia, gall bladder disease, diabetes, respiratory dysfunction, joint diseases, deep venous thrombosis and endometrial carcinoma. The dangers of obesity are also seen during anaesthesia and may be associated with psychiatric problems. Respiratory problems are due to an increased oxygen consumption and increased carbon dioxide production. A reduced functional residual capacity results in airway closure during normal tidal breathing, promoting anoxia. Severe cases give rise to sleep apnoea, cyanosis, polycythaemia and, eventually, right ventricular hypertrophy and heart failure.

Anaesthetic problems include respiratory depression, cardiac disease and hypertension. Intubation may be difficult in a bull neck, there is an increased risk of aspiration of gastric contents due to hiatus hernia and delayed gastric emptying. There is altered distribution of anaesthetic drugs due to lipid binding and mild liver abnormalities from fatty infiltration. Post-operative drugs must be chosen with care to prevent respiratory depression, and measures taken to reduce the incidence of deep venous thrombosis.

Reducing weight is predominantly a dietary problem but pathological causes of obesity must be identified and treated appropriately. Regular exercise should be encouraged, aerobic activity such as jogging is more effective than short bursts such as in squash. Increasing the metabolic rate can reduce weight but as this is usually dependent on thyroid hormones, smoking or amphetamine-like drugs, such treatment is usually inappropriate.

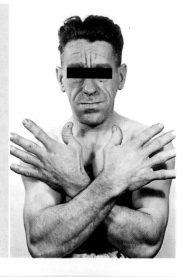

Figure 2.20.
Hands and face of acromegalic.

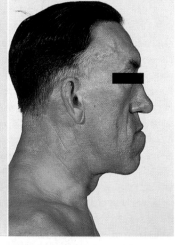

Figure 2.21.
Side view
(acromegaly).

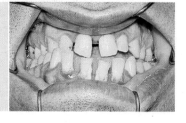

Figure 2.22.
Teeth (acromegaly).

Acromegaly

Acromegaly is produced by growth hormone secretion from a pituitary acidophilic adenoma, commencing after completion of normal growth; hyperactivity before this time results in gigantism. The clinical features of acromegaly are due to overgrowth of bony and soft tissues.

The skin is thickened and greasy due to increased sebum, and there may be hirsuties and hyperpigmentation. In the hands the bones are longer and broader, especially the distal phalanges, producing a long hand with wide fingers (*Figure 2.20*). The feet are larger, especially in width, and patients may have noticed increasing glove and shoe sizes.

The skull is enlarged, particularly the prognathic jaw (*Figures 2.21* and *2.22*) and nasal air sinuses. Skull radiograph usually shows an enlarged pituitary fossa. Increase in the soft tissues of the face include prominent lips, nose and tongue. Most patients present, or are recognized, because of these changes in their features.

There is not usually a marked growth of the long bones of the arms and legs but there are exuberant osteoarthritic changes. The spine is subject to spondylitic changes and a dorsal kyphosis can make the arms look longer. There is visceromegaly, including the liver, spleen kidneys and lungs.

The overgrowth of bone and soft tissue can induce nerve entrapment problems, particularly carpal tunnel syndrome, spinal nerve compression with sciatica and brachial neuropathy. There may be a proximal myopathy. Nerve pain, visual disturbances due to compression of the optic chiasm and headache may bring the patient to a doctor.

Associated conditions – due to an increase in basal metabolic rate – are intolerance to heat, with excess sweating. There may be diabetes mellitus, hypercalcaemia and hypophosphataemia. Hypopituitarism may give rise to a goitre and sometimes myxoedema. The condition may be part of a multiple endocrine syndrome. The patients are subject to cardiomyopathy and obesity, and there is an increase in cerebrovascular disease. In the respiratory system, soft tissue abnormalities can produce an increased lung volume and voice changes. There is an increase in malignancy in males.

Thyrotoxicosis

Thyrotoxicosis is due to excess circulating thyroid hormone in the form of thyroxine or tri-iodothyronine. This effect is on the basal metabolic rate and increased sensitivity of β-adrenergic responses and – if occurring before the end of the growth phase – early maturation and a slight increase in growth rate. Primary thyrotoxicosis (p. 223) is associated with thyroid stimulating antibodies and may occur in conjunction with autoimmune conditions such as vitiligo, myasthenia gravis and pernicious anaemia. A few rare cases may be due to drugs such as thyroxine and iodine, an increased TSH from the pituitary or gonads, or a well-differentiated thyroid carcinoma. Secondary thyrotoxicosis (p. 223) describes the development of thyrotoxicosis in a patient with a pre-existing goitre. It is seen in areas where endemic goitres occur due to deficient iodine intake.

The effects of thyrotoxicosis are seen in all systems but are most marked in the cardiovascular and neuropsychiatric responses. The onset may be precipitated by sepsis or stress but may also appear at puberty or during pregnancy. Onset is usually gradual but occasionally explosive. The metabolic effects of increased metabolic rate include a marked increase in appetite yet loss in weight. Occasionally there may be nausea and vomiting and usually a mild diarrhoea.

The excess heat production gives rise to sweating and a dislike of hot weather, there being palmar erythema and spider naevi. Skin changes also include a pre-tibial myxoedema, alopecia and onycholysis.

Cardiovascular symptoms may dominate the clinical features and patients may present with the dyspnoea of cardiac failure. There is a tachycardia – which persists through sleep – palpitations, extra-systole and, commonly, auricular fibrillation. These factors may lead to a high-output, congestive cardiac failure with extreme dyspnoea and debilitation.

Neurological features are those of agitation, nervousness, restlessness, irritability and insomnia. There is marked emotional lability, rapidly changing from an excited and manic state to anxiety, depression, melancholia, with frequent bouts of crying. Patients are often short tempered and occasionally an overt psychosis may occur.

Muscle wasting is common – accompanying the weight loss – and may be severely disabling. It particularly affects cheek facial muscles, giving hollow cheeks, the small muscles of the hands and the shoulder muscles (*Figures 2.23 and 2.24*). Fatigue is common and may mimic myasthenic symptoms. Movements are jerky and a fine tremor is usually present, particularly seen in the outstretched hand and tongue. There may be hyperaesthesia but – in spite of motor problems – there is no sensory loss.

Eye signs are the most noticeable clinical features of thyrotoxicosis (*Figures 2.25 and 2.26*) but care must be taken in their diagnosis since some of the signs are occasionally seen in normal individuals. There is lid retraction, exposing

sclera above and below the iris and giving a wide-eyed, staring look, and proptosis from retro-ocular fatty infiltration.

In other systems there may be oligomenorrhoea or amenorrhoea and loss of libido. The thyroid gland, as well as being enlarged from diffuse, or single or multiple nodules, usually has a soft systolic bruit over it.

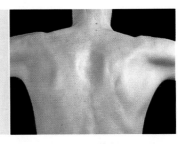

Figure 2.23.
Proximal myopathy of thyrotoxicosis.

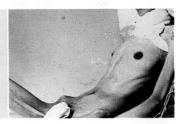

Figure 2.24.
Emaciation of severe thyrotoxicosis.

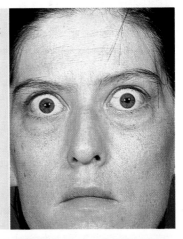

Figure 2.25.
Exophthalmos (front view).

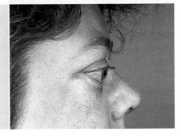

Figure 2.26.
Exophthalmos (side view).

Myxoedema

Myxoedema is a hormonal disease resulting from a reduction in circulating thyroid. In primary myxoedema the abnormality is in the thyroid gland. Examples include agenesis, atrophy, destruction by auto-immune disease, thyroiditis, malignancy, radioactive iodine, surgical excision, iodine deficiency and drug suppression. Secondary myxoedema is due to reduced thyroid stimulating hormone, resultant on tumours or infarction involving the hypothalamic–pituitary axis.

The disease can occur at any age but peaks between 56 and 60; it is commoner in female patients by a ratio of 5:1. The symptoms are due to the reduction of the basal metabolic rate and are initially insidious. They include fatigue and lethargy, tiredness and weakness. They are vague and can bring the patient to many different clinics and are thus easily missed. There may be aches and pains, cramps and stiffness, with feeling the cold and a dislike for cold weather. Constipation and menorrhagia are common.

There is usually a reduction in mental activity, with slowness of thought, speech and action. Rare complications include myxoedema madness and myxoedema coma, the latter being precipitated by cold, exposure, narcotics and analgesics. It is often seen in the aged patient living alone. It is a serious complication with a 50% mortality, it being very difficult to warm the patient without precipitating cardiac abnormalities and failure. The temperature may drop to 24°C, the patient being cold, dry and cadaveric, with no shivering.

On examination the patient is slow in communication and actions. The deposition of mucinous substance within the skin and subcutaneous tissue produces a thickening in these layers. The non-pitting, fatty tissue is prominent over the supraclavicular region, the back of the neck, the shoulders and face, the latter producing puffy eyelids and gross features. The tongue may be enlarged. The voice is deep, gruff and weak with some hoarseness.

The skin is cold, dry, scaly, thickened and pale. A malar flush, together with the pale skin colour, produces a 'strawberries-and-cream' complexion and there may also be a tinge of yellow. This has also been described as a 'peaches-and-cream' picture (*Figure 2.27*). Hair is dry, coarse, lacklustre, inelastic, brittle and falls out, producing baldness and, commonly, loss of the outer aspects of the eyebrows (*Figure 2.28*). The hands are cold and puffy (spade-like) with cyanosed tips.

The thyroid gland may be felt but this depends on the underlying pathology (p. 223). Cardiac deposition of mucinoid material can produce cardiac failure, the signs being

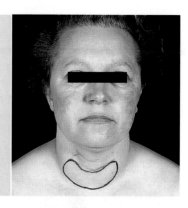

Figure 2.27.
Myxoedema of the face.

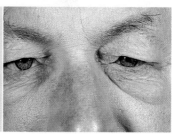

Figure 2.28.
Loss of eyebrow in myxoedema.

accentuated by a co-existent pericardial effusion, there being a weak pulse, peripheral oedema, a raised jugulovenous pressure, dyspnoea and basal creps. The ECG shows low voltage with flattening and inversion of T-waves.

In the nervous system there may be mental changes as commented on in the history, slurring of speech, ataxia, weakness, myopathy, polyneuritis, sluggish reflexes with a characteristically delayed relaxation phase of the ankle jerks.

Cretinism

Although myxoedema can occur in children, hypothyroidism in the newborn produces cretinism (*Figure 2.29*); older children may have a mixture of myxoedema and cretinism (*Figure 2.30*). In the syndrome there is reduction of growth, poor bone maturation and abnormal mental development. The clinical picture may not appear for a number of weeks and can be difficult to detect. This has important clinical implications since irreversible damage usually commences after 6 weeks, the full picture of mental and physical retardation taking some months.

Initial symptoms are feeding problems, respiratory difficulties, constipation and jaundice. The established syndrome is dwarf-like stature with a wide skull, short limbs and trunk, and

Figure 2.29.
Neonatal cretinism.

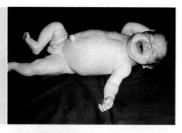

Figure 2.30.
Child cretin.

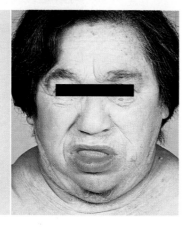

common. Pigmentation may accompany excess circulating ACTH as with pituitary tumours, particularly if adrenalectomy is undertaken. There is an increase of lanugo hair and facial hirsutism. The scalp hair is often lost.

There is characteristically an increase in weight, this being due both to oedema from fluid retention and obesity. The obesity is mostly around the face (moon face; *Figure 2.31*), the trunk and the back of the neck (buffalo hump; *Figure 2.32*). The limbs remain thin. The appearance has been likened to a central lemon with projecting matchsticks.

Associated conditions are hypertension, diabetes mellitus (30%), myopathy with proximal wasting, oligomenorrhoea, impotence and infertility. Osteoporosis is present – particularly of the axial skeleton – with occasional fractures of ribs and vertebrae. Mood lability is common, and about 20% of patients suffer from depression.

Due to the frequent associated conditions, important differential diagnoses include hypertension, diabetes, psychoses and obesity. Sudden weight gain as, for example, in pregnancy, may give rise to cutaneous striae (*Figures 2.33–2.35*).

spade-like hands. There is hypertelorism, macroglossia, the skin is dry, the abdomen is protruberant and there may be an umbilical hernia present. Mental retardation may be marked.

Most hypothyroid infants are picked up by routine screening at birth. Causes may be agenesis and ectopic thyroid. A goitre is present in a third of patients.

Cushing's syndrome

Cushing's syndrome is due to excess circulating corticosteroids. This is most commonly due to adrenal stimulation by a pituitary tumour but may be related to a primary adrenal tumour, steroid medication or an ectopic steroid source, such as an oat cell carcinoma of the bronchus. Other tumours of the lung, pancreas or thymus may also secrete corticosteroids, as can a medullary carcinoma of the thyroid. Hypersecretion in children may be accompanied by arrested growth.

The skin in Cushing's syndrome is thin with atrophy of the elastic lamina. Stretching occurs, with paper thin scars that may be pale but are usually light purplish in colour. Healing is poor. The superficial capillary network may be easily seen through the skin, giving rise to plethora, most marked on the face. Capillary fragility is accompanied by spontaneous purpura. Acne is

Figure 2.31.
Moon face of Cushing's syndrome.

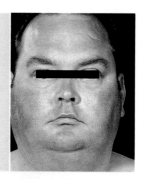

Figure 2.32.
Cushing's stature.

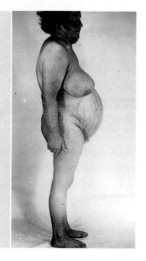

Figure 2.33.
Striae of Cushing's syndrome.

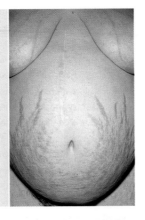

Figure 2.36.
Addison's pigmentation of the face.

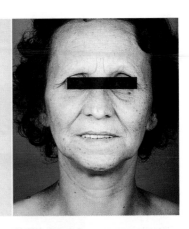

Figure 2.34.
Striae of pregnancy.

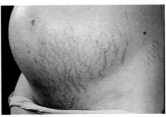

Figure 2.37.
Addison's pigmentation of the nails.

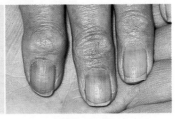

Figure 2.35.
Striae post pancreatitis.

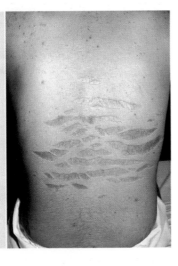

Figure 2.38.
Addison's pigmentation of the back.

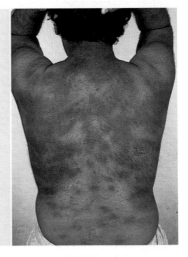

Addison's disease

Addison's disease is the clinical manifestation of adrenal failure. A variety of abnormalities can produce bilateral adrenal lesions, including tuberculosis, metastases, granulomatous lesions, autoimmune conditions, amyloid and infection. Pigmentation is a common finding, most marked in skin creases, particularly of the palm, in scars, inside the lips and cheeks and on exposed areas (*Figures 2.36–2.38*). Very occasionally depigmentation is present interspersed with pigmentation or normal skin. Skin changes may be absent in autoimmune induced disease.

Weight loss, diarrhoea and vomiting are commonly present, together with non-specific abdominal pain, colic, malaise, loss of energy, postural hypotension, muscle cramps and unexplained pyrexia. In extreme cases, hypovolaemic shock may be present, accompanied by hyponatraemia, hypertension and hyperglycaemia.

Myasthenia gravis

Myasthenia gravis is an autoimmune muscular disorder producing abnormal fatigue on exercise. Movement and power return after resting but repeated testing produces more rapid decline. Wasting and permanent weakness are a late feature of the disorder but tendon reflexes are preserved. In the initial stages the abnormality is confined to, or predominantly in, a single muscle group. The disorder is particularly marked in extraocular and bulbar muscles but extends in the later stages to involve the neck, shoulder girdle and, later still, respiratory, trunk and proximal lower limb movements.

Early symptoms are ptosis and weakness of facial and jaw movements. The ptosis may initially be uni- or bilateral (*Figure 2.39*) and is accentuated by an upward gaze. Pupillary size and responses are not affected. The orbicularis oculi are rarely spared, and weakness of these muscles and difficulty of retraction of the angles of the mouth means that a 'smile' produces more of a 'snarl'.

Weakness of the palate, pharynx, larynx and tongue produce difficulty in swallowing and chewing as a meal progresses, with fluid regurgitation up the nose. Difficulties of articulation occur with prolonged speech, there being progressively less distinct articulation and a nasal tone. In the later stages of the disease, neck muscle weakness is accompanied by dropping of the head on to the trunk, limb weakness produces difficulty in bringing the hands to the mouth and often terminal respiratory failure due to weakness of respiratory movements. An injection of anticholinesterase drugs can temporarily alleviate the symptoms and is diagnostic. Occasionally the condition is helped by thymectomy.

Ehlers–Danlos syndrome

Ehlers–Danlos syndrome is a congenital abnormality caused by lysyl hydrolase deficiency, producing defective crosslinks within collagen. It can be inherited by both dominant and recessive transmission. Patients are of short stature, the skin is smooth and velvety, demonstrating poor healing, and vascular fragility can lead to prolonged bleeding and spontaneous haemorrhage. Ligaments are lax and produce extensible joints making them susceptible to recurrent dislocation. In certain forms of the disease there may be ocular abnormalities.

Marfan's syndrome

Marfan's syndrome is a dominantly inherited disorder of connective tissue. The abnormal collagen synthesis affects the basal cement layer, particularly in the musculoskeletal, vascular and ocular systems. In the latter there is a tendency to lens dislocation with resultant blindness. Individuals are tall and thin, the span being greater than the height, and the lower segment being greater than the upper. There is arachnodactyly (spidery fingers and toes; *Figure 2.40*). The sternum may be depressed and twisted with an associated scoliosis.

Weakness of joint capsules and aponeuroses can lead to joint dislocation and hernia formation. They also influence physical tests of stretch, e.g. passing the thumb across the ulnar edge of the palm and overlap of the fingers when gripping around the opposite wrist.

Other features are a high-arched palate, dissecting aneurysms, aortic valve incompetence and mitral valve prolapse.

Klinefelter's syndrome

Klinefelter's syndrome denotes a male patient with, usually, an XXY chromosomal pattern, but many karyotypic variations also exist. Patients are often tall and there is subnormal testosterone production. The testes are small and soft, and there may be maldescent. There is no spermatogenesis, therefore the subjects are infertile.

The body hair is masculine in distribution but body fat has a female distribution around the breasts and pelvis and there may be mental retardation.

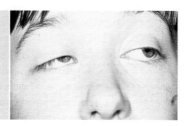

Figure 2.39.
Myasthenic ptosis.

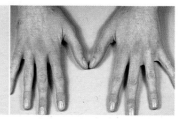

Figure 2.40.
Marfan's arachnodactyly.

Turner's syndrome

Turner's syndrome denotes a female patient with an XO chromosomal pattern resulting in mild skeletal and soft tissue abnormalities, amenorrhoea and, occasionally, associated coarctation of the aorta, horseshoe kidney and lymphoedema. Skeletal abnormalities include a masculine build, short stature, wide shoulders, cubitus valgus, a short fourth metacarpal, a high-arched palate, a wide (shield) chest with separation of the nipples and a narrow pelvis.

The breasts are underdeveloped and there is scanty axillary and pubic hair. The neck is wide and there is classically webbing of the skin from the neck to each shoulder (*Figure 2.41*).

Down's syndrome

Down's syndrome is the single most frequent cause of mental retardation, making up 20–30% of these patients. The condition is a genetic abnormality due to an extra chromosome 21 (trisomy 21). The condition occurs in all races and is equally frequent in males and females. There is a marked increase in the incidence of Down's syndrome with advancing maternal age – whereas the usual incidence is 1.5 cases per 1000 live births, at the age of 46 the incidence is 3.75 per 1000.

The syndrome comprises a number of congenital anomalies some of which are fatal. About two-thirds of foetuses do not reach term. Affected babies are floppy and hypotonic and already demonstrate recognizable adult features of the syndrome.

The outer angles of the eyes are raised, the sloping appearance, the prominent epicanthic fold and the hypertelorism giving a Mongoloid appearance (*Figure 2.42*), hence the earlier name for the condition. There may be a squint, nystagmus and myopia, keratoconus is found in adults, and there are pigment (Brushfield) spots (*Figure 2.43*) on the iris.

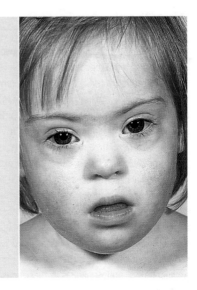

Figure 2.42.
Down's features.

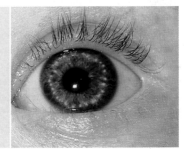

Figure 2.43.
Brushfield spots.

The head is bradycephalic with flattening of the face and a prominent fold of redundant skin is present over the nape of the neck. The tongue is large and fissured, and the ears hypoplastic. The skin and hair are smooth and fine.

The stature is short, especially the limbs, and the hands are small. There is characteristic shortening of the middle phalanx of the fifth finger and typical palmar crease markings. Mental retardation is a constant finding but extremely variable in severity. Individuals are practical, with a sense of humour, personable, with preservation of musical appreciation, but with poorly-developed numeracy and abstract thought. Speech is dysarthric and hoarse. Walking is delayed and remains broad-based throughout life. Epilepsy occurs in over 5% of cases.

A congenital cardiac anomaly is present in 40% of individuals. This is usually an atrial or ventricular septal defect but patent ductus arteriosus and Fallot's tetralogy also occur. Other congenital anomalies include duodenal atresia and imperforate anus. There is male sterility.

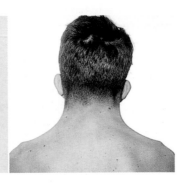

Figure 2.41.
Webbed neck of Turner's syndrome.

Dwarfism

Dwarfism can be classified into proportionate and disproportionate forms.

The **proportionate** group includes some genetic abnormalities – such as Turner's syndrome – and mucopolysaccharide deficiency. The majority of the group are related to systemic abnormalities. Examples include renal and hepatic disorders, congenital heart disease, hypothyroidism, low growth hormone and increased corticosteroid secretion.

Nutritional disturbances giving rise to dwarfism include starvation and coeliac and fibrocystic disease. The vitamin D deficiency produced by these gut abnormalities gives rise to the abnormality of **rickets** (*Figure 2.44*) This is characterized by lateral bowing of the long bones, especially the femur and tibia, scoliosis and prominent costochondral junctions. The lumps produced by the latter have been termed the 'rickety rosary'. Another chest wall abnormality is the transverse groove around the attachments of the diaphragm – Harrison's sulcus.

The **disproportionate** group is a disparate set of genetic abnormalities. The commonest is achondroplasia but there are also a number of rare abnormalities resembling achondroplasia. They have a different genetic profile but express a variety of achondroplasia-like symptoms. Severe osteogenesis imperfecta can also present with disproportionate loss of stature.

Achondroplasia (*Figure 2.45*) is the commonest form of dwarfism. It is inherited as an autosomal dominant gene, and the abnormalities are due to growth failure of epiphyseal cartilage; periosteal bone development is normal. There is a marked shortening and deformity of the long bones, the umbilicus being below the midpoint of the vertical height. The hands are trident-like with short fingers, and may only reach the iliac crest, thus giving difficulties in toiletry. The trunk is shortened

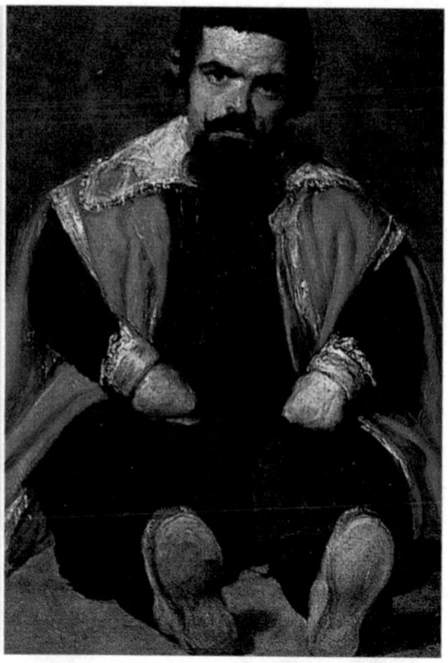

Figure 2.45.
Achondroplasia.

and there may be increased lumbar lordosis, wedging of the upper vertebrae and scoliosis. The gait is waddling. Late complications include spinal stenosis and osteoarthritic changes.

The head is relatively large with bulging of the vault. The face is short with flattening of the bridge of the nose. Intelligence is normal.

Paget's disease (osteitis deformans)

Paget's disease is a bony disorder of unknown aetiology in which there is active osteoclastic bony reabsorption. Although there is equivalent replacement by osteoblastic activity, the bone so formed is soft, deformed and lacks normal mineralization. There is a marked increase in the blood supply of the affected area which is warm and – if there is widespread bony involvement – it may lead to high-output cardiac failure.

The involved bones may be painful and in about 1% of patients there is a sarcomatous malignant change. Although very thick, the bone may be fragile and brittle and pathological fractures may occur, the commonest being the classical transverse fracture of the femur just below the lesser trochanter. Any bone may be involved in the process but typically the skull, spine, pelvis and long bones are affected. The skull vault is enlarged (*Figure 2.46*) with overgrowth above the eyes and the ears. Enlargement of the skull base may produce compression of cranial nerves, particularly producing deafness, dysphagia and dysarthria. There may be associated raised intracranial pressure. Long bones are thickened and may be bowed forwards and outwards (*Figure 2.47*).

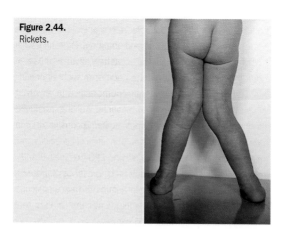

Figure 2.44.
Rickets.

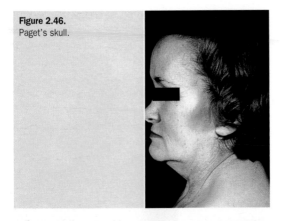

Figure 2.46.
Paget's skull.

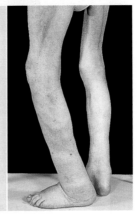

Figure 2.47.
Tibial deformity in Paget's disease.

Parkinson's disease

Parkinson's disease is a disorder of movement due to dopamine deficiency in the striatum nigra of the mid-brain. The abnormalities are rigidity, tremor, akinesia and postural changes. They are often insidious in origin.

Rigidity is most marked in the head, trunk and proximal limbs. Movements are slow and stiff. There is absence of facial expression with an unblinking, blank, mask-like stare. The volume of the voice is reduced with loss of modulation, producing a soft, monotonous tone. Eye movements are usually preserved. There is slight, 'plastic' resistance to passive movement, this being constant through the full range of movement. However, when tremor coexists, the resistance may show some 'cog-wheel' features.

Tremor may involve the hands, head, jaw or limbs. It is most common in the hands where it is of a pill-rolling form produced by wrist rotation. It is increased with emotional stress but absent in sleep. It may be unilateral.

Akinesia presents with poverty of movement. Postural changes include flexion of limbs, neck and trunk. This produces an alteration of the centre of gravity and instability when standing and walking, there being a tendency to fall forwards. Although akinesia produces difficulty in initiating walking, there is also difficulty in stopping, the short, shuffling steps taking the subject forward until a suitable obstruction is reached.

Sitting is in a flexed, motionless position, and getting out of a chair or out of bed may be impossible. Eating and swallowing become increasingly difficult as the disease progresses, there being some drooling and similar difficulties in washing and toileting. Handwriting becomes tremulous, small and untidy. Somatic and cranial nerve sensation remain intact but abnormal sensations of pain, hot and cold may be experienced in the feet. Constipation is universal and there may be lack of urinary control. The mental state remains intact but symptoms may give rise to depression and occasionally dementia does occur at the end stages of the disease.

Hysteria

Hysteria is the development of the symptoms of physical or mental disease in the absence of an equivalent physiological or pathological disorder. In primary hysteria the symptoms result from an unconscious mental process. In secondary hysteria the symptoms may be associated with organic disease of the central nervous system or an anxiety or depressive disorder. The patient's response is inappropriate and there may be over- or under-emphasis of the problem. Symptoms are often of benefit to the individual, enabling them to achieve or avoid a specific situation.

Physical symptoms may resemble disorders of the nervous system such as black-outs, fits, faints, gait abnormalities, tremors, tics, paralysis, aphonia, aphasia, globus hystericus, deafness, anaesthesia, pain and vomiting. There is usually indifference to these symptoms and a lack of concern (*la belle indifférence*), and inappropriate responses such as smiling, laughing, anger or fear. The anatomical position or physiological pattern of a symptom may be wrong, such as anaesthesia up to a joint rather than within a dermatome, or fits may have inappropriate movements, with no loss of consciousness, tongue biting or incontinence, and no EEG changes.

Diagnosis can be very difficult in the presence of pre-existing disorders such as multiple sclerosis, head injury and epilepsy. Mental symptoms include recent or long-term amnesia, wandering thought processes (fugue), multiple personalities and hysterical psychoses. The symptoms are commonly of sudden onset and are often precipitated by stress.

Congenital syphilis

Syphilitic disease is very rare in the newborn and, if present, is a fulminating infection with a poor prognosis.

Infantile syphilis appears at 10–12 months, rarely before seven. The symptoms are of a cutaneous rash, and destructive granulomatous lesions of the nasal cavities, mouth and anus. The rash is symmetrical and bullous, the bulli containing highly infectious fluid. The rash does not persist but healing produces linear scars. On the face the scars are prominent and radiate from the lateral angles of the mouth and eyes –termed rhagades (*Figure 2.48*) – producing the wrinkled 'old man' look.

Nasal granulomata produce an active rhinitis, the symptoms are termed 'snuffles'. The subsequent destruction of the nasal septum produces flattening and widening of the bridge of the nose and a typical saddle nose (*Figure 2.49*). The disease of the oral and anal mucosa produces condylomata at these sites.

Congenital syphilis in **children and young adults** occurs after the age of two. It has been summarized as producing a blind, deaf and lame subject. Blindness is due to interstitial keratitis and optic atrophy, and the deafness to atrophy of the vestibulo–cochlea nerves. The entire skeleton is underdeveloped, producing a small stature. A symmetrical, painless synovitis particularly involves the knees and produces swelling – Clutton's joints; bones are thickened but the tibia is also bowed anteriorly (sabre tibia).

Rhagades, saddle nose and nasal perforation may again be present with prominent parietal and frontal bulging – Parrot's nodes. The permanent incisors have characteristic central notching along their margins. These have been termed Hutchinson's teeth. Hutchinson's triad is interstitial keratitis, nerve deafness and the tooth abnormalities.

Figure 2.49.
Saddle nose.

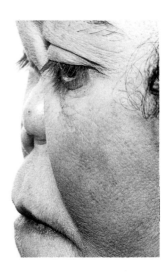

Figure 2.48.
Rhagades of
congenital syphilis.

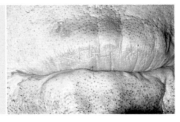

3 Lumps, ulcers, sinuses and fistulae

Lumps

History

In the history, determine as precisely as possible when the patient **first noticed** the lump and what brought it to their attention. A common history is one of minor trauma, but often the trauma merely draws attention to the lump rather than causes it. The lump may be observed or felt when washing or observed by another person, as in a thyroid swelling, or it may become apparent because of pain. Question for any changes in the lump. Rapid enlargement may imply inflammation, particularly if it is painful, whereas progressive enlargement may signify neoplasia.

It is common for patients to report a variation in size of the lump. This may be a genuine **change** but can also be due to prominence in certain movements or positions. Note whether it has ever disappeared completely. True examples of variation are the obstructed parotid gland enlarging on eating and the reduction of a hernia. Blood filled lumps – such as varicose veins and some fluid-filled lumps such as communicating bursae – can be emptied by positional changes or direct pressure. Enquire whether there is anything the patient can do to make the lump get bigger or smaller, such as tensing the abdominal wall or performing a Valsalva manoeuvre. Some lumps may discharge, in which case question the quantity, colour, consistency and smell of the contents.

Painful lumps are commonly due to trauma and inflammation but malignant lumps may also be painful when rapidly expanding, breaking down or invading nervous tissue. A **previous history** of the lump or other similar lumps may help in the diagnosis. Congenital lumps may be associated with multiple abnormalities.

Note the systemic effects that can be produced by infection, trauma or neoplastic changes. Ask the patient what they think the lump is, as they might know or suspect a cause.

The word **deformity** is frequently used by both patient and doctor but not necessarily with the same meaning. Although it can be applied to any marked deviation from the normal size or shape of the whole or part of the body and, as such, is applicable to any disease, it is usually used in relation to

Table 3.1. Features to consider in the description of lumps and ulcers.

Feature	Definition/aetiology
Pathogenesis	Tissue of origin; single/multiple; classification Incidence; age; sex; familial; ethnic; occupational; environment
Symptoms	Appearance; progress; disappearance Precipitating, exacerbating and/or relieving factors Course of symptoms: pain; discharge Systemic effects; social history
Signs*	Site: anatomy; depth; relations External: colour; temperature; tenderness; shape; size; surface; edge; mobility [Edge: sloping; punched out; undercut; raised; everted] Internal: consistency; fluctuation; transillumination; compression; reducibility; cough impulse; thrill; pulsation; resonance; bruit [Base: slough; granulation; deep tissues; fixation; discharge] Surroundings: induration; spread; fixation; penetration; perforation; lymphangitis; nodes; veins; arteries; nerves; muscle; bones; joints

* Substitute 'edge' and 'base' for 'external' and 'internal' to describe ulcers.

musculoskeletal abnormalities, particularly contractures of soft tissue, fixation of joints and bony angulation.

Lumps are commonly presented to the student, who is expected to communicate with the patient before palpating the lesion. The most important question is whether the lump is tender but also ask **how long** it has been present and whether it is **changing** in size. To these questions add 'Where is it?' if a lump you have been asked to examine is not immediately obvious (Table 3.1).

Examination

The clinical examination of a lump provides important clues as to its diagnosis; many lumps have characteristic features. The following description is of features that must be considered with every lump. Although all are not applicable in every situation, by considering them in an organized fashion, important steps will not be omitted.

It has previously been emphasized that the student and trainee must be able to describe accurately the clinical features elicited. This ensures that they remember to look for each sign and are able to give an opinion on its presence or absence. The description may have to be given to a senior colleague over the telephone. As the recipient may be basing the diagnosis and management plans on this description, it must be full and reliable.

Useful descriptive features are highlighted in bold in the following text. A later attempt is made to make these signs more memorable (p. 60) but, at this stage, remember that the examination covers four aspects: **Site**, the **External** and **Internal** features of the lump and its effect on the **Surrounding** tissues (i.e. SEIS).

Site

The position of a lump has important implications on its likely aetiology, and this must be recorded both in terms of its surface markings and its depth. The **site** (*Figure 3.1*) is measured from fixed bony prominences such as the manubriosternal angle, olecranon or tibial tubercle. The **relations** of the lump define its anatomical **origin,** its anatomical plane and the structures covering the surfaces of the lump. It may arise from the skin, subcutaneous tissues, the bones, joints or muscles, or lie within one of the body cavities. The abnormality may be due to a **deformity** (*Figure 3.2*) of one or more tissues, perhaps of congenital or post-traumatic origin. When a lump is rapidly changing size, e.g. a haematoma

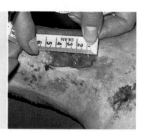

Figure 3.3.
Clinical measurement starts with a tape measure.

or an abscess, its progress can be monitored by outlining the circumference with a skin marker (p. 25, *Figure 2.12*).

Exterior of a lump
Size

First, measure the **size** (*Figure 3.3*) of the lesion. This should be carried out with a tape measure, for example, as an inaccurate estimate can lead to a false interpretation of change of size at the next visit. Lumps are three dimensional and so three measurements should be written down. It may not be possible to measure deeply placed lumps with a tape measure, so therefore learn how to estimate these sizes within 0.5–1 cm. As the hand is always available for comparison, measure the width of your thumb nail, the length of your thumb from the interphalangeal joint to its tip, the index finger from the metacarpophalangeal joint to the tip and your digital span. These measures can serve as a reference. Oranges and grapefruit, while useful for describing the shape of a lump, like walnuts and even golf balls, are subject to size variation.

Shape, surface and edge

The **shape** of a lump, like its size, is three dimensional and so descriptive terms should take this into account. Common terms – round (*Figure 3.4*); oval; flattened; triangular; rectangular; square; irregular (*Figure 3.5*) – should be used for each plane being described. Likening the lump to common objects can be helpful, and the shape may be characteristic of the organ of origin, such as an enlarged kidney, gall bladder or thyroid gland. Many lumps are poorly defined (*Figure*

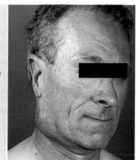

Figure 3.1.
Parotid adenoma. Parotid lesions are not necessarily restricted to the face – they can be sited behind and sometimes inferior to the angle of the mandible and can then mimic swellings of the submandibular gland or upper cervical lymph nodes.

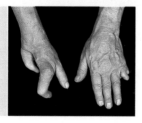

Figure 3.2.
Lobster claw deformity of the hand.

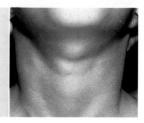

Figure 3.4.
The smooth, regular, hemispherical shape of the suprahyoid thyroglossal cyst.

Figure 3.5.
Irregular surface of keloid scar.

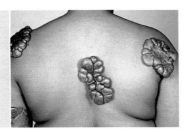

Figure 3.9.
Clearly defined, right accessory auricular appendage.

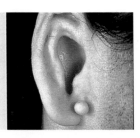

Figure 3.6.
Poorly defined neck swelling. Retropharyngeal abscess extending laterally beneath the left sternomastoid muscle.

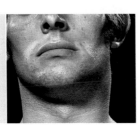

Figure 3.10.
Poorly defined thigh mass that proved to be a large subfascial lipoma.

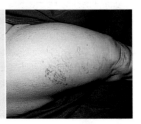

3.6) and all these features should be noted. Cutaneous lumps may be raised above the skin surface and the base may be narrowed, producing a polypoid lesion.

The **surface** of a lump can provide an indication of its aetiology. It is described in terms such as smooth and regular (*Figure 3.7*), rough and irregular (*Figure 3.8*) or any mixture of these. Lesions arising in the epidermis may exhibit a surface abnormality, such as the irregularity of a wart, and there may be a pit or punctum when the lump arises from a dermal appendage, such as a sebaceous cyst. Deeper lesions are usually covered with normal skin. There may be a specific pattern to an irregular surface, such as small or large nodules; the terms lobulated, cobblestone and bossellated are sometimes used to describe these features.

The **edge** of a flattened or projecting lump may be clearly (*Figure 3.9*) or poorly defined (*Figure 3.10*) and may be sharp, rounded, regular or irregular. The use of simple, well-known terms ensures that the description is fully understood.

Colour, temperature and tenderness

The **colour** of a lump, in the case of a cutaneous lesion, may be that of the lesion itself, but when the lump is more deeply placed, colour can be due to normal skin or changes in the overlying skin. Pigmentation (*Figure 3.11*) is an important characteristic as it can be the brown melanin of a malignant melanoma. Rodent ulcers and squamous carcinomas can also contain melanin as can a number of benign moles. Xanthelasma are the yellowish colour of their fatty content while gouty tophi are the white of their calcific content. Vascular lesions may be stained from iron pigments or may be discoloured through the excess circulating blood in surface vessels.

Figure 3.7.
Smooth, well-localized, degenerative cyst of the lateral meniscus.

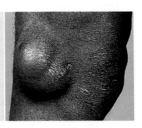

Figure 3.8.
Irregular papilliferous lesion growing out of the auricular canal.

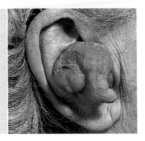

Figure 3.11.
Dark pigmentation of a malignant melanoma of the back.

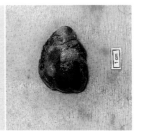

Inflammatory and necrotic tissue changes, from infiltration of the overlying skin, produce colour changes varying from the pink or red of hyperaemia to black dead tissue. The latter is further considered with the features of the base of an ulcer. The overlying skin may be pale due to tissue oedema or cyanosed due to the reduction of oxygenated haemoglobin.

Increased blood flow in the superficial tissues increases their **temperature**; this is seen in inflammatory changes (*Figure 3.12*), tumours with a rich blood supply and tumours of vascular tissue. Large masses may reduce the temperature of the overlying skin or more distal areas. In temperature assessment, compare the local temperature with that of adjacent skin and an equivalent site on the other side of the body. The examining hand is a sensitive indicator of temperature – the dorsum has the advantage over the palm in that it has fewer sweat glands and is dryer, making assessment easier. Gently draw the back of the fingers over the area being assessed and then the area being used for comparison.

Tenderness may accompany trauma, inflammation and malignant lumps that are expanding rapidly, degenerating or invading nervous tissue. It has already been emphasized that a patient must be asked whether there is any tenderness before any lump is examined. With this information, the appropriate degree of pressure can then be applied during palpation. If in doubt, always watch the patient's face when carrying out these manoeuvres.

Lump mobility

The **mobility** of a lump to a large extent depends on its tethering and fixation to surrounding tissue (this is considered in a later section). However, the local features of the lump and its site of origin can also produce characteristic signs of mobility. A lipoma, for example, is one of the commoner subcutaneous lumps and if its edge is pressed the swelling slips from under the finger, producing a characteristic 'slipping' sign.

Tension in the underlying muscles and fascia make all subcutaneous lumps more easily palpable. If, however, a lump is more deeply situated, for example within a muscle compartment, muscle contraction tenses the deep fascia and

often render the lump impalpable. Similarly, a lump beneath the deep investing fascia of the neck can become impalpable by pressing the chin on the opposite side of the neck against the examiner's hand. Lipomas, or other lumps within the muscle, may become more prominent on muscle contraction. The muscle is still mobile from side to side and is more prominent at the site of the lump. Also, muscle bulges through splits in the deep fascia; such protrusions become more prominent on muscle contraction, the patient being asked to tense the relevant muscle group.

Certain postures can make some lumps more palpable. Standing on an extended knee, for example, brings into prominence some masses in the popliteal fossa – such as a Baker's cyst – while flexion of the knee can accentuate infra- and pre-patellar bursae. Flexion of the wrist can bring ganglia of the dorsum of the hand into prominence. Movement may also produce characteristic **crepitus** when moving inflamed tendons, for example in de Quervain's disease of the wrist or osteoarthritic joints. In joints, the crepitus may be a fine, 'squeaky' sensation (from subacute or chronic infections), coarse (e.g. from contact of the irregular surface of the femur, patella and tibia in osteoarthritis) or a click of a loose body or torn cartilage. In fractures, the broken ends produce a grating sensation on testing movement. Demonstrating crepitus in this situation, however, is likely to be extremely painful and diagnosis should be by other means (p. 419). Clicking of a tendon may be seen and felt, as in trigger finger, when the tendon nodule is pulled through a narrow area of sheath.

Abdominal masses have a characteristic mobility. The kidney, gall bladder and liver typically descend longitudinally on deep inspiration. It may be possible to 'bounce' mobile abdominal lumps anteroposteriorly or from side to side – this is termed '**ballottement**'. In the supine position, a renal mass can be pushed forward with short, sharp finger movements from a hand placed under the loin, and felt anteriorly by the palm of the other hand. An enlarged spleen, untethered by adhesions, may also be ballottable.

An ovarian mass and other mobile abdominal swellings, such as a mass of secondaries in the greater omentum, can be ballotted from side to side or backwards on to the posterior abdominal wall. The sign is more prominent when ascites is also present. A pregnant uterus and a large bladder can be felt bimanually by a hand placed suprapubically when pressure is applied on the mass by a digit inserted into the pelvis through the rectum or vagina.

If an abdominal viscus is dilated with fluid and air, a splashing noise can be elicited by holding the trunk and shaking it from side to side. This is a **succussion splash.**

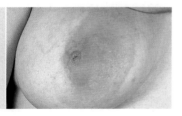

Figure 3.12.
Red, inflamed oedematous, tender breast abscess.

Interior of a lump

Contents

The **contents** of a lump can be composed of cells, fluid or gas (*Figures 3.13a, b*); the cells may be normal or abnormal. Normal cells may increase in number, as in the overgrowth of a congenital anomaly, in hyperplasia or in benign tumours. Abnormal cells may be due to alteration of the local tissues, such as a malignant change, or invasion by other cells, such as inflammation and secondary malignant deposits.

Fluid is usually extracellular as in the swelling of oedema due to inflammation and venous or lymphatic obstruction. Focal collections include encapsulated secretions, abscesses or intravascular blood retained within abnormal vessels, such as arteriovenous malformations, and some scrotal swellings.

Gas is usually within the gut, such as within an inguinal hernia, but can be within an abnormal segment of lung or within the tissues, e.g. after an incision, trauma or dental extraction damaging a nasal sinus, infection with a gas-forming organism, lung damage in rib fractures, a tension pneumothorax, trauma to the larynx, a tracheotomy and as a complication of a ruptured oesophagus. Gas in the tissues – termed subcutaneous or surgical emphysema – has a characteristic crepitus on palpation.

This 'crackling' sensation is also audible if a stethoscope is pressed on the tissues.

Consistency

Lumps range from stony hard to very soft. The simplest classification of **consistency** is the bony hardness of the forehead, the firmness of the nasal cartilages and the softness of the lip. Another useful classification is bony (stony hard), rubbery (hard, i.e. can be indented slightly), spongy (i.e. squeezable) and soft with resilience (e.g. jelly) or without (e.g. butter).

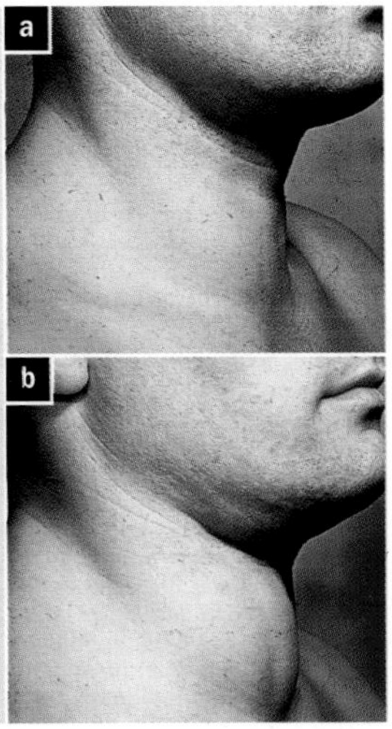

Compressibility and reducibility

Lumps are termed **compressible** when they can be emptied by squeezing but reappear on release. These features are characteristic of blood-filled lesions, such as a cavernous haemangioma, but may also be seen in lymphangioma and narrow-necked meningoceles. This sign of emptying in cavernous haemangiomas may be accompanied by blanching as blood is expressed out of the lesion. **Blanching** may also be seen by pressing a glass slide on a telangiectasia or other superficial vascular lesion, such as capillary naevi. Refilling of vascular lesions is due to arterial pressure and in some instances this can be demonstrated by pressure on the feeding artery, filling being delayed.

Reducibility indicates that a lump can be emptied by squeezing but does not return spontaneously – this requires an additional force, such as a cough or the effect of gravity. A classic example is an inguinal hernia. A hernia may also demonstrate two other important signs, those of a **cough impulse** and, by pressing on the neck of the sac, it may be possible to **control** the impulse, preventing refilling.

There is overlap between the features of compressible and reducible and, in some instances, both terms can be applied. An example is that of a saphena varix that can be compressed digitally and controlled by appropriate digital pressure. It can also be reduced by elevating the limb and will then refill with gravity. In this lesion, a cough impulse can usually be palpated as, with increased abdominal pressure, blood is expelled from the inferior vena cava and iliac vessels proximally into the heart and distally down to the first competent valve. Incompetence of the saphenofemoral junction means that blood is expelled into the great saphenous vein and a **fluid thrill** can be palpated.

Indentation and fluctuation

If the contents of a lump are solid or semi-solid and not too tense, they can be **indented** by pressure. This can be well demonstrated by compressing faeces in the palpable sigmoid colon in the left iliac fossa. It may also be possible to demonstrate this sign in a lax sebaceous cyst and in large dermoid cysts.

If pressure is applied to one side of a fluid-filled lump, the fluid tends to protrude in all other directions and, provided it cannot escape into another compartment, this bulging of the rest of the wall can be demonstrated, the sign

Figure 3.13.
a. Laryngocele. b. Laryngocele becoming apparent once the patient exhales against closed lips and palate (the Valsalva manoeuvre).

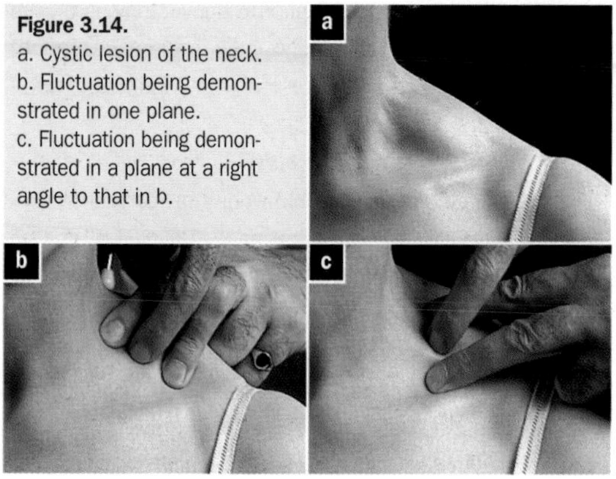

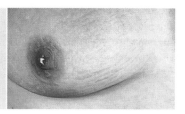

Figure 3.14.
a. Cystic lesion of the neck.
b. Fluctuation being demonstrated in one plane.
c. Fluctuation being demonstrated in a plane at a right angle to that in b.

Figure 3.15.
Nipple discharge in a patient with a galactocele prolactinoma.

Abscesses are variable in their smell, depending on the organisms involved. Faecal organisms in particular are foul smelling and this can be a useful sign when a perianal abscess is released, as a foul-smelling discharge usually indicates a fistulous connection with the anal canal.

being termed **fluctuation** (*Figures 3.14a, b, c*). The cyst is held between thumb and finger (the watching digits) of one hand and pressure applied downwards between them with a digit of the other hand (the displacing digit); the watching digits can feel the expansion.

This same expansion can be felt if a bundle of muscle fibres is held transversely, but the sign is not present if an attempt is made to hold the muscle longitudinally. Therefore, when testing for fluctuation, it is important to examine in two planes at right angles to one another. With a small cyst it may not be possible to apply three digits at the same time and in two planes, but downward digital pressure may still demonstrate the bulging if the lesion is over a firm surface. When lumps of less than 2 cm in diameter are situated over soft tissues, pressure displaces the lump and gives a false impression of fluctuation in solid masses; the test is therefore unreliable in this group.

Examples of cystic lesions are hydroceles, spermatoceles, abscesses – do not try to demonstrate the sign if there is excessive tenderness – and branchial cysts. At body temperature, fat is semi-fluid and fluctuation can be demonstrated in superficial lipomas, provided they are not too tense.

Expression and discharge

When the skin over a cystic lesion breaks down, the contents may be **discharged** (*Figure 3.15*) on to the surface; this is a common feature of sebaceous cysts and abscesses. In the former, the contents are putty-like and granular and, on **expression**, are expelled in spurts as large particles intermittently block the punctum. The **smell** of these contents can be bad, as is common when dead cutaneous elements are retained and moisturized; a putrid smell is also present in necrotic, degenerating, malignant skin lesions.

Pulsation

If a lump lies adjacent to an artery it can be felt to pulsate (*Figure 3.16*). This **transmitted pulsation** may be demonstrable in a pancreatic mass situated in front of the abdominal aorta. Other masses, for example an abdominal aortic aneurysm, are **expansile** as well as pulsatile. This can be demonstrated by gently pressing a finger of each hand on either side of the mass, the fingers being moved outwards away from each other, whereas in transmitted pulsation they both move in the same direction. The size of an aneurysm can be assessed by measuring the horizontal distance between a finger pressed on to each side of it.

Vascular malformations and the veins of arteriovenous fistulae may also be expansile. Compression of a feeding artery may reduce the size and pulsation of a focal vascular malformation. A carotid body tumour situated in the carotid bifurcation usually has a rich blood supply and is expansile as well as transmitting pulses of the external and internal carotid arteries within which it is embedded. This is an important sign since biopsy or removal of this tumour requires an experienced surgeon and, if the pre-operative diagnosis is not made, serious complications can ensue. Some other tumours, usually sarcomas, have a large enough blood supply to make them expansile.

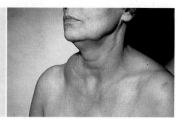

Figure 3.16.
Pulsatile right supraclavicular mass due to a subclavian aneurysm.

Transillumination

Clear fluid transmits light. This **transillumination** (*Figure 3.17*) is a valuable diagnostic sign – a lump containing such fluid glows when the beam from a pen torch is shone across it. There are, however, a number of precautions to take when demonstrating this sign. Fat transilluminates, as can be demonstrated when placing a thumb or finger over the end of the torch. Thus, pressing the end of the torch on to the skin produces a surrounding glow, which can be misinterpreted as transillumination of an underlying lump.

'Trans' means through, and the lump must be big enough to shine the beam across it for transillumination to be confirmed. A bright torch with a unidirectional beam is essential and it may also be necessary to cut out surrounding light or to demonstrate the sign in a dark room. A fine cardboard tube, such as that used to package Smarties for example, placed over the skin opposite the torch excludes outside light and helps demonstrate the sign.

Vaginal hydroceles and epididymal cysts are brilliantly transluminant; spermatoceles less so. Hydroceles with thick walls or those containing blood may not transilluminate. Cystic hygromas, ganglia and, to a lesser extent, branchial cysts and bursae, transilluminate, as does cerebrospinal fluid in a meningocele and a hydrocele of the canal of Nuck. Non-cystic lesions that can transilluminate include lipomas and, in a baby or young child, an inguinal hernia containing small intestine.

Percussion

Percussion is used routinely on the chest and abdomen to demonstrate the resonance of gas-filled organs such as the lung and gut, and the dullness of solid structures such as the heart and liver; it is also useful over some masses. An enlarged bladder, a pregnant uterus or an ovarian cyst are dull to percussion, whereas gas-distended loops of gut, such

as the stomach or an obstructed intestine, are resonant. An enlarged thyroid gland may extend deep to the sternum and this retrosternal portion may be detected by dullness to percussion over the manubrium sterni.

Ascites is dull to percussion, the fluid level being demonstrated by percussing towards each side from the central, resonant, gas-filled intestine. If these levels are marked on the skin and percussion repeated after turning the patient through 45°, the line of dullness changes since the fluid level of the ascites remains horizontal. This is a useful diagnostic sign termed '**shifting dullness**'.

Tapping fluid produces a ripple through it; this **fluid thrill** may be demonstrable, for example with ascites. With the patient lying supine, place one hand on one side of the abdomen and flick a finger against the opposite side. As the flick produces an impulse through the fat over the centre of the abdomen, the patient or a third person is asked to place the side of a hand along the midline to block out such additional movement.

Auscultation

Listening to a mass can reveal a number of characteristic diagnostic signs. Examples include bowel sounds in a hernia, bruits over vascular lesions, crepitus over a joint and **friction rubs** over pleuritic and pericardial surfaces. The **bruits** of vascular lesions include machinery murmurs of an arteriovenous fistula and also masses, such as an enlarged toxic thyroid gland, which may have an audible blood supply.

Surrounding tissues

A lump can produce characteristic signs in surrounding tissues, one of which is **induration.** Whereas most terms used to describe a lump are drawn from everyday language, induration is a specific medical term implying thickening and firmness of surrounding tissues, due to oedema or infiltrating neoplasia. If the former, it is often due to an inflammatory response. The hardness and indentability vary with the amount of fluid. To confirm oedema, sustained digital pressure must be exerted for 10–15 seconds. A positive sign is a residual, temporary denting at the pressure point that can be seen, or, for minor degrees, felt by passing a finger over it. The amount of pressure needed depends on the amount and type of oedema. Venous and lymphatic obstruction, and the oedema of systemic disease, are initially soft, pitting with gentle finger pressure. Inflammatory oedema requires increased pressure, usually with the thumb. As there may also be tenderness, watch the patient's face during this test and increase pressure very slowly.

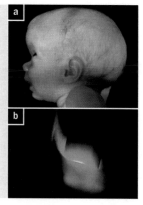

Figure 3.17.
a. Transillumination across the skull demonstrating fluid in an anencephalic infant.
b. Transillumination of the supraclavicular cystic mass in *Figure 3.14.*

The indurated area may also be tender, and bleeding within the tissues may produce bruising and pigmentation. Measure the size of the indurated area and record its shape so that progress can be mapped. If induration is due to neoplastic invasion there may be irregularity of the surface from tumour nodules, or the tumour may spread through tissue planes or along veins, and may produce satellite or distant metastatic lesions.

The **mobility** features of a lump have already received some consideration but the lump can also become tethered or fixed to surrounding tissues, for example by inflammation or neoplastic involvement. The latter carries important prognostic implications. In the early stages, tethering to skin and adjacent fascia may be difficult to demonstrate. To-and-fro movement or gentle squeezing of the skin over the lump in at least two directions at right angles to one another is necessary to exclude early signs of **pitting**, wrinkling or pulling on the skin. Gentle squeezing of the skin over a sebaceous cyst accentuates the central depression at the site of the blocked duct if this punctum is not already obvious. This sign demonstrates that the lesion is of dermal rather than subcutaneous origin.

When looking for **tethering** to deeper structures, grip the lump between finger and thumb and move it in two planes at right angles to one another. Repeat the movement once the underlying fascia has been tensed by appropriate muscle contraction, for example by asking the patient with a breast lump to place their hands on the hips and apply downward pressure. An untethered lump moves equally in both planes, whether the underlying tissues are tensed or relaxed.

As the attachment to adjacent tissues progresses, there is less independent movement of the lump and, as fixation may be to adjacent bone or other organs, further signs may develop, such as **peau d'orange** of the skin in a malignant breast lesion (p. 231). In this case, oedema stretches the skin between the dermal pegs giving the surface a pitted, orange-peel appearance. A lesion may also perforate surrounding skin and adjacent viscera, discharging its contents, or erode into a blood vessel causing haemorrhage.

The draining **lymph nodes** must always be palpated as part of examination of a lump – this usually means the axillary (*Figures 3.18–3.20*), groin and cervical nodes. Remember that the lymphatic drainage of the testis is to the para-aortic lymph nodes so the abdomen must be palpated in this instance. Inflammation may occur along the line of superficial lymphatics producing **lymphangitis**, characterized by pain, redness and swelling.

The **blood vessels** supplying or draining a lump may undergo change. The enlarged feeding arteries of vascular

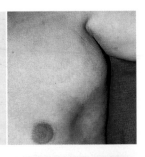

Figure 3.18.
Malignant axillary mass.

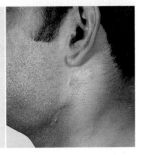

Figure 3.19.
Tuberculous lymphadenitis.

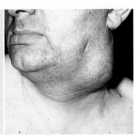

Figure 3.20.
Secondary deposits in the cervical lymph nodes, due to primary nasopharyngeal carcinoma.

malformations have already been referred to under compression. Veins may become more prominent in association with a lump and there may be local thrombosis, accompanied by pain and oedema. Large masses in the thoracic inlet, such as a retrosternal goitre or matted malignant nodes, can compress the superior vena cava; similarly, pelvic masses can cause inferior vena caval obstruction (*Figure 3.21*). In these instances, the veins over the trunk dilate to provide alternative channels for venous return to the heart. The direction of flow in these abdominal wall varices can be demonstrated by compressing a point in the vein with the index finger of the left hand, and using the right index finger to empty a segment of the vein by milking it away from the compressed point. By releasing the right index pressure, the emptied segment fills rapidly if the obstruction is in the direction of milking. Repeat the test, milking a segment of vein in the opposite direction; this will show slow refilling towards the non-obstructed direction.

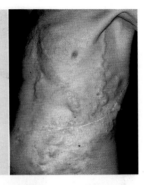

Figure 3.21.
Abdominal wall varicosities secondary to inferior vena caval obstruction.

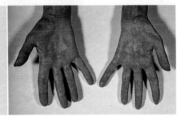

Figure 3.22.
Bilateral small muscle wasting of the hands due to T1 nerve lesions from cervical ribs.

Involvement of adjacent **nerves** by the disease process may give rise to pain or motor and sensory abnormalities (*Figure 3.22*). This usually indicates infiltration from neoplastic disease. Examine for sensory loss around and distal to the lump and the power of related muscles.

On completion of the examination of the external and internal features of a lump, and their effects on surrounding tissues, it is usually possible to formulate a diagnosis, or a differential diagnosis of possible causes. Information also has to be gained from the history and full general examination of the patient. The latter should be routine, to exclude systemic disease related or unrelated to the lump. Signs may include weight loss, malaise and increased pulse rate and temperature.

The process of formulating a differential diagnosis when there is still doubt is considered in *Table 1.1* on p. 15 and uses additional anatomical, aetiological and systemic clues. Diagnosis may be further confirmed by specific investigations such as imaging or needle biopsy. A lump may need to be excised to obtain a definitive diagnosis, for example persistently large cervical lymph nodes, but a warning has already been given (p. 52) to exclude a possible carotid body tumour before such an exploration.

Most lumps are easily diagnosed, and undergraduate and postgraduate candidates are expected to recognize lipomas, sebaceous cysts, benign and malignant skin lesions, vascular abnormalities, enlarged thyroid and salivary glands, breast lumps, hernias, scrotal swellings, abdominal masses and lymph nodes. All of these are more readily diagnosed if they have been seen before. Hence clinical experience is an essential part of medical training, but never disregard the stages of examination referred to above as a 'spot' diagnosis should not preclude the careful palpation of a lump and assessment of its mobility, and the examination for regional node enlargement.

Ulcers

History
An ulcer is a persistent discontinuity of an epithelial surface that can occur in the skin or mucosa of the alimentary and respiratory passages.

Ulcers differ from the defect of acute surgical or other trauma in their persistence, this being due to recurrent minor physical or chemical injury, ischaemia, neoplastic change and a poor healing response, such as in patients with malnutrition or other systemic disease.

Features to look for in the history and examination of an ulcer are similar to those described for a lump, and the reader is referred for more detail to the previous section. In the history, enquire when the patient first noticed the ulcer and what brought it to their attention. This latter may have been due to symptoms such as pain, discharge, bleeding or smell. Neuropathic ulcers may be painless and often out of sight, e.g. on the sole. In diabetics, this may become compounded by visual impairment. These patients must be taught how to regularly examine their feet with a mirror, by palpation or with the help of a carer, to identify early lesions and initiate therapeutic and preventive measures. The progress of the ulcer should be determined, particularly with reference to its size, shape, depth, base, discharge and response to any treatment. As with lumps, enquire about previous local or similar lesions, any systemic symptoms and what the patient thinks the lesion is.

Examination
Note the **site**, **edge**, **base** and **surrounding** tissues (i.e. SEBS – compare this with the SEIS mnemonic for a lump and note how many of the terms used are equally applicable).

Site
The site of the ulcer is usually characteristic. The three lower limb ulcers that a student can expect to see in qualifying examinations are venous, arterial and diabetic neuropathic ulcers.

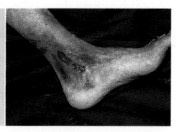

Figure 3.23.
Venous ulcer.
Healing has reduced
the size of the ulcer
to a linear defect.
Note the typical
pigmentation and
residual varicosities.

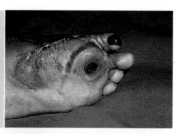

Figure 3.25.
Perforating
ischaemic ulcer of
the great toe in a
diabetic patient. Note
also the swelling of
the proximal sole
associated with this
foot abscess.

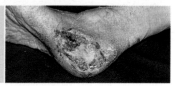

Figure 3.24.
Arterial ulcer due to
ischaemic pressure
of the heel.

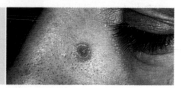

Figure 3.26.
Rodent ulcer of the
nose.

Venous ulcers (*Figure 3.23*) (p. 392) are sited just above the malleolus. They are usually medial but in the more florid states can become circumferential.

Arterial ulcers (*Figure 3.24*) (p. 371) occur when occlusive arterial disease reduces the arterial pressure in the foot to critically low levels. They are situated distally, i.e. over the tips of the toes and between the toes, where the pressure is lowest and over the malleoli and heel where minor pressure, such as lying in bed, is sufficient to abolish capillary flow and produce ischaemic skin necrosis. A bandage can have similar effects over the tendo Achilles and the tibialis anterior tendon across the ankle.

Diabetic ulcers (*Figure 3.25*) (p. 371) are of multiple aetiology. Arterial disease occurs in these patients about ten years earlier than in the rest of the population. They are also subject to microvascular disease, are more susceptible to infection and are subject to neuropathic changes, including motor, sensory and autonomic abnormalities. Diabetic arterial ulcers are similar to those already described. With peripheral neuropathy, the small muscles of the foot may be paralysed, allowing unopposed action of the powerful long flexor tendons. The shortening of the longitudinal arches means that the heads of the metatarsals are subject to an additional load during walking. The loss of the protective sensation of pain places an area such as the sole at particular risk from repetitive excessive trauma or unnoticed damage by sharp objects. The commonest site for diabetic neuropathic ulcer is, therefore, over the heads of the first and second metatarsals.

The shin is particularly susceptible to direct trauma. The tibia is subcutaneous and the lack of underlying muscle means that the skin's blood supply is reduced, with poor heal-ing potential. Skin and bony injuries at this site can give rise to longstanding ulceration.

Peptic ulcers are usually sited in the distal stomach and proximal duodenum, while malignant ulcers are common in the oesophagus, stomach, colon and rectum.

Malignant ulcers can also occur in typical locations, for example rodent ulcers occur on the upper part of the face (*Figure 3.26*).

Edge

The edge of an ulcer must be accurately drawn in the patient's record, noting the shape and measuring the size in at least two directions. As one does not wish to rest a tape measure on the ulcer surface, it may have to be gauged by the measure being held taught just above the surface. More accurate records can be made by resting a gauze on the surface and then measuring the imprint, or by placing a sheet of cellophane over the surface and tracing the edge. The cellophane can be retained, cut out or reproduced in the patient's notes. The edge may be characteristic of the underlying pathology:

- **Flat sloping** (*Figures 3.27* and *3.28*) – venous; septic; often with a transparent healing edge along part of its circumference.
- **Punched out** – syphilitic; trophic; diabetic; leprosy; ischaemic (*Figure 3.29*).
- **Undermined** – tuberculous; pressure necrosis (*Figure 3.30*), particularly over the buttocks; carbuncles.
- **Raised** – rodent ulcer (*Figure 3.31*), often of a slightly rolled appearance.
- **Raised and everted** – carcinoma (*Figure 3.32*).

Figure 3.27.
Flat, sloping ulcers of a burn lesion to leg.

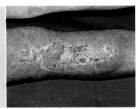

Figure 3.31.
Rodent ulcer of the face. The typical pearly, rolled edge is present at some points on its circumference.

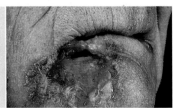

Figure 3.28.
Healing, granulating ulcer with skin islands. Epithelialization can extend from these islands as well as from the surrounding skin edge.

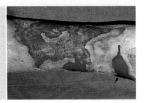

Figure 3.32.
Raised and inverted edge of a carcinoma of the forearm.

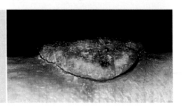

The colour of the edge may be red from inflammation, or pale or cyanosed from ischaemia, although in the later stages of ischaemia the skin has a permanent staining of blue, purple or black. Pigmentation may be present around venous ulcers and also a malignant melanoma. A basal cell carcinoma has a characteristic pearly edge, while keratinization of the edge is common in neuropathic ulcers of the sole.

Ulcers may be very tender, particularly when inflamed, when the local temperature may also be raised. Arterial ulceration is usually painful, the pain also being due to ischaemia of surrounding tissues. Neuropathic ulcers, by definition, have far less pain than one would expect, while venous ulcers are not usually very painful. Vasculitic ulcers (p. 393) can be very painful and the pain may precede the appearance of the ulcer.

Figure 3.29.
Punched-out ischaemic ulcer over the dorsum of the foot.

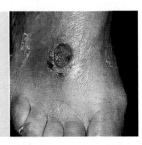

Figure 3.30.
Undermined ulcer of the buttock due to pressure necrosis.

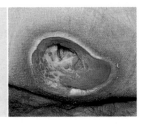

Base

In the base, note the **depth**, the **covering** (the floor) and any **discharge**. The depth can be described in millimetres and in terms of the tissue the ulcer has **penetrated**. In venous ulcers there may be full or partial thickness skin loss but the ulcer does not usually extend deeper than the subcutaneous tissues. In ischaemic ulcers it is not uncommon to see fascia, tendons, bones and joints in their base. Inflammatory ulcers usually only extend into the subcutaneous tissue but may communicate with a deep abscess cavity. Skin cancers initially spread circumferentially but as their bulk increases there is a progressive deepening through subcutaneous tissue on to deeper structures, with fixation to fascia, muscles and bone. Penetration of the wall of a viscus may lead to **perforation** into a body cavity or **fistulation** into another organ.

The base provides an indication of the progress of the ulcer; a wound may expose normal tissues. Primary healing indicates the apposition of cut edges and the establishment of continuity through the ingrowth of fibroblasts and blood vessels, with minimal inflammatory change. In secondary healing there is no initial skin cover, and capillary loops and fibroblasts grow towards the surface. Initially, there is an inflammatory response with the production of **slough**

Figure 3.33.
Slough in the base of a deep sacral ulcer.

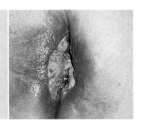

(*Figure 3.33*), a yellowish, adherent surface made up of dead tissue and inflammatory cells stimulated by trauma and subsequent infection.

Signs of a healing ulcer are when the slough is replaced by **granulation tissue** (*Figure 3.34*) and the skin creeps in over the granulating surface. Granulation is usually pink with red dots at the site of the capillary loops but it may have other characteristic appearances, such as the bluish granulation in TB and the wash-leather appearance of a syphilitic ulcer. With ischaemic ulcers, there may be no evidence of any healing or granulation formation, the underlying tissues being exposed, such as the tendons crossing the ulcer and deep fascia, or bone and joint surfaces.

Slough and small amounts of discharge may dry to become a **scab** and a layer of dead tissue may become dehydrated and form a dark brown or black **eschar** (*Figure 3.35*) such as after a burn or ischaemic necrosis. The base may be formed of **malignant** (*Figure 3.36*) tissue and this does not produce normal granulation tissue or allow skin ingrowth.

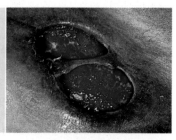

Figure 3.34.
Granulating tissue covering the floor of an ulcer produced by a dehiscent abdominal wound.

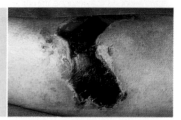

Figure 3.35.
Eschar following shin trauma.

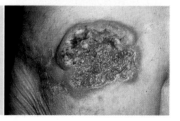

Figure 3.36.
Malignant ulcer. Note the dead tissue over its base, with no evidence of granulation formation.

Discharge may be serous, serosanguinous or purulent. Serous discharge is of normal tissue fluid as other discharges imply superadded infection. Pus requires culture to determine the causative organism though in a few cases the colour provides preliminary clues: staphylococci produce yellow, creamy pus; that from streptococci is watery and opalescent; from *Pseudomonas* it is blue/green; amoebic liver abscess produces purplish-brown pus; and actinomycosis gives yellow granules. Discharge may be more copious when associated with oedema, whether from venous or lymphatic obstruction, or generalized oedema such as in cardiac, liver and renal failure.

The smell of the discharge may provide a clue to the infecting organism, faecal organisms being particularly offensive. Dead tissue, such as that associated with a malignant ulcer, and wet gangrene may also be foul smelling. An ulcer may bleed from the initial or subsequent trauma. A healing granulating surface bleeds with minimal abrasion. Bleeding may also indicate the erosion of adjacent vessels, particularly in malignant disease.

Surrounding tissue

As with lumps, the effect of ulcers on surrounding tissues is largely dependent on their aetiology. The depth of penetration and possible perforation has already been referred to. **Induration** of surrounding tissues is seen particularly in the inflammatory response to infection, trauma and malignancy, or it may be direct invasion of a malignant process. **Blood vessels** may be prominent, with an increase of blood supply and venous drainage in an inflammatory response. Pigmentation is common around a venous ulcer, and the surrounding skin may be scarred from previous ulceration.

If the prime aetiology of the ulcer is neuropathic, there is sensory loss over the adjacent skin and reduced sweating in an autonomic neuropathy. Neuropathy may also be related to damage to adjacent **nerves** by the ulcer. The **mobility** of the ulcer depends on the degree of penetration and the effects of induration on surrounding tissues. The skin may show adherence to underlying fascia or muscle, tethering or subsequent fixation. As with lumps, it is essential to examine for local and more distant **nodal** involvement by the disease process.

Sinuses and fistulae

A **sinus** is a tract lined with granulation tissue, connecting an abnormal cavity to an epithelial surface (*Figure 3.37*). The cavity usually commences as an abscess in which the normal healing process is impaired. The granulations may be exuberant and protrude through the opening. A number of factors can lead to delayed healing and sinus formation. They include:

- Inadequate drainage of an abscess.
- Chronic inflammation. The tuberculous, syphilitic and leprosy bacteria, the fungal infection actinomycosis and some diseases, such as Crohn's, stimulate a chronic inflammatory granulomatous response from the body from which there is a slow resolution. Typical examples of sinus formation in this group are a collar-stud tuberculous abscess in the neck, the multiple sinuses of actinomycosis (*Figure 3.38*) and Crohn's sinuses along the alimentary tract.
- A foreign body in an abscess cavity stimulates a prolonged inflammatory response and recurrent infection. A foreign body may gain access through injury, such as clothing material, or at operation, such as a non-absorbable suture, or an orthopaedic or vascular prosthesis. The latter have particularly serious consequences, since it may only be possible to eradicate the sinus by removal of the prosthesis. Hair, or the bony sequestrum of osteomyelitis, may act as a foreign body, preventing healing and promoting sinus formation. A pilonidal sinus (p. 325) is an example of the former.
- Epithelium in the cavity wall prevents resolution of an abscess. This can result from congenital or acquired lesions. Examples of the former are congenital epithelial rests, such as dermoid cysts, along the embryological lines of facial fusion. It may become infected and start to discharge its contents on to the surface. Penetrating injuries to the pulp of the finger can bury surface epithelium in the subcutaneous tissue, producing an implantation dermoid and lead to sinus formation.
- Malignant disease in a cavity wall can prevent healing and precipitate sinus formation. The opening of a sinus can be on to the skin or a mucous membrane and it can be sited some way from the cavity. A sinus probe may be passed, gently negotiating the lumen of the tract, to enter the cavity and establish its depth and position.

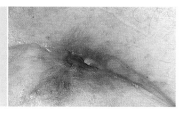

Figure 3.37.
Sinus from a septic arthritis of the shoulder due to actinomycosis.

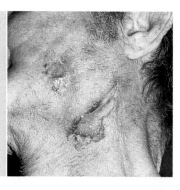

Figure 3.38.
Actinomycosis of the left side of the jaw with multiple sinus formation.

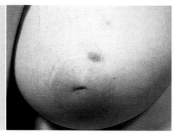

Figure 3.39.
Mammary fistula.

A sinus can give symptoms through recurrent discharge and recurrent bouts of acute infection of the abscess cavity. They are likely to persist until removal of the causative factors listed above.

A **fistula** is an abnormal tract between two epithelial surfaces (*Figure 3.39*). It is usually produced when an abscess cavity breaks into two adjacent epithelial surfaces; the aetiological factors that prevent the closure of the tract and normal healing include those listed under sinus formation. An additional factor, however, is that the epithelial surfaces may be of adjacent organs and the contents of these organs may pass through the fistulous tract and prevent healing. Examples are fistulae between adjacent loops of the gut in Crohn's disease and between the gut and the bladder in diverticulitis or malignant disease of either organ.

Perianal abscesses may communicate with the rectum and the anal canal and, in these cases, surgical drainage produces a fistula that may persist, with continued discharge. Foul-smelling pus suggests faecal organisms and the likely presence of a fistulous connection. Diseased gut may perforate and discharge its contents on to the abdominal wall. Again, there may be foul-smelling discharge, and the presence of gas bubbles is confirmation of the alimentary connection. Tracheobronchial fistulae are usually congenital anomalies, presenting soon after birth, but may follow malignant invasion of the adjacent organs in later life.

CHECK LIST FOR LUMPS AND ULCERS (*bold* type relates to *both* abnormalities)

▼ SEIS	▼ Lumps	▼ Ulcers
▷ Site	▶ **Tissue of origin** ▶ **Relations**	
▷ Exterior	▶ **Size** ▶ **Shape** ▶ **Surface** ▶ **Colour** ▶ **Temperature** ▶ **Tenderness** ▶ **Mobility**	▼ Edge: ▶ flat sloping ▶ punched out ▶ undermined ▶ raised ▶ everted
▷ Interior	▷ Consistency ▷ Compressibility ▷ Reducibility ▷ Cough impulse ▷ Fluid thrill ▷ Indentation ▷ Fluctuation ▷ Discharge ▷ Pulsation ▷ Expansion ▷ Transillumination ▷ Bruit	▽ Floor: ▷ depth ▷ covering ▷ discharge ▽ Base: ▷ penetration ▷ fistulation
▶ Surroundings	▶ **Induration** ▶ **Tetherting/fixation** ▼ **Invasion:** ▶ **nerves** ▶ **vessels** ▶ **other tissue** ▶ **Nodes** ▶ **Related disease**	

4 Inflammation

Introduction

Inflammation is the body's response to injury and is an attempt to eliminate or minimize the harmful effect. The commonest injuring agent is a micro-organism; the condition is then termed **infection**. Other harmful modalities include trauma, physical and chemical agents, and invading tumours. Three main categories of inflammatory response exist:

- The walls of all bacteria contain polymers that cause inflammation; bacteria also secrete enzymes and toxins, with similar effects.
- An inflammatory reaction can be produced by antibody–antigen complexes and sensitized lymphocytes. These immune responses include autoimmune disease, drug reactions, foreign body reactions and the response to bacteria, viruses, fungi, parasites and tumours.
- Damaged tissues, such as an infarct or dead viruses, may release endogenous inflammatory mediators.

These mechanisms activate enzyme cascades, such as the production of complement and fibrinolytic systems, and activate circulating and fixed macrophages, giving rise to the local features of inflammation. The four cardinal signs of inflammation – **redness**, **swelling**, **heat** and **pain** – were described by Celsus in the first century AD; Galen added 'loss of function' a century later. In dark-skinned individuals, the redness is masked but the stretching of the skin by oedema produces a shiny surface.

Inflammation produces **systemic responses** as well as **local responses** in a patient. Many of these are mediated through cytokines. The effects include pyrexia, pyrogens from neutrophils and macrophages having a direct effect on hypothalamic thermoregulation. General symptoms include anorexia, malaise and weight loss. Much of the wasting occurring in tuberculosis (TB) is due to a tumour necrosis factor.

The term systemic inflammatory response syndrome (SIRS) includes both sepsis and non-infective causes, such as after major surgery, trauma, burns and pancreatitis. The inflammatory response is manifested as two or more of the following features:

- Temperature of >38°C or <36°C.
- Heart rate >90 beats per minute.
- Respiratory rate of 20 breaths per minute.
- White blood cell count $>12 \times 10^9 \, L^{-1}$ or $<4 \times 10^9 \, L^{-1}$.

In turn, SIRS can progress to multiple organ dysfunction syndrome, which clinically presents as acute respiratory and renal failure, liver dysfunction, coagulopathy and shock (pp. 22 and 117).

The **tissue response** is vasodilatation, producing local redness, heat and increased capillary permeability, with extrusion of plasma and lymphocytes, and increasing extracellular fluid (**oedema**). Lymphatic capillaries also dilate, and inflammatory fluid, bacteria and other cellular debris pass to, and are filtered by, local lymph nodes. The associated lymph node enlargement is termed **lymphadenopathy** (pp. 54 and 85). Splenomegaly may occur with intracellular organisms, such as malaria; haematological changes include normochromic, normocytic anaemia.

An inflammatory response may **resolve** by phagocytosis of bacteria and dead cells by neutrophil polymorphs and macrophages. The damaged tissue is replaced by the proliferation of fibroblasts and capillary loops, and covered by an ingrowth of epithelial tissue. Scarring may be minimal. When epithelialization is delayed, healing is by **secondary intention**. Fibroblasts and capillaries grow towards the surface where dead, superficial debris (**slough**) is gradually replaced by pink **granulation** tissue, prior to epithelialization, by skin growing in from the sides; healing is accompanied by scar formation.

Unresolved, subcutaneous dead tissue, organisms and other foreign material give rise to an **abscess**, the dead material producing **pus**; the abscess cavity is surrounded by granulation tissue. When an inflammatory response lasts for a number of weeks, or longer, it is termed **chronic**. Chronic inflammation may be due to failure of an abscess to drain completely or organisms may be retained in the fibrous wall of an abscess or within necrotic bone. Such organisms are inaccessible to antibodies and antibiotics due to the poor blood supply of these areas.

Chronic inflammation may also occur as a distinct process from the outset and is seen in a variety of conditions:

- It can be due to the presence of exogenous or endogenous indigestible substances. The former include suture material, prostheses, asbestos and silica. The latter irritants include fragments of hair (pilonidal sinus), keratin (ruptured epidermoid cyst) and uric acid crystals (gout).
- Certain types of organism with a persistent but low toxicity incite a cell-mediated immune response. Of particular note are TB, leprosy, syphilis, and fungal and parasitic infections.
- Autoimmune disease – in which the body reacts against its own proteins – is characterized by a chronic inflammatory response. Examples include rheumatoid arthritis, chronic hepatitis and Hashimoto's thyroiditis.
- Some chronic inflammatory diseases are of unknown aetiology, such as Crohn's disease, sarcoid and Wegener's granulomatosis.

A wide variety of cells are involved in the chronic inflammatory response. The key mechanism is an immune response to the **persistent** damaging agent that involves interaction between the lymphocytes, plasma cells – involved in humoral and cell-mediated immunity – and macrophages, i.e. phagocytic cells involved in the development and modulation of an inflammatory response.

Lymphocytes and macrophages predominate in **granulomatous** inflammation, a form of chronic inflammation which occurs particularly with *Mycobacterium tuberculosis* but also with fungi and parasites, and in a foreign body granuloma. In the case of TB, the cheesy content of degenerating granulomas in termed **caseous** rather than purulent.

Macrophages undergo a transformation to epithelioid histiocytes and often fuse to produce multinucleated giant cells. An essential feature of all chronic inflammation is that it occurs simultaneously with tissue repair. This is in contrast to acute inflammation, where inflammation and healing are sequential. Another important feature of healing in chronic inflammation is an intense fibrous reaction; this can damage adjacent normal tissue, as seen in pulmonary fibrosis or silicosis.

Infection

The human body is covered with many bacteria and other organisms. These are particularly common in the skin of the axillae and perineum, and the mucosa of the nose, mouth, pharynx and large bowel. Many of these harmless **commensals** have the potential to become harmful **pathogens** if they breach the body surface and multiply. The portal of entry may be an abrasion or other trauma, such as surgery and instrumentation; surgical and traumatic wounds are at particular risk. A patient's general resistance to infection may be lowered by trauma, a prolonged surgical illness, malignancy, poor nutrition, immunosuppressive drugs and steroids. Such states allow minor inoculation with pathogens to produce infection. The problem is compounded in immunocompromised patients (p. 84) when the inoculation of otherwise non-pathogenic organisms can give rise to serious infective states, a condition called opportunistic infection, the organisms then being termed opportunists.

Infection from commensals is termed **endogenous**, and from elsewhere **exogenous**. Most exogenous infections are from a community source such as other humans, animals and the environment, but hospital-acquired infection is termed **nosocomial** and may be more harmful because of drug resistance. A potentially serious and troublesome example of this in current hospital practice is a methicillin-resistant *Staphylococcus aureus*. This organism can be acquired by cross-infection from another patient and the problem may be accentuated if a member of a hospital staff becomes a 'carrier'.

In general, the size of an inflammatory response is related to the number of bacteria and their ability to multiply. Several million organisms are required to produce an inflammatory response and many millions for abscess formation. The virulence of an organism is, therefore, related to its ability to cross resistant surfaces and to overcome non-specific tissue defences and specific immune responses. To combat these body defences, bacteria produce various enzymes and a number of toxins – such toxins may be **exotoxins**, when secreted by the organism, and **endotoxins**, when released on the death of the organism. Harmful mechanisms include the enzymes hyaluronidase and streptokinase promoting tissue invasion, leukocidins inhibiting phagocytosis, haemolysins destroying blood cells and neurotoxins such as those of polio, diphtheria and tetanus.

Gram-positive organisms produce **peptidoglycan** and **teichoic acid**, giving rise to fever and general malaise. They do not usually have the lethal consequences of the endotoxin of Gram-negative organisms, which, in high doses, can induce the marked abnormalities of tissue permeability and disseminated intravascular coagulopathies of endotoxic shock (p. 23). The importance of the number of bacteria present, rather than their physical and chemical properties and pathogenicity, is further demonstrated in immunologically compromised patients in which acute and chronic infective conditions often do not have organ-specific signs or symptoms, the diagnosis being made by bacteriological culture.

The terms bacteraemia and septicaemia are often used interchangeably; however, bacteraemia implies the culture of bacteria from the blood of an asymptomatic patient and does not necessarily carry any serious clinical significance. Septicaemia denotes a systemic disturbance due to organisms or their toxins disseminated throughout the blood stream, as in septicaemic shock. The term pyaemia is best avoided.

Cellulitis

Inflammation of cellular tissue can be superficial or deep. Superficial – i.e. cutaneous and subcutaneous – is the more common and easier to diagnose. The part affected is swollen, tense and tender. Later it becomes red, shiny and boggy. From the point of view of differential diagnosis, superficial cellulitis may be said to have no edge, no fluctuation, no pus and no limit.

Cellulitis frequently commences in an infected wound (*Figure 4.1*). If the wound is not obvious, look for a small puncture, blister or abrasion where organisms could have gained entrance. In the absence of a breach in continuity of the skin, a common site of origin for cellulitis is an infected anatomical bursa, e.g. olecranon or pre-patellar, or adventitious bursae, e.g. the bunion over a hallux valgus.

In children, when no obvious abrasion is found, bear in mind Morison's aphorism: 'Cellulitis occurring in children is never primarily in the cellular tissues but secondary to an underlying bone infection'.

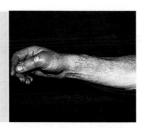

Figure 4.2.
Lymphangitis on the arm and forearm following an infection of the thumb.

Cellulitis is commonly accompanied by a pyrexia and general malaise. Examine for regional node enlargement; inflamed superficial lymphatic vessels (**acute lymphangitis**) (*Figure 4.2*) may be seen coursing from the site of infection to the regional lymph node. The tell-tale red lines are principally seen on the arm or leg. Occasionally the initiating lesion is difficult to find.

Erysipelas

Streptococcal cellulitis has a characteristic rosy or crimson colour. It is peculiarly smooth and has a characteristically shiny appearance.

The face is the most common site of origin in cellulitis (*Figure 4.3*) and oedema is prominent and may completely close the eyelids. The cellulitis has a distinct, raised surrounding edge. Regional lymph nodes are usually moderately swollen. The eruption reaches its peak on the fifth day, the brilliant erythema then changes to a livid hue after which it turns to brown and later yellow. Sometimes an exudate occurs beneath the cutis to form vesicles, later turning to pustules. Other sites involved include the hands, genitalia, the umbilicus of young infants and the lower limb, particularly associated with lymphoedema.

Milian's ear sign differentiates non-specific cellulitis from erysipelas in that the latter involves the pinna because it is a cuticular lymphangitis. On the other hand, subcutaneous inflammation stops short of the pinna because of the close adherence of the skin to the cartilage.

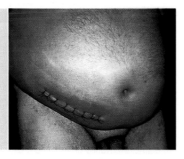

Figure 4.1.
Cellulitis. An infected appendix wound is a potential complication in any patient undergoing surgery for suppurative appendicitis.

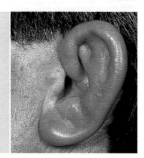

Figure 4.3.
Erysipelas of the left ear.

Orbital cellulitis

Orbital cellulitis (p. 180) may arise from hair follicles and other facial infections, or penetrating orbital wounds. It most commonly follows infection of the nasal sinuses, especially the ethmoidal and frontal. It is not surprising that ethmoiditis is the commonest cause of orbital cellulitis as the paper-like lamina papyracea of the ethmoid bone forms the major part of the medial wall of the orbit. In infants, the infection may follow infection of the gums and teeth.

The condition is accompanied by prominent swelling of the eyelids and, on parting the lids, the proptosis and frequent chemosis become apparent. Because of pressure on, or involvement of, the optic nerve, acuity of vision is often reduced. The condition carries two dangerous complications – cavernous sinus thrombosis and infection of the globe of the eye (p. 180).

Ludwig's angina

Ludwig's angina is cellulitis involving the sublingual and submandibular spaces beneath the deep cervical fascia; it is almost invariably due to dental sepsis. In many instances the floor of the mouth becomes oedematous.

Other examples of superficial and deep cellulitis occur in:

- Layers of the abdominal wall.
- The scrotum.
- Spreading subcutaneous gangrene in the diabetic patient.
- Pelvic cellulitis, e.g. parametritis, occurring in the connective tissue around the uterus.

These conditions result from an infection with a mixture of aerobic and anaerobic organisms and are termed **synergistic**. The spread is along tissue planes and is accompanied by a great deal of oedema, tissue necrosis and gangrene. Frequently, gas-forming organisms are present.

Meleney's synergistic gangrene or ulceration

The condition is usually of the abdominal or chest wall, following surgery for septic conditions. An area of cellulitis appears that progresses rapidly with the formation of a central purplish zone surrounded by angry, red inflammation. The whole area is exquisitely tender with gross oedema of the surrounding skin. Soon the purplish zone becomes gangrenous and, unchecked, the gangrene spreads widely. At first the general signs are mild, unless the patient is already debilitated from underlying disease. The gangrene and skin slough, producing an ulcer with an undermined edge.

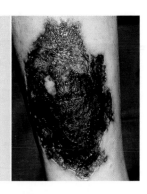

Figure 4.4.
Pyoderma gangrenosa.

Pyoderma gangrenosum

Pyoderma gangrenosum (*Figure 4.4*) has a similar acute pathology to synergistic gangrene but is related to recent wounds. Tender blue nodules progress to skin necrosis with undermining multiple sinuses and exuberant granulation. Half of the patients have depression of the immune system; associated diseases include Crohn's disease, ulcerative colitis, rheumatoid arthritis, plasma cell dyscrasia and leukaemia.

Fournier's gangrene of the scrotum

This rare condition is notable for its rapidity of onset and absence of precipitating causes. It commences as an acute inflammatory oedema of the scrotum followed, in a matter of hours or days, by sloughing gangrene. Diabetes should be excluded and a search made for perianal sepsis.

Diabetic gangrene

Diabetic gangrene is similar to Meleney's and Fournier's gangrene and is seen particularly at needle injection sites. Malignant otitis externa is a form of diabetic gangrene seen in the elderly and requiring urgent debridement.

Abscesses

An abscess (*Figure 4.5*) is the end product of unresolved inflammation. It consists of a collection of pus surrounded by an inflammatory zone and a lining of granulation tissue. The production of pus is termed suppuration. Pus is a fluid composed of living and dead bacteria, dead fixed and free cells (the latter representing the body's phagocytic response) and foreign material such as sutures, implants and splinters. The granulation tissue seals off the cavity from surrounding structures. The natural history of an abscess is to discharge through an epithelial covering or into a body cavity. The fibroblasts and

Figure 4.5.
Suppurative inguinal nodes may be secondary to infection in the leg, the abdominal wall, penis, scrotum or perineum.

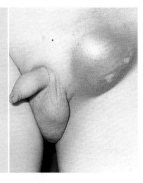

Figure 4.7.
Sequestrum of the right tibia.

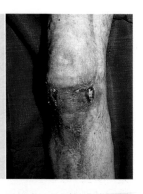

Figure 4.8.
Osteomyelitis of the jaw secondary to a tooth abscess.

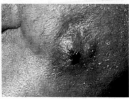

capillary in-growth of the wall then proceed to heal the cavity. If the contents cannot discharge, they may become a sterile collection which is gradually reabsorbed, particularly if antibiotics have sterilized the pus. In this case, the residual collection is termed an **antibioma**. Organisms may continue to proliferate with expansion and further destruction of the abscess wall. This may be seen, for example, in a deep breast abscess. Abscess formation is particularly common with staphylococcal infections and, to a lesser extent, pneumococci and streptococci. Abscesses of the large bowel commonly contain coliforms and *Bacteroides*.

Superficial abscesses are often associated with hair follicles, nail beds and wounds. Intra-abdominal abscesses are commonly associated with the appendix, the colon and tubo-ovarian disease, producing paracolic, subphrenic and pelvic abscesses. Less frequently, intra-abdominal abscesses are located around the kidney (perinephric) and liver (related to biliary and portal infection, and amoebic and hydatid organisms). Perianal abscesses are relatively common.

Infection related to bones (*Figure 4.6*) and joints is difficult to eradicate, as evidenced by subperiosteal sequestration (*Figure 4.7*) of bone and prolonged infection in joint prostheses. Abscesses of the head and neck include styes, those of the teeth (*Figure 4.8*), tonsil, mastoid, retropharyngeal space and of the intracranial cavity.

Figure 4.6.
Pus from a vertebral infection, particularly TB, can track within the psoas sheath and a psoas abscess may therefore present as a lump in the groin.
Associated spasm causes hip flexion.

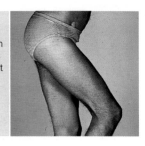

The local symptoms and signs of an abscess are those of inflammation, there being redness, swelling, heat and tenderness, with regional node involvement. At this stage, the lesion may be effectively combated by the body's own defences or by the addition of antibiotics. If the infection progresses, the swelling becomes soft centrally and the abscess cavity spherical. If large enough, fluctuation may be demonstrated. The pain becomes more intense and throbs, particularly on dependency and at night. The entry of bacteria and toxic products into the blood stream gives rise to pyrexia, which is characteristically swinging in variety. The pyrexia and raised white blood count may be the only signs of a deep-seated abscess, and the aphorism 'pus somewhere, pus nowhere, pus under the diaphragm' should always be heeded.

Septicaemia may develop and be accompanied by the complications of endotoxic shock. The natural discharge of an abscess, for example, through the skin, gut or bronchus, or by surgical drainage, is accompanied by rapid resolution of pain and pyrexia. The abscess **points** after the destruction of a pathway to the surface; this pathway is termed a **sinus** (*Figure 4.9*). If discharge is complete, the cavity fibroses and the sinus opening heals as a scar. If discharge is incomplete, recurrent symptoms and recurrent, multiple sinuses can be expected. Chronic abscesses of this form, and sterile collections as described above, only resolve after adequate drainage and debridement; this healing does not occur if foreign bodies, such as prostheses, mesh, bone sequestra or necrotic tendon, remain.

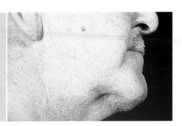

Figure 4.9.
Sinus from a tooth abscess.

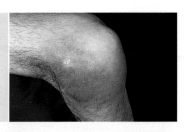

Figure 4.10.
Tuberculosis of the tibia.

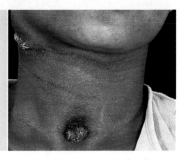

Figure 4.11.
Cervical TB.

The physical characteristics of a purulent discharge are of limited value in suggesting the cause of the organism, bacteriological examination always being required. Streptococcal pus from newly infected tissues is watery and slightly opalescent. Sometimes it is blood stained. Staphylococcal pus is yellow and of a creamy consistency. Blue or bluish-green pus is typical of *Pseudomonas* infection. The purplish-brown coloured pus from an amoebic abscess of the liver is very characteristic.

Pus resulting from the activity of certain micro-organisms emits a characteristic odour. This is particularly true of coliform bacteria, producing abdominal abscesses or sinuses, and perianal abscesses which are in communication with the anal canal. *Bacteroides*, also common in intra-abdominal suppuration and infections of the abdominal wall, gives rise to an odour similar to that of over-ripe Camembert cheese. The smell of gas gangrene infection of *Clostridium perfringens* emits a peculiar, sickly-sweet odour like decaying apples.

Chronic abscesses

Chronic abscesses (p. 218), as well as being due to foreign bodies and inadequate drainage, may be due to communication with a hollow viscus. If the abscess cavity communicates with a second epithelial surface, such as another loop of gut or to the surface, a **fistula** develops. Other causes of chronic abscess, which must be excluded, are an associated malignancy and the presence of epithelium in the wall of the abscess cavity, such as a sebaceous cyst, which prevents healing.

Certain types of infection, such as TB (*Figure 4.10*), leprosy and syphilis, produce a granulomatous response. Liquefaction of caseous material produces a thin, creamy discharge, as opposed to purulent. Tuberculous abscesses are termed cold abscesses since they do not produce the local heat and redness and do not have an associated, marked pyrexia. The neck is a common site due to degenerative nodes and is termed **scrofula** (*Figure 4.11*). There may be collections superficial and deep to the deep fascia, producing a **collar stud abscess**. The reactions of specific bacteria are included in *Table 4.1*.

Boils and carbuncles

Boils (*Figure 4.12*) – folliculitis; furuncles – and carbuncles (*Figure 4.13*) are staphylococcal skin infections commencing in hair follicles. They are common in diabetics, and urine examination is essential. Initial inflammation progresses to a pustule and, with the carbuncle, this infection spreads subcutaneously due to coagulase activity. The subcutaneous tissue dies with the production of a core of hard, adherent slough with multiple, overlying, discharging sinuses. The lesions are very painful and may be accompanied by systemic symptoms of malaise and pyrexia.

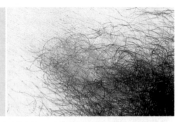

Figure 4.12.
Inguinal folliculitis.

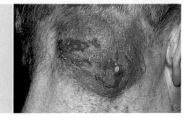

Figure 4.13.
Cervical carbuncle.

Table 4.1. Surgical bacterial infections.

Organism	Clinical features
Cocci	
Gram-positive aerobic	
Staphylococcus (in bunches)	
aureus	Common commensal of the skin, nose and perineum. Resistant to dehydration, therefore viable in dust. Boils, carbuncles, wound infections, deep and superficial abscesses, osteomyelitis. Produces coagulase that clots plasma and limits access of neutrophils. Problem of antibiotic resistance, particularly in hospital, because of methicillin-resistant *S. aureus*. Danger in intensive care units, surgical and neonatal wards.
epididymus *(albus)*	Usual skin commensal; increasing awareness of infections of intravascular lines and prosthetic implants.
Streptococcus (in chains)	
pyogenes	Common nasal commensal in children. Throat infections, cellulitis, erisypelas, wound infections, lymphangitis, lymphadenitis, septicaemia.
viridans	Oral commensal but potential of endocarditis after dentistry in susceptible individuals.
pneumoniae	Pneumonia, meningitis, peritonitis in susceptible and occasionally fit individuals.
faecalis	Gut commensal. Pathogen in urogenital and biliary tracts and endocarditis.
Anaerobic staphylococci and streptococci	Commensals in the gut. Commonly found in the mixed growth of intra-abdominal abscesses. Can be gas forming and therefore an important differential diagnosis of *Clostridium perfringens*.
Gram-negative	
Neisseria	Aerobic intracellular diplococci
gonorrhoeae	One of the commonest sexually transmitted diseases.
meningitidis	May be a commensal. Epidemic meningitis in children and young adults, endemic in infants. The endotoxin is capable of producing fulminating septicaemia and meningitis.
Bacilli	
Gram-positive	
Clostridium	Anaerobes, gut commensal, resistant spores proliferate in devitalized tissue
tetani	In soil, particularly horse droppings. Powerful exotoxin producing neuromuscular excitation.
perfringens *(welchii)*	Powerful, lethal exotoxin, producing myositis and gas gangrene.
difficile	Endotoxin may give rise to pseudomembranous colitis.
botulinum	Powerful exotoxin from contaminated foodstuffs. Mild gastroenteric symptoms followed by progressive symmetrical paralysis of cranial and spinal nerves. Autonomic dysfunction but no sensory loss.
Actinomycosis	Branching mycelial network spreading infection, abscess formation, yellow granules in pus.
Anthrax	Spore-forming, highly resistant. Animal carriers, in wool, hides, bones. Cutaneous lesions, boil-like but no pus and coal black centre. Pulmonary and intestinal manifestations.
Acid fast	
Mycobacterium	
tuberculosis	Primary lymphadenopathy, meningeal infection, secondary and tertiary pulmonary, urinary tract infection (p. 343).
leprae	'Tuberculoid' variety localized to skin and peripheral nerves 'Lepromatous' generalized bacteraemia, lesions also involving many systems.
Gram-negative	
Enterobacteria (coliform)	Normal gut flora, non-spore bearing, both anaerobic and aerobic. Capable of gut infection and opportunistic infection of host. Produce Gram-negative septicaemia, especially in immunocompromised patients and neonates.
Escherichia coli	Gut and urinary tract infection.
Salmonella	Typhoid and paratyphoid fevers commencing as gut infection but becoming widespread; potentially lethal infections affecting many organs.
enteritidis/typhimurium	Salmonella food poisoning producing 2–3 days acute diarrhoea, tenesmus, bloody stool, malaise, fever, abdominal pain. Continues to secrete organisms for 4–8 weeks. One of the leading causes of intestinal perforation in Africa and Asia.
Shigella	Bacillary dystentry, ranging from mild to fulminating infection, fever, malaise, headache, diarrhoea.
Yersinia	Mesenteric adenitis with or without terminal ileitis. Also produces plague, 'bubonic' from rats via flea vector, massive discharging lymphadenopathy. 'Pneumonic' human cross-infection from pulmonary involvement.

Table 4.1. Surgical bacterial infections/continued.

Organism	Clinical features
Enterobacter	Gut infections and common organism in post-infective malabsorption (also *E. coli* and *Klebsiella*).
Klebsiella	Gut infection and common opportunistic pneumonia.
Proteus	Common urinary tract infection.
Pseudomonas aeruginosa	Common, hospital-acquired infection, resistant to many chemical disinfectants, antiseptics and antibiotics. Important pathogen in burns, producing blue-green discharge. Problems in ophthalmic surgery and potential fatal septicaemia as opportunistic organism.
Haemophilus	Common upper respiratory tract commensal. Acute epiglottitis, pneumonia, meningitis.
Coccobacilli *Brucella*	Primarily an animal parasite, infection from close contact with cattle and carcasses. High, swinging fevers, dramatic sweating, severe, generalized aches and pains.
Bacteroides	Common synergistic organism in bowel infections and intra-abdominal abscesses.
Curved bacilli *Vibro cholera*	Epidemic in Indian sub-continent. Colonizes small bowel. Enterotoxin impairs reabsorption from the gut, producing severe, extra-cellular fluid depletion. Characteristic 'rice water stool'.
Campylobacter	Acute, self-limiting infectious diarrhoea.
Spiral bacteria *Treponema pallidum*	Syphilis, veneral disease, demonstrated by dark field illumination, as size is on the limits of light microscopy. World-wide distribution, no geographical or racial barriers. Profoundly influenced by the discovery of penicillin. Capable of congenital transmission (p. 45).

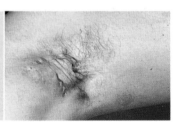

Figure 4.14. Suppurative hydradenitis of the right axillae.

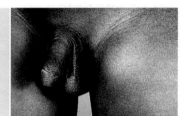

Figure 4.15. Left inguinal lymph adenopathy from unsuspected cat scratch disease.

Hydradenitis suppurativum

Suppurative hydradenitis (*Figure 4.14*) – apocrinitis – is an infection of the sweat glands and usually occurs in the axillae, often bilaterally. The condition may also involve the groins, the back of the neck and the perineum; the last must be differentiated from perianal fistulae. The infection is usually recurrent and persistent with multiple abscess and sinus formation occurring over many years. It can be very disabling.

Cat-scratch disease

Cat-scratch disease (*Figure 4.15*) is due to a cat bite or scratch and is frequently misdiagnosed. Surprisingly, the aetiology is in doubt but an intercellular bacillus may be responsible. The disease occurs about 10 days after inoculation by which time a minor breach in the skin has usually healed. Although one should search for a primary lesion, the initial sign is considerable lymphadenitis without visible intervening lymphangitis, the axillary and inguinal nodes being affected almost exclusively. The constitutional symptoms are often considerable. The diagnosis is supported by findings of an enlarged spleen and confirmation is by specific intradermal testing or node biopsy.

Phlebitis

This is thrombosis of a superficial vein accompanied by marked pain and an inflammatory response of the overlying tissues. The thrombus is palpable as a tender, hard cord following the line of the varicose or superficial vein; propagation can be mapped by the cord and the inflammatory response (p. 383).

Tuberculosis

Mycobacterium tuberculosis infections occur in three stages: the primary complex, secondary dissemination and tertiary focal disease.

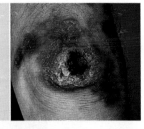

Figure 4.16.
Lupus vulgaris.

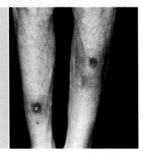

Figure 4.17.
Tuberculosis ulcer of the shin.

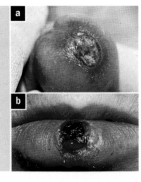

Figure 4.18.
a. Primary syphilitic infection of the penis. b. Primary chancre of the lower lip.

a

b

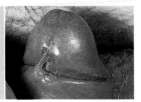

Figure 4.19.
Chancroid of the penis.

The primary lesion is usually a Ghon's focus sited in the lungs, spreading to hilar lymph nodes, but the portal of entry may be through the skin or alimentary tract. The infection is usually subclinical, residual evidence being a pulmonary scar, calcified lymph nodes and a positive skin test.

Secondary dissemination may occur months or many years later and causes widespread and haematogenous spread with multiple lesions. Any organ may be involved but commonly it is the lungs, bones and kidneys; tuberculous meningitis is common in some localities, particularly across Asia. Systemic resistance develops, or the condition is treated.

Tertiary lesions are usually focal and granulomatous with extensive cellular destruction and possible abscess formation. Again the lungs, bones and kidneys are common target organs. The cutaneous manifestation of TB is lupus vulgaris (*Figure 4.16*) which commences as a hyperaemic nodule and proceeds to a spreading, undermined ulcer (*Figure 4.17*), healing with extensive, pale scarring.

Syphilis

Infections caused by the spirochaete *Treponema pallidum* follow a similar pathological course to TB: a primary lesion, secondary haematogenous spread and tertiary local tissue destruction. The primary lesion is a solitary, painless, erythematous nodule occurring 9–90 days, usually about 21, after exposure (p. 201). The lesion breaks down to form a hard ulcer, a chancre, usually of the penis (*Figures 4.18a, b*) but it may occur on the lips, anus, nipples or fingers. It has a

sloping edge and a blood-stained discharge. The ulcer is accompanied by regional non-suppurative lymphadenopathy. Inguinal nodes from a penile lesion are hard and shotty but the nodes are usually much larger when associated with extragenital lesions.

A penile lesion (p. 355) has to be differentiated from carcinoma of the penis and **chancroid** (*Figure 4.19*) – this is a softer, less indurated, painful lesion that may be multiple. It is due to the Gram-negative bacillus *Haemophilus ducreyi*. Regional lymph node involvement may suppurate.

Secondary syphilis is a generalized disease accompanied by fever, malaise, a skin rash and generalized lymphadenopathy. There may be glossitis and pharyngitis, and oedematous papules of the mouth, penis, anus and vulva.

The tertiary focal granulomatous stage of syphilis is the gummatous ulcer. The lesion never reaches a large size. At first it is firm but soon the centre softens and the overlying skin becomes infiltrated and reddish-purple. Finally, there is central necrosis with ulcer formation. It is punched out and painless. The base is covered with a characteristic wet-wash leather ('chamois leather') slough, which contains one or more 'islands' of normal tissue that have escaped the necrosis. The healed gumma gives a circular, characteristic, paper-thin scar with surrounding pigmentation; although the scar of yaws is a similar lesion there are usually other manifestations of a previous syphilitic infection.

Any organ may be affected by tertiary syphilis, hence its name as the great imitator. Classic gummatous lesions are

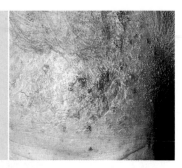

Figure 4.20.
Gummatous syphilitic lesion of the skull.

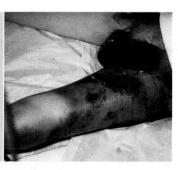

Figure 4.21.
Gas gangrene of the upper thigh with skin staining from muscle destruction.

found in the skull (*Figure 4.20*). The syphilitic lesions of the ascending aorta may produce superior mediastinal aneurysms; neurosyphilis comprises general paralysis of the insane, tabes dorsalis and meningovascular disease.

Actinomycosis

Actinomyces is a branching, filamentous, Gram-positive bacteria. It gives rise to a chronic, spreading infection with indurated, woody lesions. The subcutaneous involvement gives the overlying skin a dusky appearance (p. 218). Abscess formation is common, with multiple discharging sinuses, the pus containing characteristic 'sulphur-like' granules. Spread is directly through the blood stream without lymph node involvement. Common sites involved are the jaw (from dental infection), neck, lungs, caecum and liver.

Tetanus

Tetanus is a lethal condition produced by the powerful neurotoxic exotoxin of the Gram-positive, anaerobic spore-bearing bacillus, *Clostridium tetani*. The bacillus is a commensal of the gut, found in human and animal faeces, and in soil. It is, therefore, a common contaminant of dirty wounds and can multiply in dead and ischaemic tissue.

Widespread programmes of anti-tetanus prophylaxis have rendered tetanus an uncommon disease in western civilization. However, tetanus is still a major health problem in the developing world, neonatal tetanus being a particularly lethal condition. The incubation period ranges from a few days to a few weeks but it is usually 10–14 days. The initial symptoms are of lassitude, irritability, dysphagia and muscle spasm. Spasm of the facial muscles – trismus – produces the characteristic painful smile, risus sardonicus. This is followed by rigidity – lockjaw – and generalized tonic and clonic spasm. Prognosis is worst with short incubation and a short interval between the onset of symptoms and the first convulsions.

Gas gangrene

A number of anaerobic infections can produce gas and crepitus within tissues; examples of gas producing synergistic gangrene have already been discussed. However, the term 'gas gangrene' usually refers to infection with *Clostridium perfringens/welchii*, the condition being a toxic myositis with myonecrosis produced by an exotoxin. The organism is a commensal of the alimentary tract and a potential infective agent in gangrenous bowel. Gas gangrene can follow septic abortion, and ischaemic muscle injuries are particularly at risk (*Figure 4.21*).

The diagnosis is based on clinical grounds because *Clostridium* sp. may be contaminants of wounds, producing mild cellulitis or more lethal myositis, depending on local conditions. Pain is frequently the first indication of something amiss. An anxious look and a rising pulse, out of proportion to the temperature, increase suspicion and require inspection of the wound. The characteristic odour is a sickly-sweet smell suggestive of decaying apples, and the wound shows a surrounding area of red, brawny swelling with a distended limb, due to gas spreading along the muscle planes. Crepitus may be elicited at some distance from the wound.

Later, general signs suggesting the possibility of clostridial septicaemia include hypersensitivity and irritability, dyspnoea, and tachycardia out of proportion to the pyrexia. By this time there are profound systemic symptoms of shock, obvious crepitus, bluish-brown skin discoloration, bullous formation with a watery discharge and pronounced odour. The fluid from bullae provides a heavy growth of the causative organism.

Viral diseases

Virus-related diseases are common world-wide and affect every system. Although they require less surgical involvement than the pus-forming bacteria, surgical patients are suscep-

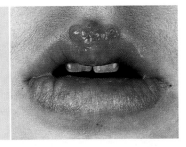

Figure 4.22.
Herpes simplex
infection of the lip.

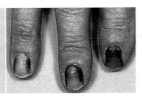

Figure 4.24.
Candidial infection of the
nails.

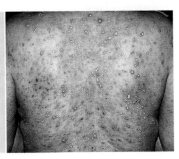

Figure 4.23.
Cutaneous lesions
of chicken pox.

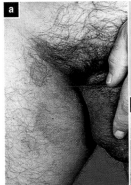

Figure 4.25.
a. Tinea cruris. b. Tinea
corporis.

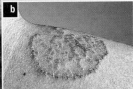

tible to viral infection, and viral diseases may require surgical intervention, often because of secondary bacterial infection. The surgeon is also at risk of contracting certain viral infections such as hepatitis and HIV (p. 83) from patients.

Classification of viral disease can be based on physical properties, protein coat or nucleic acid core, but a more practical division is based on the prime organ of involvement. Systemic effects are also common, and the incidence of multi-organ pathology is increased in immunocompromised patients, a specific example being **cytomegalovirus** which has serious consequences after organ transplantation. Some viruses are endemic, such as **plague**, which is transmitted through wild animals, and many are tropical in their distribution, such as the mosquito-born **alphaviruses**. Other groups may become epidemic, such as the influenza viruses, while plague and **typhus** are prevalent in malnourished refugee populations.

In the respiratory tract, the common cold is produced by **rhinoviruses**, while specific virus groups also affect the lungs, e.g. influenza viruses. Other organs commonly involved include the CNS, e.g. **poliomyelitis** and **rabies**, and the gut, e.g. **hepatitis** and **yellow fever**. Many viral infections have cutaneous manifestations, examples being **herpes simplex** (*Figure 4.22*), **herpes zoster** (p. 167, *Figures 10.9 and 10.11*), **measles**, **mumps** and **chicken pox** (*Figure 4.23*); a few viruses are largely restricted to cutaneous manifestations such as warts on the hands and the plantar aspects of the feet, and molluscum contagiosum (p. 136, *Figure 8.26*).

Fungal infections (mycoses)

Fungi affect humans in a number of ways. They can destroy crops, thereby promoting starvation in tropical areas; some fungi, such as certain mushrooms, are poisonous; they can act as allergens, producing asthma and hypersensitivity pneumonitis; and some fungi are invasive. The latter may be subdivided into those invading the skin, the subcutaneous tissues and the deep tissues.

Superficial infections of the skin include thrush (*Candida albicans*) (*Figure 4.24*) and ringworm (tinea cruris and tinea capitis) (*Figure 4.25a, b*). Subcutaneous fungal infections are usually tropical in distribution, the prime example being mycetoma (p. 79). Deep visceral fungal infections are often opportunistic, occurring in immunocompromised individuals, for example *Cryptococcus* which affects the lungs and produces meningitis.

Protozoa and worms

These parasitic infections are common in the tropics (p. 105) but are also widely distributed in temperate zones. The majority pass their life cycle in more than one host, producing millions of eggs to ensure survival and reaching humans by way of a vector. Many of these diseases involve surgical management, particularly those affecting the alimentary tract.

Protozoal infections include **amoebiasis**, **malaria** (the mosquito being the vector), **trypanosomiasis** (carried by the tsetse fly in Africa), **toxoplasmosis** (usually contracted from household pets) and **leishmaniasis** (carried by the sand fly) (p. 111). See also Chapter 6.

Amoebiasis

Amoebiasis is a gut infection, producing inflammatory dysentery and caused by **Entamoeba histolytica**. Occasionally there is systemic involvement which usually takes the form of inflammatory amoebomas of the large bowel – this mass occurs most commonly in the caecum. Portal venous invasion can lead to a liver abscess, which is usually solitary; rupture through the diaphragm into the bronchial tree produces the characteristic purplish-brown sputum from red-brown necrotic liver tissue. The disease is endemic and sometimes epidemic in the tropics, but sporadic cases occur elsewhere. Cysts are excreted in the stool, the disease being contracted through poor hygiene or insect transfer.

Malaria (*Plasmodium falciparum*; *P. vivax*; *P. ovale*; *P. malariae*)

Malaria (*Figures 4.26a, b*) is the pre-eminent tropical disease, with 200 000 000 sufferers and probably an annual mortality of 2 000 000. It is transmitted by the blood-sucking female *Anopheles* mosquito. Parasites are trapped by the liver within 30 minutes of infection and the symptoms then usually occur within one month but may be within five days or, rarely, after one year. The diagnosis is suspected on clinical grounds and confirmed by the presence of parasites within red blood cells viewed on a thick blood film. The importance of malaria to the surgeon is mainly in its differential diagnosis. Fever, headache, nausea and myalgia occur in many tropical conditions, but the rigors may be diagnostic in their timing (p. 106), and the intense shivering. Anaemia, abdominal pain, jaundice and diarrhoea are also common, together with splenomegaly, particularly with *P. malariae*. The large spleen is fragile, rupturing with minor trauma and having a high mortality. Most deaths are from *P. falciparum*, patients usually suffering from cerebral malaria, accompanied by shock, hypoglycaemia and renal failure.

Trypanosomiasis

In **African trypanosomiasis** the first sign is the nodule at the site of the tsetse fly bite. This is followed by fever and lymphadenopathy. Central nervous system involvement, with the onset of the characteristic mental changes of sleeping sickness, may take a month or over a year to appear. **American trypanosomiasis** is located in North and South America and is transmitted by the house bug. The disease was initially described, and is now named, after Chagas. There is local swelling at the site of the bite but the chronic symptoms may take many decades to appear – these involve chronic inflammation of cardiac muscle, producing a cardiomyopathy, and involvement of the smooth muscle and nerve plexuses of the gut, producing a megaoesophagus and megacolon, causing dysphagia and constipation.

Toxoplasmosis

Toxoplasmosis is a world-wide infection, usually carried from infected mice by household cats. The majority of infections go unnoticed, but patients may present with painless lymphadenopathy. The disease, however, has serious implications in the immunocompromised patient where fatal encephalitis can develop. Neonatal infections may also be accompanied by fatal cerebral involvement and chorioretinitis (*Figure 4.27*).

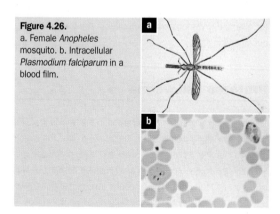

Figure 4.26.
a. Female *Anopheles* mosquito. b. Intracellular *Plasmodium falciparum* in a blood film.

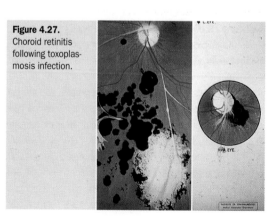

Figure 4.27.
Choroid retinitis following toxoplasmosis infection.

Worms

Worms include **roundworms** (nematodes), **tapeworms** (cestodes) and **flukes** (trematodes); a common finding in an eosinophilic response to their foreign protein. In the roundworms, **hookworm** is one of the most prevalent diseases in the world. The larvae migrate to the top of blades of grass and enter humans through skin abrasions. They pass through the lungs and then to the small intestine. The head becomes firmly attached to the intestinal wall and, although each worm is small – less than 2 cm long – as they are present in their thousands, a chronic, debilitating anaemia results.

The **Ascaris** worm (*Figure 4.28*) is the common roundworm that resembles the earthworm in shape but may be 20–30 cm long. Large collections of these worms can produce intestinal obstruction, especially in children. They also produce systemic disturbances, as larvae that are ingested penetrate the gut wall and pass to the lungs via the circulation. They then break into the bronchi, migrate to the epiglottis and are again swallowed; they mature in the small intestine. Very occasionally, and usually after irritation by drugs or manipulation during surgery, a worm may migrate into the appendix, or the common bile or pancreatic ducts, giving rise to obstruction and secondary infection. **Filarial** (**Wuncheria bancrofti**) infections are also produced by round worms of 6–8 cm that are transported in their larval form by the mosquito. The adult worms migrate into human lymphatics, producing gross secondary lymphoedema of the legs and scrotum (*Figures 2.29a, b*), termed elephantiasis. Obstruction of the thoracic duct may give rise to chylous ascites, and subcutaneous nodules may be produced by an inflammatory response surrounding a local worm. **Pinworms** or **threadworms** are up to 1 cm long and are common in children. Their presence in the perianal area produces intractable itching.

Guinea worm and larvae migrans

Guinea worm, *Dracunculus medinensis* (*Figures 4.30* and *4.31*), is extensively distributed across central Africa and Asia. The secondary host is the water flea, and transfer to humans is in contaminated water. The worm migrates from the gut to the surface. The male worm usually dies after mating but the adult female can grow to 70–120 cm in length and 2 mm wide. The local inflammatory response may be intense. It is sometimes possible to extract the full length of the worm once it has surfaced.

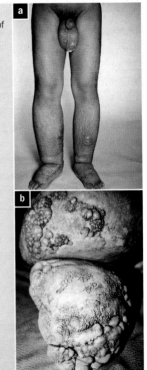

Figure 4.29.
a. Secondary lymphoedema of the leg and scrotum from filarial infection. b. Severe secondary lymphoedema of the lower leg due to filarial infection.

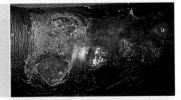

Figure 4.30.
Extensive skin inflammation and ulceration following guinea worm infection.

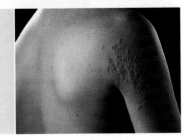

Figure 4.31.
Cutaneous larvae migrans.

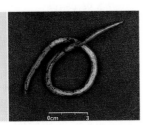

Figure 4.28.
Common roundworm. *Ascaris.*

Cutaneous larvae migrans, ***Strongyloides stercoralis***, occurs in the West Indies and central Asia. The worm is about 3 mm long and is atypical in that it can produce several generations within the same human host, leading to heavy infestation and prolonged symptoms. Its cutaneous migration is accompanied by a marked inflammatory response.

Flat tapeworms

The flat tapeworms have a wide distribution. In those where the secondary host is cattle (*Taenia saginatum*) (*Figure 4.32*), pig (*T. solium*) and fish (*Diphyllobothrium latum*), the adult tapeworm is found in the alimentary tract of the human. Some grow to many metres in length. Symptoms are usually mild, although occasionally a severe anaemia occurs in the Chinese fish tapeworm and, rarely, bile duct adenocarcinoma can develop (p. 287). If the eggs of *T. solium* are transferred directly from one human to another, the cysticercus stage may occur in man. The symptoms of cysticercosis are usually severe neurological problems due to invasion of the CNS.

The **hydatid tapeworm** *Echinococcus granulosus* differs from the others in that the cystic stage occurs in man, the other hosts being the dog and the sheep. The ingested eggs penetrate the bowel wall and are carried by the portal vein to the liver and thence around the body; cysts develop mainly in the liver, lung (*Figure 4.33*), kidneys and brain. The cysts cause pressure as well as toxic effects in many systems.

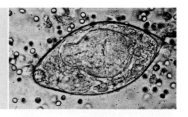

Figure 4.34.
Bilharzia eggs in blood film.

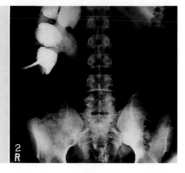

Figure 4.35.
Hydronephrosis due to ureteric stenosis from bilharzial infection.

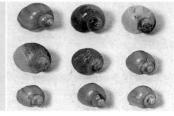

Figure 4.36.
Snail *Bulinus physopsis*. The intermediate host in bilharzia infection.

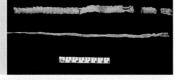

Figure 4.32.
Tapeworm. *Taenia saginatum.*

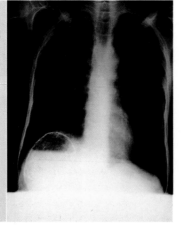

Figure 4.33.
Chest X-ray showing calcified hydatid lung abscess.

Liver flukes

Liver flukes are prevalent in China, and **lung flukes** are common parasites in Japan and China. The most important disease caused by flukes, however, is **schistosomiasis** (bilharzia) (*Figure 4.34*). The *Schistosoma* organism produces granulomas, particularly of the bladder and liver, and causes bladder dysfunction, recurrent infections (*Figure 4.35*) and, in the late stages, transitional cell carcinoma. The intermediate host of the flukes is the water snail (*Figure 4.36*) – larvae enter the human through skin abrasions and mature in the liver.

External parasites

Common external parasites include scabies (*Figures 4.37a, b*), lice (*Figures 4.48a, b*) and fleas (*Figure 4.39*); they belong to the jointed arthropods. Their bites may be painful and cause hypersensitivity and itching. They may also carry diseases, particularly epidemic typhus and relapsing fever. The reactions to insect bites vary from mild hyperaemia to acute allergic local or systemic effects (*Figures 4.40a, b*).

Figure 4.37.
Scabies is carried by the itch mite *Sarcoptes scabiei*. a. The female burrows into the skin to lay her eggs, producing a papule, the site of the lesion commonly on the dorsum of the web space. b. This produces intense itching.

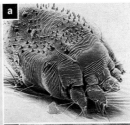

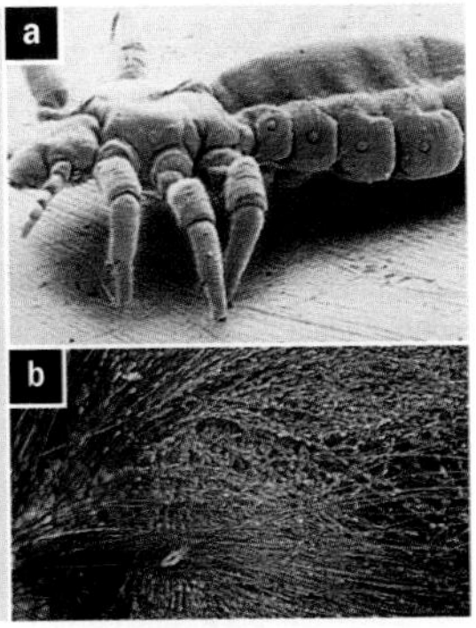

Figure 4.38.
a. Head louse. b. Head lice *in situ*.

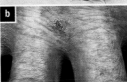

Figure 4.39.
There are more than 20 species of flea that attack humans, the commonest variety in the UK is *Pulex irritans*. The bites can cause irritation and erythema. These effects vary remarkably between individuals.

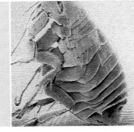

Figure 4.40.
a. Insect bite. b. Acute allergic response secondary to insect bite.

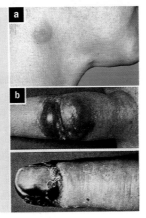

Hand infections

Hand infections have become less common in the UK over the last two decades. This is due to the mandatory wearing of protective apparel, including gloves, at the work place, and to the automation of many industries, with a consequent reduction in manual labour. Nevertheless, hand infections still make up 0.7% of accident and emergency attendances in the UK, and the early recognition and treatment of these lesions are important to prevent prolonged loss of work and hand deformity. Those particularly at risk include manual workers and patients with diabetes or who are immunosuppressed. Patients with ischaemia, whether from large or small vessel disease, such as scleroderma, are subject to recurrent infection with necrosis and tissue loss.

When describing hand conditions it is important to document the digits as the thumb, and the index, middle, ring and little fingers as numbered digits leads to confusion, with disastrous results if an amputation is being undertaken. The infected hand is held in the position of rest, this being with all joints flexed to 5–25° and a flexed elbow. Oedema is usually prominent, this being most evident on the dorsum of the hand, irrespective of the site of the lesion, due to the greater laxity of the skin and fascia over the dorsal aspect. Cellulitis is common with superficial lesions. Lymphangitis may present as red streaks along the arm, and is accompanied by axillary lymphadenopathy, the supratrochlear node being enlarged with infection of the medial aspect of the forearm and hand. Focal tenderness is the cardinal sign of pus, and demonstration of this tenderness is a very important diagnostic tool, particularly when searching for deep infection such as in a tendon sheath. There may be an associated pyrexia and general malaise.

Streptococci (50%) and staphylococci are the commonest infecting organisms but wounds may become infected with coliforms (19%), and *Bacteroides* and other anaerobes. Viral infections, e.g. herpes simplex, can occur and opportunistic organisms should be considered in immunosuppressed individuals.

Paronychia

Paronychia (*Figures 4.41a, b*) is the commonest hand infection (30%), encountered in every walk of life, affecting both sexes in all age groups. Infection arises underneath torn nails or damaged cuticles, being a sub-eponychial suppuration, spreading around the nail fold, often to the collateral side. In 60% of cases, pus burrows beneath the nail (subungual abscess) (*Figure 4.41c*). In this case, pressure on the nail

Figure 4.41.
Acute paronychia.

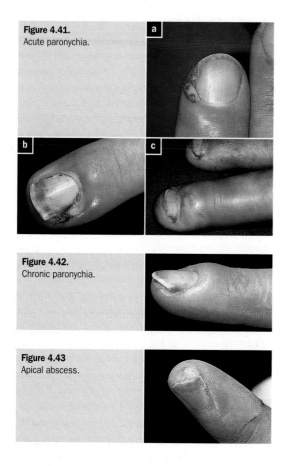

Figure 4.42.
Chronic paronychia.

Figure 4.43
Apical abscess.

evokes exquisite pain. The infection may persist as a chronic inflammation around the nail fold (*Figure 4.42*). Chronic lesion may also be secondary to fungal infection such as candidiasis.

Apical abscess

An apical abscess (*Figure 4.43*) lies beneath the free edge of the nail following a sharp injury, such as by a splinter. Pus may burst through the subungual epithelium to lie in the distal nail bed.

Pulp space infection

Pulp space infection (*Figure 4.44*) is a common (14%) and potentially serious infection following penetrating injury, the index finger and thumb being most susceptible. The space is filled with compact fat, partly partitioned by septa and separated from the rest of the finger by a distinct transverse septum at the level of the epiphyseal line of the terminal phalanx. A dull ache and swelling are initially present, with cellulitis. With pus formation there is severe nocturnal

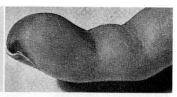

Figure 4.44.
Pulp space infection.

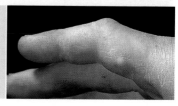

Figure 4.45.
Septic arthritis following pulp space infection.

exacerbation of throbbing pain interfering with sleep, and marked local tenderness. The subcutaneous abscess may break through and spread under the dermis, or extend deeply to involve the bone (*Figure 4.45*). In the former (collar stud abscess), the deeper component may only be recognized after deroofing the subcuticular abscess.

Infection over the middle and proximal phalanges

These infections have a similar aetiology and clinical course to terminal pulp space infections but oedema is more marked, due to greater skin laxity. Infection over the middle phalanx is localized by proximal and distal septa but over the proximal (*Figure 4.46*), pus can communicate freely with the adjacent web space of the hand.

Web space infections produce gross oedema of the space and extend over the dorsum of the hand. The infection may be poorly localized with marked systemic symptoms. The differential diagnosis of tendon sheath infection is difficult until local pus formation, when the redness becomes more focal. Pus can track across the palmar surface of the base of the fingers from one web space to the next and into the proximal digital compartment of the adjacent fingers.

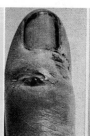 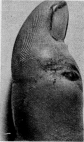

Figure 4.46.
Infection over proximal phalynx.

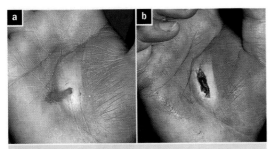

Figure 4.47.
a. Palmar infection. b. On excision. The superficial component proved to be a collar stud abscess involving the mid-palmar space.

Thenar space infection

The thenar compartment encloses the short thenar muscles and long tendons to the thumb. There is marked ballooning of the thenar eminence; flexion of the distal phalanx may be pronounced but it lacks the resistance to extension that is present in infection of the sheath of the flexor pollicis longus. The **hypothenar** space may be similarly affected but it is less common.

Mid-palmar space infection

Infection of the mid-palmar space containing the long digital flexor tendons deep to the palmar fascia (*Figures 4.47a, b* and *4.48*) usually follows penetrating injuries but can follow rupture of an infected tendon sheath. There is obliteration of the concavity of the palm, with bulging, and extreme swelling of the dorsum, giving the characteristic 'frog hand' appearance (*Figure 4.49*).

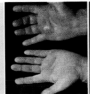

Figure 4.48.
Mid-palmar infection accompanied by extensive oedema.

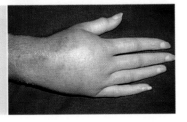

Figure 4.49.
'Frog hand' showing extensive oedema over the dorsum of the hand. The prime focus may be situated on the palmar aspect.

Infection of the tendon sheaths

Infection of the tendon sheaths usually follows penetration by a sharp pointed object such as a needle or thorn, particularly over digital flexor creases where the sheath is near the surface. Very occasionally, the infection may spread from the more superficial abscesses. The whole sheath is rapidly involved and, within a few hours of the injury, throbbing pain is felt in the affected digit, with an accompanying pyrexia. The involved finger is held in a flexed position and, as the infection proceeds, there is symmetrical swelling of the whole finger, with puffy swelling on the dorsum of the hand. Although the finger can be moved back and forth, by lumbrical action, active finger flexion is absent. Passive extension produces extreme pain. There is marked tenderness along the tendon sheath, this being extreme at the proximal and distal limits of the sheath where it extrudes outside the fibrous containing bands.

The little finger communicates with the ulnar bursa, and the thenar flexor sheath with the radial bursa. The proximal limit of tenderness with bursal involvement extends proximal to the flexor retinaculum. As there is usually a communication between the radial and ulnar bursae, it may be difficult to distinguish infection of one bursa from the other. Associated palmar and dorsal swelling can make differential diagnosis with other palmar infection difficult but the absence of extension and the extreme pain on movement are usually diagnostic.

Other infections of the palm include barber's pilonidal sinus (p. 326) and penetrating injuries from spray guns dispensing oils, solvents and paints (grease gun injuries). These are serious injuries and the damage can be underestimated in the early stages due to small entry wounds, lack of bleeding, numbness masking pain and the part feeling cold rather than demonstrating the classical signs of inflammation. Debridement can thus be delayed, with subsequent extensive subcutaneous necrosis, which may involve tendons and tendon sheaths.

Infection of the dorsal space

This is unusual but may accompany boils and carbuncles, and extensions of these lesions can involve extensor tendon sheaths. Focal tenderness over the infected area differentiates it from dorsal swelling associated with palmar lesions.

Animal and human bites may also cause a variety of superficial and deep infections from a range of pathogenic organisms. Healing of penetrating injuries may be followed by implantation dermoid cysts, most commonly seen in the pulps of the fingers.

For **warts** and *Candida* infection of the nail see p. 80.

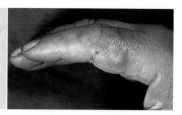

Figure 4.50.
Erysipeloid infection.

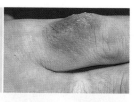

Figure 4.53.
Fish tank granuloma.

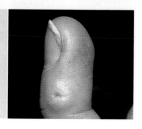

Figure 4.54.
Herpetic whitlow.

Uncommon hand infections

In addition to the infection described above, the hand is subject to a number of other characteristic lesions. **Cutaneous erysipeloid** (*Figure 4.50*) is due to infection with *Erysipelothrix* sp. bacteria, which contaminate meat, game and fish; it is seen particularly in butchers.

Orf and anthrax

Orf and anthrax are acquired from animal contact; orf (*Figure 4.51*) is a poxvirus carried by sheep, cattle and goats, and occurs in shepherds, farmers, abattoir workers and veterinary surgeons. The vesicular macular lesions break down and are usually painless until secondary infection occurs. Generalized disease is very rare.

Anthrax (*Figure 4.52*) is a Gram-positive bacteria whose resistant spores can be transported in hides, wool, hair and bone. The latter is ground down in the preparation of gelatin and glue. The lesions are found in those coming into direct contact with infected animals or animal products. They consist of a black, firmly adherent scab surrounded by oedematous, purplish vesicles. There is surprisingly little pain from these aggressive-looking lesions. Systemic infection may follow, typically affecting the lungs, intestines and, more rarely, the meninges.

Fish tank granuloma

Fish tank granuloma (*Figure 4.53*) is acquired in an abrasion from a fish tank that is infected with atypical mycobacteria. A soft, subcutaneous nodular lesion is produced, which becomes secondarily infected. There is often associated lymphangitis.

Herpetic whitlows

Herpetic whitlows (*Figure 4.54*) occur in medical and other health professionals in contact with infected patients. The digital lesions are painful blisters, initially containing clear fluid, but later exuding pus and debris. The lesions take a number of weeks to heal.

Systemic infection

Cutaneous infection may be secondary to systemic disease as seen in the gonococcal lesion in *Figure 4.55*. The dissemination of septic emboli may produce deep or superficial lesions such as the septic lesion on the thumb shown in *Figure 4.56*.

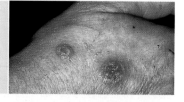

Figure 4.51.
Orf infection.

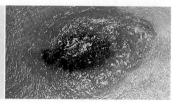

Figure 4.52.
Anthrax infection.

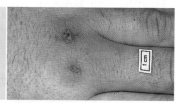

Figure 4.55.
Cutaneous infection may be secondary to systemic disease as seen in this gonococcal lesion.

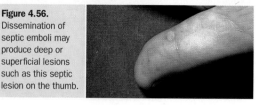

Figure 4.56.
Dissemination of septic emboli may produce deep or superficial lesions such as this septic lesion on the thumb.

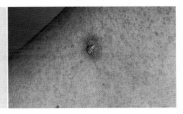

Figure 4.57.
Foreign body
granuloma.

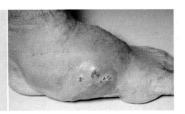

Figure 4.58.
Madura foot.

Foreign body granulomas

Foreign body granulomas (*Figure 4.57*) are produced by sub-cutaneous implantation of external debris and bacteria.

Tropical infections are considered in Chapter 6.

Foot infections

Infection of the sole of the foot is common among those who walk barefooted and so is seen mostly in the tropics. Tight, rigid footwear can produce blisters over the heel and prominent joints, and pressure on the great toenail can precipitate the problem of an ingrowing toenail. Neuropathic feet are prone to unnoticed injury, with secondary infection; this is particularly common in diabetic patients (p. 371).

The dense fascial layers of the foot and their various septa tend to localize infection, spread from one compartment to another being slow. Pus within a compartment produces extreme local tenderness and throbbing pain that may interfere with sleep. As in the hand, associated oedema may appear over the dorsum or lateral aspects of the foot, rather than over the sole. If the infection is in the **heel space**, the patient dare not put the foot to the ground. Infection of the **deep fascial spaces** of the sole may track along neurovascular bundles or into tendon sheaths. Penetrating injuries may allow **subcutaneous infection** to produce collar stud abscesses and **web space** infection to spread through tissue planes and track into the plantar or dorsal aspects of the foot.

Mycetoma (Madura foot)

This fungal infection is endemic in tropical Africa, India, and South and Central America. It is almost confined to individuals who walk barefoot and are liable to contamination of mild abrasions with road dust. The first manifestation is a firm, painless, rather pale nodule, usually on the foot. This increases in size, and others appear. In the early stage, especially if the sole is involved, a malignant melanoma may be suspected. In about a week, vesicles appear on the surface of the nodules and these soon burst to reveal the mouth of

a sinus, which discharges purulent, mucoid fluid. The fluid contains black, red or yellow granules, depending on the species. The black variety spreads mainly subcutaneously but the red and yellow varieties spread early to the muscles and underlying bone. Nerves and tendons are resistant and neurological signs are conspicuously absent; there is no associated lymphadenitis or blood-born dissemination. Sooner or later secondary infection supervenes, producing gross swelling of the foot with obliteration of the concavity of the instep (*Figure 4.58*).

Differential diagnosis of multiple sinuses in the foot

A large number of tropical infections can cause foot ulceration and sinus formation. The diagnosis depends on a knowledge of the local endemic infections and isolating the causative organisms. Tuberculosis is common in the tropics and is often long untreated. Kaposi's sarcoma (p. 86), in which soft nodules often become infected, can resemble Madura foot (above). Tropical ulcer (p. 110) may also occur in the foot.

Ingrowing toenail (onychocryptosis)

An ingrowing toenail usually affects the great toe (*Figure 4.59*), particularly on the lateral side. It develops when there is excessive outward growth of the nail into the nail fold. It may be precipitated by tight shoes or cutting the corner off the nail, the sharp residual edge then penetrating the nail fold as it grows forward, rather than growing clear of the skin.

Figure 4.59.
Ingrowing toenail.

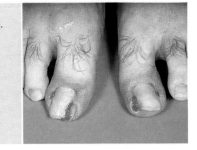

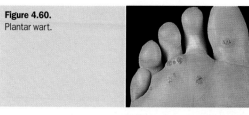

Figure 4.60.
Plantar wart.

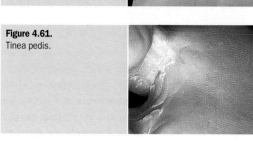

Figure 4.61.
Tinea pedis.

The laceration produced allows entry of bacteria and a painful infection. In chronic cases there can be protuberant granulation tissue. The lesion is very tender and the patient wears capacious shoes or sandals to prevent a painful limp.

Plantar wart

Plantar warts or verrucae (*Figure 4.60*) are produced by infection with the human papillomavirus. They occur on the weight-bearing areas of the ball of the foot or the heel. Pressure of walking inverts the warty lesion, so that it is surrounded by a rim of cornified skin, there being a central red or black pitted area. They may have adjacent satellite lesions. Verrucae are usually found in children and can be exquisitely tender.

Tinea pedis

This fungal infection produces maceration between the toes, usually the fourth interspace, and often itching (*Figure 4.61*). In its more aggressive form it produces purplish-red, raised skin around the web, which may blister. Interdigital infection of the fungus *Candida albicans* can mimic these symptoms. It can also infect the nailfold and nail, producing chronic paronychia and a ridged and brown pigmented nail.

Wounds

Injuries may be open or closed, the former implying a break in the epithelial covering and thus having a potential for bacterial invasion. The terms are not synonymous with minor and major since a lethal injury, e.g. cardiac or cerebral trauma, may occur in either group.

The term 'wound' usually implies a break in the skin, irrespective of its aetiology, e.g. surgery or accidental injury, or of the amount of underlying tissue damage. There are a number of different classifications of wounds related to their position, their depth and the amount of tissue damage, e.g. incision, laceration and contusion. A practical subdivision, however, is into tidy and untidy injuries.

Tidy injuries are when tissue damage and contamination are minimal; they include surgical incisions undertaken under aseptic techniques, and clean knife and glass injuries. Direct closure by suture, staple or clips can usually be undertaken, although tetanus prophylaxis and the need for antibiotic cover must be considered. Possible injury to deeper structures, e.g. blood vessels, nerves and viscera, have also to be taken into account. Surgical incisions are placed along tension lines or skin creases and aim to avoid underlying vessels, nerves and organs.

Untidy injuries indicate irregular skin damage, with possible skin loss, external contamination and damage to underlying tissue, such as blood vessels, nerves, muscles and fractures. Tearing of the skin produces haemorrhage, contusion and haematoma formation, and lifting flaps, e.g. de-gloving or scalping, may denervate the skin or render it ischaemic. Managing such wounds involves the removal of foreign material and dead tissue, and closure may need to be delayed or the wound left open.

Although division into tidy and untidy wounds is of practical value, each wound has to be assessed independently for associated problems, since even a small insect bite may result in a lethal anaphylactic response or be followed by marked cellulitis. The body responds to all injuries with an inflammatory response, this being capillary dilatation and the production of an inflammatory exudate, incorporating both cellular and humoral responses to damaged tissue.

In a sutured wound, the opposed edges are sealed with the exudate and fibrin clot, and there is a firm union in 3–4 days. This is the first phase of **primary repair**. In the second phase, there is capillary proliferation with outgrowth of capillary buds and fibroblast migration, collagen deposition and epithelial ingrowth from each edge. This stage lasts from 4–15 days during which there is increasing strength across the wound, such that in the absence of tension, e.g. on the face and neck, stitches can be removed in 3–4 days. In the abdomen, where there can be tension – coughing, straining and distension – stitches are left in for 10–14 days. In the third phase of healing there is contraction and maturation of the scar, normal strength returning by approximately 3 months.

In non-opposed wounds, healing is by **secondary intention**, the inflammatory response producing a slough of damaged and dead tissue, foreign material and organisms. The capillary growth and fibroblast activity is towards the surface and gradually replaces the green slough with pink granulating tissue, epithelial ingrowth being from the surrounding edge.

Drains are placed in wounds to remove existing or anticipated blood, pus or body fluids, or to drain dead spaces where such collections may occur. They are removed when they stop draining, usually after 24–48 hours post injury but, when draining a potentially infected anastomotic leak, they may be left for 3–8 days to allow the development of a fibrous tract.

Complications

Postoperative healing is promoted by delicate handling of tissues, minimizing tissue damage, removing foreign or dead material, obliterating dead space and the meticulous alignment of skin edges, opposing the tissues without tension. Conversely, delayed healing occurs when there is residual dead, damaged or ischaemic tissue, foreign material or when undrained dead space and haematoma prevent tissue apposition. Foreign material, such as synthetic vascular grafts and joint prostheses delay tissue ingrowth. Prophylactic antibiotic treatment must be considered to prevent infection of tissue fluids and haematoma around prostheses until tissue incorporation is complete.

Infection is one of the commonest complications of wound healing, occurring in 6–8% of cases. The incidence is 1–2% in clean wounds, such as those encountered in plastic surgery and neurosurgery, being higher in abdominal incisions and occurring in up to 40% of cases when there is pre-existing infection or when large bowel organisms contaminate the field. Signs of cellulitis are redness and discharge, which may become purulent. Staphylococci and streptococci are the usual organisms but gut flora may be involved, or opportunistic infection in immunocompromised patients. The effects in the majority of patients are trivial discomfort and delayed healing. However, infection of haematoma, or serious collections with abscess formation, carry a more serious prognosis. Persistent dead tissue or foreign bodies can result in sinus formation and leaks from gut anastomoses may result in a fistula. A number of factors have been implicated in **delayed healing**. These include malignancy, old age, hormonal abnormalities, steroid therapy, anaemia, diabetes and obesity. However, controlled studies of these factors are not well documented. Malnutrition, particularly hypoproteinaemia and vitamin C deficiency, does produce fragile wounds and poor healing but the degree of deficiency necessary to delay healing is unusual in western society.

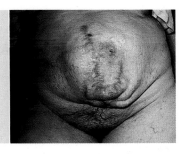

Figure 4.62.
Incisional hernia.

Vertical abdominal wounds are liable to stretch due to the tension from abdominal distension, trunk movements and coughing. Such wounds are prone to late development of **incisional herniae** (*Figure 4.62*), particularly if multiple incisions are present. The powerful forces of coughing, vomiting and distension can occasionally give rise to a **burst abdomen**. This may be linked with inadequate incorporation of the layers of the rectus sheath or early removal of sutures. The burst may be heralded by a pink discharge of serous peritoneal fluid, indicating disruption of deeper layers, before the skin gives way. Although the presentation of loops of small gut can be dramatic, there is remarkably little systemic disturbance and the patient often appears the least concerned. Covering the gut with saline packs and a tension bandage, followed by re-suture is accompanied by rapid recovery.

Hypertrophic scars and keloids

Some wounds are accompanied by a fibrous overgrowth and enlargement of the scar. In a **hypertrophic scar** (*Figure 4.63*) this fibrous reaction is limited to the scar, which is pink,

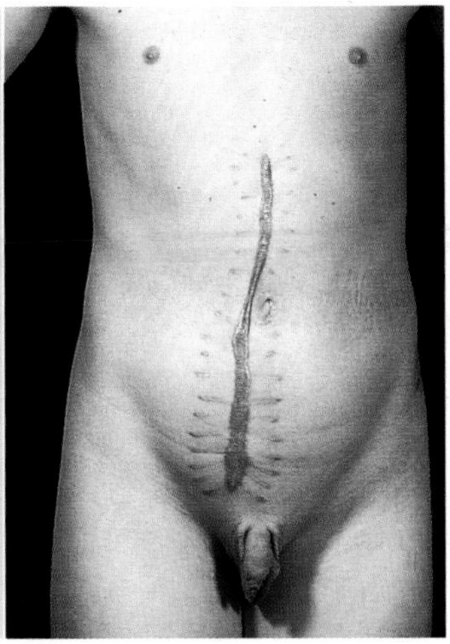

Figure 4.63.
Hypotrophic abdominal scar.

may be tender and may itch. The scar can continue to enlarge for about 6 months but regresses after a year to pale, thin, stretched scar tissue. The heaping-up and overgrowth of the scar in **keloid** (*Figures 4.64a, b, c*) formation is composed of hyperplastic vascular collagen fibres, which can extend in a claw-like fashion into adjacent tissues. The process can continue for a number of years. It is common in individuals with pigmented skin, in children, in pregnancy, and it may be familial. Keloid is distributed more commonly in the midline over the face and the neck, the sternum and the anterior abdominal wall. It can be copious after burns, radiotherapy, scarification and puncture wounds, such as BCG (bacillus Calmette–Guérin) inoculation sites and pierced ears.

Hypertrophic tissue in a wound may be due to a foreign body response to a suture or other foreign material (*Figure 4.65*).

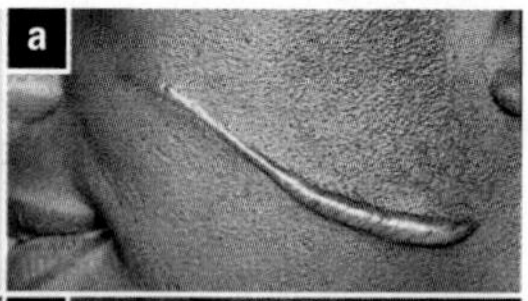

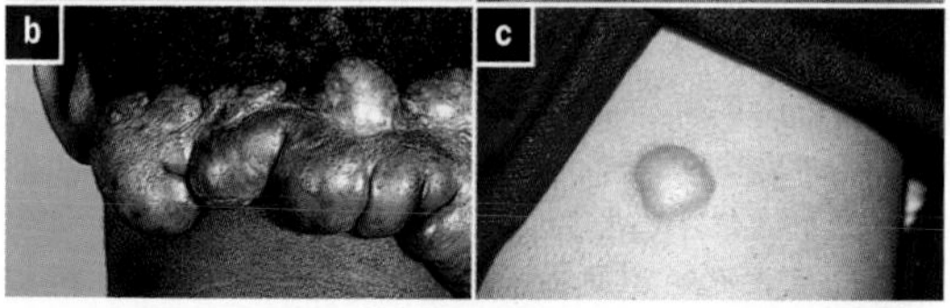

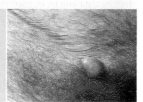

Figure 4.64.
a. Facial keloid. b. Cervical keloid. c. Keloid at vaccination site.

Figure 4.65.
Hypertrophic tissue at the medial end of an inguinal hernia wound due to a foreign body response to a suture.

5 HIV and AIDS

Introduction

In recent years the human immunodeficiency virus (HIV) has had a major impact on surgical practice with the emergence of a new spectrum of surgical pathology. This is often **unique to the geographical location** of the surgical practice and, as ever, there is no substitute for knowledge of the local range of pathology. It is vital to recognize that HIV and acquired immunodeficiency syndrome (AIDS) patients also develop the same surgical conditions as an age, sex and race matched non-HIV population (*Figure 5.1*). With advancing immunodeficiency their presentation may differ due to a relative lack of inflammatory response.

History

States of immunodeficiency have long been recognized. The newest syndrome to emerge was noted in previously healthy young homosexual men in 1981. The virus presumed responsible for this acquired immune deficiency was originally named human T-cell lymphoma virus III (HTLV-III) because it was distinct from the already known retroviruses HTLV-I and HTLV-II. It was later renamed the human immunodeficiency virus. A different strain of HIV is common in West Africa, so the two subtypes were classified into HIV-I and HIV-2. A probable third subtype is currently under investigation. All the known subtypes result in chronic HIV infection and AIDS. By 1993 the World Health Organization had documented 2.5 million AIDS cases and estimated that 14 million people were HIV positive. Worldwide it is estimated that by the year 2000 AD, 40 million people will be HIV positive. This figure fails to take into account the many unreported cases in less developed countries, where seroprevalence may be as high as 85% in some areas.

No medical speciality is exempt from the impact of HIV-positive patients. An index of suspicion for HIV disease is important for **both** patient care and health worker protection. In this chapter a brief synopsis of the immune deficiencies found in HIV infection is given and the physical manifestations of HIV infection that the surgical specialities might be

exposed to are reviewed. In doing so, no prior knowledge of the HIV status of the patient is assumed. In the final section of the chapter special issues relating to the preparation of an HIV-positive person for surgery are raised. Considerations for HIV-positive surgeons and legal aspects for all health-care workers are briefly discussed.

Natural History

Once infection with HIV has occurred it may take several weeks for the body to mount an immune response. Routine current HIV tests detect the presence of antibodies to the virus. Therefore, before immune activation the patient has a negative HIV test even though they are infected (the 'window period', *Figure 5.2*). Recognition by the immune system of the presence of the virus and the subsequent production of antibodies results in seroconversion, i.e. the person is now antibody positive on testing, or HIV positive. In the majority of cases seroconversion is subclinical. However in about 10%

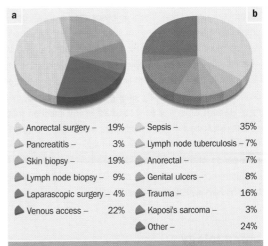

a		b	
Anorectal surgery –	19%	Sepsis –	35%
Pancreatitis –	3%	Lymph node tuberculosis –	7%
Skin biopsy –	19%	Anorectal –	7%
Lymph node biopsy –	9%	Genital ulcers –	8%
Laparascopic surgery –	4%	Trauma –	16%
Venous access –	22%	Kaposi's sarcoma –	3%
		Other –	24%

Figure 5.1.
Pie charts illustrating the distribution of surgical pathology in two geographically distinct and morphologically dissimilar groups of HIV positive patients: a. St Mary's Hospital, London (AG Tanner, 1994); b. Female rural Zambian cohort (Rev. Dr AC Bayley, 1991).

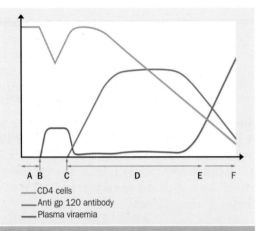

_____ CD4 cells
_____ Anti gp 120 antibody
_____ Plasma viraemia

Figure 5.2.
The events following infection with HIV. **A**, Not infected, truly HIV negative. **B**, infection with HIV and a rise in viral titre. **C**, immune system recognition with an antibody response (seroconversion) and a subsequent decrease in viral load. The period **B–C** is the window period in which the individual is infected, but does not test HIV antibody positive as there are insufficient antibodies to be detected by current laboratory tests – this lasts for 3–6 weeks. Once seroconversion occurs, the patient tests antibody positive, i.e. HIV positive. **D–E** is a variable period of clinical latency (2–8 years) which ends with symptoms of HIV infection and ultimately an AIDS-defining event, **E**. From AIDS to death, **F**, may be 0–2 years, but occasionally is longer.

of cases a glandular fever-like illness with lymphadenopathy, sore throat and a maculopapular rash may be noted. There is increasing evidence to suggest that the occurrence of a severe seroconversion illness is associated with a poorer prognosis in terms of long-term survival. Following seroconversion most individuals enter a clinically latent phase in which they are relatively asymptomatic despite rapid viral multiplication in their tissues and lymph nodes. The duration of clinical latency varies widely among individuals and may last for 2–8 years. Gradually, early stigmata of HIV infection such as oral candidiasis, thrombocytopenia, seborrhoeic dermatitis and oral hairy leukoplakia become apparent. After a variable period of time patients develop one or more of the designated unusual infections or malignancies which define them as having AIDS (see Appendix 1).

Immunology

An understanding of the basic immune defects caused by HIV augments early recognition of the presenting pathologies. Subsequent appropriate management increases both survival and the quality of life. Both the **cell-mediated** and **humoral** (antibody) arms of the human immune system are affected by HIV. Defects of cell-mediated immunity (CMI) appear ultimately to be the most important. As HIV is a ribonucleic acid (RNA) retrovirus it utilizes a reverse transcriptase enzyme for proliferation. It is trophic to CD4 receptor-bearing T-lymphocytes (helper cells). These CD4 positive cells play a pivotal role in the orchestration of an effective immune response. The subsequent decline in their functional ability and number forms the basis of the immune abnormality. Also, HIV interferes with B-cell production and regulation, and directly infects other nonimmune cell lines. Disruption of T- and B-cell function with direct infection of other nonimmune cell lines results in the heterogeneous spectrum of diseases in HIV.

Cell mediated immunity

The principal immune defect in HIV is the progressive dysfunction and depletion of CD4 positive T-lymphocytes. Depletion occurs by an average of 60×10^6 cells/L per year. B-lymphocyte cell growth and therefore antibody synthesis is also defective. In a healthy immune system, CD4 positive T-cell function includes:

- Production of cytokine interleukin-2, which activates cytotoxic T-cells to kill viruses.
- Production of cytokine interferon gamma, which stimulates and augments macrophage and monocyte function. The latter two cell types are responsible for killing intracellular facultative organisms, e.g. _Pneumocystis carinii_, mycobacteria and salmonella species.

The loss of CD4 positive cell function in HIV infection therefore renders the individual particularly susceptible to both viral and **intracellular** pathogen infection.

Humoral immunity

Stimulation of the humoral immune system by HIV results in a **global** increase in antibodies. This is an expansion of **nonspecific** antibodies already present in the body and is known as hypergammaglobulinaemia. Other defects noted include an inability to form antibodies to **new** antigens (neoantigens) and a specific immunoglobulin G2 (IgG2) subclass deficiency. The latter plays an important role in the prevention of infection with encapsulated organisms, including _Streptococcus pneumoniae_ and _Haemophilus influenzae_. Excessive IgE production, as part of the hypergammaglobulinaemia, results in an increased sensitivity which is exhibited by eczema, seborrhoeic dermatitis

(*Figure 5.3*) and urticaria. Vasculitis (*Figure 5.4*), fixed drug eruptions (*Figure 5.5*) and Stevens–Johnson syndrome (*Figure 5.6*) are all more common in HIV positive patients compared to controls. The adverse drug reactions may occur to **previously tolerated** antibiotics and drugs, thus making routine medical management strategies fraught with difficulties.

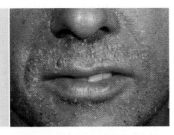

Figure 5.3.
Severe seborrhoeic dermatitis.

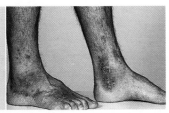

Figure 5.4.
Vasculitic rash. Classically seen on the lower limbs, with residual pigmentation as healing occurs.

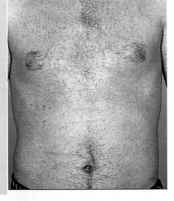

Figure 5.5.
Acute drug reaction. A nonspecific maculopapular rash.

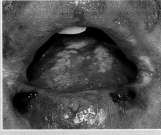

Figure 5.6.
Stevens–Johnson syndrome. Severe mucosal involvement of the whole gastrointestinal tract as well as of the conjunctiva may occur. Drugs are not the only agents responsible for this syndrome, but are the most common cause in the presence of HIV.

Disease progression

As the CD4-positive lymphocyte cell count falls (*Figure 5.7*), patients become increasingly susceptible to opportunist infections by organisms which require CMI for their eradication. 'Opportunist' implies that in the normal immune system these organisms would not result in pathological disease. It is imperative to understand that **multiple** infectious agents can **coexist**, so isolation of one organism does not exclude the presence of other opportunists. Multiple specimens for microbiology, virology, cytology and histopathology are of paramount importance. In the more developed countries, the introduction of prophylactic agents at various levels of declining CD4-positive lymphocytes [e.g. *P. carinii* pneumonia (PCP) prophylaxis at a CD4-positive level of approximately 200×10^6 cells/L] has changed the natural history of HIV and AIDS. Thus, HIV positive individuals now have a longer life expectancy and clinicians are faced with a new spectrum of terminal diseases.

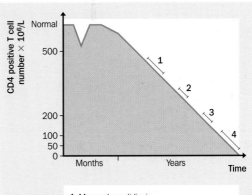

1 Mucosal candidiasis
  Hairy oral leukoplakia
  Ulcerative herpes simplex
  Thrombocytopenia

2 *Mycobacterium tuberculosis*

3 *Pneumocystis carinii* pneumonia

4 Cryptococcosis
  Toxoplasmosis
  Cytomegalovirus
  Mycobacterium avium-intracellulare

Figure 5.7.
Progressive decline in CD4 positive T-helper cells from the time of HIV infection. Different clinical conditions and infections manifest themselves at varying levels of immunosuppression. On average, the CD4 cell count drops by 60×10^6 cells/L/ year. The initial sharp decline (up to 30%) of the total CD4 cell population, which accompanies seroconversion, is usually rapidly restored once the developing antibodies mount a partial response to the virus.

Pointers to Possible HIV Infection

The majority of patients present to the on-call surgeon with no knowledge of their HIV status. A high index of suspicion facilitates the diagnosis and can radically alter management, resulting in life-saving decisions in the acute stage.

General examination

Lymph Nodes

Peripheral generalized lymphadenopathy
Lymph nodes of less than 2 cm in diameter which are bilaterally symmetrical, smooth, rubbery, mobile and nontender are characteristic of peripheral generalized lymphadenopathy (PGL, *Figure 5.8*). By definition the syndrome requires that the lymph nodes be present at two or more extrainguinal sites for a minimum of 3–6 months with no other explanation for their presence. The most frequently involved node groups are the posterior and anterior cervical, occipital, axillary and submandibular. As PGL is a highly sensitive marker for HIV it, in the absence of any other reason for lymphadenopathy, should prompt an evaluation of HIV status. Histology of lymph nodes reveals follicular hyperplasia.

Differential diagnosis includes:

- Sarcoid.
- Hodgkin's disease.
- Secondary syphilis.
- Toxoplasmosis.
- Infectious mononucleosis.

Isolated lymphadenopathy
Isolated, tender, rapidly expanding or thoracic lymphadenopathies are more suggestive of underlying malignancy or infection. Fine needle aspiration or, preferably, open biopsy are required to exclude conditions such as lymphoma, *Mycobacterium avium-intracellulare* (MAI), *M. tuberculosis* (TB) and Kaposi's sarcoma (KS).

Cutaneous

Kaposi's sarcoma

It should be noted that cutaneous KS is not pathognomonic of HIV infection. However, in the 'epidemic' form seen in AIDS the cutaneous lesions, if present, are more widely distributed over the skin than in the endemic form. These subcutaneous tumours are painless, nonpruritic and vary in colour from brownish red to dark purple (*Figures 5.9* and *5.10*). They occur as solitary or multiple lesions and range from a few millimetres to several centimetres in diameter. Cutaneous KS may exhibit Koebner's phenomenon and be found at the site of old scars (surgical or infective, such as varicella-zoster). The clinical diagnosis of cutaneous KS is fortunately usually easily made. Occasionally biopsy may be required to differentiate KS from other lesions, e.g. bacillary angiomatoses. Massive lymphoedema (seemingly out of proportion to the extent of the cutaneous KS) and overlying skin breakdown are two common complications that necessitate medical intervention.

Herpes simplex virus and varicella-zoster virus

Chronic recurrent herpes simplex eruptions (*Figure 5.11*), or nonhealing, ulcerating, herpetic lesions commonly seen in the genital area, may be the first indicator of immunosuppression. Varicella-zoster virus causing shingles may leave characteristic dermatomal scarring (*Figure 5.12*), particularly on individuals of dark skin. The typical unidermatomal, vesicular lesion on an erythematous base seen in an otherwise healthy individual may, in HIV, be replaced with multidermatomal, haemorrhagic or necrotic lesions (*Figure 5.13*).

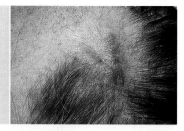

Figure 5.9. Kaposi's sarcoma. This scalp lesion is typically raised and not painful. Recent evidence implicates human herpesvirus 8 as the causative agent.

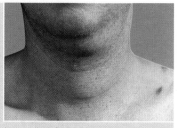

Figure 5.8. Peripheral generalized lymphadenopathy. Enlarged submandibular, submental and cervical lymph nodes – note the two cutaneous Kaposi's sarcoma lesions on the left shoulder.

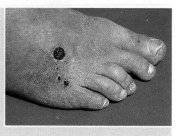

Figure 5.10. Kaposi's sarcoma. The raised lesions are surrounded by less obvious subcutaneous lesions that give a purple hue to the dorsal aspect of the foot and cause lymphoedema by lymphatic obstruction.

Figure 5.11.
Sacral herpetic lesion. Caused by the herpes simplex virus, these lesions are painful and, as shown here, commonly secondarily infected with bacteria. The typical blisters are often absent, leaving a widely sloughed ulcerated appearance.

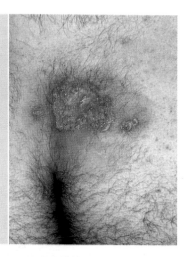

Figure 5.12.
Multidermatomal shingles.

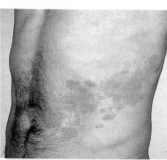

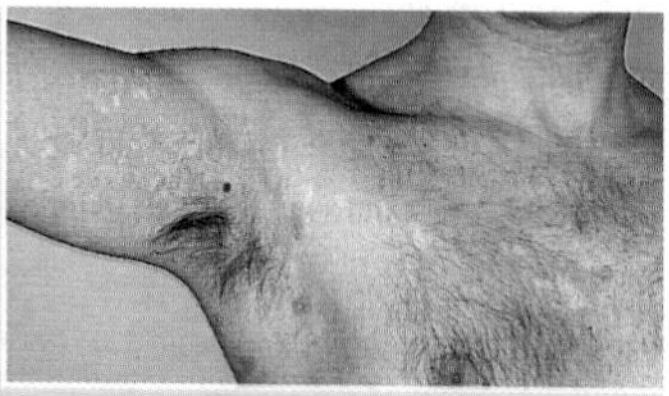

Figure 5.13.
Scars of varicella-zoster infection. The multidermatomal distribution is classic in the presence of HIV. Note the scattered lesions of seborrhoeic dermatitis across the chest and in the axilla.

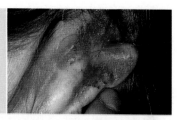

Figure 5.14.
Postauricular seborrhoeic dermatitis. Secondary bacterial infection is common.

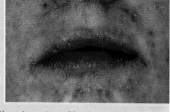

Figure 5.15.
Seborrhoeic dermatitis in a nasolabial and perioral distribution. Patients often complain of 'burning' of the skin in the affected areas, particularly if there is contact with sweat.

Figure 5.16.
Molluscum contagiosum. Trauma from shaving exacerbates the spread of molluscum across the beard area. In individuals with no immunodeficiency, such large extensive lesions in this distribution would be highly unusual.

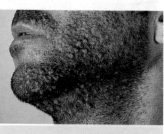

Figure 5.17.
Molluscum contagiosum. The umbilication on these large coalescing lesions on the right cheek helps to confirm the diagnosis.

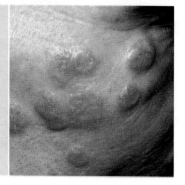

Seborrhoeic dermatitis

About 60–80% of HIV positive individuals develop seborrhoeic dermatitis, although it also occurs with moderate frequency in HIV negative individuals. It is often extensive, erythematous and may be psoriasiform in nature (*Figures 5.14* and *5.15*). It is commonly the first clinical manifestation of HIV disease.

Molluscum contagiosum

Molluscum contagiosum is a benign condition caused by an as yet unidentified poxvirus. It is not confined to immunocompromised individuals. In healthy individuals (most commonly children), the characteristic small, pearly, firm, umbilicated papules are found on epithelial surfaces, usually the thigh and genital area. The papules generally resolve spontaneously with no sequelae. In HIV positive individuals, the papules have a predilection for the face and tend to increase in size, number and severity (*Figures 5.16* and *5.17*), requiring active and aggressive treatment for their containment. Large and/or traumatized lesions may become secondarily infected.

The Oral Cavity

Kaposi's sarcoma

Kaposi's sarcoma of the oral cavity, particularly the palate (*Figure 5.18*), may occur in isolation. It more commonly indicates that systemic KS, with its consequent problems, is also present. The lesions may be flat or raised – in the latter case they may interfere with normal oral function (*Figures 5.19–5.21*). Unlike cutaneous KS, it is not always easy to make a definitive clinical diagnosis from lesions of the oral cavity. Biopsy may be required to exclude lymphoma or infections, e.g. fungal, mycobacterial or syphilitic gummata.

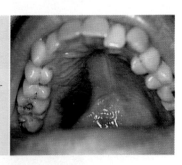

Figure 5.18.
Palatal Kaposi's sarcoma. This particular asymptomatic raised lesion was found coincidentally. Note the early flat KS lesions on the left side of the hard palate.

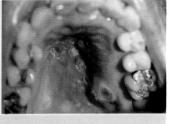

Figure 5.19.
Ulcerated palatal Kaposi's sarcoma. Trauma from eating with subsequent secondary infection may result in severe pain and weight loss. Chemotherapy may be the only option for treatment as it effectively flattens the lesions. Antibiotics to treat infection and topical analgesic gels are useful in controlling pain and thus encouraging adequate dietary intake.

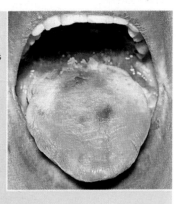

Figure 5.20.
Lingual Kaposi's sarcoma. The purple–brown lesions are present on a coated tongue. The coating may be due to poor oral hygiene and smoking, but consider swabs to exclude candidal infection. (Courtesy of Rev. Dr A. Bayley.)

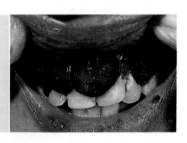

Figure 5.21.
Gingival Kaposi's sarcoma.

Hairy oral leukoplakia

Hairy oral leukoplakia (HOL) is not pathognomonic of HIV infection, but its presence in an HIV positive individual is a marker of symptomatic HIV disease and a poor prognostic indicator for progression to AIDS. The lesion is painless, white, raised and striated that, unlike candidiasis, cannot be scraped off easily with a spatula. It occurs most commonly on the lateral borders of the tongue (*Figure 5.22*), but may also be seen on the tongue's surface (*Figure 5.23*), in the buccal mucosa or in the oesophagus (commonly the middle third), in all of which the lesion may have a more plaque-like appearance. There appears to be a relationship between HOL and the uncontrolled replication of the Epstein–Barr virus (EBV). Although the lesions are generally symptomless, they may impair taste or cause discomfort; they are not premalignant.

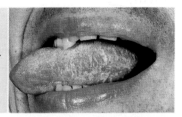

Figure 5.22.
Hairy oral leukoplakia on the lateral border of the tongue.

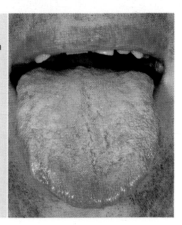

Figure 5.23.
Hairy oral leukoplakia on the dorsum of the tongue. If the tongue is painful, swabs to exclude candidal infection are required. Yellow–brown discoloration of the lesion may be present in smokers.

Oral candidiasis

Oral candidiasis (OC) is most commonly seen as an erythematous base from which white curd may be easily scraped (*Figures 5.24–5.26*). However, candidal infection may also form flat, erythematous plaques. Since this atrophic form does not have the classic white exudate, it is often not recognized by clinicians so an important pointer to an immuno-compromised state of health is missed. Also, OC exists in a hypertrophic form which manifests as a lesion similar to the plaque form of HOL (*Figure 5.27*). In this form, OC may be distributed in similar locations to HOL, e.g. the lateral margin of the tongue, and may not be easily scraped off. Angular cheilitis lesions (*Figure 5.28*) may be the result of vitamin and mineral deficiencies as well as of candidal infection.

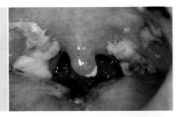

Figure 5.27. Hypertrophic oral candidiasis. This presentation is most commonly seen when drug-resistant strains of *Candida* are present.

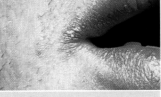

Figure 5.28. Angular cheilitis. Lesions such as this may be the result of vitamin and mineral deficiencies as well as of candidal infection. Topical treatment in the latter case is highly effective. (Courtesy of Dr M. Nathan.)

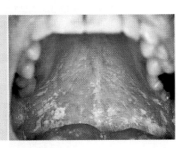

Figure 5.24. Psuedomembranous oral candidal infection of the hard palate.

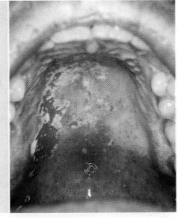

Figure 5.25. Oral candidiasis. The typical erythematous base from which the white plaques have sloughed off is often painful. This is the form most often seen in the oral cavity.

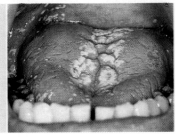

Figure 5.26. Oral candidiasis on the dorsum of the tongue. The raised curd-like lesions may be scraped off easily.

Evidence of lifestyle
Cutaneous

Careful examination of the skin may provide evidence of 'high-risk' behaviour that increases the likelihood of HIV infection (*Figures 5.29* and *5.30*). Evidence of other sexually transmitted diseases may be significant.

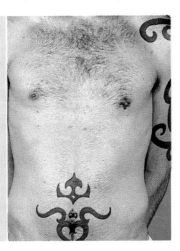

Figure 5.29. Intravenous mainline scarring. Repeated femoral stabs have caused a large single scar. Tracking of multiple small scars along the course of veins and arteries is also commonly seen in the forearms and feet.

Figure 5.30. Tattoos and body piercing. Although traditionally associated with the acquisition of contagious viral infections, the presence of tattoos and piercing is not sufficient to make assumptions about HIV status. Changes in fashion mean that such body art is now frequently seen in individuals who have no risk factors for the acquisition of HIV.

High-Risk Behaviour

With a tactful enquiry made in private conditions, patients may freely reveal that they have engaged in 'high-risk' activities:

- Use of injected drugs and crack cocaine.
- Unprotected sex with individuals who practise the above.
- Unprotected male sex with other males.
- Recipients of blood and other human products.

Physical Signs in HIV Infection

In this section the physical signs that a surgeon may encounter in HIV disease are described. In tertiary centres the majority of HIV cases seen by surgeons are referred by a specialist physician. In most instances this is for procedures such as diagnostic biopsies or central venous access. This is not true in other centres or countries where there may not be a designated HIV unit or medical team.

Patients may present with no knowledge of their HIV status. In other cases, HIV-positive patients may not report their status. Tolerance of surgical procedures is always a matter for consideration, as it is proportional to the CD4-positive lymphocyte count of the patient. Surgical procedures should be discussed (where possible) with colleagues who are experienced in the management of HIV infection. The following descriptions are confined to the physical manifestations that a surgical practice is most likely to encounter.

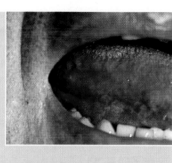

Figure 5.31.
The single ulcer on the lateral border of the tongue was due to CMV infection. This diagnosis was made following a biopsy, requested because the lesion failed to respond to conventional antiherpetic medication.

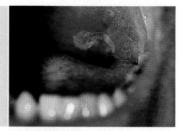

Figure 5.32.
Severe aphthous ulceration. This is a diagnosis of exclusion.

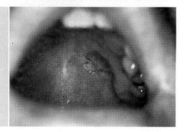

Figure 5.33.
Ulceration of the hard palate. A high-grade B-cell lymphoma was demonstrated on histology.

Oropharyngeal

Oral lesions are often an early sign of HIV infection – up to 90% of AIDS patients have at least one kind of lesion. However, none are pathognomonic of infection with HIV; their presentation and natural course may vary considerably, depending on the level of immune compromise present. Most are medically managed, but ominous lesions such as lymphomas may masquerade in a variety of ways, e.g. as ulcers. Biopsies for diagnostic purposes are frequently indicated to exclude a sinister lesion.

Both KS and tonsillar lesions are mentioned in the preceding section.

Oral Ulceration

Oral ulcers are commonly caused by herpes simplex virus (HSV). Recurrent severe aphthous ulceration, also common, may, like HSV and cytomegalovirus (CMV), cause significant pain (*Figures 5.31–5.33*). Difficulties with swallowing and speech may occur and significant weight loss is a serious problem. Failure of treatment with acyclovir and other medical therapy necessitates biopsy to exclude lymphoma and guide further therapy. A drug history is important as both foscarnet and zalcitabine (DDC), both commonly used antiviral agents, may cause oral ulceration. Neutropenia, a well-recognized cause of oral ulceration, needs to be excluded.

Oesophageal

Up to 90% of patients with AIDS complain of odynophagia (painful swallowing), dysphagia or retrosternal chest pain at some point during the course of their illness. Oesophageal candidiasis is the most common cause of these symptoms – a trial of therapy is considered to be appropriate initial management. Failure to respond to simple medical therapy warrants further investigation to exclude other pathologies. Although a barium swallow may be a useful procedure, oesophagoscopy is the procedure of choice as a definitive diagnosis (or diagnoses) may be obtained by biopsies and brushings. As 10% of patients have multiple pathologies, specimens must be sent for mycobacterial, viral, fungal and histological diagnosis.

Differential diagnosis includes:

- Oesophageal candidiasis.
- CMV.
- EBV (uncommon).
- KS.
- Aphthous ulceration.
- Neutropenia-associated ulceration.
- Ulcerating lymphoma.

Oesophageal Candidiasis

Although oesophageal candidiasis (*Figure 5.34*) may cause no symptoms, it invariably presents with dysphagia. Nausea and epigastric pain commonly accompany the dysphagia, but may occur independently. The upper half of the oesophagus is the most common site of involvement. In up to 30% of cases there is no concomitant oral candidiasis. Barium swallow typically shows extensive, fine ulceration with plaques (*Figure 5.35*). Oesophageal stricture and rupture are uncommon.

Cytomegalovirus

Cytomegalovirus is more common in homosexually acquired HIV than in either African or heterosexually acquired HIV. Lesions tend to involve the lower third of the oesophagus and are typically large, single, deep ulcers. Barium swallow typically shows one or more discreet linear ulcers.

Herpes Simplex Virus

Herpes simplex virus forms multiple small, shallow ulcers.

Ebstein–Barr Virus

Ulceration due to EBV is relatively uncommon and occurs in the midoesophageal region.

Superinfection

Any of the lesions described above may have bacterial super-infection (*Figure 5.36*). Although uncommon in the oesophagus, MAI and *M. tuberculosis* may also be isolated.

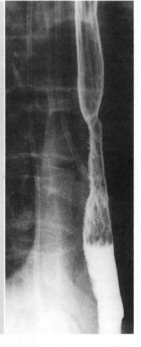

Figure 5.35.
Film from a barium swallow study. This shows a relatively long segment stricture in the midoesophagus and fine ulceration – biopsy proved candidiasis. Raised KS lesions may appear as nodular filling defects when barium swallows are performed and must be differentiated from submucosal metastases.

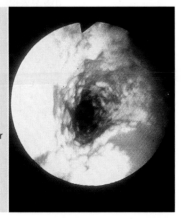

Figure 5.34.
Oesophagoscopy demonstrating moderately severe oesophageal candidiasis macroscopically. Histological specimens confirmed the diagnosis and further identified CMV inclusion bodies.

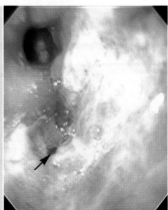

Figure 5.36.
Oesophagoscopy demonstrating a large single ulcer at 40 cm. Viral stains for CMV and EBV were negative, but a high grade B-cell lymphoma was diagnosed histologically. A mild degree of oesophageal candidiasis was visible macroscopically.

Thoracic

The thorax and bowel are perhaps the best examples of where 'opportunists hunt in packs'. Pathology in these areas is commonly the result of infection with several coexisting organisms – the need for multiple specimens cannot be overemphasized. Specimens should be sent for virological, microbiological (including mycobacterial), fungal and histopathological studies. Bacterial infections are more common in HIV positive females and intravenous drug users. Often PCP presents with a normal chest radiograph and few, if any, signs on examination (*Figures 5.37* and *5.38*). Focal signs therefore raise the suspicion of alternative pathologies, such as tumours, mycobacteria, fungi, CMV and aggressive bacterial infection (*Figures 5.39–5.41*).

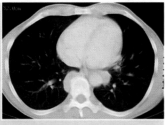

Figure 5.37.
Computed tomography (CT) of the chest. A right-sided paravertebral mass with surrounding clear lungs and left perihilar lymphadenopathy can be seen. The presumptive differential diagnosis was of lymphoma or TB; however, interestingly, this was biopsy proved PCP.

Figure 5.38.
Interstitial process typical of PCP.
a. Chest radiograph.
b. High resolution CT scan. Both show an extensive mid and lower zone perihilar interstitial process typical of PCP.

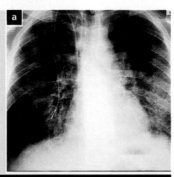

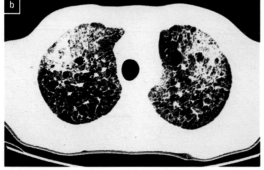

Figure 5.39.
Bacterial empyema and parenchymal abscess.
a. The chest radiograph shows extensive consolidation, with a lozenge-shaped air collection and a smaller, more irregular air collection inferiorly.
b. The CT scan shows the lozenge-shaped collection as a pleural empyema and the more medial smaller intraparenchymal abscess lying within the consolidated left lower lobe. Pneumococci were grown from the aspirate.

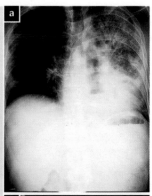

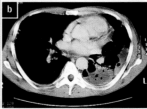

Figure 5.40.
Invasive sinonasal aspergillosis.
a. A coronal CT scan showing extensive opacification of the right maxillary and ethmoid air cells. b. Erosive aspergillus filling the right frontal sinus and eroding through the roof into the anterior cranial fossa.
c. An axial T2-weighted magnetic resonance image (MRI) scan showing retained material in the right frontal sinus with invasion through the bone and an associated extradural abscess extending through the dura into the right frontal lobe with surrounding vasogenic oedema. Invasive aspergillus infections are associated with neutropenia.

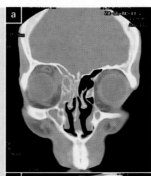

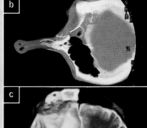

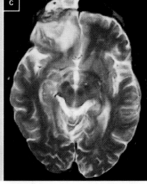

Figure 5.41.

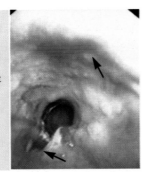

Kaposi's sarcoma. Two flat lesions visible at bronchoscopy. Raised lesions may cause obstruction with wheezing, cough and recurrent bacterial infections. Sputum production may be minimal in the absence of intercurrent infection; it often resembles marmalade rather than appearing as frank blood.

Stomach and intestinal

HIV infection manifests as disease throughout the gastrointestinal (GI) system. Individuals present with routine surgical conditions of the abdomen, as well as with conditions unique to HIV infection that require surgical intervention. Tolerance to surgical procedures is always a matter for consideration (see 'Perioperative considerations', p. 102). Frequent causes of surgical review and intervention are HIV-related abdominal pain, GI bleeds, obstruction, peritonitis and toxic megacolon. The physical signs expected to accompany these conditions are frequently absent or altered because of the reduced inflammatory response in HIV.

Pain is one of the more common presentations of HIV-related GI disease. Both KS and lymphoma are relatively common causes of abdominal pain and may cause obstruction, intussusception, bleeding and perforation (*Figures 5.42–5.45*). Both may be seen on endoscopy. Lymphomas often present while the patient still has a relatively preserved CD4 count, whereas abdominal KS tends to cause problems later in the course of HIV disease. Abdominal KS is also usually accompanied by obvious KS lesions of the palate. With appropriate chemotherapy given in the early stages, patients may be completely cured of the lymphoma and have total resolution of symptoms from both lymphoma and KS.

Figure 5.42.

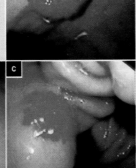

Gastric Kaposi's sarcoma. a–c. These three lesions caused early fullness and epigastric pain consistent with moderately severe gastritis. Note that one lesion is raised (a) and the other two flat.

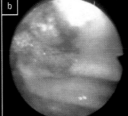

Figure 5.43.
Duodenal Kaposi's sarcoma. a. Presented as diffuse upper abdominal pain and chronic pathogen-negative diarrhoea; palatal KS was present. b. Complete resolution of lesion and symptoms followed chemotherapy.

Figure 5.44.

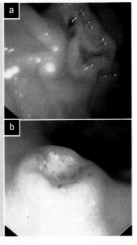

Gastric lymphoma. a and b. Both depict biopsy-proved, EBV-driven B-cell lymphomas, typical in immunocompromised HIV positive individuals.

Figure 5.45.

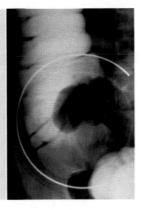

Ileocaecal intussusception secondary to lymphoma. Radiograph from a barium enema study showing the ileocaecal intussusception as a filling defect in the barium-filled caecum. Kaposi's sarcoma may also cause intussusception, particularly if the lesions are raised.

Abdominal pain may also be caused by retroperitoneal lymphadenopathy (*Figure 5.46*). Biopsy is usually required to differentiate between MAI, TB and lymphoma, each of which is potentially treatable but fatal if left to progress. Kaposi's sarcoma may also invade lymph nodes and cause debilitating abdominal pain.

Acute ischaemic colitis may result in severe pain, massive haemorrhage, toxic megacolon and perforation. It is the second most common presentation of CMV (retinitis being the most common). Cytomegalovirus colitis typically presents with left iliac fossa rebound tenderness. It may also affect the caecum and terminal ileum.

A further surgically related HIV symptom in the GI tract is bleeding. In a study of 37 GI bleeds, thirteen were from the upper and 24 from the lower GI tracts. The distribution of the causative pathology is shown in *Table 5.1*.

It is vital to remember that standard surgical problems, such as appendicitis, cholecystitis, perforated duodenal ulcers and complications of secondary adhesions, also occur in HIV positive patients, as do the common medical causes of abdominal pain. Small bowel and biliary tract disease caused by opportunist infections is common and debilitating. Endoscopic retrograde cholangiopancreatography (ERCP), biopsies and duodenal aspirates provide essential definitive diagnosis where pathogens (or HIV itself) have invaded the mucosa.

Hepatobiliary

Hepatic and biliary tract disease manifests as right upper quadrant pain with an elevated alkaline phosphatase. It may be accompanied by fever and jaundice, but this is not invariable. The most common infective organisms found in the liver are TB and MAI, but hepatitis B and C infections must not be forgotten (especially in sexually and intravenous drug acquired HIV infections). In the biliary tract, *Cryptosporidium*, microsporidan and CMV are more common, but MAI is a frequent isolate. All these organisms may be found in conjunction with one another. **Acalculous cholecystitis**, an increasingly frequently diagnosed condition, causes symptoms indistinguishable from symptomatic gallstone disease. It is usually a result of CMV, *Cryptosporidium* or *Campylobacter* infection. Severe right upper quadrant colicky abdominal pain, nausea, vomiting, pyrexia and a thickened gallbladder wall, but no gallstones on ultrasound study, are the hallmarks of this condition (*Figure 5.47*). HIDA scan may confirm the diagnosis. **Emergency cholecystectomy** is often required to prevent fatal peritonitis following rupture of the gallbladder. **Sclerosing cholangitis** causes debilitating pain and may be suspected when ultrasound shows dilatation and thickening of the bile duct walls (*Figure 5.48*). Confirmation is by ERCP, which shows beading of the bile ducts. Biopsies provide diagnostic and therapeutic guidelines. Also, ERCP may show an

Figure 5.46. Abdominal CT scan showing marked retroperitoneal lymphadenopathy secondary to biopsy-proved MAI infection.

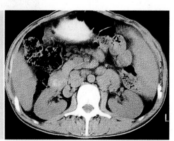

Table 5.1. Distribution of causative pathology in GI bleeds.

Upper gastrointestinal tract		Lower gastrointestinal tract	
Pathology	*Number*	*Pathology*	*Number*
KS	4	KS	2
CMV	2	CMV	5
Lymphoma	2	HSV	2
Non-HIV	5	Idiopathic ulcers	2
		Haemorrhoids	4
		Idiopathic proctitis	2
		Behavioural trauma	4
		Other	3

Figure 5.47. Ultrasound showing a dilated gallbladder with intramural oedema consistent with acalculous cholecystitis. No definitive diagnosis was obtained, but the patient responded to a combination of anti-MAI and *Cryptosporidium* therapy.

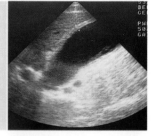

Figure 5.48. Sclerosing cholangitis. Note the dilatation and beading of the intra- and extra-hepatic biliary tree. HIV cholangiopathy is most commonly caused by *Cryptosporidium*, but MAI and CMV need to be excluded. (Courtesy of J.M. Parkin.)

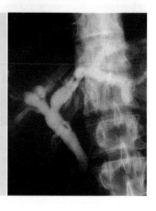

oedematous and swollen ampulla that causes **papillary stenosis** (*Figure 5.49*). Sphincterotomy may allow biliary drainage and pain relief, but biopsy is required to isolate the causative agent.

Pancreatitis is a common cause of abdominal pain in HIV positive individuals. It is commonly caused by excessive alcohol, calculi, high lipid levels (a feature of HIV disease) and drugs such as pentamidine (*P. carinii* treatment) and didanosine (an antiretroviral).

Other opportunists and malignancies that cause ampullary mass lesions need to be excluded.

Anal and perianal

Anorectal pathology is the leading cause of surgical intervention in an HIV population. It causes considerable morbidity. The spectrum of anorectal and perineal disease includes tumours, fissures, fistulae, abscesses and ulceration (*Figures 5.50–5.59*). Faecal incontinence as a result of infection, neoplasm, perineal neuropathy or mechanical damage to the sphincter may require a defunctioning colostomy. Perineal neuropathy with subsequent mucosal prolapse may lead to

the 'solitary rectal ulcer syndrome'. Rapid, effective management relies on accurate diagnosis via biopsy and appropriate swabs. It is common to isolate several **coexisting** pathogens and diagnose concomitant pathogenic processes. Failure of resolution with appropriate antimicrobials must prompt a repeat and thorough search for the presence of underlying neoplasms or previously unidentified organisms.

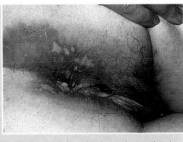

Figure 5.51. Superficial perianal ulceration. This occurs most commonly secondary to HSV. The classic vesicles caused by the virus are usually replaced by extensive, shallow painful ulceration with tissue destruction. In the presence of a normal immune system, acute exacerbations of herpes simplex are self-limiting. In an HIV positive individual aggressive treatment and secondary prophylaxis is required. (Courtesy of Dr P. Simmons.)

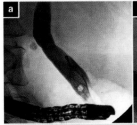 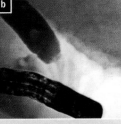

Figure 5.49. HIV-induced papillary stenosis with a retained calculus in the dilated common bile duct. a. Endoscopic removal of the calculus with a basket device. b. After removal – biopsy of the stenosis revealed CMV histologically. (Courtesy of Dr P. Fairclough.)

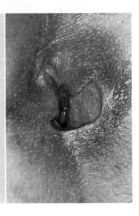

Figure 5.52. Deep perianal ulceration. Recurrent nonhealing ulcers require biopsy to exclude pathology such as lymphoma (as shown here), squamous cell carcinoma or infections other than HSV, e.g. CMV. (Courtesy of Mr A. Tanner.)

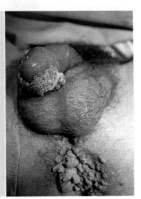

Figure 5.50. Penile and perianal warts. Such extensive human papilloma virus infection is unlikely to be contained by conventional therapy and requires surgical or laser intervention. (Courtesy of Mr A. Tanner.)

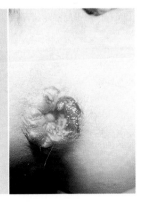

Figure 5.53. Squamous cell carcinoma of the anus. The ulceration in this lesion suggests a more invasive pathology, but in its absence both condylomata acuminata (wart virus) and condylomata lata (secondary syphilis) are included in the differential diagnosis. (Courtesy of Mr A. Tanner.)

Figure 5.54.
Condylomata lata.
(Courtesy of Dr P.
Simmons.)

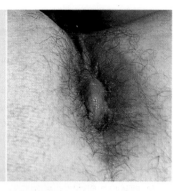

Figure 5.55.
Primary syphilitic
ulceration of the
vulva. (Courtesy of
Dr P. Simmons.)

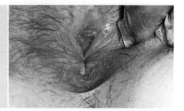

Figure 5.56.
Rectal mucosal
prolapse secondary
to HIV-related
perineal neuropathy.
(Courtesy of Mr A.
Tanner.)

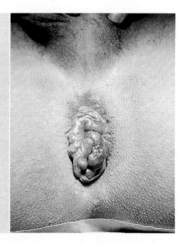

Figure 5.57.
Perianal abscess
with several under-
lying fistulae tracts
and superficial ulcer-
ation. Specimens
from the superficial
ulcers grew HSV, but
biopsy specimens
from the tracts were
CMV positive.
*Staphyloccocus
aureus* and
*Enterococcus.
faecalis* were
isolated from the
abscess swabs. MRI
of the pelvis delin-
eated the multiple
fistulae tracts and
defined a further
ischiorectal abscess

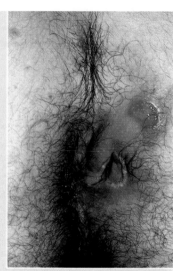

which required surgical drainage. Defunctioning colostomy was
performed.

Figure 5.58.
Low, complex fistula
in ano. (Courtesy of
Mr A. Tanner.)

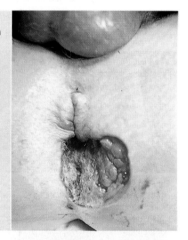

Differential diagnosis of infective lesions includes:

- HSV.
- CMV.
- HIV.
- Amoebiasis.
- Tuberculosis.
- Syphilis.
- Gonorrhoea.
- Chancroid.
- Lymphogranuloma venereum.

Figure 5.59.
High fistula in ano
secondary to
mycobacterial
infection.

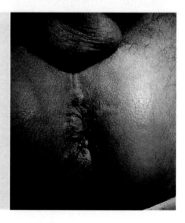

Musculoskeletal

HIV infection has changed the epidemiology, presentation and management of several musculoskeletal disorders.

Haematogenous Osteomyelitis

Haematogenous osteomyelitis (*Figures 5.60* and *5,61*) was previously considered a paediatric disease with only sporadic presentation in adults who tended to be immunosuppressed (diabetic, transplantation patients, patients with cancer, drug addicts). In these sporadic adult cases haematogenous osteomyelitis rarely affected the long bones and confined itself to the spine, pelvis and flat bones. In addition, in both paediatric and adult cases, there was rarely bilateral involvement. It is now common in adults with HIV infection. It may be subacute or chronic, but is typically the former. There is a predilection for the upper tibial and lower femoral metaphyses and the disease is often bilateral. In most cases, despite extensive necrosis of the bone with spread along the diaphyses, there is an incongruous lack of periosteal new bone formation. Clinically, pain, localized swelling and heat over the affected area are the most common findings. Fluctuant subfascial abscesses may be present. The content of the bone at

surgery has been described as faeculent. *Staphyloccocus aureus*, nontyphoid salmonella species and other gram-negative organisms have all been isolated from aspiration or incision specimens, but the presence of anaerobic organisms has not been documented. Blood cultures are usually sterile.

Tuberculosis

An increasing number of patients present with bone and joint tuberculosis (particularly of the lumbar spine). Pointers to the presence of tuberculosis, such as Mantoux, Heaf and typical radiographic findings, are unreliable and difficult to interpret in the presence of HIV infection.

Tropical Pyomyositis

Tropical pyomyositis, the incidence of which was decreasing, is now a common and serious consequence of advanced HIV disease. Single or multiple abscesses are found at unusual sites. Bowel flora are isolated in up to 10% of affected patients, but the most commonest cause remains *Staph. aureus*.

Orthopaedic Complications

Orthopaedic complications associated with the management of fractures and insertion of surgical prosthesis in HIV positive individuals continue to alter established orthopaedic practices. Closed fractures usually heal normally, but open fractures have a poor prognosis with a high incidence of nonunion and sepsis. Internal fixation carries considerable risk of sepsis (up to 30% increase over HIV negative individuals) and sepsis around implanted metal from surgery performed many years previously is well documented.

Reactive Arthritis

Reactive arthritis is a common condition in HIV disease, probably caused by an immune phenomenon. Differentiation from septic arthritis (*Figure 5.62*) can be difficult clinically – aspirated effusions may contain significant numbers of both neutrophils and lymphocytes. Cultures are sterile. Drugs such as rifabutin may also cause reactive arthritis.

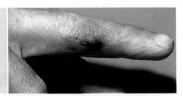

Figure 5.60.
Osteomyelitis of the phalanx.

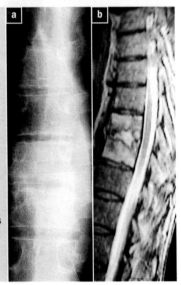

Figure 5.61.
Candidal discitis and abscess.
a. Plain radiograph of the thoracic spine showing loss of cortical outline of the T9–T10 disc end plates with erosion and associated paravertebral swelling.
b. T2-weighted sagittal MRI showing increased signal in the T9 and T10 vertebral bodies with features of discitis and abscess formation. Biopsy proved candidal infection.

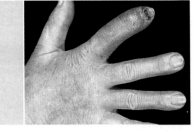

Figure 5.62.
Septic arthritis.

Central nervous system

Practically all HIV positive individuals develop some degree of neurological dysfunction as part of their illness. The manifestations of HIV in the central, peripheral and autonomic nervous systems are legion. While seroconversion to HIV positive status may be accompanied by an acute encephalitis or meningitis, the conditions of interest to the neurosurgeons tend to occur **later** in the history of the disease. Neoplastic conditions and opportunist infections cannot always be adequately differentiated on CT and MRI. Identification by brain biopsy should be considered because, while most infections respond well to appropriate therapy, the present management of cerebral neoplasms is not as successful. Confidence in the diagnosis allows the patient the informed option of active or palliative care.

Cerebral Toxoplasmosis

Cerebral toxoplasmosis is the most common brain mass lesion in patients with advanced HIV disease and is easily treatable. In most instances it results from reactivation of latent infection rather than from acute infection. It classically presents with headaches, low grade pyrexia and focal neurological signs. The onset of symptoms is often rapid. Single or multiple ring-enhancing lesions may be seen on both contrast CT scans (*Figure 5.63*) and MRI of the brain. Cerebral toxoplasmosis has a predilection for the posterior fossa. In the presence of clinical neurological abnormality suggestive of cerebellar involvement MRI is preferable to CT, as CT scans do not depict the posterior fossa adequately in a significant proportion of studies. The ring-enhancing multifocal abscesses are characteristic enough that, in the absence of other diagnostic pointers, e.g. intravenous drug use or negative *Toxoplasma* serology, a trial of *Toxoplasma* therapy

should be commenced. If *Toxoplasma* serology is negative the diagnosis is highly questionable, so brain biopsy becomes mandatory to identify other pathogens.

Progressive Multifocal Leukoencephalopathy

Progressive multifocal leukoencephalopathy (PML; *Figure 5.64*) is a demyelinating condition caused by the polyoma JC virus. The condition is found in approximately 4% of AIDS patients, although postmortem studies report a higher incidence. Clinical presentation depends on the area and extent of the brain affected. However, the most common presentation is with visual symptoms, slurred speech, pyramidal signs and confusion. Onset is far more insidious than that of *Toxoplasma* infection and MTRI scans usually distinguish between the two conditions At present there is no effective therapy for PML.

Cerebral Lymphoma

The presence of a **primary** cerebral lymphoma (*Figure 5.65*) in an adult under 60 years of age is diagnostic of AIDS as primary cerebral lymphomas have not been reported in such patients without HIV infection. Cerebral lymphomas may be difficult to differentiate from toxoplasmosis, both clinically and radiologically. Toxoplasmosis usually presents with multiple lesions and cerebral lymphoma as a single lesion, but, this is not invariable. As toxoplasmosis is an easily and successfully treatable disease while lymphomas have a poor prognosis, if

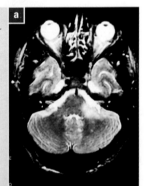
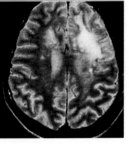
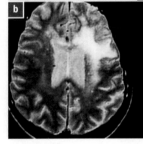

Figure 5.64.
Progressive multifocal leukoencephalopathy.
a. T2-weighted MRI showing increased signal in the left middle cerebellar peduncle.
b. T2-weighted MRI showing focal increased signal in the left frontal white matter and to a lesser extent on the right side. Note that PML can be focal or diffuse, but in the latter it is usually asymmetrically distributed.

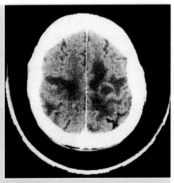

Figure 5.63.
Cerebral toxoplasmosis.
Contrast-enhanced CT scan showing a ring-enhancing abscess with prominent vasogenic oedema in the left posterior frontal and parietal lobes, and oedema in the right frontal white matter. This proved to be toxoplasmosis. Note that in patients with a very low CD4 T-cell count, contrast enhancement and vasogenic oedema may be absent due to an inhibited inflammatory response.

Figure 5.65.

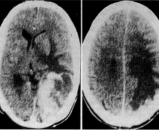

Cerebral lymphoma. Contrast-enhanced CT scan showing a large enhancing mass in the left parieto-occipital region creeping around the left trigone with prominent vasogenic oedema. This proved to be AIDS-related lymphoma, which in an immune competent patient needs to be distinguished from secondary lymphoma, where the disease is usually leptomeningeal.

Figure 5.66.

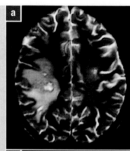
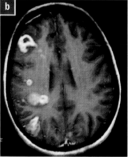

Cerebral candidiasis.
a. T2-weighted MRI showing a right posterior frontal lobe abscess surrounded by prominent vasogenic oedema.
b. T1-weighted MRI with Gd-DTPA (diethylenetriamine penta-acetic acid) enhancement showing multiple predominantly ring-enhancing candidal abscesses. This case occurred in an intravenous drug user who also developed infective endocarditis. Brain biopsy is essential to exclude other pathogens, such as bacteria, mycobacteria, *Toxoplasma*, cysticercus (particularly in African patients) and *Nocardia*.

there is any doubt about the diagnosis or if a course of empirical toxoplasmosis treatment has failed rapid definitive diagnosis is made by stereotactic brain biopsy. Of HIV-associated lymphomas 99% are EBV-driven lesions, usually of B-cell origin. Patients tend to present with signs of late-stage HIV disease and B symptoms (night sweats, unexplained fever of more than 38°C, more than 10% weight loss in 6 months). Radiotherapy may relieve symptoms initially but, up to the present, chemotherapy has been of little value.

Candidal Brain Abscesses

Candidal brain abscesses are a rare cause of cerebral mass lesions in HIV and are usually only found in intravenous drug users. They are typically seen as multiple ring-enhancing lesions on cerebral CT scans and MRI (*Figure 5.66*). Their differential diagnosis includes infection caused by:

- *Toxoplasma*.
- *Nocardia*.
- *M. tuberculosis* (tuberculoma).
- *Cryptococcus* (cryptococcoma).
- Pyogenic organisms.

Mycobacterium tuberculosis

M. tuberculosis brain infection may cause meningitis, abscesses or isolated cranial nerve palsies. Infection tends to occur with a higher CD4 count than with other brain opportunists. The incidence of neurological complications are increased in the presence of HIV infection. High swinging fevers are normally found. Respiratory involvement with abnormal chest radiographs provide important clues to the diagnosis, but their absence or the lack of a positive Mantoux (requires competent CMI) does not exclude the diagnosis of cerebral tuberculosis.

Ophthalmic

The ophthalmic manifestations of HIV may be classified as microvasculopathy, infections, neoplasms and neuro-ophthalmic manifestations.

Microvasculopathy

Conjunctival microvasculopathy

Conjunctival microvasculopathy is associated with findings such as capillary dilatation, vascular fragmentation, calibre irregularity, microaneurysms and red blood cell clumping.

Retinal microvasculopathy

Retinal microvasculopathy is the most common ophthalmological manifestation of HIV infection (*Figure 5.67*). It is usually a self-limiting condition but may occasionally precede the development of CMV retinitis in the same location.

Figure 5.67.

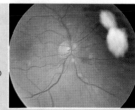

HIV retinopathy and artefact. Features include cotton wool spots, microaneurysms, intra- and pre-retinal haemorrhages and capillary abnormalities. No treatment is required for this condition, but patients who present with extensive retinal microvasculopathy should be monitored carefully as they have an increased risk of CMV retinitis, which may commence in the same retinal area. (Note the large artefact in the right superior aspect.)

Infections

Cytomegalovirus retinitis (*Figure 5.68*) is by far the most common ocular infection in AIDS patients and is the leading cause of blindness in this population. Complaints of visual blurring or distortion, visual field loss or increased floaters necessitate urgent pupil dilatation and retinal examination by an ophthalmologist. The sclera are white, without discomfort, pain or photophobia. Clinical CMV retinitis affects 15–45% of adult AIDS patients, but is rare in children. It occurs in advanced HIV disease, when the CD4 count is usually well below 100×10^6 cells/L, and previously implied a life expectancy of less than 9 months. However, with better diagnosis, follow-up and medication many patients now survive up to 2 years after their first presentation with CMV retinitis. Preventing blindness is therefore of paramount importance. In up to 15% of HIV positive individuals retinitis is the AIDS-defining diagnosis.

Untreated CMV retinitis progresses in all cases. It leads to involvement of the optic disc or macula by retinitis (*Figure 5.69*), or retinal detachment and total loss of vision in that eye. Intravenous and intraocular antiviral agents are used for the treatment and secondary prophylaxis of CMV retinitis. Ideally, all lesions should be photographed and monitored by slit-lamp examination on a regular basis.

Toxoplasma retinochoroiditis (*Figure 5.70*) should be considered if a lesion is initially thought to be CMV, but appears atypical or does not respond to conventional CMV therapy.

Other ocular conditions related to secondary infections in AIDS include molluscum contagiosum (*Figure 5.71*), herpes zoster ophthalmicus, progressive outer retinal necrosis (due to Herpes zoster), acute retinal necrosis (due to Herpes zoster or simplex) and multifocal choroiditis which may be a manifestation of disseminated infection, such as tuberculosis, *M. avium-intracellulare*, *P. carinii*, *Cryptococcus neoformans*, *Histoplasma capsulatum*, candidiasis (particularly in intravenous drug abusers) or syphilis.

Suspicion of any of these infections should lead to prompt referral to an ophthalmologist.

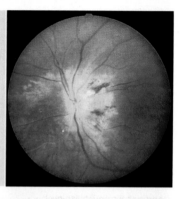

Figure 5.69. CMV papillitis. Involvement of the posterior pole (macula or, as seen here, optic disc) causes extensive visual loss, and is associated with more severe immunodeficiency and higher mortality. (Courtesy of Dr Pavesio.)

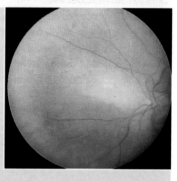

Figure 5.70. *Toxoplasma* retinochoroiditis. In contrast to CMV retinitis, *Toxoplasma* retinochoroiditis is much less common, is more often found in patients with a CD4 count greater than 50, shows more intraocular inflammation (sometimes with pain), shows dense retinal infiltrates with smooth borders and has minimal or no haemorrhage. In immunocompetent patients the pigmentation typical of *Toxoplasma* retinochoroiditis is not usually seen. (Courtesy of Dr Pavesio.)

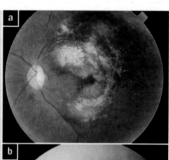
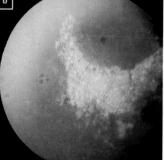

Figure 5.68. CMV retinitis.
a. Greyish white granular lesions with exudates and retinal opacification are visible. Retinal haemorrhage usually occurs, giving the classic 'pizza' appearance. There is usually little or no evidence of vitritis. (Courtesy of Dr Pavesio.)
b. Absence of haemorrhage is more common in peripheral lesions as opposed to lesions within the vascular arcades. (Courtesy of Dr Pavesio.)

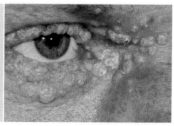

Figure 5.71. Multiple molluscum contagiosum along the palpebral fissure. These lesions may cause marked irritation and are difficult to treat in this area.

Figure 5.72.
Kaposi's sarcoma.
a and b. Discrete
vascular lesions
deep red in colour in
skin or conjunctiva.
The latter may
resemble a subcon-
junctival
haemorrhage.
(Courtesy of Elsevier
Science Ltd, Oxford.)

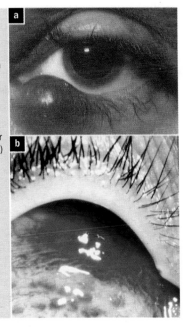

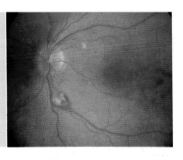

Figure 5.73.
Ocular lymphoma.

Neoplasms

Kaposi's sarcoma occurs in 25% of AIDS patients, and 20% of these have periocular involvement usually on the lid margin or conjunctiva (*Figure 5.72*).

Lymphoma (*Figure 5.73*) may be intraocular or orbital – the former is rare and notoriously difficult to diagnose. It may present as a chronic uveitis and diagnosis is dependent on vitreous biopsy.

Neuro-ophthalmic Manifestations

Neurological features are due either to a direct effect of HIV or to opportunistic infections (producing meningitis, encephalitis, cerebral abscess, vasculitis or toxoplasma cysts), central nervous system (CNS) neoplasms (most commonly lymphoma), cerebrovascular complications (i.e. stroke) or central or peripheral neuropathies.

Intracranial space-occupying lesions in patients with HIV are most commonly due to *Toxoplasma gondii* or lymphoma. In the absence of a mass lesion on CT or MRI, direct involvement of the CNS by HIV, CMV, Herpes zoster or Herpes simplex are the most important diagnostic considerations. Since any part of the nervous system can be affected the features are many and varied. The most common are syndromes due to damage of the midbrain (e.g. internuclear ophthalmoplegia, Parinaud's syndrome), cranial nerve palsies and homonymous field defects or cortical blindness.

Vascular

Intravenous access for the administration of therapeutic agents is required in many patients with advanced HIV disease. The majority are able to administer their own antimicrobial and other agents and can be managed in the community if they have permanent venous access. The choice between a Portacath® or Hickman Line® is usually a personal one. While the former has the disadvantage that the skin must be punctured for access, the Hickman Line® is more visible and in some studies marginally more prone to infection. Positioning of the Portacath® is an important consideration. Patients with CMV retinitis who have visual field defects must have the intended position of their Portacath checked to ensure they can visualize it adequately prior to surgical insertion.

HIV Testing

HIV may be transmitted by exposure to blood products, blood-stained body fluids, sexual intercourse or vertical transmission via the placenta. The risk of transmission from faeces, nasal secretions, sputum, saliva, sweat, tears, urine and vomitus is very low unless they contain blood. Infection of an individual is usually established by the detection of antibodies to HIV (except in paediatric cases for which viral culture may be necessary).

There is much debate about routinely testing patients for the presence of HIV. In many countries it is a legal requirement to obtain informed consent prior to testing, whereas in others it is considered an ethical requirement. Testing should not occur without pre- and post-test counselling. The controversy about routine testing revolves around the arguments for 'need to know' versus the adverse emotional and subsequent discrimination such knowledge may bring. Doctors experienced in the management of HIV positive individuals argue that good clinical skills and life-saving treatment should always be instituted immediately without laboratory confirmation of HIV status. There is **no** role for **urgent** HIV testing.

Universal precautions based on the premise that all patients are potentially infectious should apply. Presumptions of negative HIV, hepatitis B and C status based on a patient's age, race or sexual orientation are as potentially dangerous for health workers as for the patient. A 60-year-old grandmother may well have received a contaminated transfusion or be sexually active with an HIV positive partner. Complacency may be lethal for the patient and the health workers.

The application of universal precautions to all patients does not negate the responsibility of hospitals to protect health workers, particularly when in the operating and emergency rooms. All staff should be familiar with procedures for the handling of sharp instruments and for protection from dissemination of body fluids. Theatres and examination areas should be organized so as to minimize the risk of accidental exposure to hepatitis B, hepatitis C or HIV.

The risk of seroconversion following a single parenteral occupational exposure, according to ten prospective studies, is 0.37%. Factors which influence this are related to the type and extent of the exposure and also to the immunological characteristics of the patient and recipient of the exposure. Approximately 80% of seroconversion in health workers followed percutaneous exposure, which emphasizes the need for good sharp-instrument management. Protocols that clearly define procedures to be followed in the event of needlestick or other exposure must be readily available.

Patient Protection

The HIV positive surgeon

The risk of acquiring blood-borne infection occupationally is proportional to the prevalence of HIV in the population under treatment and to the risk of inoculation injuries in the procedures undertaken. A surgeon may acquire HIV through occupational or other exposure. **Confidential advice** offered by leading HIV services should be sought in the **first instance** to protect the surgeon, both medically and professionally. Hospital protocols, such as taking serum samples and azidothymidine (AZT, zidovudine), should be adhered to. Decisions regarding HIV testing should take into account both the professional and nonprofessional considerations of the surgeon involved.

However, it is unethical to knowingly put patients at risk. The risk can be minimized by modifying professional practice. In all instances the surgeon involved should act on the appropriate advice from his/her governing body.

Perioperative considerations

The postoperative tolerance of surgical procedures is proportional to the patient's CD4 count. There is no value in measuring the CD4 count when a patient is ill, since the CD4 cells migrate from the blood stream to the tissue source of infection, so their measurement in the peripheral blood gives a falsely low reading. In all instances it is preferable to discuss the patients with doctors who are knowledgeable in the management of HIV disease.

It is important to note in the workup prior to surgery some considerations, described below, that are particular to HIV patients, even when their CD4 count is high or normal.

Haematology

Thrombocytopenia (*Figure 5.74*) is one of the first signs of immunological dysfunction in HIV, so all patients should have their platelet levels and clotting ability tested. Note that an abnormal adjusted partial thromboplastin time is common and is related to the presence of antiphospholipid antibodies (cf. anticardiolipin antibodies in systemic lupus erythematosus).

Neutropenia must be excluded prior to surgery or invasive clinical procedures, such as rectal examination or central line insertion. Scrupulous aseptic technique is required at all times. It is probably easier for health carers to pass infection to immunocompromised patients than vice versa!

Confidentiality

Confidentiality is the right of every individual under medical care. Before information is passed to **any** person who does not 'need to know', including relatives and health workers, or to other services, permission should be sought from the patient.

Nutrition

Many patients with advanced HIV disease are malnourished. If surgical intervention or the presenting complaint place the patient in a further increased catabolic state,

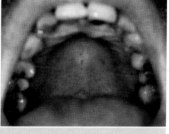

Figure 5.74.
Palatal thrombocytopenic purpura in a HIV positive individual who had no other stigmata of HIV disease. The patient had been admitted for routine surgical naevus removal when this abnormality was noted. (Platelet count, 6×10^9/L.)

early interventional feeding should be considered. The risks of parenteral feeding should always be weighed against the risks of further malnutrition.

Ethical Issues

The HIV positive person has the right to equal health care and treatment that non-HIV positive people receive.

Appendix 1

AIDS indicator diseases

In the presence of an HIV-positive blood test, the following conditions (adapted from CDSC) are currently considered to be AIDS-defining diagnoses in Europe (the criteria differ slightly in the US):

- Bacterial infections, multiple or recurrent in a child aged less than 13 years.
- Candidiasis, trachea, bronchi or lungs.
- Cervical carcinoma, invasive.
- Coccidioidomycosis, extrapulmonary or disseminated.
- Cryptosporidiosis, with diarrhoea for over 1 month.
- Cytomegalovirus retinitis.

- Cytomegalovirus disease (onset after 1 month) not in liver, spleen or nodes.
- Encephalopathy (dementia) due to HIV.
- Herpes simplex: ulcers for 1 month or bronchitis, pneumonitis, oesophagitis (onset after age 1 month).
- Histoplasmosis, disseminated or extrapulmonary.
- Isosporiasis, with diarrhoea for over 1 month.
- Kaposi's sarcoma.
- Lymphoid interstitial pneumonia and/or pulmonary lymphoid hyperplasia in a child aged less than 13 years.
- Lymphoma: Burkitt's, immunoblastic or primary in brain.*
- Mycobacteriosis disseminated (including extrapulmonary TB)* *P. carinii* pneumonia.
- Pneumonia recurrent within a 12-month period.
- Progressive multifocal leukoencephalopathy.
- Salmonella (nontyphoid) septicaemia, recurrent.
- Toxoplasmosis of brain after age 1 month.
- Wasting syndrome due to HIV.

Full case definitions, notes on AIDS indicator diseases for neoplasms, mycobacteriosis and indicator diseases in children are available from the Communicable Disease Surveillance Centre (CDSC), London, UK.

6 Tropical surgery

Introduction

Surgery in the tropics is, to a large extent, similar to that in temperate zones, with the addition of infections and parasitic lesions that are peculiar to these areas. The high intensity of international air travel and population migrations has, however, resulted in the internationalization of disease patterns that were once confined to tropical or subtropical zones.

Tropical diseases are caused by a wide spectrum of organisms and are often produced by more than one agent; they may also involve a number of organ systems. Nevertheless, they do have common forms of presentation and in this chapter emphasis is given to the differential diagnoses of some common presenting symptoms. These include fever, gastrointestinal abnormalities, hepatosplenomegaly, cutaneous manifestations and the common malignancies encountered in the tropics. Some diseases have a well-defined geographical distribution (see also protozoa and worms, p.71).

Fever

Fever is a cardinal symptom of infection. In the tropics it may present a difficult diagnostic problem, especially in the presence of limited investigative facilities.

The mechanism of fever

Exogenous pyrogens, usually infective e.g. bacterial, viral, protozoal and fungal stimulate second line lymphoreticular cells i.e. monocytes, tissue histocytes, liver Kupffer cells, alveolar macrophages and splenic sinusoidal cells to release endogenous pyrogens. They are released by the other cell groups of the lymphoreticular system.

The endogenous pyrogens in turn stimulate the release of prostaglandin in the hypothalamus, which resets the thermoregulatory centre to sense a normal surrounding temperature as above normal. The action of antipyretics is to interfere with prostaglandin synthesis and thus prevent its hypothalamic activity.

Patterns of fever

Four main patterns of fever are illustrated in *Figure 6.1*. Seven fever patterns are listed as follows:

- Abrupt onset. Often accompanied by rigors; a frequent feature of malaria and pyogenic and viral infections.
- Gradual, slow onset. Characteristic of subacute or prolonged infections, e.g. TB and brucellosis.
- Continuous. The temperature does not remit but may fluctuate between morning and evening, e.g. typhoid and typhus.
- Pyrexia occurring every 2–4 days. A characteristic feature of established malaria (hence its old terminology of tertian and quartan forms) (geographical pattern shown in *Figure 6.2*).
- Relapsing fever. A pattern typically displayed by *Borrelia recurrentis*, tick- and louse-borne, infection but also occurs in brucellosis, subacute bacterial endocarditis, malaria, African trypanosomiasis, ascending cholangitis, filariasis, visceral leishmaniasis, lymphomas and pyogenic infections.
- Remittent fever. The temperature remains elevated and does not return to normal. This occurs in severe falciparum malaria, typhoid fever, septicaemia and osteomyelitis.
- Intermittent fevers. In which there is a characteristic periodicity of the temperature, fluctuating between febrile and afebrile states and possibly falling to normal levels. These are classically seen in severe pyogenic infections (e.g. amoebic liver abscess; ascending cholangitis; brain abscess), lymphomas, malaria (early stages) and TB.

Common causes of fevers in the tropics are presented in *Table 6.1* and common gastrointestinal problems in *Table 6.2*. Dysphagia and jaundice are presented in *Tables 6.3* and *6.4* respectively.

Figure 6.1.
Fever patterns. a. Malaria. Fever patterns of tertiary and quartan forms of the disease. b. Typhoid. The fever is of gradual onset over a few days accompanied by malaise, headache and epistaxis. The high fever continues with some morning or evening fluctuation for a further 6–7 days accompanied by diarrhoea and distension. The typhoid state of confusion and gut complications occurs in the established disease accompanied by leukoplakia. c. Relapsing fever typically occurs in tick- and lice-borne *Borrelia* infections, the parasite being recoverable from the blood during the febrile episodes. d. Intermittent fevers occurring in a patient with an amoebic liver abscess. In this patient the fever was accompanied by profuse sweating, the temperature not returning to normal between attacks.

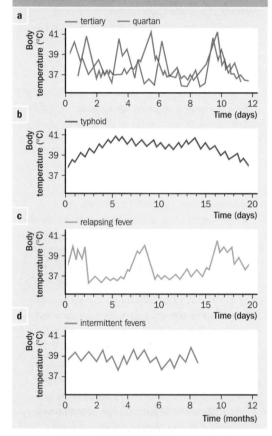

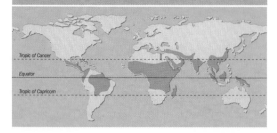

Figure 6.2. Geographical distribution of malaria.

Table 6.1. Common causes of fevers in the tropics.	
Viral	Influenza Mumps Measles Epstein–Barr virus (infectious mononucleosis) Hepatitis A, B, C Lymphogranuloma venereum/inguinale Viral haemorrhagic fevers caused by the arbovirus group: Lassa; Ebola; yellow; Rift Valley; HIV-related disease (p. 000) Dengue fever typically displays a biphasic pattern with double humps, one that occurs due to viraemia while the other corresponds to an antigen/antibody reaction with the virus and/or host cells harbouring the virus.
Bacterial	Pneumococcal pneumonia Typhoid fever (salmonellosis) Bacillary dysentery (shigellosis) Whooping cough (*Bordetella pertussis*) Undulant fever (brucellosis) Legionnaire's disease Relapsing fevers (tick- and louse-borne) Plague (*Yersinia pestis*) TB (pulmonary and extrapulmonary) Rickettsial (typhus) fevers Coxiella (Q fever)
Parasitic and protozoal	Malaria Invasive (toxaemic) *Fasciola hepatica* Invasive (hepatic disease) *Entamoeba histolytica* Visceral leishmaniasis (*kala-azar*) Invasive *Schistosoma mansoni* and *S. japonicum* infections African trypanosomiasis Toxoplasmosis Acute filaria lymphangitis (*Wuchereria bancrofti*) Endemic treponematoses and treponemal infections, e.g. syphilis, yaws and pinta Borreliosis (tick- and louse-borne) Leptospiral infections (*Leptospira interrogans* and *L. biflexa*) Intestinal cryptosporidiosis *Pneumocystis carinii* pneumonia
Fungal	Candidiasis Cryptococcosis (disseminated) Histoplasmosis (disseminated) Aspergillosis
Symptoms commonly associated with fever	Rash (haemorrhagic or non-haemorrhagic) Generalized or locoregional lymphadenopathy Spleno-/hepatomegaly or hepatosplenomegaly Jaundice Polyarthralgia Ascites Anaemia
Conditions commonly associated with fever	Bacterial endocarditis (acute or subacute) Septicaemia Erythema nodosum Decompensated liver cirrhosis Pneumococcal peritonitis Tuberculous peritonitis Ascending cholangitis Deep sepsis, e.g. pelvic sepsis; amoebic liver abscess Pyelonephritis Lower abdominal pain and bloody diarrhoea Malignancy Systemic lupus erythematosus
Some causes of Pyrexia of 'unknown' origin	Tuberculous peritonitis Cold abscess Systemic lupus erythematosus Drug reaction Malaria Typhus Toxoplasmosis HIV-related diseases

Table 6.2. Common gastrointestinal problems in the tropics.

Small intestine	Large intestine	Liver	Biliary
Hookworm (can cause in isolation or collectively: blood loss; anaemia; intestinal obstruction; gastroenteritis)	Amoebic dysentery/colitis Schistosomal colitis	Hydatid cyst Amoebic liver abscess	Ascariasis → luminal obstruction Clonorchiasis
Strongyloides stercoralis	Trichuriasis → rectal prolapse in children		Opisthorchiasis Salmonellosis – cholecystitis
Giardia lamblia *Ascaris lumbricoides* Typhoid fever	Cholera → severe debilitating diarrhoea		

Table 6.3. Dysphagia.

Chagas' disease (South American trypanosomiasis)
Candidiasis
Mucormycosis (*Rhizopus* sp.; *Absidia* sp.)
Extrinsic pressure from endemic goitre
Oesophageal carcinoma

Table 6.4. Jaundice.

Viruses	Hepatitis A, B, C and E → cirrhosis → portal hypertension Epstein–Barr virus (Burkitt's lymphoma) Cytomegalovirus (surgical complications of AIDS-related infection)
Bacteria	Leptospirosis Typhoid fever Syphilis Bartonellosis Acute bacterial infection, e.g. pneumococcal lobar pneumonia and pyomyositis
Parasites and protozoa	Acute malaria Schistosomiasis Toxoplasmosis (eye complications) Trichinellosis Fascioliasis (*Fasciola hepatica*) ⎤ → liver abscess Clonorchiasis (*Clonorchis sinensis*) ⎦ (malignancies?) Opisthorchiasis Ascariasis (biliary and bowel obstruction) Hydatidosis (rarely) Amoebiasis (rarely): differential diagnosis of rectal bleeding
Miscellaneous	Sickle cell disease Glucose-6-phosphate dehydrogenase deficiency Dubin–Johnson syndrome Thallassaemia

Causes of diarrhoea in the tropics

Acute diarrhoea

Watery diarrhoea

Acute infective diarrhoea is very common in the tropics. It is characteristically large volume and watery (secretory). It is still a major problem in the tropics and subtropics, accounting for significant mortality and morbidity, especially in small children. It is caused by enteropathogens that produce an enterotoxin, which operates via cyclic adenosine monophosphate reversing the transportation of water and electrolytes across small intestinal membranes, with the end result of secretion rather than absorption. (Ulcerative colitis, Crohn's disease and diverticulitis are very uncommon in the tropics and are, therefore, only considered in expatriates.)

Common examples are as follows:

- Travellers diarrhoea (turista) caused by enterotoxigenic *Escherichia coli* (ETEC).
- Enterotoxic *Vibrio cholerae* (and other Vibrios, e.g. *V. parahaemolyticus*).

Food poisoning bacteria include:

- *Salmonella typhimurium* and enteritidis enterotoxin.
- *Campylobacter jejuni*.
- Staphylococcal gastroenteritis.
- *Clostridium perfringens*, which produces an exotoxin that eventually produces small intestinal haemorrhage and possibly perforation and peritonitis (pigbel disease)

Bloody diarrhoea (dysentery syndromes)

In this group the enteropathogen invades the lining of the bowel by acting through a cytotoxin. There is increased passage of the mucus, blood and pus, associated with the formation of immune complexes, large joint arthropathy and haemolytic uraemic syndromes. It can have a poor prognosis if treatment is delayed.

Common examples are as follows:

- Bacillary dysentery caused by *Shigella dysenteriae* and other *Shigella* species, e.g. *S. sonnei*, *S. flexneri* and *S. boydi*.

- Enteroinvasive *Escherichia coli* (EIEC) or enteropathogenic *E. coli* (EPEC) caused by certain strains of atypical *E. coli*.
- *Campylobacter jejuni* infection which causes chronic mucosal damage; the jejunum and ileum are involved to a lesser extent.
- *Yersinia enterocolitica* which produces colonic ulceration and acute bloody diarrhoea. This must be differentiated from appendicitis, Crohn's disease and TB.
- Amoebiasis caused by *Entamoeba histolytica* which presents with a gradual onset of watery diarrhoea associated with abdominal pain and the passage of blood and mucus. It resembles the toxic megacolon of ulcerative colitis and must be differentiated from this condition.
- Pseudomembranous colitis is an antibiotic-associated colitis caused by toxins from *Clostridium difficile*.

Fatty diarrhoea (malabsorption syndrome)

This must be distinguished from pancreatic insufficiency. There are characteristically large, pale and offensive stools with a high level of fat on examination of faecal smears. The commonest examples are infective, caused by:

- *Giardia lamblia*.
- *Strongyloides stercoralis*.
- *Capillaria philippinensis*.
- *Klebsiella pneumoniae*.
- *Enterobacter cloacae*.
- Coccidia: *Isopora belli*; *Cryptosporidium* sp.

Chronic diarrhoea

Tuberculosis syndromes are caused by infection with *Mycobacterium tuberculosis* and *M. bovis*. These include:

- **Ileocaecal TB**. This may present as an acute abdomen with diarrhoea, pyrexia of unknown or uncertain origin (PUO) and abdominal pain. It must be differentiated from Crohn's disease, lymphoma and *Yersinia enterocolitica*.
- **Tuberculous peritonitis**. This presents with diarrhoea, an acute abdomen and rapidly developing ascites. It must be differentiated from hepatoma with peritoneal seeding and carcinomatosis.

Schistosomiasis (*Figure 6.3*). This may present with mild diarrhoea or severe dysentery, together with the other symptoms of schistosomal infection.

Parasitic infestation with *Strongyloides* and *Ascaris* worms may present with an acute abdomen, diarrhoea, blood loss and anaemia, as well as the passage of the worms per rectum. *Trichuris trichiuria* infection causes bloody diarrhoea and rectal prolapse, especially in malnourished children.

Chagas' disease (South American trypanosomiasis; *Figure 6.4*) is caused by infection with *Trypanosoma cruzi* and can present with changes in bowel habit due to the destruction of Auerbach's plexus, affecting bowel motility.

Lymphomas. Burkitt's and Mediterranean lymphoma can present with an acute abdomen, PUO and diarrhoea. They must be differentiated from other causes of glandular enlargement.

Common causes of hepatomegaly and hepatic granulomas in the tropics

These are presented in *Tables 6.5* and *6.6*.

Figure 6.3. Geographical distribution of schistosomiasis.

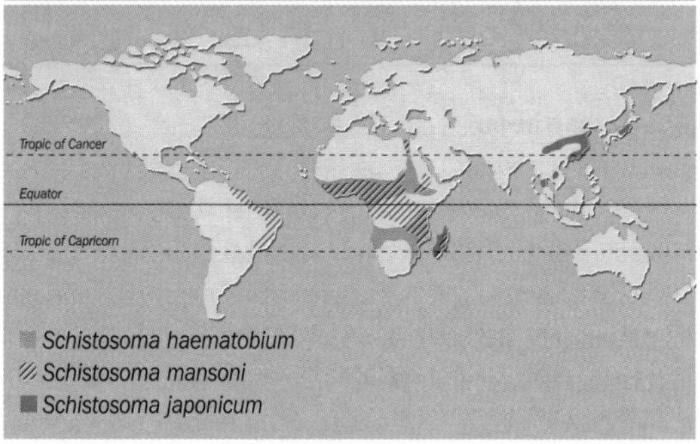

Tropic of Cancer
Equator
Tropic of Capricorn

▓ *Schistosoma haematobium*
▨ *Schistosoma mansoni*
▊ *Schistosoma japonicum*

Figure 6.4. Geographical distribution of trypanosomiasis.

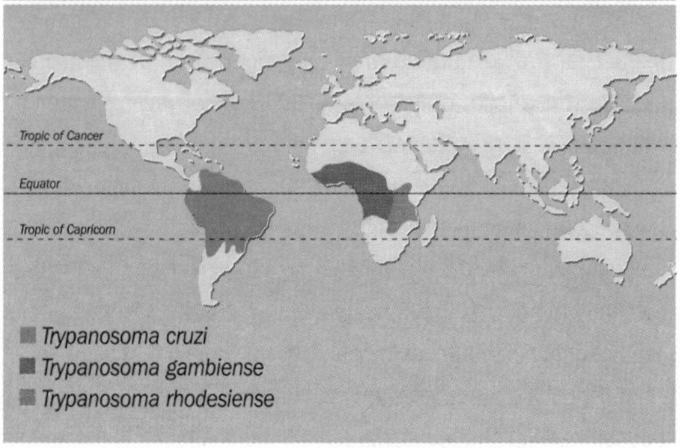

Tropic of Cancer
Equator
Tropic of Capricorn

▓ *Trypanosoma cruzi*
▊ *Trypanosoma gambiense*
▨ *Trypanosoma rhodesiense*

Table 6.5. Common causes of tender hepatomegaly and hepatic granulomas in the tropics.

Infections	
Viral	Cytomegalovirus; hepatitis A; Epstein–Barr virus; yellow fever
Bacterial	TB; leprosy; syphilis; brucellosis; leptospirosis; relapsing fever
Protozoal/ parasitic	Malaria; amoebic liver abscess; South American trypanosomiasis (Chagas' disease); helminthiasis (*Ascaris lumbricoides* and *Toxocara canis* infection); strongyloidiasis; visceral leishmaniasis
Fungal	Aspergillosis; coccidiomycosis; actinomycosis; candidiasis
Miscellaneous	
Sickle cell anaemia; thalassaemia	
Beri beri	
Veno-occlusive disease	
Budd–Chiari syndrome (from drinking 'bush tea')	

Table 6.6. Common causes of non-tender hepatomegaly and hepatic granulomas in the tropics.

Infections	
Viral	Hepatitis B and C
Bacterial	Brucellosis; plague
Protozoal/ parasitic	Schistosomiasis; African trypanosomiasis; *kala-azar*; hydatid liver disease; liver fluke infestations (i.e. fascioliasis; clonorchiasis; opisthorchiasis)
Miscellaneous	
Liver cirrhosis (micronodular and macronodular)	
Hepatocellular carcinoma	
Portal hypertension	
Haemosiderosis	
Kwashiorkor	

Table 6.7. Common causes of tender splenomegaly in the tropics.

Infections	
Viral	Epstein–Barr virus; viral hepatitis; cytomegalovirus
Bacterial	Brucellosis; typhoid fever; borreliosis (relapsing fever); bartonellosis; amoebic liver abscess
Parasitic/ protozoal	Malaria (acute malaria); trypanosomiasis
Miscellaneous	
Sickle cell disease	
Thalassaemia	
Portal hypertension	

Table 6.8. Common causes of non-tender splenomegaly in the tropics.

Infections	
Viral	Viral hepatitis
Bacterial	Tuberculosis; leprosy (*Figure 6.7*)
Parasitic/ protozoal	Visceral Leishmaniasis (*kalar-azar*), schistosomiasis, leptospirosis, endemic malaria (tropical splenomegaly), hydatid liver disease (ecchinococcosis)
Miscellaneous	
Reticuloendothelial diseases: lymphomas, leukaemias, reticulosis	
Amyloid disease	

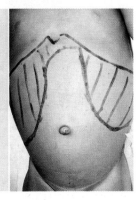

Figure 6.5. Massive hepatosplenomegaly in a patient with visceral leishmaniasis (*kala-azar*).

Common causes of splenomegaly in the tropics

These are presented in *Tables 6.7* and *6.8*, and the geographical distribution in *Figure 6.5*.

Cutaneous manifestations of tropical diseases

Peripheral gangrene of typhus

This is caused by *Rickettsia rickettsii* (Rocky Mountain spotted fever). It invades the endothelial cells of the blood vessels causing vascular damage with resultant mural thrombi (Frenkel's nodules). This is associated with perivascular infiltration and occasionally produces gangrene of the feet and hands.

Ainhum (little toe autoamputation)

A slowly progressive fibrous stricture (*Figure 6.6*) that encircles the little toe at the level of the metatarsal joint, leading eventually to spontaneous amputation. It may be attributed to abnormal fibrogenesis with the overproduction of fibrous tissue in response to multiple infection in Africans who habitually walk with bare feet. Obstruction of the posterior tibial artery, together with angiodysplasia of the plantar arch and its branches, have been demonstrated in some cases.

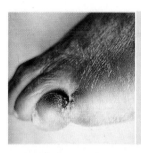

Figure 6.6. Ainhum.

Figure 6.7. Geographical distribution of leprosy.

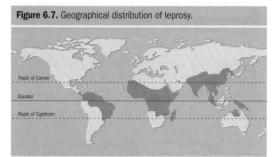

Tropic of Cancer

Equator

Tropic of Capricorn

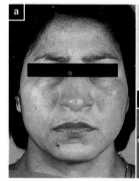

Figure 6.8. Leprosy.
a. Cutaneous facial lesion.
b. Neural muscle wasting in hand demonstrating the neurological sequelae of the disease.

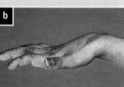

Lepromatous deformities that are correctable by surgery

Damage to the ulnar nerve in tuberculous leprosy occurs early in the course of the disease. The affected nerve is thickened and progressive damage leads to weakness and wasting of all the intrinsic muscles of the hand, with relative sparing of the flexors and extensors, causing flexion and separation of the ring and little fingers. This results in the characteristic picture of the *main de preditateur* (*Figure 6.8*).

Nerve thickening

This occurs in leprosy, associated with sensory or motor dysfunction of the progressive disease. The nerve thickening, like skin involvement, tends to be bilateral and symmetrical, with

Figure 6.9.
Tropical ulcer.

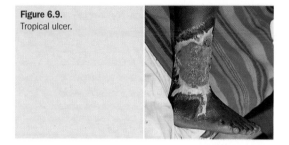

slight difference in the degree in the two sides. It is found in the superficial portion of peripheral nerves, e.g. the ulnar nerve above the elbow, the great auricular nerve in the neck and the radial and median nerves at the wrists.

Tropical ulcer

Shown in *Figure 6.9*. This is endemic in the monsoon-ridden, humid zones of Africa, India and tropical America; it also is seen as seasonal epidemics. The ulcer occurs almost exclusively in the lower leg and foot and is due to infections by two organisms, *Fusobacterium fusiformis* and *Borrelia vincenti*. Other constant organisms, i.e. pseudomonas, proteus and diphtheroids, are probably contaminants. Other aetiological factors involved are possibly nutritional deficiency and trauma.

The skin infection develops due to trauma or an insect bite. It commences as a papulopustule which, within hours, becomes surrounded by a zone of acute inflammation with induration and accompanying painful, tender lymphadenitis. In 2 to 3 days the pustule bursts and by a process of necrobiosis an ulcer forms and extends rapidly. Its interior is brown, its edges are undermined and a zone of skin in the immediate vicinity is infiltrated and raised. There is copious serosanguineous discharge and considerable pain.

Untreated, the ulcer remains practically the same size for months, sometimes even for a year or two. It can then become of such dimensions and with so great a destruction of the soft parts of the leg and foot as to require amputation. The constant pain, profuse serosanguineous discharge, the offensive odour, the extreme tenacity of the contained slough and comparatively mild constitutional symptoms suggest the diagnosis. If healing occurs, a permanent scar is left that is characteristically circular, thin and faintly pigmented.

Tropical ulcer must also be distinguished from yaws, veld sore, Buruli ulcer, venous ulcers and malignant melanoma. Occasionally squamous cell carcinoma may supervene producing a rolled everted edge with bone destruction and lymphadenopathy.

Veld sore (cutaneous diphtheria) or diphtheric desert sore

Diphtheric infection of the skin by *Corynebacterium diphtheriae* is peculiar to the hot, parched desert wastes of the world, in all of which it is fairly common. The infection enters through a skin breach, producing a painful vesicle full of straw-coloured fluid, which bursts, leaving a shallow ulcer with a thin grey pedicle and a very tender, raw surface. After 23 weeks the ulcer becomes chronic, characteristically punched out with undermined edges, thick margins and a base covered with grey, scaly debris. The organism multiplies in the ulcer, producing an exotoxin that circulates in the blood, causing toxic manifestations, especially in the heart (myocarditis) and the peripheral nerves (peripheral neuropathy).

Cutaneous leishmaniasis (Figure 6.10): two forms

Old World cutaneous leishmaniasis (*Figure 6.11a, b, c*) (oriental sore; Delhi boil) is caused by *Leishmania tropica*, *L. major* and *L. aethiopica*. It is transmitted by a sandfly bite. The infection is confined to the skin, with no visceral or mucosal spread. The lesions, localized to the site of the sandfly bites, may be single or multiple, warty or papular and may ulcerate; they may be complicated by secondary infection and regional lymphadenopathy. Lesions occur mostly on the uncovered parts of the body, hands, feet, arms, legs and especially the face. They are rare on the trunk and are never seen on the palms, soles or hairy scalp.

New World cutaneous leishmaniasis (American leishmaniasis) is caused by *Leishmania mexicana* and *L. brasiliensis*.

L. mexicana causes chiclero ulcer, which is an ear lesion with necrosis and erosion of the auricular cartilage. *L.*

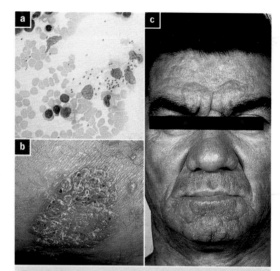

Figure 6.11.
Leishmaniasis. a. Blood film demonstrating the organism. b. Cutaneous lesion. c. Chronic cutaneous sequelae of disseminated leishmaniasis.

brasiliensis begins as a small, painless nodule which may itch when it ulcerates after 12months. The ulcer is round and shallow with prominent, raised borders. Frequently the condition presents with a large ulcer on the lower leg. In multiple lesions involving many sites, e.g. the hip, elbow, head or nasal mucosa, mucosal lesions tend to develop. The process usually starts at the upper lip and nose junction and may proceed to destruction of the whole front of the face (espundia).

Buruli ulcer

This is a chronic ulcerating condition caused by *Mycobacterium ulcerans*, an acid-fast bacillus whose common name comes from the part of Uganda where it was found and studied; Uganda and New Guinea are the major foci of infection. The lesion starts as a subcutaneous nodule attached to the skin and then spreads by non-caseous necrosis of the subcutaneous tissue. It heals with granulation tissue and non-caseating epithelioid granuloma, which may calcify. Healing may take months or years, producing severe scarring.

Yaws

Shown in *Figure 6.12a, b*. Yaws is a non-venereal, treponemal infection caused by *Treponema pertenue* and restricted to tropical areas with coastal distributions in South America; it is limited to the population of African descent. Although it persists in Africa it is showing considerable recrudescence.

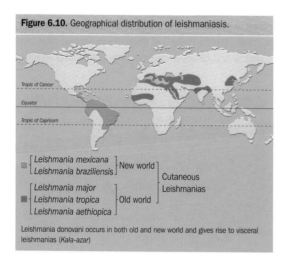

Figure 6.10. Geographical distribution of leishmaniasis.

Tropic of Cancer
Equator
Tropic of Capricorn

$\left.\begin{array}{l}\text{Leishmania mexicana}\\\text{Leishmania braziliensis}\end{array}\right\}$ New world $\left.\begin{array}{l}\quad\\\text{Cutaneous}\\\text{Leishmanias}\end{array}\right.$
$\left.\begin{array}{l}\text{Leishmania major}\\\text{Leishmania tropica}\\\text{Leishmania aethiopica}\end{array}\right\}$ Old world

Leishmania donovani occurs in both old and new world and gives rise to visceral leishmanias (Kala-azar)

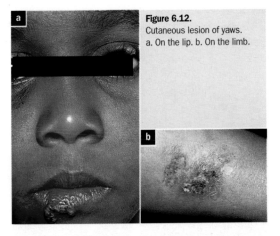

Figure 6.12.
Cutaneous lesion of yaws.
a. On the lip. b. On the limb.

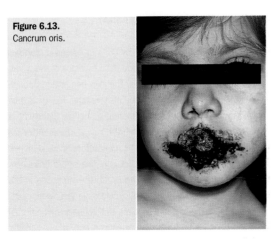

Figure 6.13.
Cancrum oris.

Transmission is by direct contact with an infective lesion, probably entering through skin breaches and producing a variety of cutaneous lesions.

The primary (initial) lesion is round or oval and papillomatous, occurring on exposed areas and usually healing spontaneously. Secondary (disseminated) lesions include:

- Cutaneous papillomatous or papular lesions, healing spontaneously with little or no scarring.
- Plantar lesions are common in those who walk barefoot and hence are subject to trauma and hyperkeratosis. They are often painful.
- Goundou is a form of yaws osteitis involving the maxilla bilaterally, leading to the formation of bony swellings on either side of the nose, not involving the cartilages. The swellings persist and can grow to a large size, tending to obstruct the nostrils; they sometimes involve the hard palate.

The **late lesions** are characteristically solitary destructive lesions that heal, leaving scars and depigmented skin:

- The skin lesions are gummas, which may be localized or spreading.
- The bone lesions are due to periosteitis, gummatous osteitis or a combination of both, e.g. gangosa, an advanced destructive ulcer affecting the maxillary bones and hard palate or nasal septum, spreading to perforation of the turbinates as well as extending to the pharynx, causing dysphagia.

Cancrum oris

This is a rapidly spreading, unilateral, necrotic ulceration of the cheek. It is caused by infection with organisms of Vincent's stomatitis, namely *Fusobacterium fusiforme* and *Borrelia vincenti*. It is common in Africa, Asia and South America, predominantly in malnourished children. The commonest predisposing factor or cause is measles but gastroenteritis, typhoid, bronchopneumonia and *kala-azar* may act as antecedents.

It may involve the lips (*Figure 6.13*), exposing the underlying bone, leading to a well-defined slough and a large defect in the cheek or lip. Soon bone and teeth sequestrate.

Calabar swelling

Calabar swelling is a subcutaneous swelling caused by infection with the filarial worm loa loa (*Figure 6.14*). The swelling itself is caused by antigenic material released by the wandering worm, resulting in a type I immediate hypersensitivity reaction. The swellings are about 8 cm across, appearing suddenly and disappearing gradually over 3 days. It forms

Figure 6.14. Geographical distribution of filariasis.

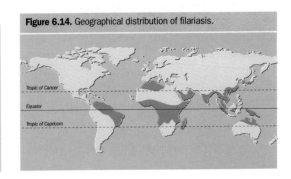

cyst-like swellings resembling ganglia which cause pain on movement. Dying worms under the skin may cause a chronic abscess followed by a granulomatous reaction and fibrosis.

Common cancers in the tropics

Squamous cell carcinoma of the mucosa of the oral cavity and the oesophagus

The condition is associated with the cultural practice of chewing betel quid and/or the smoking of locally made cheroots called bidi.

Squamous cell carcinoma of the middle or lower third of the oesophagus

The lesion develops in the susceptible epithelial lining after exposure to exogenous ingested agents, e.g. home-brewed beers, drinking bootleg whisky brewed in tar barrels and coexistent dietary deficiencies of trace elements and vitamins such as Zn, Mg, riboflavin and nicotinic acid.

Nasopharyngeal carcinoma (squamous cell carcinoma)

The spectrum ranges from poorly differentiated or non-keratinizing squamous cell carcinoma (lymphoepithelioma) to well-differentiated squamous cell carcinoma.

The lesions are associated with the Epstein–Barr virus, carcinogenic factors, e.g. inhaling thatch smoke of huts, and the high intake of salted marine fish and pork using sodium nitrate as a preservative, the carcinogenic agents being the nitrosamines.

Primary hepatocellular carcinoma arising from parenchymal cells of the liver

This disease is more frequently of macronodular than micronodular type; it is also associated with hepatitis B infection and mycotoxins, e.g. aflatoxin, a product of the fungus *Aspergillus flavus*, which contaminates foodstuffs such as peanuts and can cause liver cirrhosis and hepatoma. Cirrhosis is uncommon in the tropics except following infection with the hepatitis B virus; the incidence of associated carcinoma is therefore low.

Bile duct adenocarcinoma (cholangiocarcinoma) that may arise from the intra- or extrahepatic bile ducts

This lesion is associated with infection with liver flukes: clonorchiasis and opisthorchiasis. Patients present over 50 years, usually with jaundice.

Well-differentiated transitional cell carcinoma of the urinary bladder

In some areas this is the predominant type of squamous cell carcinoma. It is associated with severe infection of *Schistosoma haematobi*. The non-schistosomal type is associated with urethral stricture which produces bladder dysfunction and recurrent infections. Imperfect bladder emptying gives rise to further recurrent infection and conversion of ingested nitrates to nitrosamines.

Carcinoma of the cervix

Epidemiologically, this lesion is related to sexually transmitted herpes simplex virus type 2 and human papilloma virus (HPV).

Carcinoma of the penis (squamous cell carcinoma)

The incidence of this lesion is closely related to poor socioeconomic conditions and poor personal hygiene. It is associated with sexually transmitted viral infection and DNA virus of human papilloma virus type 2 (HPV II). It has been reported in patients with verrucous carcinoma. Carcinoma of the penis is less frequent in populations that practise circumcision.

Malignant tumours of connective tissue, i.e. Kaposi's sarcoma

This is a malignant, undifferentiated angiosarcoma that is usually a cutaneous manifestation but may involve other organs in the body. (See AIDS p.88).

Malignant tumours of the skin

Squamous cell carcinoma and **basal cell carcinoma** may arise in an area of damaged skin, most frequently in long-standing tropical ulcers, epithelialized skin sinuses, scars of old burns and self-inflicted skin damage. Deeply pigmented or light-brown skins are resistant to the effect but albino people are more prone to develop multiple squamous cell carcinomas than others.

Malignant melanoma of the skin is less common in deeply pigmented skin and differs from that of white people in that it is not usually on sun-exposed areas and occurs in the older population. It often occurs on the palmar aspect of the hands and fingers and is more common in those who walk with bare feet and are subjected to continuous trauma; 90% of the leg lesions occur below the ankle.

Malignant lymphomas (leukaemias)

Burkitt's lymphoma is a non-Hodgkin's lymphoma originating from B-lymphocytes and endemic across sub-Saharan Africa.

It is caused by the Epstein–Barr virus, mostly affecting children of 4–7 years old, with a declining incidence between 8 and 16. It is found to be more common in immunosuppressed children, especially those who develop recurrent malarial infection.

Mediterranean lymphoma (primary upper small intestinal lymphoma) develops in the upper part of the small intestinal mucosa and is endemic in areas of Lebanon, Israel, Iraq, Algeria, Syria and Tunisia, as well as in some countries in South America and southern Africa. It must be distinguished from the primary intestinal lymphoma seen in temperate climates.

Histocytic medullary reticulosis occurs in an unusual frequency in some countries of sub-Saharan Africa including Uganda, Kenya, Zambia and Malawi. It presents clinically with anorexia, fever, weakness, abdominal swelling and haemolytic anaemia. Deterioration is rapid and diagnosis is rarely made in life.

7 Management of the multiply injured patient

Introduction

The primary aim of this text is the demonstration of symptoms and signs, and there is minimal reference to treatment. However, in multiple injuries resuscitative measures begin simultaneously with assessment, and, in this chapter, primary evaluation and resuscitation are considered together, followed by a more detailed secondary survey.

When dealing with multiple casualties it is essential to categorize patients so that optimal use is made of medical resources. The system used is termed 'triage' (from the French word for sorting) and this is considered first. The subsequent sections on the management of individual patients follow a similar approach to that of the advanced trauma life support system (ATLS).

Triage

Triage is a system for sorting patients, based on the severity of their injuries and their need for treatment. This sorting should begin in the field, ensuring that each patient ends up in a facility appropriate to their needs. When adequate facilities are available, severe injuries are treated first. In disasters, when the number of patients and the severity of their injuries exceeds the capability of available facilities and staff, the patients with the greatest chance of survival, and with the least expenditure of time, equipment, supplies and personnel, are treated first.

Patients must be categorized uniformly, based on valid, reliable and feasible criteria. Two systems of triage are in common use.

The **P** (for **Priority**) system colour codes patients into three priorities:

- P1 – immediate (red) – patients who require immediate life-saving procedures.
- P2 – urgent (yellow) – patients who require resuscitation then early and specific treatment.
- P3 – delayed (green) – patients who do not require resuscitation or early and specific treatment.

The **T** (for **Treatment**) system is used when categorizing large numbers of casualties that have overwhelmed the available medical facilities. It is similar to the P system but adds a fourth expectant group – T4 (blue) – which is judged irrecoverable or to require considerable use of inadequate resources.

Triage is a dynamic and continuous process. Patients can rapidly change their category, as can the level of skill and available time for assessment changes, as the patient progresses from the site of the accident to the receiving area and on to an Accident and Emergency (A & E) department.

In the 'first look' **primary assessment**, walking wounded are separated from the incident (P3). The ABC (airway, breathing, circulation) criterion is used to categorize P1, P2 and dead patients. If apnoea is present, in spite of the application of a chin lift or jaw thrust, a patient is triaged as dead. P1 is given to patients with respiratory rates greater than 29 or less than 10, and when there is a capillary refill time of greater than 2 seconds. In cold conditions or bad light, capillary refill is replaced by a pulse rate of greater than 120 beats per minute. **Secondary triage**, at an ambulance point or at the A & E department entry, categorizes patients using the triage revised trauma score, in which coded values are given to the Glasgow Coma Scale, systolic blood pressure and respiratory rate.

Table 7.1 is used to calculate the triage revised trauma score (Champion, 1989) and categorizes patients as follows: Dead: 0; P1: 1–10; P2: 11; P3: 12, i.e. serious injuries have the lowest scores.

An anatomical assessment of the patient's injuries is added to the initial physiological assessment on arrival in the A & E department and is carried out as the primary and secondary surveys, considered below.

Table 7.1. Revised trauma score.

Coded value	Respiratory rate	Systolic blood pressure	Glasgow Coma Scale
4	10–29	>89	13–15
3	>20	76–89	9–12
2	6–9	50–75	6–8
1	1–5	1–49	4–5
Zero	Zero	Zero	3

Management of the individual patient

The widespread introduction of the ATLS system for the management of the severely injured patient has provided a well-tried and unified team approach. It is based on the rapid assessment of injuries and the institution of life-preserving therapy. The overall ethos of the ATLS system is 'to supply oxygenated blood to the brain and vital organs and to do no further harm'.

The ATLS scheme firstly considers the pre-hospital phase of rapid assessment of ABC, immobilization of the patient and immediate transfer to the closest appropriate facility.

The history must include the time of the injury and the events of the injury, and its mechanism, whether blunt, penetrating or blast, as this can influence the degree and type of injury sustained. The receiving hospital's facilities should be prepared and able to respond with immediate airway control, appropriate monitoring equipment and investigatory services.

As clinicians concerned with the assessment may come into contact with the patient's body fluids – and as the patient's hepatitis and HIV status are usually unknown – face-masks, eye protection, water-impervious aprons, leggings and gloves – collectively known as universal protection – should be worn.

Primary survey

The aim of the primary survey is to rapidly identify existing or potentially life-threatening conditions, and simultaneously to treat and continually reassess until the patient is stable. The headings used to remember these items included in the primary survey are conveniently remembered by the letters A to E:

A – **airway maintenance**, with cervical spine control.

B – **breathing and ventilation**.

C – **circulation**, with haemorrhage control.

D – **disability** (neurological status).

E – **exposure/environmental control** (completely undress the patient but prevent hypothermia).

Airway maintenance and cervical spine fractures are assessed together as they may be produced by similar injuries and, therefore, may co-exist.

A cervical spine injury should be assumed to be present in every patient with multiple injuries, particularly in blunt trauma above the clavicle and in any altered level of consciousness. Spinal cord injury is not an inevitable consequence of cervical spine fractures but the potential is always present. The neck must, therefore, be immobilized until a

cervical fracture is later excluded by radiological studies. Temporary control is achieved by holding the head in the anatomical position until a hard collar can be applied, preferably with the addition of sandbags at either side of the head. The head can be further secured with the use of strong sticky tape firmly applied across the patient's forehead and secured at either side to the hard structure of the trolley or stretcher. When moving the patient, the in-line immobilization is maintained by one member of the team thus avoiding movement of the cervical spine.

Airway obstruction may be complete or partial, intermittent, sudden or insidious. It may be due to secretions, vomit, blood, bone or a foreign body. One of the commonest causes is the patient's own soft tissues falling back during unconsciousness. Less common causes include laryngeal or tracheal disruption and fractures of the facial bones. Airway obstruction is assessed by observation of respiratory distress and cyanosis, listening for noisy breathing, particularly stridor, and by palpation to feel primarily movement of air and respiratory effort. This is followed by palpation of the neck, mandible, face and then, with a finger in the mouth, examination for foreign bodies and abnormal mobility of the upper jaw and mandible.

Mid-face fractures can cause airway obstruction by external pressure, blood and secretions. A gloved finger in the mouth, holding the mandible forward to relieve obstruction, may be a life-saving manoeuvre. In all cases of suspected airway obstruction, the chin lift or jaw thrust maneouvres are used early to pull soft tissues forward; this alone relieves many cases of airway obstruction in the unconscious trauma patient. To establish and maintain a patent airway, a nasopharyngeal airway may be required. If the patient is unconscious and has no gag reflex, an oropharyngeal airway may be used, but with caution, since the absence of a gag reflex in a trauma patient almost certainly means that the airway is unprotected lower down, i.e. there are impaired laryngeal reflexes. Such a patient should be strongly considered for early endotracheal intubation to be certain of a safe, secure and patent airway.

Breathing and ventilation involves the lungs, chest wall and diaphragm. It is assessed by exposing the chest, to inspect and palpate the front, back and sides of the chest wall for the presence and equality of movements, looking for any evidence of a flail segment and for open wounds or 'sucking chest wounds'. Bruising may be observed and surgical emphysema may be felt. Auscultation assesses air entry throughout the lung fields; percussion may demonstrate increased dullness over a haemothorax.

Immediately life-threatening chest injuries are looked for and managed during the primary survey. These include:

- Airway obstruction.
- Tension pneumothorax.
- Open pneumothorax.
- Massive haemothorax; this is defined as the presence within the chest cavity of over 1500 mL of blood, or continuous loss through a drain of more than 200 mL h^{-1}.
- Flail chest.
- Cardiac tamponade.

A tension pneumothorax requires immediate needle decompression. In unilateral cases there is tracheal deviation away from the lesion, reduced chest movement and the absence of breath sounds. In severe cases, increased intrathoracic pressure prevents cardiac filling; this can result in hypotension. The overall reduction in movement and breath sounds in the very rare bilateral case is accompanied by severe respiratory distress and significant cardiovascular compromise. An open pneumothorax requires the wound to be covered by a sterile dressing but secured only on three sides to allow the dressing to form a closed flap on inspiration and to open on expiration, thus allowing air to be released from the chest and to prevent the development of a tension pneumothorax. Flail chest segments do not usually require active compression; the main significance of the finding of a flail chest is that there is severe underlying pulmonary contusion caused at the time of injury. Such patients usually need ventilation to allow the pulmonary contusion to resolve and to aid breathing in the presence of multiple fractures and the associated pain. A massive haemothorax requires adequate fluid resuscitation before placement of a large chest drain. Failure to resuscitate the patient prior to drainage leads to sudden, severe decompensation.

Serious ventilatory problems in unconscious patients require the control of a patient's airway and, often, artificial ventilation. Airway control is initially as described above but endotracheal intubation, either nasally or orally, may be required. The cervical spine must be controlled during these procedures. If nasal and oral intubation are precluded by facial injuries, a surgical airway through the trachea or larynx is needed. Every seriously injured patient should receive supplementary oxygen at a flow rate of 10–12 L min^{-1} by a tight-fitting reservoir oxygen mask.

Circulation: haemorrhage is the predominantly reversible cause of post-injury death and needs rapid identification and

treatment. If haemorrhage is untreated it leads to the clinical state of shock, which is defined as 'inadequate organ perfusion and tissue oxygenation'. The physical signs of shock or impending shock can be subtle. The early signs of compensation for blood loss need to be detected to allow early resuscitation. The physiological classification of haemorrhage is a useful theoretical model on which to base treatment (*Table 7.2*).

In summary, Class 1 haemorrhage represents a 'blood donor', where the blood loss is 500–750 mL; this is not significant and is usually well compensated for, particularly in the young and fit. At the other extreme, Class 4 haemorrhage is severe and surgical intervention is usually required – more than 50% of the circulating volume is lost and the patient is rapidly unconscious and moribund.

Class 2 haemorrhage is the difficult, subtle state that *must* be appreciated clinically. This is usually blood loss of 750–1500 mL; note that the blood pressure is often normal at this stage but that pulse pressure is decreased, due to a rise in the diastolic pressure.

Class 3 haemorrhage is the classic 'shock', the familiar signs of a pale, anxious, shut-down patient with a tachycardia, tachypnoea and a decreased systolic blood pressure. This is the smallest amount of blood loss that consistently causes a decrease in blood pressure, therefore, from the point of view of physical signs, a patient who is already hypotensive is a patient who has had a significant loss of fluid and requires urgent resuscitation.

This is a very didactic model and its application must be modified to take into account the age of the patient and other conditions. For example, a young, fit patient compensates very well for a significant blood loss and then suddenly decompensates, i.e. move from Class 2 to Class 3 rapidly. An elderly

Table 7.2. The physiological effect of haemorrhage.

Haem-orrhage	% Blood loss	Vol. of blood loss (mL)	Pulse rate	Blood pressure	Pulse pressure	Respira-tory rate
Class 1	Up to 15	Up to 750	<100	Normal	Normal or increased	14–20
Class 2	15–30	750–1500	>100	Normal	Decreased	20–30
Class 3	30–40	1500–2200	>120	Decreased	Decreased	30–40
Class 4	>40	>2000	>140	Decreased	Decreased	>35

This can easily be remembered as the 'tennis score classification' with the % blood losses being approximately 15, 30, 40 and over 40.

patient, particularly one on beta-blockers or with a diabetic autonomic neuropathy, may compensate much less well.

In the assessment of a patient's circulatory status, the pulse rate, skin perfusion, level of consciousness and pulse pressure are the main diagnostic features. Urine output and respiratory rate should also be noted.

To examine the pulse, choose an accessible central vessel such as the femoral or carotid artery and compare the two sides to exclude any local abnormality. Note the volume, rate and regularity. A good volume, regular, slow pulse usually indicates normality. Hypovolaemia produces a thready, rapid pulse, while irregularity carries a warning of cardiac impairment. An impalpable pulse is a sign of existing or imminent cardiac arrest, requiring immediate restoration of blood volume if death is to be avoided.

An individual with pink skin is rarely critically hypovolaemic whereas pale mucous membranes, an ashen grey face and exanguinated, white extremities are indicative of a greater than 30% loss of blood volume – these are ominous signs. A critical reduction in cerebral perfusion produces an altered level of consciousness. This is a useful sign in the absence of head injuries; however, a normal conscious level or a normal blood pressure, especially in the young, does not exclude severe blood loss.

Hypovolaemia is treated by the control of haemorrhage and immediate fluid replacement, with careful observation of the response.

There are three patterns of response to an initial bolus of 2000 mL of fluid. They are:

- Responders – those patients who respond to fluid resuscitation are those who have lost less than 2000 mL and in whom there is no continuing significant loss.
- Transient responders – those patients having continuing haemorrhage, which needs to be identified and stopped.
- Non-responders – those patients with severe, on-going blood loss. They require continuing aggressive resuscitation and, usually, require surgical intervention.

Severe external bleeding is managed by manual compression over the bleeding site. Pneumatic compression devices can be of value and, if transparent, the injured area can be kept under surveillance. Arterial tourniquets can crush underlying tissue and render a limb totally ischaemic. In general they are best avoided but can be life-saving in extensive vascular limb lacerations. When used, the responsibility for removal must not be delegated and the tourniquet should be released hourly until definitive treatment is available.

Concealed blood loss may be within the thoracic or peritoneal or retroperitoneal cavities, around deep arterial and venous damage from penetrating injuries and around fractures, particularly those of the pelvic ring and major long bones. Severe thoracic and abdominal haemorrhage require urgent surgical intervention.

Fluid replacement is through a minimum of two wide-bore, intravenous cannulae. The sites depend on accessibility and the skills of the attending clinician. On obtaining vascular access, blood is taken for cross match, baseline full blood count, urea, electrolytes, liver function tests, and a pregnancy test in women of child-bearing age. Balanced electrolyte solution is rapidly infused and warmed O negative or type-specific blood considered if resuscitation is not keeping pace with blood loss. Fluid warmers should be used to reduce the chances of hypothermia. Balancing high-volume fluid replacement requires continuous monitoring of pulse, blood pressure, temperature, respiratory rate, arterial blood gases and urine output.

Urinary outflow is a sensitive measure of a patient's volume status. However, rectal and genital examination should be undertaken to exclude traumatic urethral rupture before attempting passage of a catheter. A nasogastric tube is inserted to reduce gastric distension and fluid accumulation, and reduces the risk of aspiration. ECG monitoring should be undertaken in all major trauma patients. Cardiac contusion may give rise to dysrhythmias and ST segment changes. Electromechanical dissociation – defined as 'the absence of a cardiac output in the presence of a rhythm that is normally consistent with a normal cardiac output' – may be associated with cardiac tamponade, tension pneumothorax or profound hypovolaemia. It is also seen specifically in aortic or cardiac rupture, pulmonary embolism, hypothermia and occasionally in electrolyte disturbance.

Disability (in the A–E mnemonic) is used as a reminder to assess neurological function at the end of the primary survey. The Glasgow Coma Scale (see below) is used, or the simpler AVPU method. The latter mnemonic represents four grades of consciousness: **A**lert; responds to **V**ocal stimuli; responds to **P**ainful stimuli; and **U**nresponsive. An altered level of consciousness may be due to a head injury but also occurs in hypoxia and hypovolaemia, or may be due to alcohol and other drugs.

Exposure/environmental control reminds the clinician to completely undress victims of major trauma, usually by cutting clothing, in order not to miss any diagnostic signs. Due consideration must, therefore, be given to the temperature of the environment and the use of warm blankets and high-flow warmers for infusion fluids to prevent hypothermia.

Powerful analgesics may be required in the control of the pain of multiple injury but these agents can depress cerebral and pulmonary function, as well as mask important physical signs. Analgesia should, therefore, be withheld until at least a primary survey has been undertaken by a skilled clinician. In the case of mass casualties, patients should be marked as having received analgesics during or after triage, to avoid double dosage. Small, incremental doses of intravenous opiates, titrated against pain and the condition of the patient, are appropriate. There is no place for intramuscular analgesia in major trauma patients. Naloxone should be readily available.

Secondary survey

The previous sections have been concerned with the rapid assessment of the multiply injured patient in order to identify and treat reversible life-threatening conditions. In this respect the airway, breathing and circulation were seen to be of prime importance, and these vital areas must be constantly re-evaluated until the patient's condition is stable.

Once life-threatening injuries have been managed, a detailed examination of the patient is undertaken. This secondary survey examines the patient from top to toe. It includes every part of the body and every system, as even major injuries can be overlooked in the severely injured patient, who may be unconscious or in whom immediate attention has had to be concentrated on a life-threatening problem.

Up to this time, any radiological investigation taken in the resuscitation area has been essential to immediate treatment, e.g. anteroposterior views (AP) of the chest and pelvis, and lateral cervical spine, and it must not have interfered with or delayed any aspect of resuscitation. During the secondary survey, systematic radiological assessment is undertaken, together with specific haematological or other diagnostic procedures, e.g. peritoneal lavage.

History

A detailed history is obtained from the patient or, if this is not possible, from relatives and witnesses of the incident. It is particularly important to speak to the paramedics before they leave the department. A description of the event and details of the environment related to the injury provide important background information. The mechanism of the injury and the force and direction of the impact provide information on the type of injury to expect. For instance, the presence of an explosion, the involvement of guns or knives or, in the case of a vehicle, the use of seat-belts, head-rests and airbags, and the extent of cabin space deformity.

Injuries can be broadly categorized into blunt, penetrating or blast, or be due to exposure to extreme temperatures and hazardous substances, one of the most hazardous being water. Any history of drowning, particularly associated with hypothermia, creates particular problems with resuscitation. Prolonged resuscitation is necessary following drowning associated with hypothermia, particularly in the case of children, as some spectacular recoveries have been documented.

Blunt injuries are commonly caused by falls or by road and other traffic accidents, or sustained in the workplace or during recreational activities. Penetrating injuries are due to firearms and knives, and may be from explosive fragments. The speed of a bullet or missile at the point of impact and the area involved, have a marked influence on the degree of injury. For example, high velocity missiles can fragment bone and produce extensive shock effects on soft tissues. The trajectory and entry and exit wounds may also indicate likely organ damage.

Burns may occur alone or be coupled with blunt and penetrating trauma, for example in burning vehicles or with explosions; they may also be associated with inhalation injuries. Burns are considered on p. 122, cold injuries on p. 125 and hazardous substances on p. 126.

The past history and current medication may reveal a connection with the incident, such as a history of blackouts and epilepsy, and, like allergy, may influence subsequent management. The social history indicates prior independence and family commitments; a history of alcohol abuse may be relevant. Systemic enquiry identifies other clinical problems that could influence management. The length of time from the last meal to the trauma should be noted; this is more important than the time since the last meal as gastric emptying can be delayed or impaired by trauma. This is particularly true in children.

Physical examination

The examination of the head starts by inspecting and palpating the entire scalp. Lacerations and contusions are easily missed and may indicate underlying bony or cerebral damage. Eye opening may be difficult because of orbital oedema but the lids should be retracted to observe the pupils and eyeballs and, where possible, visual fields and acuity.

Inspection and palpation of the face and jaw has already been considered (in the primary survey) because of potential airway obstruction from a fractured mandible or a mobile fracture of the upper jaw. More detailed examination should include observation for missing teeth, since these may have been aspirated. The chest radiograph should be examined for the presence of teeth in the large airways. Further examination of the face is for depressed facial fractures that can affect bite and visual axes (zygomatic fractures affecting the suspensory ligament of the eyeball), infraorbital nerve paraesthesia (zygomatic fracture) and damage to the lachrymal apparatus and nasal bones. Soft tissue injuries may damage branches of the facial nerve. Fractures may damage the main trunk either primarily (which is irreversible) or secondarily by oedema (which undergoes slow recovery). The ears should be examined with an oroscope to look for evidence of haemotympanum, which is associated with basal skull fractures. The nasal secretions should be examined for rhinorrhoea. The patient may demonstrate Battle's sign, which is bruising at the base of the mastoid, or periorbital haematomas – 'racoon eyes' – all of which are associated with basal skull fractures.

The importance of in-line cervical spine immobilization for suspected cervical spine fractures has been repeatedly emphasized; the spinal cord is at risk in any lifting or carrying procedures. This is especially true during extraction from a vehicle or removing a motorcycle helmet. Hyperextension and rotation movements must be guarded against when maintaining the airway, particularly if endotracheal intubation is required. Once the patient's condition is stable, a full radiological assessment of the cervical spine is made, to exclude fracture and initiate appropriate management.

Penetrating wounds of the neck may be divided into three zones:

- Zone 1 may involve structures at the thoracic outlet.
- Zone 2 may involve structures between the clavicle and the mandible.
- Zone 3 is from the angle of the mandible to the base of the skull.

One of the key questions to be answered when assessing a penetrating wound of the neck is whether the platysma has been penetrated or not. If so, most people would advise surgical exploration since penetrating wounds of the neck can produce unsuspected injuries. These may be of the large vessels of the carotid sheath, the larynx, trachea, pharynx or oesophagus. The internal carotid artery is subject to traumatic dissection with or without thrombosis and not necessarily accompanied by neurological sequelae, while tracheal disruption may be accompanied by palpable emphysema. In view of the potentially serious nature of these injuries, penetrating neck wounds should always be explored in the operating room.

The chest, in the primary survey, was fully exposed and examined by observation, palpation, auscultation and percussion, to exclude a flail chest, open, tension and simple pneumothoraces and a haemothorax. Now, more detailed examination includes observation of the entire chest wall, palpating all ribs and applying sternal and lateral pressure to identify rib fractures and costochondral separation. Rib fractures may be conveniently grouped into three: ribs 1–3 may be associated with major vessel damage; ribs 4–9 may be associated with chest problems; and ribs 10–12 may be associated with abdominal perforations or contusions. The finding of rib fractures in these groups should alert you to the possibility of associated injuries. Sternal fractures should be considered as these may be associated with underlying mediastinal and particularly cardiac damage. Auscultation of breath sounds can be difficult in a noisy environment, though the resuscitation room should be as quiet as possible. Absent or reduced sounds are important diagnostic criteria, as is percussion dullness of a haemothorax. Distended neck veins may indicate cardiac tamponade, though this should have been identified in the primary survey. A chest radiograph confirms pulmonary and cardiac problems. Particular note should be made of the width of the mediastinum, while remembering that in a resuscitation setting, the chest radiograph is likely to be an AP view, which magnifies the mediastinal structures to some degree. Deviation of the nasogastric tube to the right, with mediastinal widening, may be suggestive of traumatic aortic dissection, which has tamponaded. Minor bony abnormalities are more reliably detected clinically.

Major intra-abdominal haemorrhage may have presented with problems of hypovolaemia in the earlier assessment. However, the majority of abdominal wounds can only be identified during the second survey and, even then, the signs may be minimal. Repeated examination is needed to identify changing signs such as increasing tenderness, guarding, an abdominal mass, shifting dullness or absent bowel sounds. Particular note must be taken when there is tenderness, suggesting fracture of the lower ribs or when there is known to have been rapid deceleration when wearing seat-belts. Intraperitoneal lavage can be useful in identifying haemorrhage from the liver, spleen or major vessels, although it may also be positive with less specific retroperitoneal bleeding and multiple pelvic fractures. Renal injury is accompanied by microscopic or frank haematuria. If visceral injuries, such as perforation of a hollow viscus or pancreatic trauma, are suspected because of penetrating abdominal wounds or changing signs, early laparotomy is indicated.

In the primary survey a warning was given that, prior to urethral catheterization, it was essential to examine for perineal bruising and to undertake a rectal examination to exclude a high-riding prostate. Examination also identifies rectal tears and the quality of sphincter tone. In the female, vaginal tears must be excluded and also the diagnosis of pregnancy.

Musculoskeletal injuries produce pain and interfere with function and may be associated with significant blood loss. The identification of fractures, so that they can be splinted for comfort and to reduce blood loss, is important in the secondary survey. Early diagnosis and reduction of dislocations, particularly of the hip, to avoid avascular necrosis, is also important. In the severely injured patient, however, with widespread contusion and lacerations, and who may be unresponsive, clinical signs and a radiological assessment are usually more informative. The signs of fractures, dislocations and ligamentous injuries include bruising, deformity and, on palpation, local tenderness and possibly abnormal mobility and crepitus. Each bone deserves attention as, for example, digital and clavicular fractures are easily missed. Anteroposterior and side-to-side pressure on the chest and pelvis elicit pain from rib and pelvic fractures in a conscious patient but, like the thoracic and lumbar spine, should be examined by appropriate radiographs if the physical findings and mechanism of the injury suggest that these areas could be damaged.

Vascular injuries may be incurred in blunt and penetrating wounds, presenting as haemorrhage and ischaemia (p. 368). All peripheral pulses should be palpated, particularly those distal to injuries around major vessels. The signs of ischaemia, however, may be difficult to detect because of bruising and associated nerve damage. Nevertheless, ischaemia must be identified in the secondary survey as urgent revascularization may have to be undertaken to prevent permanent soft tissue damage. The severe pain of a compartment syndrome should also be noted; this is made worse on passive stretching of muscles. It may be seen particularly in association with long bone fractures, e.g. of the tibia, and supracondylar fractures of the humerus. But it is also seen in the palm and the foot, wherever tight fascial spaces exist. The pain of a compartment syndrome is due to ischaemia at tissue level and is caused when tissue perfusion pressure is elevated above 30 mmHg. The presence of a palpable arterial pulse within the compartment does not exclude a compartment syndrome. It is primarily a clinical diagnosis. However, although some people advocate the use of compartment pressure probes, these can only confirm a clinical suspicion and are not reliable in excluding a compartment syndrome if the clinical findings are present.

Preliminary assessment of the CNS has already been undertaken by the AVPU or the Glasgow Coma Scale; the latter should now be either initiated or repeated. A deteriorating or impaired consciousness level is defined as 'a reduction in the Glasgow Coma Scale of 2 points or more'. This is associated with significant neurological deterioration and requires urgent computed tomography (CT) scanning and a neurological opinion. Depressed fractures, extradural, subdural and intracerebral haemorrhage require specialized care.

Any degree of paralysis suggesting a spinal cord injury necessitates immobilization of the entire patient, and this must be maintained until spinal injury has been excluded radiologically or until the patient is being managed by the appropriate specialist team. Peripheral nerve injuries related to blunt or penetrating wounds should be identified in the secondary survey. They are usually managed after the acute event has settled but transected nerve endings may be identified and marked during any early wound exploration.

Continuing care

This is the stage of planning and prioritizing care. Overall responsibility for the patient must be established with one consultant but communication between specialists is vital.

The primary and secondary surveys identify immediately life-threatening complications of trauma and allow management of these problems and the planned long-term management of less urgent conditions such as fractures and nerve injuries. Nevertheless, the multiply injured patient is, for many days and possibly longer, still at risk of further life-threatening conditions such as reactionary and secondary haemorrhage, sepsis from a perforated viscus, a contused lung, adult respiratory distress syndrome (ARDS), renal failure, myoglobinuria and clotting problems. Monitoring and a high index of suspicion must, therefore, be continued, possibly in an intensive care unit, until the patient's condition is stable for 24–48 hours. Basic requirements include pulse, blood pressure, respiration, temperature, ECG, urinary output and arterial blood gas analysis.

Records must never be neglected during an emergency resuscitation. Precise documentation is an essential part of management, both for patient treatment, for medicolegal reasons and for the purposes of audit, e.g. a major trauma outcome study. Chronological flow charts of vital signs can detect early deterioration and stimulate immediate action. The task should, therefore, be the responsibility of a designated member of the management team. Documentation of the primary and secondary survey also provides a clinical base line against which changing signs can be recognized, ensuring that new events are managed appropriately. Clinical photography is also very valuable as an adjunct to the notes.

Multiple injuries are often subject to subsequent medicolegal problems and may be the basis of criminal action. Accurate records are needed, with full documentation of all injuries and all results filed, such as blood alcohol and other drug levels. In criminal cases, all clothing and other items, such as bullets and missile fragments, must be retained for examination by law enforcement agencies.

Physical injury

Burns

Burns may be thermal, electrical (including lightning) or chemical.

Thermal injury may take the form of a flame burn, a burn from contact heat or radiated heat, a scald from hot liquid or steam, or an electrical burn.

Smoke inhalation in household or industrial fires, or the inhalation of hot gases, injures the respiratory tract both from the inhaled heat and the toxicity of the inhaled gases, particularly carbon monoxide (CO) and toxic gases such as cyanide.

Electrical burns and cold injury are also a form of burn and are described on pp. 125 and 126.

Chemicals (p. 127) may cause burns on coming into contact with skin or mucosal surfaces by their corrosive or combustible properties.

Radiation burns are considered on p. 127.

Burns are usually accidental, except for those caused by warfare, terrorism and arson. Disturbingly, burns caused by non-accidental injury to children, self-immolation and torture are increasingly encountered in many parts of the world.

Survival following a burn injury is dependent on the patient's age as well as the burn area and depth. In the very young, the very old and the ill, the morbidity is high from complications.

Clinical assessment

The arrival of a burned patient to the A & E department is usually dramatic due to the visual impact of the injuries and the accompanying distress of relatives and bystanders.

When the burned area is extensive, the urgent need for resuscitation, ABC, pain relief and wound management take precedence over the history and physical examination. However, the mechanism of injury must be ascertained early as it may have therapeutic and prognostic significance, for example the patient may have other co-existing trauma. A detailed enquiry and examination must be carried out as soon as the patient's condition permits.

The area of burn surface is estimated by the 'Rule of Nines'. This takes into account the burned area but excludes simple erythema. This is used as a guide to the body surface area. In the adult, head and neck accounts for 9%, front and back of the trunk 18% each, the upper limb 9% and the lower limb 18%. As a useful guide, the palm of the hand, i.e. not including the fingers, and the groin are 1% each. In children the area of the head and neck is amended to 18% and the lower limb to 12% (*Figure 7.1*).

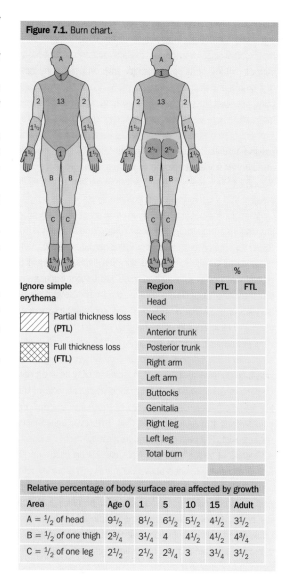

Figure 7.1. Burn chart.

Ignore simple erythema

▨ Partial thickness loss (PTL)

▧ Full thickness loss (FTL)

		%	
Region		PTL	FTL
Head			
Neck			
Anterior trunk			
Posterior trunk			
Right arm			
Left arm			
Buttocks			
Genitalia			
Right leg			
Left leg			
Total burn			

Relative percentage of body surface area affected by growth						
Area	Age 0	1	5	10	15	Adult
A = $^1/_2$ of head	$9^1/_2$	$8^1/_2$	$6^1/_2$	$5^1/_2$	$4^1/_2$	$3^1/_2$
B = $^1/_2$ of one thigh	$2^3/_4$	$3^1/_4$	4	$4^1/_2$	$4^1/_2$	$4^3/_4$
C = $^1/_2$ of one leg	$2^1/_2$	$2^1/_2$	$2^3/_4$	3	$3^1/_4$	$3^1/_2$

Table 7.3 Classification of burns.

Partial thickness		Full thickness
Superficial partial thickness	Deep dermal	
Red blisters, weepy, very painful	Patchy white, decreased sensation	Leathery hard, no sensation
	May need grafting, particularly if it becomes infected	Needs grafting

The common classification of burns in the UK is shown in *Table 7.3*. There can be a significant overlap between the clinical findings of deep dermal (*Figure 7.2*) and full thickness burns (*Figure 7.3*) but the classification here is useful and clear. The American classification is into first, second and third degrees: first degree is erythema without blistering, third degree equates to full thickness (as in *Table 7.3*) and second degree incorporates the remaining varieties.

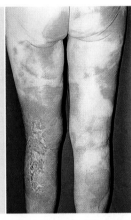

Figure 7.2.
Partial thickness burns over the posterior aspect of thigh and legs (recovery phase).

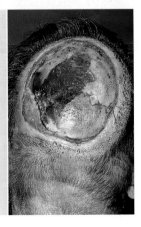

Figure 7.3.
Full thickness burn of the posterior aspect of the scalp.

The best indication of the depth of a burn is the sensation to pin prick, but this is sometimes equivocal and may require reassessment after 24 hours following the use of non-stick dressings or open wound management.

The extent of tissue injury that determines prognosis is influenced by the temperature, the duration of contact and the type of burning agent. The severity of a scald is largely determined by the duration of contact with the hot water or steam as neither exceeds 100°C except in pressure cookers and scalds from hot cooking oil (approx. 180°C). As scalds are common in toddlers and children, it is important to obtain details of the liquid involved and its approximate temperature, the duration of contact, whether the area was covered with clothing at the time of injury and whether the area was cooled immediately with tap water or cold milk. Non-accidental injury in a child should always be considered when managing burns.

Clinical features

The psychological trauma caused by the injury manifests initially as fear and acute anxiety, which may progress to profound depression and listlessness. The mental and emotional state of the patient must, therefore, be included in the initial and continuing clinical assessment so that the patient may be counselled through the various stages of recovery.

Pain is severe with superficial burns but deep burns, in contrast, are numb due to the destruction of the cutaneous nerve network; in the latter the loss of extracellular fluid rapidly leads to dehydration, anaemia and circulatory collapse.

The extent of tissue damage is estimated from the depth and surface area involved. In superficial burns the surface is reddened with blistering (*Figure 7.4*) and is exquisitely tender to the touch. A straw-coloured or blood-stained fluid oozes from the capillaries to form blisters on the surface. In deep burns the

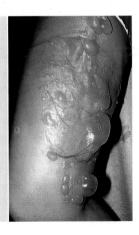

Figure 7.4.
Blistering of superficial thigh burns.

surface is insensitive and is of a pale yellow or dark brown colour due to exposed fat or muscle. The extensive inflammatory response in deep burns leads to oedema of the underlying tissue planes which, if severe, may compromise the airway in the neck or the circulation in a limb. Beware of circumferential burns, particularly of the chest, neck, limbs and digits, as these may be associated with impaired ventilation, airway obstruction or ischaemia. They may in some cases require emergency escharotomy, particularly to allow chest expansion. Perineal burns may be associated with urethral obstruction, secondary to oedema. Early urinary catheterization is required.

An unconscious patient rescued from a fire is of special concern. This may be due to asphyxia from smoke inhalation and may involve primarily CO poisoning, or may be due to a severe head injury from falling masonry and require urgent resuscitatory measures. It is also important to exclude other internal injuries.

Pulmonary injuries

Fires in confined spaces produce injury to the respiratory tract from heat, chemicals or blast. The nose, mouth and throat must be inspected for mucosal injury. Toxic products of combustion from burning fabrics and furniture release CO which binds haemoglobin, preventing oxygen transport. Lung function may require frequent monitoring with repeated chest auscultation, radiographs and arterial blood gas estimations over the ensuing days. Laryngeal oedema or respiratory distress syndrome from pulmonary oedema may develop rapidly, leading to acute respiratory failure. Facilities for endotracheal intubation and assisted ventilation must be immediately accessible.

Local effects of burns

Heat results in cell injury which, when severe, leads to cell death and tissue matrix denaturization with thrombosis of the microcirculation. In lesser injuries, the inflammatory response produces an erythematous induration with increased capillary permeability, leading to subcutaneous oedema. Bacterial colonization of the burned surface is usually complete within 24–48 hours. This may remain a local infection or may give rise to systemic spread, with fever and rigors from a septicaemia.

Regional effects of burns

These vary with the anatomic site of the burn injury. The initial tissue swelling may compromise underlying vital structures and later, when the overlying burn tissue hardens into an unyielding eschar, further restriction of function may develop. Contractures are a late manifestation of burns and may lead to deformities and loss of function (*Figure 7.5*).

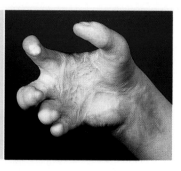

Figure 7.5. Contracture and deformity following deep burn of right hand.

Systemic effects of burns

Fluid is lost from the circulatory volume in a burn injury in the form of surface evaporation, local tissue oedema and, in more extensive injuries, from generalized oedema from the cytokine-mediated effects on the microcirculation.

Following a major burn, the patient develops hypovolaemic shock due to the passage of fluid from the intravascular space to the intercellular space due to generalized capillary leakage. Some of this fluid is lost to the exterior from the burned surface but the bulk is sequestered as generalized oedema involving all organs, including the lungs and brain. This phase lasts 24–48 hours when diuresis commences and the capillary wall integrity is regained.

Heat is lost from the body due to the loss of thermoregulatory function of the damaged skin and heat loss from evaporation of extracellular fluids.

Red cells are damaged and haemolyse in the region of the burn, and, in general, have a reduced life span resulting in progressive anaemia in the days following a significant burn injury. Haemoconcentration from fluid loss may, however, mask the anaemia and may even result in a raised haematocrit.

Cardiac output falls following a major burn and is due in part to the effect of vasoactive agents on the myocardium.

Vomiting following a burn is due to gastric dilatation and ileus due to mesenteric vasoconstriction. Systemic infections from burn wound sepsis also cause vomiting.

Urinary output falls after a severe burn due to the renin–angiotensin effect on the kidney, with sodium retention and potassium excretion. Acute renal tubular necrosis may result from extracellular fluid loss or be due to haemoglobin and myoglobin released from damaged red cells and muscle.

Multiple organ failure is a poorly understood complication of extensive burn injury and involves the kidney, liver, lungs and heart. It has been variously attributed to electrolyte and fluid derangement, systemic infection or an uncontrolled inflammatory response.

Specific systemic complications are stress ulcers of the stomach and duodenum, which may result in significant bleeding or perforation. Later, the effects of tissue protein breakdown lead to a catabolic phase with severe weight loss and protein/calorie malnutrition.

Electrical burns

Electrical injury occurs when the body becomes part of an electrical circuit. The degree of injury depends on the type of current, the duration of contact and the part of the body involved. Alternating current is generally more harmful than direct current. Unfortunately, the most effective frequency for power transmission is also within the most harmful range to the human body. Generally, high voltage is more harmful than domestic levels although the latter injuries are far more common.

Two forms of injury are produced. The first is an electric shock, which depolarizes cell membranes. The clinical effect is on cardiac muscle, producing cardiac arrest and arrhythmias, and on skeletal muscle producing tetanic spasm. When the latter occurs in the back muscles it can produce compression fractures of the vertebrae and the subject may also receive injuries from being catapulted by the muscle contraction. An ECG is essential for all electrical burns.

The second effect is a thermal injury, principally seen after high voltage contact. Skin is a good insulator, especially when dry, but once its threshold has been exceeded, the current follows the line of least resistance through the tissue planes. A severe local burn is sustained at the point of contact, especially if this is of small circumference, such as the hand or the foot. A core of deep burn occurs as the power is dissipated along the electrical path, producing extensive damage remote from the entry and exit wounds. Bone is of high resistance but the surrounding deep muscles are of low resistance and sustain maximum damage.

The muscle damage gives rise to a raised serum potassium and myoglobinaemia. Deep muscle necrosis causes myoglobinuria, which may cause renal failure. It is important to identify this and to maintain a good diuresis, often using mannitol. A urine output of more than 100 mL h^{-1} should be maintained. A raised potassium level may lead to arrhythmias, so monitoring is required. Oedema in the muscle compartments produces vascular compression if it is not relieved by fasciotomy, and the resultant ischaemia is accentuated by any arterial damage and associated thrombosis. If the head is the point of contact, as well as an extensive scalp injury there may be delayed onset cataract. Other visceral injuries, e.g. to the gut and liver, can occur but are rare.

Lightning can be considered as a high voltage, direct current injury. Death is usually due to cardiac arrest but this can be prevented if resuscitation is at hand. Neurological damage, including coma and nerve injuries, is often reversible. Burns are usually superficial and spreading spider fashion across the skin. Deep burns and myoglobinaemia are rare.

Flash burns, following arcing across a metal tool, produce a characteristic appearance of blackened hands and face and singed eyebrows and hair. Although the appearances can be quite dramatic, this is a superficial cutaneous burn (*Figure 7.6*) and is replaced by pink skin within a few weeks, provided there is not a deeper component from ignited clothing. The blinking response to the flash is fast enough to protect the eyeball.

Response to cold

A uniform body temperature of 37°C is required to maintain normal cellular function. This is achieved by a thermal balance between heat production and heat loss, involving physiological and behavioural activity. Heat is produced by normal metabolism and increased by shivering and physical activity. Physiological responses can increase heat production more than twentyfold in response to a cold stimulus. Heat is conserved by peripheral vasoconstriction, with opening of proximal arteriovenous shunts. Skin blood flow can be decreased a hundredfold, this being highest in the fingers, but vasoconstriction is poor over the face and scalp.

Behavioural activities are more important than physiological, heat being preserved by appropriate clothing and shelter from the cold and wind. The body exchanges heat with its environment by evaporation, conduction, convection and radiation. A quarter of heat loss is by the evaporation of water vapour from the respiratory tract and the evaporation of sweat. Heat loss through conduction is dependent on clothing. This should be warm, windproof and waterproof yet permeable to water vapour to prevent it becoming sodden, since wet clothing loses 80% of its insulating value. The head and face

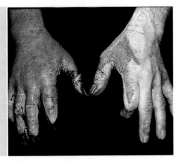

Figure 7.6. Electrical flash burn of hands following separation of superficial burnt epithelium.

should be covered. Lying in snow or immersion in cold water are accompanied by a rapid heat loss. Wind chill plays an important role in convection losses. Radiation from the sun is critical in maintaining thermal balance at altitude, exceeding metabolic heat production by a factor of two or three.

The temperature falls approximately 1°C for every 1000 ft (approx. 305 m) above sea level; the effect of altitude is further complicated by the reduced partial pressure of oxygen. The lack of oxygen reduces metabolic heat production, there is an increased ventilatory rate and, therefore, evaporation of water vapour from the respiratory tract and heat loss increases, and exhaustion occurs more readily, thus preventing heat production from exercise. The body has no cold acclimatization equivalent to altitude acclimatization.

Cold injury

Hypothermia is defined as a reduction of core temperature to below 35°C. The condition is severe below 32°C and, below 28°C, lethal cardiac arrhythmias occur. Intense widespread vasoconstriction produces a relative increase in circulatory volume, there being hypertension and a cold diuresis, the latter probably accounting for much of the weight loss encountered on cold exposure. There may also be pulmonary hypertension and right heart failure ('Eskimo lung'). The blood viscosity and packed cell volume are increased and there may be thrombosis of peripheral vessels. Cold reduces nerve conduction, with reduced sensation and motor power. There is a loss of dexterity, this also being limited by stiffness of joints due to the increased viscosity of synovial fluid. Muscles stiffen and can rupture.

Hypothermia alters mental function with loss of insight, poor judgement, unnatural acts – such as paradoxical undressing and trying to kill companions – and hallucinations deteriorating to coma. Death must not be diagnosed until the core temperature has returned to normal.

Local pathological responses to cold include frost nip and superficial and deep frostbite. **Frost nip** is a blanching of the skin, with sensory loss, but the tissue remains pliable. There is rewarming, painful hyperaemia and there may be minor superficial skin desquamation. In **superficial frostbite** there is superficial skin death. Rewarming of the white blanched skin is accompanied by blotchy, purplish discoloration and blistering. This is gradually converted to a black carapace. This takes many weeks to separate but a thin, new epithelial layer is in place when it falls off. **Deep frostbite** (*Figure 7.7*) is accompanied by crystal formation of interstitial fluid, with cell death and associated thrombosis of small vessels. The tissues are rigid and the extent of tissue loss is difficult to

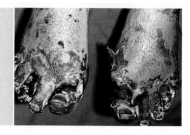

Figure 7.7.
Frostbite of feet.

determine. The gangrenous area shrivels and the inflammatory response of the adjacent viable tissue eventually provides a line of demarcation.

Trench foot (*Figure 7.8*) is a non-freezing injury due to prolonged exposure to cold, but not necessarily freezing, temperatures. The injury can occur up to 15–20°C. The cold is often accompanied by immersion and, as water is a good conductor, there is continued heat loss through the feet. There is sensory loss, patients feeling as if they are walking on cotton wool. The skin is initially red but later pales and may progress to superficial gangrene accompanied by systemic malaise, fever and weight loss. On rewarming, viable skin blisters and ulcerates. There may be marked pain during nerve recovery, and sometimes late hyperaesthesia. Other long-term sequelae are thin, pigmented skin, loss of subcutaneous tissue, wasting of the small muscles of the feet and joint stiffness. The condition may also involve the hands under such conditions as trench warfare and survival after shipwreck.

Hazardous substances

Harmful substances include physical agents such as radiation sources and a number of chemical groups, e.g. toxic, corrosive, inflammable and explosive compounds. The danger of these substances is well understood in the countries manufacturing them and there are usually stringent laws strictly controlling their use, storage and transport. The public are, therefore, rarely put at risk but accidents causing spills and leakage, and deliberate acts such as terrorism, can give rise to large scale civilian casualties and extensive economic damage. These incidents usually only involve one or two indi-

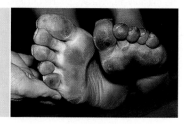

Figure 7.8.
Trench foot.

viduals but they carry the potential for disasters such as an explosion in a chemical plant or a nuclear reactor or the leakage of toxic waste. Nuclear material and chemicals are also manufactured as military weapons.

An affected individual may require sophisticated treatment but is also a potential source of contamination to carers and emergency departments. Thought must, therefore, be given to isolation and handling techniques prior to the arrival of an affected individual at an emergency centre.

This section mainly considers the problems of hazardous substances in relation to surgical practice. It does not consider abnormal drug reactions or the wide variety of poisons used in suicide attempts. Physical injuries and burns are considered elsewhere.

Radiation injury

Radiation can be from alpha, beta and gamma particles, X-rays and solar energy. Alpha, beta and gamma particles are emitted from nuclear power sources and nuclear weapons, and in radiotherapy. Alpha particles can be inhaled or injected and may remain in the body for considerable periods, producing irradiation tissue damage. Beta particles can penetrate the skin and produce superficial burns, while gamma particles pass through the body and damage cell structure.

The immediate local effect of radiation is to the skin and lungs, and these areas require close assessment. The effects depend on the power of the source, the length of exposure and the amount of shielding. Skin injury through exposure and contact with radiation sources takes the form of burns resembling those of thermal, chemical and electrical aetiology (p. 125; *Figure 7.9*). However, there may be additional problems of decontamination, usually by water irrigation, and a need for protective and appropriate clothing for the management team. Lung damage produces pulmonary oedema, giving rise to dyspnoea and progressing to respiratory and cardiac failure. Deeper radiation produces cell damage and denatures enzyme

pathways (*Figure 7.10*). It may also alter DNA structure, producing long-term malignant transformation.

Chemical burns

Chemical burns vary widely and cause, in addition to skin damage, a wide spectrum of systemic insults from the absorption of poisonous chemicals.

Acids that damage the skin on contact are hydrochloric, nitric (*Figure 7.11*) and sulphuric and, to a lesser extent, chromic, tannic, formic and picric.

Alkalis are more destructive and penetrate more deeply. Those commonly encountered are sodium, potassium and ammonium hydroxide and calcium oxide. Cement burns are commonly seen. Metabolic acidosis or alkalosis results if sufficient amounts of these substances are absorbed into the circulation.

Phosphorus burns on contact with the air, while metallic sodium, potassium and lithium ignite on contact with water. They produce deep burns if the combustion occurs on the skin surface.

Organic chemicals, such as phenol, cresol and trilene, produce minor skin burns but are lethal if swallowed due to oesophageal injury and grave systemic effects.

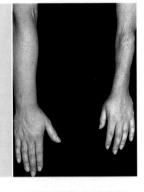

Figure 7.10.
Shortening of a limb due to radiation damage of the epiphysis of the left elbow.

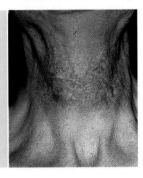

Figure 7.9.
Post-radiotherapy scarring of the skin.

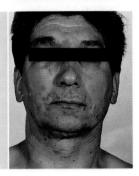

Figure 7.11.
Superficial facial burn due to nitric acid.

Bleaching agents, such as sodium hypochlorite and potassium permanganate, burn skin by oxidation while hot bitumen used in road surfacing burns by adhering to the skin.

Poisoning by drugs and chemicals

Drugs and chemicals can damage the human body. Access of these agents may be by self-poisoning, accident or through criminal intent. The effects may be acute or chronic and depend on the toxicity of the reagent, the dosage, the time span of administration and any therapeutic measures undertaken.

Self-poisoning in suicide attempts makes up a substantial proportion of emergency hospital admissions in western civilization. In the USA, for example, this figure exceeds 2 million a year. The actual number of attempts may be two or three times greater as many cases recover rapidly at home or die before reaching hospital.

The agents used in suicides are usually those that have been prescribed for the patient or a relative. In approximately half the cases, alcohol has been taken in addition to the overdose. Suicide attempts are predominantly in the third decade and more commonly in women. In contrast, accidental overdose of drugs and chemicals is usually in toddlers. It is due to accessible tablets being left around the home, together with toxic agents such as cleaning fluids, herbicides and pesticides. Iron tablets often cause tragic deaths in toddlers.

Accidental overdose of recreational drugs primarily occurs in the teens and twenties. Poisoning in older age groups is uncommon. Workers handling chemicals, or populations near factories manufacturing hazardous materials, e.g. asbestos, are at risk.

Certain trades carry recognized dangers. For example, the cerebral effects of mercury gave rise to the term 'mad as a hatter' since hot mercuric nitrate was used in preparing felt. The link between harmful chemicals and specific symptoms may not be well recognized or employers may choose to ignore potential risks. Chronic poisoning from unsuspected sources such as lead, zinc and chromium may, therefore, be very difficult to diagnose.

Poisoning with criminal intent carries similar difficulties. The most important factor is to be aware of such a possibility as, once considered, chemical analysis can usually rapidly confirm the diagnosis and the agent involved. Arsenic, strychnine, phosphorus and cyanide have all retained a place in criminal fiction. In practice, however, commonly available poisons such as weedkillers (paraquat) and rat poison (warfarin) are more likely sources.

The effect of poisons may be acute or may occur over many years, such as the onset of mesothelioma after exposure to asbestos. In general, care of the poisoned involves identification of the agent, removing free agent from the body and supporting injured systems until natural recovery takes place, or the use of specific antidotes, for example acetylcysteine for paracetamol overdose. In view of the potential and medicolegal consequences, a detailed history, including drug history and chemical exposure, must be documented. All suicide notes and contaminated clothing must be retained, together with the results of all investigations on the blood and body fluids.

Corrosive substances are of particular note to the surgeon. They produce burns and subsequent scarring can produce strictures, e.g. in the oesophagus. Commonly encountered fluids are strong acids and alkalis; of the former, hydrochloric, sulphuric, nitric and carbolic acids are used in batteries and as descaling fluids around the home. Harmful alkalis include bleach and paint thinners and strippers. Drinking of these fluids is usually by children and produces burns of the lips, mouth, larynx, pharynx, oesophagus and stomach. The effects may be mild erythema but may progress to inflammation, blistering and ulceration, and penetration necrosis may produce perforation of the oesophagus or stomach.

The use of chemical weapons accounted for high fatalities and morbidity in the First World War and remain a lethal threat in terrorism and modern warfare. Chemical weapons may be delivered in bombs and shells or sprayed from an aircraft, often in liquid form, that may become gaseous on exposure. They can dramatically affect the morale of an army and involve the donning of restrictive, protective clothing. They also produce a large number of casualties, ranging from trivial to lethal problems, and involve a large manpower in their care. The damage is primarily to the skin and mucous membranes but, if absorbed, can give rise to systemic problems.

Sulphur mustard (nitrogen mustard) and phosgene are examples of chemicals used in the First World War. The former produces skin burns, inflammation and blistering and has potentially lethal effects on the pulmonary mucosa through pulmonary oedema and ARDS. It also damages rapidly dividing cells, producing gut symptoms and bone marrow suppression. Phosgene is a heavy, colourless gas, that does not affect the skin but has lethal effects through pulmonary oedema, leading to cardiac failure.

Current chemical weapons are usually nerve agents that produce irreversible cholinesterase inhibition. Symptoms and signs include increased sweating and salivation, nausea, vomiting and abdominal cramps. Their effects on muscle produces weakness and respiratory paralysis; increasing toxicity is accompanied by confusion and convulsions.

8 The skin

Introduction

The skin functions as a barrier against potentially harmful physical, chemical, osmotic, thermal and photic agents, and against micro-organisms. It is important in heat preservation and provides an extensive sensory surface area. It plays a minor role in excretion, absorption and metabolism.

This chapter considers the principles of the history and examination of skin conditions, then concentrates on the diseases of surgical relevance. No attempt is made to be comprehensive. Lists are used to cover a number of important differential diagnoses, these include the cutaneous manifestations of malignant and systemic disease (*Tables 8.1* and *8.2*), skin pigmentation (*Tables 8.3* and *8.4*), purpura, pruritus (*Table 8.5*) and abnormalities of the hair (*Table 8.6*).

A number of conditions have a spectrum of cutaneous signs and these are generally considered with the relevant system. They include liver and renal failure, cutaneous disorders of the gut, and vasculitis. Some local diseases have serious or life-threatening consequences and the specific features of these conditions are covered in this chapter. Many of these conditions are instantly recognizable but making the diagnosis in the early stage of the disease can be difficult and is complicated by the great similarity between some disorders. A detailed history and examination are therefore essential. The factors that describe lumps and ulcers (Chapter 3) are particularly relevant to the skin.

Classification of skin disorders

A broad but useful classification of skin diseases is into hereditary, contact, infective and psychological causes.

The distribution of a number of skin diseases suggests a developmental origin and, in some of these **genodermatoses**, a family history is present. *Table 8.7* lists some of the large number in this group; they include atopic states, in which individuals are born with a sensitivity to certain allergens. The group does not contain many conditions with specific surgical relevance. Common problems include atopic eczema (*Figure 8.1*) and psoriasis (*Figures 8.2–8.4*).

Table 8.1. Skin manifestations of non-malignant systemic disease.

Manifestation	Disease
Erythema	Collagen disease
	Carcinoid
	Mitral valve (malar flush)
	Polycythaemia
	Superior vena caval obstruction
	Liver disease
	Hyperviscosity syndrome
Erythema multiforme	Fever
	Inflammatory bowel disease
	Rheumatoid arthritis
	Thyrotoxicosis
	Virus and microplasma infections
Urticaria	Collagen disorders
	Xanthomatoses
	Hereditary angioneurotic oedema
	Urticaria pigmentosa
	Henoch–Schönlein purpura
	Cold agglutinins
Scaling	Vitamin deficiencies
	Hypothyroidism
	Acromegaly
	Malabsorption
	Refsum's and Reiter's diseases
Papules and nodules	Behçet's disease
	Erythema nodosum
	Erythema induratum
	Gardner's syndrome
	Necrobiosis lipoidica
	Neurofibromatosis
	Polyarteritis nodosa
	Pseudoxanthoma elasticum
	Sarcoid
	Tuberous sclerosis
	Xanthoma
Blisters	Dermatitis herpetiformis
	Drugs
	Glucagonoma
	Pemphigus
	Porphyria
	Vascular disease
Angiomas	Multiple vascular formations
Pruritus	See p. 132
Purpura	See p. 26

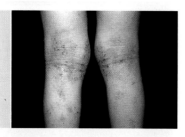

Figure 8.1.
Atopic eczema.

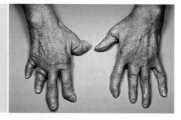

Figure 8.2.
Psoriatic skin lesions.

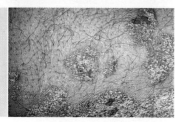

Figure 8.3.
Psoriatic nails.

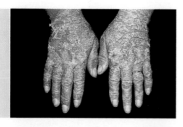

Figure 8.4.
Psoriatic arthritis.

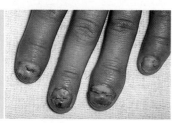

Figure 8.5.
Contact dermatitis.

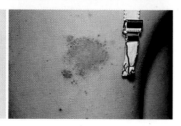

Figure 8.6.
Nickel dermatitis.

Contact skin disorders may be related to exposure to physical and chemical agents. Examples of physical agents are exposure to cold, producing cold urticaria, and chilblains. Heat and sweating produce some dermatoses, aggravate infective lesions and increase itching. Ultraviolet (UV) light from the sun and sunbeds can produce severe burns and other reactions in sunbathers.

Irritant and allergic chemical agents may be encountered in the home or industrial environment (*Figure 8.5*). Examples may be found in exposure to new clothing (*Figure 8.6*), jewellery, soaps, cosmetics, hair dyes, products for

Table 8.2. Cutaneous manifestations of malignancy.

Cutaneous manifestation	Malignancy and/or site
Primary skin malignancy	
Secondary malignant deposits or infiltration – leukaemia; lung;	
Paget's disease of the breast	
Weight loss and cachexia	Loss of subcutaneous tissue in the skin
Pruritus, particularly associated with lymphoreticular disease	
Clubbing and hypertrophic pulmonary osteoarthropathy	Lung
Superficial or deep venous thrombosis	Sometimes an occult primary, e.g. lung; gastric; pancreas
Dermatomyositis	50% associated with malignancy
Acanthosis nigricans	Gut and bronchus
Ichthyosis	Commonly gut
Alopecia	Gastric
Purpura	Thrombocytopenia
Exfoliative erythroderma	Lymphoma
Erythema gyratum repens	Breast; lung
Erythema nodosum; erythema multiforme	
Eczematous dermatitis	
Herpes zoster	Lymphoreticular disease
Flushing of carcinoid syndrome	
Skin lesions	Genodermatoses; Gardner's syndrome
Pyoderma gangrenosum	Leukaemia and multiple myeloma
Palmar keratosis	Bladder and lung
Disseminating intravascular coagulation	Leukaemia; lymphoma; cancer of the pancreas; also as a generalized terminal malignant event
Hypertrichosis langinosa	Gut

use in the garden and drugs. In industry, offending substances include vinyl chloride adhesives, fluorides and soluble cutting oils.

Infective causes include common staphylococcal infections (*Figure 8.7*), producing pus forming lesions such as boils (*Figure 8.8*), carbuncles (*see p. 66 Figure 4.13*) and industrial acne (*Figure 8.9*). Streptococcal infection produces a more cellulitic lesion such as erysipelas (*Figure 8.10*). Pets may give rise to urticaria (*Figure 8.11*) and scabies, while farm animals are associated with ringworm, milker's nodes and orf (*Figure 8.12*). Communal sports activities facilitate

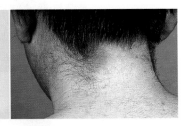

Figure 8.7.
Furuncle.

Table 8.3. Local skin discoloration.

Colour change	Cause
Haemorrhage/bruising	Trauma; blood dyscrasias; increased capillary fragility; old age; lower limb venous hypertension
Brown pigmentation	Freckles; moles; melanoma; basal cell carcinoma
	Café-au-lait spots – neurofibromatosis
	Oral spots – Peutz–Jeghers syndrome with small gut polyps
	Erythema ab igne – fires and hot water bottles
	Pregnancy – areolar and midline abdominal
	UV light
	Radiotherapy
	Warts; senile keratosis; keratoacanthoma; callosities
Black pigmentation	Eschar; burns and other scabs Gangrene Anthrax Pyoderma gangrenosum
Yellow pigmentation	Xanthelasma; pus
Purple pigmentation	Campbell de Morgan Capillary naevus – port wine; strawberry Spider naevi Telangiectasia Pyogenic granuloma Stria – pregnancy; Cushing's; sudden weight loss

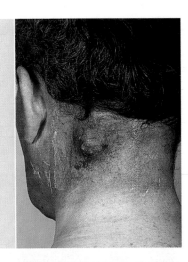

Figure 8.8.
Boil on the neck.

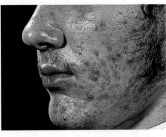

Figure 8.9.
Acne vulgaris.

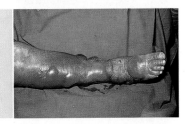

Figure 8.10.
Erysipelas.

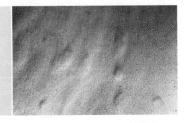

Figure 8.11.
Urticaria.

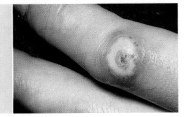

Figure 8.12.
Orf.

Figure 8.13.
Tuberculosis of the skin.

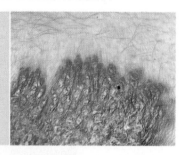

the transfer of fungal infections, while sexually transmitted diseases include scabies as well as gonorrhoea, syphilis and AIDS, all of which may have cutaneous manifestations. In tropical areas infections also include worms, cutaneous leishmaniasis, tuberculosis (*Figure 8.13*) and leprosy (p. 110).

The **psychological** group includes eczema and alopecia areata (*Figures 8.14* and *8.15*), the onset of which may follow stress.

Table 8.4. Diffuse skin discoloration.

Colour change	Cause
Brown pigmentation	UV light Acanthosis nigricans (suspected malignancy) Addison's disease Nelson's syndrome Cushing's disease ACTH secretion Haemochromatosis (bronze diabetes) Arsenic and silver poisoning Gardner's syndrome Pellagra – nicotinic acid deficiency Rheumatoid arthritis Gaucher's syndrome Lichen planus Fixed drug reaction
Pallor	Anaemia; hypoalbuminaemia
Cyanosis	Deoxygenated haemoglobin
Blue pigmentation	Methaemoglobin
Jaundice	Liver disease
Purplish pigmentation	Polycythemia
Pale brown/yellow pigmentation	Chronic renal failure
Orange pigmentation	Carotenaemia
Yellow pigmentation	Mepacrine
Purpura	Bleeding disorders Vasculitides – collagen diseases; diabetes Septicaemia – especially meningococcal Systemic malignancy Cushing's disease Ehlers–Danlos syndrome
Depigmentation	Albinism – absence of melanocytes Vitiligo – destruction of melanocytes Idiopathic Pernicious anaemia Gastric cancer Hypo- and hyperthyroidism Addison's disease Late onset diabetes Autoimmune disease (Hashimoto's) Scleroderma Syphilis Leprosy

Figure 8.14.
Alopecia areata.

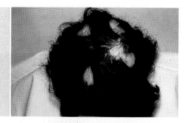

Figure 8.15.
Alopecia areata.

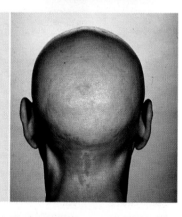

Table 8.5. Pruritus.

Association	Cause
Secondary to local skin conditions	Parasites – fleas; scabies; bites; pediculoses Eczema – local irritants; clothing; washing powder Urticaria Rectal and vaginal discharge Lichen planus Dermatitis herpetiformes Miliaria rubra (prickly heat)

Secondary to systemic disease	Neoplasia – Hodgkin's disease; leukaemia
	Chronic cholestasis – typically biliary
	  cirrhosis and obstructive jaundice
	Chronic renal failure, particularly late stage
	  and dialysis patients
	Drug reactions and food sensitivity
	Polycythemia, anaemia
	Psychological
	Endocrine – hyper- and hypoparathyroidism
	Heroin addicts

History in skin disorders

Onset

The time of onset of the skin disorder is of critical importance. Atopic conditions are those present from birth, although not necessarily presenting in their florid state until later. A family history of similar problems may also be elicited. Note the relation of the onset to exposure to physical and chemical agents, and remember that exposure may antedate the skin disorder by a number of months.

Question for exposure to possible agents in the home, work or other environments visited. Similarly, a search is made for a source of infective lesions, including human and animal contacts at home and abroad. Enquire whether the onset of the disorder coincided with times of stress. The rate of onset and progression to other sites can indicate the degree of reaction to the precipitating cause and continued exposure.

Distribution

The distribution is characteristic for many disorders, specific examples being Paget's disease of the nipple (p. 231) where the eczema overlies a deep malignancy. In contact disorders the infective skin may be limited to a ring finger or an earlobe. Wider areas of potential contact include the hands, feet and axillae. Contact disorders are commonly unilateral or asymmetrical while endogenous disease, e.g. psoriasis, is more symmetrical in its distribution.

The mode of spread provides further clues to diagnosis. Annular spread should be considered in erythema annulare (*Figure 8.16*), erythema multiforme (*Figure 8.17*) and fungal

Table 8.6. Hair changes.

Decrease/increase	Cause/reason
Decrease (alopecia)	Age
	Genetic – myotonia
	Damage from chemical treatment
	Severe illness; malnutrition
	Immunosuppressive drugs
	Radiotherapy
	Lichen planus
	Psoriasis
	Systemic lupus erythematosus
	Fungal
Increase	Racial
	Endocrine – virilizing of ovarian tumours; precocious puberty; adrenogenital syndrome; Cushing's disease; acromegaly; drugs
	Steroids; anabolic steroids
	Anti-epileptic
	Minoxidil; diazoxide
	Anorexia nervosa

Table 8.7. Genodermatoses – inherited skin disorders.

Type of disorder	Condition
Chromosomal	Down's syndrome – alopecia; ichthyosis
	Klinefelter's syndrome – leg ulcers; altered hair distribution
	Turner's syndrome – lymphoedema
	XYY – acne
Autosomal dominant	Ehlers–Danlos syndrome
	Erythropoietic protoporphyria
	Gardner's syndrome
	Gorlin's syndrome
	Hereditary haemorrhagic telangiectasia
	Ichthyosis vulgaris
	Neurofibromatosis
	Peutz–Jeghers syndrome
	Tuberous sclerosis
	Tylosis
	Urticaria pigmentosa
Autosomal recessive	Acrodermatitis enteropathica
	Albinism
	Ataxia–telangiectasia
	Lipoid proteinosis
	Pseudoxanthoma elasticum
	Xeroderma pigmentosum

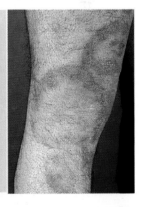

Figure 8.16.
Erythema annulare centrifugum.

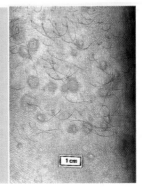

Figure 8.17.
Erythema multiforme.

infections (*Figures 8.18* and *8.19*), whereas other diseases spread in a much more irregular fashion, such as malignancy and pyoderma gangrenosum (*Figure 8.20*).

Other common symptoms include itching – which is seen in atopic states – and scabies (*Table 8.5*). Pain is a feature of inflammation – seen particularly in infective lesions – while exudation indicates superficial skin loss, as seen in acute dermatitis. Locally associated symptoms include regional lymph node tenderness and swelling. General symptoms include fever and malaise, and possibly those of the underlying associated disease (*Tables 8.1* and *8.2*).

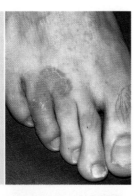

Figure 8.18.
Tinea pedis.

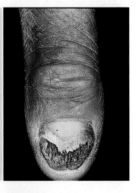

Figure 8.19.
Fungal infection of the nail.

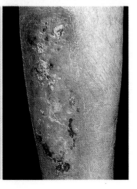

Figure 8.20.
Pyoderma gangrenosum.

Characteristics of skin lesions

Rashes may be discrete or continuous – i.e. confluent – and the lesions may be primary or secondary.

Primary lesions have specific features:

- Macules are flat, circumscribed areas of abnormal skin colour; they may also have characteristic texture or markings.
- Papules are circumscribed, raised areas of abnormal skin. Larger papules are termed nodules or tumours where, if greater than 1 cm across, raised abnormal areas may be referred to as plaques. They may be due to increased cellular content or oedema.
- Vesicles are raised papules containing clear fluid. Larger collections are termed blisters or bullae.
- Pustules are raised papules containing pus.
- Wheals are raised papules with pale centres.
- Purpura indicates haemorrhage within the skin.
- Annular lesions may indicate spreading and infiltration or may have a healing centre.

Secondary lesions develop from the expansion or decline of primary lesions, or may be related to their mechanical effect. Examples are desquamation or crusting, infiltration, ulceration and scarring. Ichthyosis is thickening of the skin, lichenification is depigmentation and there may be atrophy. Scratching produces specific longitudinal, reddened areas and there may be some associated skin thickening.

Although there are very many and diverse cutaneous lesions, only are few are commonly seen. These include acne, dermatitis, psoriasis, urticaria, warts, skin cancers and leg ulcers. The subsequent sections cover those lesions most likely to be encountered in surgical practice.

Structure of the skin

The skin is composed of an outer layer of stratified squamous epithelium – the epidermis – and a deeper layer of moderately dense connective tissue – the dermis. The epidermis has a deep, single layer of actively dividing stem cells and melanocytes attached to the basal membrane. The derivatives of these cells become progressively flattened as they pass through the stratum spinosum (the prickle cell layer), stratum granulosum and the stratum corneum. The outer layer is made up of closely packed, flattened, dead keratin cells that desquamate.

The dermis gives considerable strength to the skin, due to an extensive interweaving collagen meshwork, and some resilience due to its elastic component. A rich network of vessels and nerves lies superficially within the dermis and, more deeply, are the skin appendages, hair follicles and sebaceous and sweat glands. The dermis is divided into the outer, thinner papillary dermis (the stratum papillare) and the deeper reticular dermis (the stratum reticulare). The parallel collagen bundles in the latter are sited along lines of skin cleavage. There is great regional variation in the amount of keratin, hair, pigment, vessels, arteriovenous fistulae, nerves and glands. At most sites the skin is freely mobile over the underlying, subcutaneous fatty tissue.

The skin is subject to a large number and variety of focal and generalized diseases, many of which are cutaneous manifestations of systemic disorders. They can usually be diagnosed on the history and physical findings alone although a great diversity of signs can make this diagnosis very difficult.

The diversity of structures making up the skin and subcutaneous tissue gives rise to a variety of lumps, which are difficult to classify. Most of these do have characteristic features and it is important to make a diagnosis, to confirm or exclude premalignant and early malignant conditions. Carefully apply the system for examining lumps (p. 60) and particularly note whether the lump is in the skin or attached to it, or whether the skin is mobile over it. Abnormalities of the skin surface and colour changes are particularly helpful and remember to examine for enlarged regional lymph nodes.

The following sections consider benign and malignant lesions arising from the skin, its appendages and the subcutaneous tissues. Pigmented lesions are considered separately in view of the importance of diagnosing a malignant melanoma; ulcers are considered on p. 55 and inflammation on p. 61.

The description of cutaneous and subcutaneous lesions follows the order given in *Table 1.1*, including all applicable features. The table is based on the description of lumps and ulcers and is considered in Chapter 4.

Benign lesions of the skin and its appendages

Benign papilloma – skin tags
Papillomas (*Figure 8.21*) are hamartomas consisting of an overgrowth of all skin layers and its appendages; they have a central core and normal sensation. The lesions can occur at any age but are usually in the elderly. The symptoms are

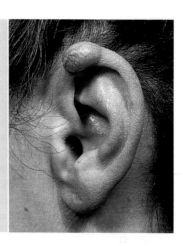

Figure 8.21.
Papilloma of left pinna.

mostly cosmetic, particularly on exposed areas, but they may catch in clothing and, if repeatedly traumatized, they may bleed and become inflamed, swollen and painful, and, on some occasions, may ulcerate.

Papillomas can be sited anywhere on the body. They are well defined, usually pedunculated, ranging from a few millimetres to a few centimetres in size, commonly 5 millimetres across. The stalk is of variable thickness. The surface may be grooved or deeply fissured, and the latter may be associated with pigmentation and keratosis. The lesions are solid, usually firm, but may be soft if there is a large, central, fatty component. They are non-invasive and not indurated unless there is associated inflammation and ulceration, in which case they may be mistaken for malignant lesions.

Seborrhoeic keratosis – seborrhoeic warts; senile warts; verucca senilis; basal cell papilloma
Seborrhoeic keratoses (*Figure 8.22*) are overgrowths of the basal layers of the epidermis. They are very common and usually multiple in the elderly of both sexes, but are occasionally

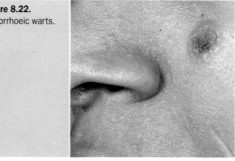

Figure 8.22.
Seborrhoeic warts.

seen in the young. The lesions slowly increase in size but not thickness over many years and may fall or be rubbed off. They give rise to cosmetic problems and can catch on clothing. Although they rarely bleed, bleeding into the lesion can produce the appearance of a pyogenic granuloma or of an epithelioma. The lesion may become infected.

Seborrhoeic keratoses are predominantly over the trunk, particularly over the back, which does not receive regular scrubbing, but also over the arms and neck. They are well-defined, firm, slightly raised, plaque-like lesions growing to 2–3 cm across. The surface is rough and hyperkeratotic and has a waxy look and feel. They are usually light brown in colour but may become deeply pigmented and mistaken for a malignant melanoma. The lesions can be peeled or scraped off, leaving a pale pink patch of underlying skin with, sometimes, a few fine bleeding points.

Warts

Warts are epidermal tumours due to infection with the papilloma virus of the papovavirus group. A number of different viruses are involved, the common and plantar warts (*Figure 8.23*) – verucca vulgaris and verucca plantaris respectively – are produced by a single virus and differ from verucca planus, genital warts (p. 355; *Figure 8.24*) and the papilloma of the larynx and oral cavity. Warts are contagious, the virus probably entering through minor abrasions. They occur at all ages but are commonest in children between 12 and 16 years old. They develop to their full size within a few weeks but there is probably an incubation period of several months. Approximately one-third disappear spontaneously within 6 months and two-thirds within 2 years. Warts cause cosmetic problems and,

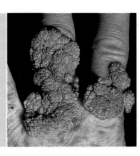

Figure 8.25.
Warts on the knuckles in a leukaemic patient.

when on the fingers, they interfere with fine movements of the hand, and can cause pain and irritation. Associated inflammation is usually due to attempts to pick them off.

Warts commonly occur over the knuckles (*Figure 8.25*) and nail folds of the fingers, the backs of hands, over the knees and on the face. They are usually multiple and may coalesce. The pigmented lesions are heavily keratinized and deeply pitted, with a frond-like surface. They are hard, 3–8 millimetres in diameter and raised 1–2 millimetres. Facial warts are often of the smoother – plain/juvenile – variety and plantar warts are inverted into the skin and, due to the pressure of walking, are often painful.

Molluscum contagiosum

Molluscum contagiosum (*Figure 8.26*) are produced by the poxvirus, the lesion being smooth, pearly white, 1–5 millimetres in diameter and umbilicated. They occur on the abdomen, genitalia, the face and arms, and undergo spontaneous regression after several months.

Keratoacanthoma – molluscum sebacium

Keratoacanthoma (*Figure 8.27*) is an overgrowth of a sebaceous gland of possible viral aetiology. It has a characteristic rapid development to its full size in 3–5 weeks and spontaneous regression occurs in 2–12 months. The lesions are usually single and occur anywhere on the body where sebaceous glands exist but particularly on exposed areas such as the arms and around the nose.

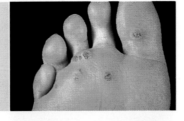

Figure 8.23.
Plantar warts.

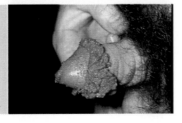

Figure 8.24.
Genital warts.

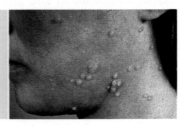

Figure 8.26.
Mollusca contagiosum.

Figure 8.27.
Keratoacanthoma.

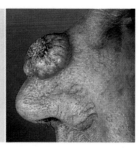

The lesion is a discrete, domed nodule 1–2 cm in diameter and 2–3 millimetres high. The firm, smooth, outer rim is skin coloured but the central core is of hard, irregular, keratinized black material. The major problems of the lesion are disfigurement, difficulty in differentiating it from squamous cell carcinoma and occasionally a residual deep pitted scar. For these reasons keratoacanthomas are sometimes excised, although histologically they can also be mistaken for squamous cell carcinomas.

Hypertropic scars and keloids

Hypertropic scars and keloids (p. 81; *Figure 8.28*) are due to the overproduction of collagen tissue in a wound. In the former this is often due to abnormal local conditions such as infection, a foreign body, undue tension across the wound and incisions across the skin creases. The scar continues increasing in width and thickness for up to 2 to 3 months. However, within a year there is often shrinkage and the initial browny-red discoloration has faded. The abnormality does not necessarily include the whole length of the scar and excision is not usually followed by a recurrence.

Keloid is often familial and commonly in black-skinned individuals. The hypertrophy includes the wound and also the tissues on either side. Proliferation continues for 6 to 12 months and can produce a tumour-like overgrowth. The scar is often itchy, tender and painful. Keloid is rare in infancy and in old age, and reduces in its severity from about 30 years onwards. In extreme examples, the overgrowth can

be pedunculated; the epithelial covering is normal. Excision of the lesion is likely to be followed by recurrence.

Histiocytoma – dermatofibroma

Histiocytomas (*Figure 8.29*) are benign, dermal tumours, predominantly of fibrous origin, covered with normal epithelium. They are asymptomatic and take a number of years to grow to their full size, which can be 5–20 mm across. They are sited predominantly on the limbs and are well-circumscribed, red-brown, smooth-surfaced lesions. Their main importance is that, as the lesions increase in size, their pigmentation can be mistaken for a malignant melanoma. A sclerosing angioma is a variant containing prominent vascular elements.

Pyogenic granuloma

Pyogenic granuloma (*Figure 8.30*) is an exuberant overgrowth of granulation tissue producing a polypoid lesion typically 7–10 millimetres across. The abnormal inflammatory response is usually in response to a foreign body, such as a splinter, and develops within a few days. The trauma may be minor and not remembered by the patient. Resolution is very slow and excision is sometimes necessary.

The lesions are single and sited over exposed areas such as the hands, arms and face. Initially they are soft, friable and red, and bleed easily. They become firmer and less friable once surface epithelialization is complete, after which they are skin coloured. Later, ulceration can make the differential diagnosis from malignant lesions more difficult. If superadded

Figure 8.29.
Histiocytoma.

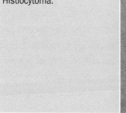

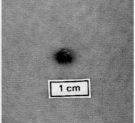

1 cm

Figure 8.28.
Keloid of the neck.

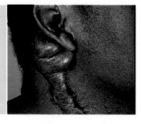

Figure 8.30.
Pyogenic granuloma.

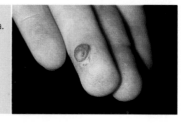

Figure 8.31.
Hyperkeratotic heel.

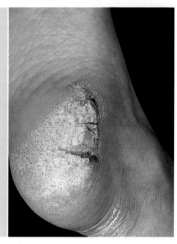

Figure 8.32.
Corn.

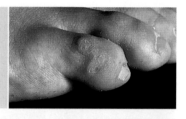

Figure 8.33.
Dermoid cyst.

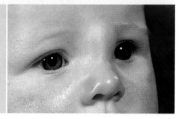

infection becomes a prominent feature, local lymph nodes may be enlarged. In this situation there may be associated pain, but this is unusual.

Callosities and corns

Callosities (*Figure 8.31*) are due to excessive skin keratinization and occur as a protective measure over an area of intermittent pressure. This is commonly in the feet – especially the inframedial aspect of the great toe and the heel – but may also occur over the dorsal aspect of deformed toes and pressure sites in other limb deformities.

Corns (*Figure 8.32*) are callosities over focal pressure points, usually over a bony prominence. A central core of keratin is compressed into the skin in the same way as a plantar wart, producing pain.

On examination the keratin of callosities marks out the pressure area and is continuous around its margins with normal skin. The callosities surrounding neuropathic ulcers can be particularly prominent. The central core of a corn is palpable as a nodule of whitish degenerate cells.

Dermoid cysts

Dermoid cysts (*Figure 8.33*) are due to the sequestration of epithelial elements deep to the skin surface. Congenital dermoid cysts occur along the lines of embryological skin fusion. Common sites are the medial and lateral ends of the eyebrow (internal and external angular dermoids), sublingual (deep or superficial to the mylohyoid muscle), post-auricular, and pre- and post-sacral. The latter may expand within the spinal canal, causing compression of the cauda equina. The lesions may be present at birth but are usually noted in the first two years; they may occasionally be first seen in adulthood. Their prime symptom is their unsightly appearance but they rarely give rise to pain, infection or discharge.

The lesions are usually single and slow growing. They are smooth, spherical and mobile, enlarging to 1–2 cm in diameter; sublingual cysts can reach 3–5 cm. The cysts are lined with keratinized, stratified squamous epithelium and may contain other epithelial elements such as hair and sebaceous material. These influence their physical signs since they do not usually transilluminate and may indent rather than fluctuate.

Implanted, acquired, dermoid cysts occur post injury. The injury is usually remembered and the overlying scar is visible. They typically occur on the fingers, are 4–6 millimetres in diameter and firm in consistency. They contain keratinized, squamous epithelium but not usually sebaceous material. They may be confused with a sebaceous cyst but, although there is often skin tethering, no punctum is present.

Sebaceous cysts – epidermoid cyst; wen

Sebaceous cysts (*Figures 8.34, 8.35*) are derived from hair follicles, their contents being altered keratin. They represent one of the commonest skin lesions, occurring at any age after childhood. They are often multiple and occur in any hair-bearing site on the body, commonly the trunk, face and neck, and particularly the scalp and scrotum; they do not occur on the palms and soles. They are associated with osteomas and intestinal polyps in Gardner's syndrome. They are unsightly and may become painful if there is superadded inflammation or abscess formation. The inflammatory response is usually a foreign body, granulomatous reaction. They can discharge toothpaste-like, whitish, granular material with an unpleasant smell.

Figure 8.34.
Sebaceous cyst.

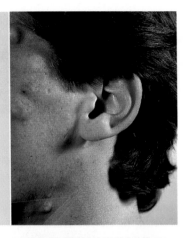

Figure 8.35.
Scalp sebaceous cyst.

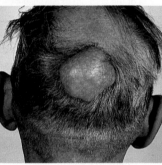

Figure 8.36.
Sebaceous horn.

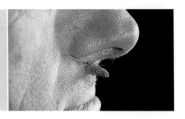

fluctuate or indent. They are rarely malignant. Hidradenomas are one of the causes of turban tumours of the scalp, the deformity being better known for its title than for its incidence. Other causes are multiple nodal basal cell carcinomas, plexiform neurofibromas and multiple cylindromas.

The lesions are well defined and hemispherical, growing slowly from 1–2 cm across. They lie in the subcutaneous tissue but are tethered to the skin by the blocked duct, there being a pit on the surface at the site of the hair follicle. Gentle squeezing of the skin over the cyst demonstrates this point of tethering though the punctum is sometimes difficult to demonstrate, particularly over the scalp; when present, it is diagnostic.

Sebaceous cysts may occasionally ulcerate and, in these circumstances, can look very much like a malignant skin lesion. They are then termed a Cock's peculiar tumour. The concretions of a sebaceous cyst can be gradually excreted and build up into a hard, conical sebaceous horn (*Figure 8.36*).

Other tumours of skin appendages

These are rare – they include leiomyomas from the smooth erector pili muscle of the hair, hidradenomas, sebaceous adenomas, cylindromas and trichoepitheliomas, these being benign tumours of the gland and lining of the hair follicle.

Hidradenomas are tumours of sweat glands, frequently multiple and commonly on the scalp. They can be from a few millimetres to a number of cm across, the latter producing disfigurement. They are soft, boggy swellings but they do not

Premalignant and malignant lesions of the skin

Sun-induced lesions

Exposure to sunlight can produce a number of skin disorders and aggravate many existing conditions. Scantily clad sun-worshippers are at risk; blond and red-headed individuals are particularly susceptible. There is a high incidence of skin disorders in Australia, South Africa and the southern states of the USA. Also at risk are outdoor workers such as fishermen, farmers and labourers.

Sunburn can occur within an hour of exposure in sensitive-skinned individuals, producing erythema, blistering and, later, peeling. Continued exposure may give rise to severe, permanent skin damage even at an early age although changes are usually degenerative and age related. The signs of ageing are a fragile skin with loss of elasticity, increased keratosis, vascular changes such as spider naevi and angioma, telangiectasia, venous lakes, and pronounced sebaceous glands. Of particular concern is the predisposition to premalignant and malignant skin lesions including solar keratosis, Bowen's disease, basal cell carcinoma, squamous cell carcinoma and malignant melanoma. Fortunately solar-induced malignant lesions do not usually metastasize.

Solar keratosis

Solar keratoses (*Figure 8.37*) are hyperkeratotic skin lesions related to prolonged exposure to sunlight. They may undergo malignant change. The lesions usually occur in the elderly and out-of-door workers and are sited over the tops of the ears, the face and the backs of the hands and fingers. The lesions are usually painless but scratching or minor trauma may produce bleeding.

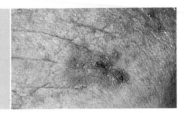

Figure 8.37.
Solar keratosis.

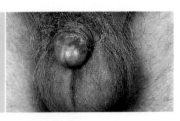

Figure 8.38.
Bowen's disease of
the penis.

Solar keratotic skin lesions are discrete, scaly, irregular patches. The keratinized surface may project occasionally, producing a grey-brown cutaneous horn. These lesions can catch on clothing and bleed. A lesion is said to have undergone malignant change once cellular dysplasia involves the full thickness of the epithelium.

Bowen's disease and erythroplasia of Queyrat

The lesions of Bowen's disease (*Figure 8.38*) are irregularly shaped but well-defined plaques that may be mistaken for a patch of eczema. They therefore present late, and any such lesion which does not respond to topical steroids should be biopsied.

The lesions vary in size from 5 millimetres to a few cm across. They are beefy red, erythematous areas, slightly raised, with a scaly crust on the surface. The skin beneath the crust is moist and papilliform. Malignant changes produce papules and nodules.

Dysplastic changes may extend from the basal layer to the surface, and the lesion is then defined as malignant. The terms carcinoma *in situ* and intraepidermal carcinoma are also applied at this stage.

Erythroplasia of Queyrat (p. 354) has identical features to Bowen's disease but is situated on the penis.

Leukoplakia

Leukoplakia can occur along the margins of the lips (p. 195) and on the vulva, although is most common in the oral cavity. It is a white coating of the mucous membrane which does not rub off, as opposed to candida and some other infections. The lesions are the result of multiple trauma such as from sharp teeth and dentures, spicy foods, sepsis, syphilis, pipe smoking and betel-nut (areca-nut) chewing.

The majority of lesions are benign but some may show dysplastic changes and there is an incidence of 13% change to squamous cell carcinoma. This incidence rises to two-thirds in the floor of the mouth where all lesions must be biopsied and carefully monitored. **Erythroplasia** is a pink coating, the cellular abnormality in this instance showing *in situ* or invasive squamous cell carcinoma in all cases.

Squamous cell carcinoma

Squamous cell carcinoma (*Figures 8.39* and *8.40*) is the commonest primary skin malignancy, usually occurring in the elderly. There are a number of predisposing factors including chemical hydrocarbons, tar and mineral oils. One of the most important hydrocarbons is soot – the development of carcinoma of the scrotum in chimney sweeps was the first recognized carcinogenic agent. There is a high incidence of skin cancer in patients living in tropical countries, the carcinoma sometimes being preceded by an area of solar keratosis. Skin cancer can be induced by exposure to X-rays; this was much commoner before the realization of the harmful effects of X-rays and appropriate preventive measures being introduced. Arsenic and chrome compounds are also carcinogenic agents.

Squamous cell carcinoma may follow chronic infection, an example being the malignant change in the edge of a chronic ulcer – **Marjolin's ulcer**. These changes can be easily missed since there is less invasion or skin eversion, and the clinician must always be on the lookout for nodular appearances and

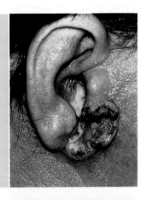

Figure 8.39.
Squamous carcinoma of the
ear.

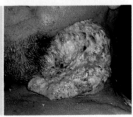

Figure 8.40.
Squamous carcinoma of the
neck.

any changes in the skin edge in venous ulcers or post-burns scarring and chronic discharging sinuses, such as osteo-myelitis. Malignant changes of this form are not uncommon over the shin in central Africa. Malignant change can occur in the tuberculous skin scarring of lupus vulgaris.

Histologically there is proliferation of the prickle cell layer – acanthosis – and keratosis. Keratin is often arranged in onion-like, concentric layers, termed epithelial pearls – not to be confused with the pearly edge of basal cell carcinoma. Lesions are usually well differentiated; they occur in the skin and the stratified squamous epithelium of the lips, mouth, pharynx, oesophagus and anal canal, the glans penis, uterine cervix and in metaplastic changes in respiratory epithelium.

Initial signs are of a round nodule. With progressive enlargement this becomes irregular and craggy and soon ulcerates. Enlargement is usually over a few months. The ulcer has a crusty or horny covering but as it becomes deeper it penetrates the dermis exposing underlying tissues such as tendon, bone, cartilage and joints; the base bleeds easily and is very necrotic. The discharge may be copious, purulent, bloody, foul smelling and debilitating. The ulcer edge is everted and local invasion of the surrounding tissues produces induration which is visible beyond the ulcer margin.

The rate of onset, progressive deepening and increased eversion are typical of malignant change. There may be associated thrombosis and the ulcer may penetrate adjacent vessels, producing severe and possibly fatal haemorrhage. Metastasis is usually by lymphatics and local nodes are commonly involved. However, one-third of these prove to be due to infection rather than secondary malignancy. Metastases can occur through the bloodstream but this is uncommon.

The differential diagnoses of squamous cell carcinoma include solar keratosis, keratoacanthoma, pyogenic granuloma, seborrhoeic warts, basal cell carcinoma and malignant melanoma.

Basal cell carcinoma

Basal cell carcinomas (*Figures 8.41* and *8.42*) are due to a malignant change in the basal layer of the epidermis. They are

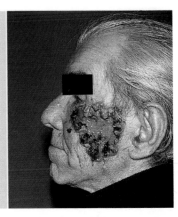

Figure 8.42.
Extensive basal cell carcinoma of the left side of the cheek.

locally malignant and undergo slow, steady enlargement, invading adjacent skin and being very destructive if left untreated. They do not metastasize. Lesions are commonest in the elderly, being twice as common in males as in females. There is also a high incidence in sun-worshippers. The slow rate of growth of basal cell carcinomas often delays medical consultation and the lesions have usually grown to a centimetre across before advice is sought. They are not usually painful.

Although the lesions are commonly sited above a line drawn from the angle of the mouth to the ear lobe, they may occur anywhere, particularly on exposed skin and therefore are common in such people as farm workers, fishermen and labourers. The lesions start as a nodule with a slightly transparent, superficial epidermal layer giving a cystic appearance. Occasionally a lesion may be pigmented. The next stage is central erosion. Although there may be some healing, ulceration recurs and progresses to scab formation, the scab falling off intermittently and with slight bleeding.

The edge is characteristic and diagnostic, being raised and rolled, with a pearly appearance. It may be also slightly pinkish due to telangiectasia running over the surface. If untreated, local invasion progresses both into the underlying tissues and circumferentially; the edge becoming irregular. It is often termed a geographic edge, this irregularity giving rise to the original nomenclature of a rodent ulcer. There is no tendency to nodal metastases. The lesions can be differentiated from squamous cell carcinoma by their original nodularity and cystic appearance with or without pigmentation and by their early superficial ulceration. The rolled pearly edge and the late geographic spread are also diagnostic.

Paget's disease

Paget's disease (p. 43) is an eczema-like skin lesion due to intraduct carcinoma invading the lymphatics of the epithelium.

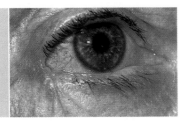

Figure 8.41.
Basal cell carcinoma. Right lower eyelid, lateral aspect.

It is usually seen in the nipple but very occasionally occurs in the glans penis.

The lesions are red, weeping, crusty and scaly plaques, involving the nipple and surrounding areola. Because of its eczema-like appearance, the lesion may be disregarded by the patient until there is retraction, ulceration and destruction of the nipple or until an underlying mass or regional lymph nodes become palpable.

Kaposi's sarcoma

Kaposi's sarcoma (*Figure 8.43*) is a neoplastic proliferation of fibroblasts accompanied by chronic inflammatory changes, endothelial proliferation and haemorrhage. The typical skin lesions are purple–brown, discrete nodules or plaques and as they progress they may become elevated and form an angiomatous tumour that may ulcerate and bleed. The condition may also progress to nodal and visceral involvement.

Before the advent of AIDS, Kaposi's sarcoma was very rare in Europe and usually involved the skin of the lower limb in males over the age of 60 years. It ran a relatively benign course. An African form of the disease occurred in young children, with widespread involvement of the lymphatic system and usually running a slow, fatal course. Its geographical distribution was similar to that of Burkitt's lymphoma (p. 000). With the advent of AIDS it is now the commonest opportunistic neoplastic lesion.

Cutaneous lymphoma

Lymphomas may affect every organ in the body but some forms predominantly affect the skin. Examples are mycosis fungoides and Sézary syndrome, which are both related to infiltration with T-cell lymphoma, producing similar lesions. Some of these features may be related to the skin response to tumour cells rather than tumour mass.

Mycosis fungoides is found in middle-aged men, early lesions being non-specific, flat, red, scaly eruptions suggestive

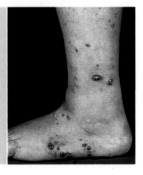

Figure 8.43.
Kaposi's sarcoma. Left lower leg.

of chronic eczema or psoriasis. However, they have a typical distribution, often over non-exposed areas, and are often pruritic. Progression may take up to 20 years before larger, multiple, irregular and ulcerated lesions appear with varied tumour formation, lymphadenopathy and visceral involvement.

Secondary skin tumours

The skin may be infiltrated by cutaneous and deep secondary tumours. Examples of the latter are sarcomas of the subcutaneous tissue, muscle and bone, perforating through to the surface. Tumour cells may be implanted in the skin at the time of surgical incision and theoretically during percutaneous skin biopsy of deeper lesions. Recurrent tumour masses may also have skin involvement. Skin infiltration by lymphomas has been considered in the previous section, and systemic Hodgkin's disease can present in this way.

Satellite tumours along lymphatic channels are seen in malignant melanoma and, occasionally, tumours from bloodstream spread, examples being from the breast, lung, kidney and parts of the gut. These nodules are usually within the dermis; histological examination of biopsy material may diagnose an unsuspected primary lesion.

Melanotic skin lesions

The pigment melanin is produced by melanocytes. These are derived from neural crest cells that migrate during development and are scattered throughout the basal layer of the skin epidermis. Although the number of melanocytes is similar in all races, the amount of melanin produced varies between black- and white-skinned individuals and also increases in response to UV light.

Benign overgrowth of melanocytes – i.e. hamartomatous lesions – are termed moles or pigmented naevi. Pigmented lesions may also be produced by an overproduction of melanin from a normal number and distribution of melanocytes – e.g. a freckle – or by an increased number of melanocytes within the basal layer of epidermis, as seen in lentigo and the pigmentation of Peutz–Jeghers syndrome.

In order to diagnose and treat malignant melanoma as early as possible it is important to recognize typical benign lesions and to examine all doubtful lesions histologically.

Pigmented naevi – moles

Moles (*Figures 8.44* and *8.45*) are very common and most Caucasians have at least one at birth, the number increasing throughout life. Moles may regress or disappear during

Figure 8.44.
Pigmented polyp.

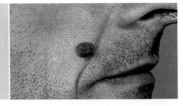

Figure 8.45.
Pigmented warty papilloma.

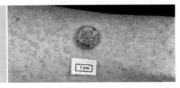

Figure 8.46.
Junctional naevus.

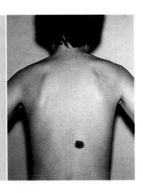

Figure 8.47.
Compound naevus.

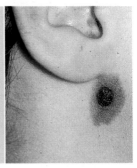

childhood; pigmentation may also increase but malignant change is very rare before puberty. Moles are less obvious in black-skinned individuals but are seen on palms and soles. Malignancy is uncommon in these races.

The lesions may occur anywhere on the body and are usually discrete, 2–4 millimetres in diameter. The colour varies from very pale to black, as does the amount of hair. Symptoms are usually cosmetic but rough and protruding lesions may catch clothing. Although pain can occur because of trauma to the lesion or due to inflammation of sebaceous glands within it, it is an unusual symptom, as are bleeding or itching. The clinician must always be on the lookout for any changes in a lesion suggesting malignant change. Lymphadenopathy is not a feature of pigmented naevi.

Proliferating melanocytic lesions can be divided histologically into three groups by the position of the melanocytes:

- **Junctional** (*Figure 8.46*) when the proliferation is within the basal epithelial layer.
- **Intradermal** when the proliferation is deep to the basal layer within the dermis.
- **Compound** (*Figure 8.47*) consisting of both junctional and intradermal components.

Junctional naevi often occur at or around puberty and are usually darkly pigmented because of their proximity to the surface. They are usually slightly raised lesions. The cells of most migrate into the dermis after puberty, accompanied by some paling of the lesion.

Intradermal naevi are paler than junctional naevi due to the thickness of the overlying epidermis. A **blue naevus** is an example of this type where clumps of heavily pigmented melanocytes are covered by a normal, smooth, shiny, epidermal layer. The lesion can grow to over a centimetre across,

is commonest in the young – but can occur at any age – and has no malignant potential.

Hairy moles (*Figure 8.48*) are another example of intradermal naevi. The associated sebaceous glands may become infected and cause minor inflammatory symptoms and signs, mimicking malignant change, although the lesions do not have any malignant potential.

Compound naevi are probably due to migration of junctional melanocytes into the dermis. The junctional melanocytes are less mature than intradermal melanocytes and have a higher malignant potential. **Smooth moles** may originate from any of the three categories.

Junctional activity in melanocytes is suggestive of malignant change. This includes cell mitoses and pleomorphism, invasion of the epidermis and dermis by the lesion and lymphocytic infiltration. An exception to this rule is when these

Figure 8.48.
Hairy mole.

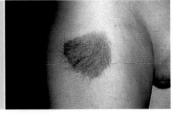

changes occur in the naevus before puberty. A specific example is the **juvenile naevus** (*Figure 8.49*) in which junctional activity is present in a compound naevus with particularly large-celled pleomorphism. As these lesions may present in later life, their characteristics must be recognized to avoid misdiagnosis of malignancy.

Freckles

A freckle is an overproduction of melanin from a normal population of melanocytes. Freckles are common and occur particularly on exposed areas such as the face and dorsum of the hands. They are pale brown lesions, 2–4 millimetres in diameter, and are usually multiple. They have no malignant potential.

Lentigo

A Hutchinson's lentigo (*Figure 8.50*) is due to an increased number of melanocytes within the basal layer of epidermis. It is usually found in the elderly, grows slowly and is darkly pigmented. The irregular area may be a number of cm across, usually flat, but may be a slightly raised plaque or have flat nodules within it. Lentigenes are usually found on the neck and the back of the hand. Although lentigenes are benign they do have the potential for malignant change into the superficial spreading variety of malignant melanoma.

Café-au-lait spots

These pale brown, flat, multiple lesions are usually a few millimetres in diameter but may be larger patches; they are present at birth. The lesions can be associated with neurofibromatosis – particularly if greater than five in number – and, occasionally, phaeochromocytomas. Histologically, the lesion can be either due to increased melanin production or an increased number of basal melanocytes. However, they have no malignant potential.

Pigmented lesions in the Peutz–Jeghers syndrome

These lesions (p. 290; *Figure 23.25*) – associated with multiple intestinal polyposis – are usually found over the mucous membrane of the lips and circumorally. They are 1–2 mm across and asymptomatic. Although they are due to an increased number of basal melanocytes they have no malignant potential.

Malignant melanoma

Malignant melanomas are highly malignant tumours of melanocytes. Approximately half develop in a pre-existing benign lesion, particularly compound naevi and lentigenes, the histological signs of junctional activity (see above) being present. The remaining lesions occur spontaneously in previously normal skin.

Melanoma occurs predominantly in Caucasians, particularly those exposed to the sunlight of subtropical zones. The highest incidence is in northern Australia but it is increasing in northern Europe. They are unusual in black-skinned individuals although Africans are susceptible to malignant melanomas of the palms and soles.

Short, sharp, repeated exposure to UV light is more harmful than an accumulated effect. This suggests a possible immunological carcinogenic response. Also, in keeping with this, is the fact that the lesions can occur anywhere on the body. They may occur at any age but are very rare before puberty and are unusual under 20; they are commonest between 20 and 30 years of age. The lentigenous group occur in the elderly (*Figure 8.50*). There is often a family history of atypical or multiple pigmented naevi, or malignant melanoma, and it is essential that individuals with this history avoid the sun or use appropriate screening agents.

Although the lesions can occur anywhere, they are commoner over the limbs, head and neck. Be suspicious of pigmented lesions on palms and soles and under the nail. Among common presentations are choroidal melanoma in the eye and lesions in the oral or anal mucosa. The incidence in males and females is approximately equal, but in males trunk lesions are commoner; in females the lower limbs. The latter also have the best prognosis of malignant melanoma. Multiple lesions are rare.

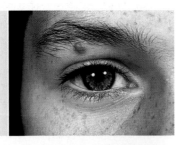

Figure 8.49.
Juvenile naevus.

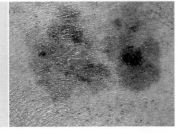

Figure 8.50.
Hutchinson's lentigo.

Figure 8.51.
Nodular malignant melanoma.

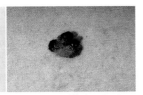

Figure 8.53.
Secondary malignant deposits following removal of a distal primary malignant melanoma.

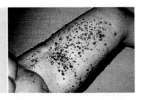

Figure 8.52.
Malignant melanoma with involvement of cervical lymph nodes.

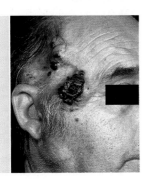

Figure 8.54.
Recurrence of a malignant melanoma, post excision.

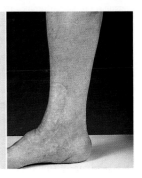

Clinically two main varieties of lesions occur: superficial spreading melanoma, which is the least aggressive, and nodular melanoma (*Figure 8.51*), these lesions being more invasive, producing early nodal involvement (*Figure 8.52*) and having the worst prognosis. There can be an element of both these varieties in a lesion. Some authorities classify lentigo maligna melanoma as a separate entity and lentigenes as a form of *in situ* malignancy. Acral lentiginous melanoma is a rare form that occurs beneath a nail and is the form seen in Afro-Asian races, often on the palms and soles.

The lesions are generally poorly differentiated with abundant mitotic figures and can increase rapidly in size over a few weeks. They are highly malignant and usually relentlessly progressive, yet they can also be unpredictable and occasionally spontaneous regression, even of nodal metastases, has been recorded. Secondary spread may become evident after the removal of the primary lesion (*Figures 8.53* and *8.54*).

A number of clinical features should alert the clinician to suspect primary malignant melanoma or malignant change in a pre-existing naevus. Its rapid growth both in size and thickness is typical, the patient presenting on cosmetic grounds or being suspicious that the lesion is malignant. The surface becomes irregular, crusted and ulcerated, with possibly some bleeding. Pigmentation is usually increased and there may be a halo of pigmentation around the lesion. Occasionally an amelanotic variety of melanoma is encountered, and these lesions still can produce melanin, the cells being dopamine positive. A pink halo is suggestive of an inflammatory response to a developing malignant lesion. The edge of the pigmentation becomes irregular and notched and

there may be satellite pigmented lesions beyond the central area (*Figure 8.55*). The surface is likely to become nodular.

Pain is a late sign but itching is not uncommon, together with bleeding, once ulceration has occurred. Nodal involvement is highly suggestive of malignant change, as are systemic symptoms such as weight loss, the dyspnoea of pulmonary involvement and pleural effusions and jaundice, suggesting liver secondaries. A number of attempts have been made at classifying malignant melanomas on clinical grounds. Stage I is defined when the lesion and any satellites are less than 5 cm across; Stage II indicates additional nodal involvement and Stage III visceral spread. More useful classifications take into account the thickness of the lesion, either measured directly or related to the depth of cutaneous involvement. Clark describes five levels:

1. Lesion confined to epidermis.
2. Lesion extending into the superficial papillary dermis.
3. Lesion reaching the junction of the reticular dermis.
4. Lesion reaching the base of the reticular dermis.
5. Subcutaneous spread.

Spread to layer 3 and beyond carries the worst prognosis, this being equivalent to a thickness of 0.76 millimetres.

Figure 8.55.
Malignant melanoma with satellites.

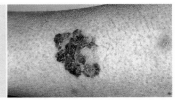

Cutaneous vascular lesions

Cutaneous vascular lesions comprise any one or combinations of arteries, capillaries, veins and lymphatics. Combinations are often termed haemangiomas or lymphangiomas although they are actually overgrowths of embryonic tissue – i.e. hamartomas – rather than neoplasms. Vascular malformations (p. 389) are developmental anomalies. They may also comprise more than one vascular element and may have an associated arteriovenous shunt.

Glomus tumours have vascular and neural elements. The term 'naevus' implies a congenital pigmented lesion and is used whether the coloration is from melanin or blood. Acquired cutaneous vascular lesions include a number of forms of capillary telangiectasia and a few, rare sarcomas. Vascular lesions can usually be emptied of their blood content and are, therefore, compressible. On emptying they blanch although there may be some fixed haemorrhagic brown staining. Telangiectasia can be blanched and observed by compression with a glass slide.

Telangiectasia

Telangiectases (*Figure 8.56*) are dilated, single arterioles, capillaries or venules. One or two are found in most individuals but greater than six is abnormal. They can be congenital and familial, examples being Fabry's disease – lysosomal storage disease, where the lesions appear after puberty over the lower trunk and thighs – and Rendu–Osler–Weber syndrome (hereditary haemorrhagic telangiectasia). The latter is transmitted as an inherited dominant trait, the telangiectases are sited periorally and along the length of the gut. The latter lesions occasionally give rise to haemorrhagic problems.

Telangiectases are common in collagen disorders (lupus erythematosus; scleroderma; dermatomyositis; post-radiotherapy), but worse in blushing (rosacea; carcinoid; oestrogen imbalance; pregnancy; liver disease) and with loss of supporting tissues (steroid atrophy; Cushing's; exposure to sun and wind; solar elastosis; ageing).

The abnormality is of the supporting tissue rather than the endothelial lining of the vessel. The lesions are flat and red or red–purple in colour. They vary in size from pin-point to pin-head and may be punctate, linear or spider-like in form. Spider naevi are particularly common in liver disease. Occasionally telangiectases are larger, raised and scaling. They do not thrombose and rarely ulcerate or bleed. They persist into old age.

Strawberry naevus

Strawberry naevi (*Figure 8.57*) are congenital intradermal collections of blood vessels that usually present within a few days of birth. They then grow rapidly and often alarmingly for 4–6 weeks and eventually stabilize at 6–12 months. The majority of lesions regress spontaneously but this may take from 2–6 years. They are usually 1–2 cm in diameter but may be much larger. As they are often visible in the head, neck and limbs, they cause much parental concern.

The lesions are covered with smooth epidermis and their pink, red and pitted surface provides the typical strawberry appearance; they may be multiple. Strawberry naevi are well demarcated, mobile over the subcutaneous tissue and compressible. The lesions can bleed with minor trauma – e.g. if under a nappy – but this can be controlled by gentle pressure. The bleeding tendency can be accentuated by platelet sequestration in some larger lesions. There is no nodal involvement. On resolution there may be some wrinkling of the skin but only a few residual telangiectases.

Port wine stain

This is a deep purple, irregular area of disfiguring discoloration occurring in early childhood and persisting throughout life (*Figure 8.58*). The lesion may become darker but does not enlarge relative to the rest of the body unless there is an associated arterial shunt. The latter may accompany other vascular malformations (p. 391). The lesions are usually flat, and compression produces blanching. There may be some surrounding prominent veins.

Campbell de Morgan spots

Campbell de Morgan spots (*Figure 8.59*) are bright red, well-circumscribed capillary abnormalities of 2–3 millimetres in

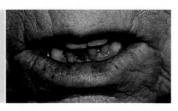

Figure 8.56.
Telangiectasia of the lips in a patient with scleroderma.

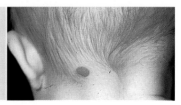

Figure 8.57.
Strawberry naevi.

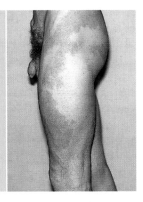

Figure 8.58.
Port wine staining over the lateral aspect of the left thigh.

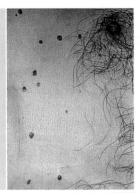

Figure 8.59.
Campbell de Morgan spots on the trunk.

diameter. They occur in most individuals after middle age and are usually on the trunk, occasionally on the limbs but rarely on the face. Although they arrive individually they are usually multiple. The aetiology of the spots is unknown and they have no clinical significance.

Lymphangiomas

Lymphatic abnormalities can be divided into cystic, solid and cutaneous; they may also be a mixture of these forms and can contribute to larger vascular malformations.

Cysts – cystic hygromas (p. 217; *Figure 16.6*) – are subcutaneous, multilocular, non-communicating lymph channels that contain clear, colourless fluid. They occur in babies, particularly in the neck and across the groins and axillae. They can grow to a large size and, in the neck, produce tracheal compression. The lesions fluctuate and are brilliantly transilluminant. Although it may be possible to squeeze fluid from one lobule to another, lesions cannot be compressed. Lesions are painless and have no lymph node involvement. They tend to regress over the course of a few years.

Solid lymphangiomas are collections of lymphatic tissue with a variable amount of fibrosis and lymphocytic infiltration. Although they contain endothelium-lined channels, they do not transilluminate or fluctuate. They appear soon after birth and extend diffusely through the tissues of a region, making complete excision impossible. They tend to grow with the child and show little regression.

Subcutaneous lymphangiomas – lymphangioma circumscripta – are vesicular lesions, resembling a poorly spread spoonful of pale or red–brown caviare. They appear soon after birth and show little tendency to regress. The lesions are situated at the junction of the limbs with the trunk but can spread extensively. The vesicles contain clear, yellowish fluid that is not compressible. The vesicles may become secon-

darily infected with some associated lymphadenopathy. Although the vesicles appear superficial, excision has to include the full depth of the skin, to the subcutaneous tissue, to avoid recurrence.

Glomus tumours

A glomus is a specialized arteriovenous anastomosis found particularly around the nail beds and concerned with heat regulation. It is surrounded by large, pale cells and is heavily innervated. Glomus tumours (*Figure 8.60*) are small, discrete, firm, benign nodules rarely greater than 1 cm across and made up of the same components. They would go unnoticed if it were not for the extreme sensitivity of some lesions in which even gentle trauma or temperature change can precipitate severe, sharp or throbbing pain. The pain may radiate and persist.

The tumours are subcutaneous, they can occur anywhere over the body – but are usually at the extremities of the limbs – and are often in a subunguinal position. The lesions have a bluish tinge because of their blood content and subunguinal lesions – which are only 1–2 millimetres across – can be seen as a bluish area or silhouetted on transillumination. The symptoms are dramatically abolished by tumour excision. An unusual and rare variant of the glomus tumour is a 5–10 cm benign, submucosal lesion presenting in the pyloric end of the stomach.

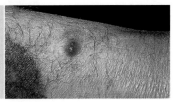

Figure 8.60.
Glomus tumour on right forearm.

Lymphangiosarcoma; angiosarcoma

These are highly malignant, rare tumours (*Figures 8.61* and *8.62*). Their relevance to the skin is that either may develop in long-standing, massive lymphoedema, whether primary or secondary, including upper limb, post-radical mastectomy. The course of the tumours is massive, relentless enlargement. They are very vascular and may bleed, producing early pulmonary metastases. Although radiosensitive, radical amputation is the only curative option, when this is possible. Angiosarcomas may also produce massive tumours within the liver, the spleen or in bone. Both tumours are usually seen in young adults.

Subcutaneous lesions

Lipoma

Lipomas (*Figure 8.63*) are very common, benign, subcutaneous tumours. They occur at any age but are less common in children. They are usually asymptomatic but large lesions can present with cosmetic problems. The lesions grow slowly and, as they have similar features to the surrounding fat, they have usually reached 2–3 cm across before a patient presents. Most lesions remain less than 5 cm across but occasionally can be four or five times this size and become more hemispherical or pedunculated, rather than the usual dome shape.

Lipomas have characteristic signs. They are smooth, soft and slightly lobulated, due to thin fibrous septa. The edge slips away from the examining finger – slippage sign. They transilluminate, fluctuate and are mobile with no attachments to skin or deep fascia. They are non-tender and non-reducible and have no associated lymphadenopathy. The overlying skin is generally normal but there may be stretch marks, thinning or prominent veins with large lesions. Lipomas may be multiple; a rare condition of painful lipomatosis is known as Dercum's disease. The lesions show no malignant potential, liposarcomas occurring *de novo*, usually retroperitoneally or in the mediastinum.

Fat necrosis can occur in lipomas if they are situated over a prominent area and subjected to repeated trauma. It is also seen after trauma to the breast and after subcutaneous injection, such as insulin. The necrotic area is a hard, irregular, tender plaque that may be tethered to the skin or deep fascia. In the breast, the lesion can be misdiagnosed as malignant change.

Xanthoma

Xanthomas (*Figure 8.64*) are yellow cutaneous polypoid lesions of lipid-filled macrophages sited within the dermis. They commonly occur in the upper eyelid and are particularly prominent in patients with hyperlipidaemia.

Neurofibromas

Neurofibromas are common, benign tumours containing both fibrous and neuromatous tissue elements but neuromas (p. 418) and fibromas are surprisingly uncommon. Other fibroid lesions are occasionally encountered. More than one neurofibroma may be present but multiple lesions

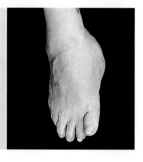

Figure 8.62.
Angiosarcoma within the right foot.

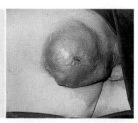

Figure 8.61.
Lymphangiosarcoma.

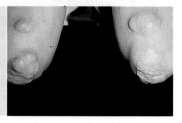

Figure 8.64.
Xanthomatosis on the posterior aspect of both elbows.

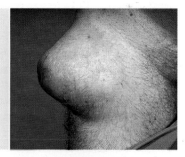

Figure 8.63.
Lipoma over the lateral aspect of the right thigh.

usually indicate the existence of von Recklinghausen's disease (below).

Isolated neurofibromas usually occur in adults and can be anywhere over the body but are attached to a nerve sheath. They are usually asymptomatic but pressure applied to the lesion may produce distal tingling and, if they are sited in a confined space such as an intervertebral foramen, they may produce nerve compression and symptoms from the damaged nerve. Single lesions are often fusiform and 4–6 millimetres across. Because of the nerve attachment mobility is from side to side but not longitudinally. There is no tethering to skin or deep fascia. There is no nodal involvement and no malignant potential.

Neurofibromatosis

Von Recklinghausen's disease – type 1 neurofibromatosis – is a congenital and familial disease, inherited as an autosomal dominant trait. Any patient seen is likely to have one parent and siblings with the disease. However, different members of the family may display a wide range of abnormalities ranging from a few nodules or pigmented areas to gross deformity. The degree of parental involvement is not a good predictor for the degree of expression in the next generation.

The neurofibromas are present at birth and increase in number. Lesions vary from a few millimetres to a few centimetres. They may be pedunculated (*Figure 8.65*). They are usually softer than single lesions and squashable. They are not usually painful and there is no nodal involvement.

There are a number of associated abnormalities. Café-au-lait spots (*Figure 8.66*) are characteristic and diagnostic of von Recklinghausen's disease if more than six in number or a patch more than 1.5 cm across. Fibroepithelial skin tags are common.

About 5% of patients develop neurofibrosarcoma. Other associated tumours are ganglioneuromas, phaeochromocytomas, gliomas and meningiomas. The phaeochromocytomas present in 1% of von Recklinghausen's disease, making up 5% of the total; any unexplained hypertensive patients should be examined for café-au-lait spots. There is diffuse, cerebral dysgenesis in 10% of patients, accompanied by a varying degree of mental retardation.

Central neurofibromatosis – type 2 neurofibromatosis – is characterized by bilateral acoustic and spinal neuromas. Hearing should be checked and the possibility of nerve root compression considered since spinal tumours may be dumbbell shaped and partly inside and partly outside the vertebral canal. This condition also shows autosomal dominant inheritance.

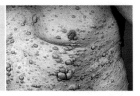

Figure 8.65.
Multiple neurofibromatosis.

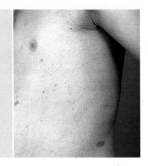

Figure 8.66.
Café-au-lait spots.

Plexiform neurofibromatosis

Plexiform neurofibromatosis is a primary abnormality in which an area of the body is involved in a diffuse and often very extensive subcutaneous enlargement (*Figure 8.67*). The overlying skin is thickened and pigmented and the deformity may resemble lymphoedema, although in severe cases the overgrowth gives a picture of the classic 'Elephant Man' (*Figure 8.68*).

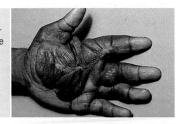

Figure 8.67.
Plexiform neurofibromatosis involving the left palm.

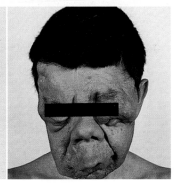

Figure 8.68.
Severe case of neurofibromatosis involving facial tissues.

Schwannomas

Schwannomas are benign, painless, firm nodules 1–2 cm across that develop from the Schwann cells of peripheral nerve sheaths. They are usually tethered to a nerve and therefore mobile only from side to side. They are asymptomatic, not tender and with no nodal involvement or malignant potential. The diagnosis is usually made histologically after excision of an asymptomatic lump.

Ganglia; bursae; synovial protrusions

These benign lesions are lined with synovial membrane and present in characteristic sites.

A ganglion (*Figure 8.69*) is produced by cystic myxomatous degeneration of fibrous tissue. It lies adjacent to a joint or tendon sheath but debate exists as to whether it has any communication with these structures or whether it has arisen as an embryonal remnant.

Ganglia occur at any age but are unusual in children. The lesions grow slowly over a number of years, usually reaching 1–2 cm across. They are painless unless knocked and asymptomatic unless they get in the way of some activity. They may disappear spontaneously or after a sharp blow but return in 50% of cases.

Ganglia are usually sited over the dorsum of the hands or feet and are tethered to the site of origin. In certain movements they may disappear underneath adjacent tendons. The lesions are smooth, spherical and may be loculated. They contain a clear, colourless, gelatinous fluid that does not empty on pressure, shows some fluctuation if the lesion is not too tense, and transilluminates.

Bursae (*Figure 8.70*) occur in relation to joints but may also develop over pressure points that are subject to repeated trauma; the latter are termed adventitious bursae. The bursae and synovial protrusions around joints are sited beneath adjacent structures such as muscles and tendons, and prevent friction during joint movement. They often communicate with the joint and are not usually mobile. They become symptomatic if the synovial fluid is increased due to joint disease such as rheumatoid and osteoarthritis, in which case the lesions are often symmetrical, and other joint abnormalities are present. They usually occur in middle age.

When the lesions are sited in the subcutaneous position, a fluid thrill – due to movement of synovial fluid between the bursa and the joint cavity – can be demonstrated. Transillumination and fluctuation may also be present. If the bursae contain loose bodies or if there is marked surrounding fibrosis, there may be palpable and audible crepitus on joint movement. Other symptoms are usually those of the underlying joint problem but there may be pain because of superadded infection, this being blood borne or due to local trauma; pain may also be due to other conditions such as gout.

Examples of adventitious bursae are: pre-patellar ('housemaid's knee'), infra-patellar ('clergyman's knee'), olecranon ('student's elbow') (*Figure 8.71*), the bunion lateral to the deformed head of the first metatarsal in hallux valgus and an ischial bursa over the ischial tuberosity. The repeated trauma producing symptomatic adventitious bursae also produces changes in the overlying skin. This may be dry, wrinkled and keratinized and there may be superadded inflammation, eczema and cracking. The bursa is well circumscribed, hemispherical and tethered to the skin and deep tissues. The diameter and fluid content are variable depending on the duration, extent of the stimulus producing it and associated infection. Fluctuation and transillumination may be demonstrable. If infection is present there may be signs of inflammation and abscess formation.

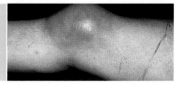

Figure 8.70.
Inflamed prepatellar bursa.

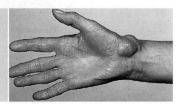

Figure 8.69.
Ganglion of the right wrist.

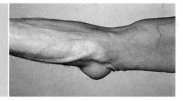

Figure 8.71.
Olecranon bursa.

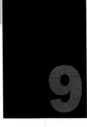

9 The head

The scalp

Meningoceles and **meningo-encephaloceles** are congenital midline swellings usually in the occipital region (p. 403). **Capillary malformations** (p. 390) appear as a red-purple skin discoloration and **venous malformations** (p. 391) appear as swellings which show the sign of emptying as do other fluid-containing communicating swellings such as the meningocele. A **sinus pericranii** also shows this sign. It appears as a soft swelling that communicates with a venous sinus through a defect in the skull.

Sebaceous cysts (*Figure 9.1*) commonly occur on the scalp and **lipomas** may also occur. **Turban tumours** (*Figure 9.2*) are rare tumours of the skin of the scalp which hang in lobulated festoons and are devoid of hair. **Plexiform neurofibromas** (p.149) may occur on the head; these may also hang in festoons but are hair bearing.

Basal cell carcinomas (*Figures 9.3* and *9.4*; p.141) and **squamous cell carcinomas** (p. 140) can arise on the scalp but are more common on the face. Examination of the draining lymph nodes is important, particularly in the case of squamous carcinoma (*Figure 9.5*). Rare tumours may be diagnosed only after biopsy and histological examination.

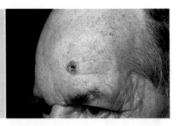

Figure 9.3. Basal cell carcinoma (rodent ulcer) of the forehead.

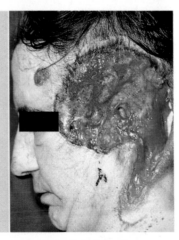

Figure 9.4. Extensive basal cell carcinoma.

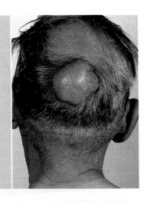

Figure 9.1. Sebaceous cyst.

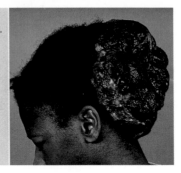

Figure 9.5. Rhabdomyosarcoma.

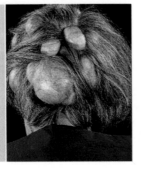

Figure 9.2. Turban tumours.

Cirsoid aneurysms (*Figure 9.6*) are pulsatile swellings over the scalp; there may be a bruit on auscultation. These so-called aneurysms are in fact traumatic arteriovenous fistulae which arise from a birth injury or from a later blow to the head. Pressure atrophy can result in erosion of underlying bone. Similarly, **carotid** and **cavernous sinus aneurysms** can arise from fractures of the base of the skull; these cause engorgement of the orbital veins resulting in oedema of the orbit and conjunctiva. **Temporal arteritis** (*Figure 9.7*) presents with headache and pain on chewing. Visual disturbance and even blindness may result from retinal artery involvement. Some localized tenderness may be present over the artery. Occasionally occipital and posterior auricular arteries may be affected.

Lacerations and **haematomas** may result from trauma. Wounds usually only gape if the underlying galea has been divided and in such cases the exposed skull should be palpated for fractures. Birth injury may result in a **cephalhaematoma** (*Figure 9.8*) in the newborn. Clinically, haematomas may give the false appearance of a depressed fracture with a soft central area surrounded by firm haematoma.

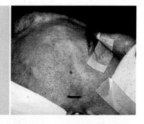

Figure 9.6.
Cirsoid aneurysm.

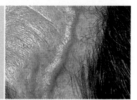

Figure 9.7.
Temporal arteritis.

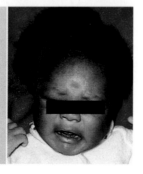

Figure 9.8. Cephalhaematoma on the right side.

The skull

Congenital and developmental abnormalities

The vault grows rapidly in the first year and reaches almost adult size by the seventh year; the sutures do not close until 30–40 years of age. The fibrous membrane that initially formed the skull remains unossified in the angles between the bones, the fontanelles. The **anterior fontanelle** is the most prominent and is palpable as a soft area at the junction of the sagittal, frontal and coronal sutures. The **posterior fontanelle** is between the parietal and occipital bones. These fontanelles later become ossified. The posterior closes at about 6 months and the anterior by about 18 months of age; tension in the fontanelles is increased during crying and reduced in dehydration. In the hydrocephalic infant they are wide and bulging. Closure of the fontanelles is delayed by metabolic diseases such as rickets.

Microcephaly (*Figure 9.9*) is defined as a head circumference of more than 3 standard deviations below the mean for age and sex. It is seen in the mentally retarded population. In **anencephaly** (*Figure 9.10*) the infant is still-born with a large defect in the skull and meninges with absent hemispheres and cerebellum.

Neural tube defects may affect the cranium and result from failure of the neural tube to close in the third or fourth week of intra-uterine development. They take the form of protrusion of tissue through a midline bony defect, a cranium bifidum. A **meningocele** (*Figure 9.11*) is a meningeal protrusion containing only cerebrospinal fluid (CSF). It is fluctuant, translucent and transmits a cough impulse on crying; it may be covered by scalp or only a thin epithelial layer. The

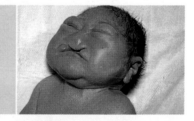

Figure 9.9.
Microcephaly.

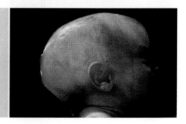

Figure 9.10.
Transillumination in an anencephalic infant.

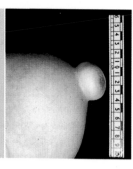

Figure 9.11. Occipital meningocele.

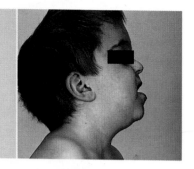

Figure 9.13. Crouzon's syndrome.

meningomyelocele and **encephalocele** (*Figure 9.12*) also contain brain. These defects most commonly occur in the occipital region but frontal and nasofrontal encephaloceles also occur. Neural tube defects of the spine are ten times more common than cranial defects.

Craniofacial deformities may result from premature sutural fusion, craniosynostosis and craniofacial dysplasia, or from developmental defects of the nasal capsule, hypertelorism or hypertelorbitism.

Craniosynostosis occurs when there is premature sutural fusion in the vault. The skull enlarges rapidly in the first 2 years of life and thus premature fusion results in skull deformities and sometimes raised intracranial pressure. A variety of abnormal skull shapes can result depending upon which sutures are involved. Premature fusion of all sutures – pansynostosis – results in severely raised intracranial pressure causing developmental delay or visual loss.

Craniofacial dysplasia occurs when vault stenosis extends into the base of the skull. As the name implies, the deformity involves not only the cranium but also the face. These deformities occur as part of a variety of syndromes such as Crouzon's and Apert's. **Crouzon's syndrome** (*Figure 9.13*) is characterized by exophthalmos, hypertelorism, beaked nose and low-set ears. Atresia of the external auditory meatus and middle ear abnormalities result in conductive deafness. There is raised intracranial pressure with mental retardation, progressive worsening of exophthalmos and visual loss. In **Apert's**

syndrome (*Figure 9.14*) the middle third of the face is underdeveloped with a small nose, hypertelorism, shallow orbits, proptosis and strabismus. There is syndactyly with complete fusion of all digits of the hands and feet, skeletal defects, congenital heart disease and anal atresia.

Hypertelorism (*Figure 9.15*) – hypertelorbitism – refers to abnormally widely separated orbits. It may be associated with craniosynostosis, clefting defects and meningo-encephaloceles.

Other disease processes can also result in craniofacial deformities. **Fibrous dysplasia** of the frontal bone may result in inferior displacement of the globe and optic nerve compression. **Haemolymphangiomas** may occur in the orbit and communicate intracranially. Localized craniofacial plexiform neurofibromas may occur in **neurofibromatosis**.

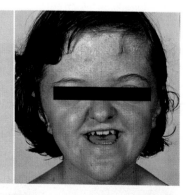

Figure 9.14. Apert's syndrome.

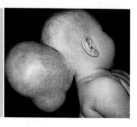

Figure 9.12. Encephalocele.

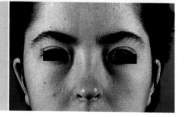

Figure 9.15. Hypertelorism with epicanthic folds.

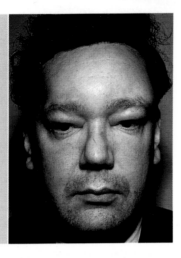

Figure 9.16.
Osteomyelitis of the frontal bone.

appear as radiopaque protuberances. **Chordomas** are malignant destructive tumours that affect the base of the skull and appear radiologically as lytic lesions. **Multiple myeloma** causes multiple 'punched-out' lytic lesions in the skull: the 'pepperpot skull'. **Fibrous dysplasia** and **eosinophilic granulomas** are tumour-like lesions that also appear, radiologically, as lytic areas.

Paget's disease of the bone – osteitis deformans (p.43) – most frequently affects the long bones of the lower extremity and the skull, and occurs in middle or later life. The skull becomes thickened and its circumference enlarges. Deafness, vertigo and failing vision may result from compression of the brain and of the cranial nerves at their foramina. Sarcoma complicates 1% of cases.

Osteomyelitis

Osteomyelitis of the skull may develop secondary to infection in the air sinuses or mastoid air cells. **Pott's puffy tumour** (*Figure 9.16*) is a localized area of oedema that forms over an area of osteomyelitis. It usually occurs in the frontal region due to incompletely treated frontal sinusitis.

Skull tumours

Metastatic deposits (*Figure 9.17*) are the commonest type of skull tumour. They may appear either as hard lumps or be soft to palpation; very vascular deposits may even be pulsatile. **Osteomas** (*Figure 9.18*) are benign tumours that

Skull injuries

A **cephalhaematoma** (p. 152; *Figure 9.8*) is a subperiosteal bleed occurring in about 2% of neonates. It presents as a soft scalp swelling and is rarely associated with fractures.

Linear vault fractures may not be apparent externally except for a history of significant injury or the presence of contusion or laceration of the scalp. Radiologically they may be visible in one plane only. Fractures crossing the **temporal bone** may result in **middle meningeal artery** injury which can give rise to **extradural haematoma**. Fractures through **air sinuses** may lead to **aeroceles** or **meningitis**.

Depressed fractures result from a relatively focused source of trauma, for example a blow from a hammer. Clinically they may appear as a depressed area surrounded by a boggy haematoma. In a **compound depressed fracture** there is an overlying laceration or an area of tissue loss and the fracture may be directly palpable. It is therefore good practice to palpate the skull through a scalp laceration while the patient is locally anaesthetized prior to wound closure. The severity of the depressed area can be assessed radiologically, preferably with computed tomography (CT) scanning. Patients with depressed fractures have a greater incidence of underlying brain injury and a greater risk of subsequent epilepsy. In compound fractures there is a risk of meningitis. **Pond fractures** are depressed areas of the skull in the neonate resulting from moulding in the birth canal or from forceps deliveries.

A **basal skull fracture** is difficult to diagnose clinically and radiologically. It should be suspected in severe head injuries but a number of specific signs help to identify less obvious cases. **Anterior fossa** fractures may pass through the paranasal sinuses and therefore be internally compound; CSF may escape through the nose – **CSF rhinorrhoea** – and

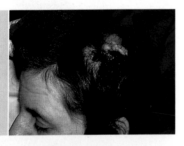

Figure 9.17.
Scalp metastases.

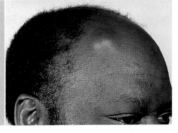

Figure 9.18.
Osteoma. Right side of the skull

there is a risk of meningitis. Bloodstained CSF may be distinguished from blood by placing a drop on filter paper: blood produces only a single ring whereas bloodstained CSF separates into two rings. Sneezing or blowing the nose can result in air being forced into the cranium beneath the dura producing an **aerocele**. The presence of a 'black eye' without direct injury also raises the suspicion of such a fracture. The discoloration is due to blood tracking through the tissues and is limited by the attachments of the orbicularis oculi, whereas in a true 'black eye' there is no such limitation. In addition, in a traumatic 'black eye' there may be intraconjunctival haemorrhage which moves with the conjunctiva when the eyelid is moved with the examiner's finger. In a fracture, blood can track into the subconjunctival space forming a fan of blood extending from the iris with no outer limit: a subconjunctival haemorrhage (*Figure 9.19*). Bilateral 'black eyes', without direct trauma, is a fairly certain sign of an anterior fossa fracture: the '**panda sign**' (*Figure 9.20*).

Middle cranial fossa fractures may result in blood and CSF escaping from the external auditory meatus. Rupture of the tympanic membrane may also result in such bleeding but here the blood tends to clot in the meatus as it is not mixed with CSF. Facial paralysis, nystagmus or deafness may result from cranial nerve entrapment. A late sign is the appearance of bruising over the mastoid process two days after the injury; this is **Battle's sign. Posterior fossa** fractures are associated with injury to the venous sinuses and brain stem. The patient is usually deeply unconscious and the outcome fatal.

Intracranial conditions

Hydrocephalus

Hydrocephalus (*Figure 9.21*) is a state where there is an increase in CSF volume. The CSF is formed in the ventricular system by the choroid plexus and exits through foramina in the fourth ventricle into cisterns at the base of the brain. It then flows over the brain and is reabsorbed by the arachnoid villi. Hydrocephalus can thus result from obstruction within the ventricular system – obstructive or non-communicating hydrocephalus – or from impaired reabsorption of CSF due to malfunction of the arachnoid villi – non-obstructive or communicating hydrocephalus.

Obstructive hydrocephalus develops because of stenosis of the aqueduct of Sylvius or fourth ventricle lesions. These include posterior fossa brain tumours and the Chiari Type II and Dandy–Walker malformations. The **Chiari Type II malformation** is an abnormal flexure of the hindbrain. The **Dandy–Walker malformation** is a cystic expansion of the fourth ventricle. Note that the **Chiari Type I malformation**, which is herniation of the cerebellar tonsils into the spinal canal, is not usually associated with hydrocephalus.

Communicating hydrocephalus may follow a subarachnoid haemorrhage in a premature infant or may result from pneumococcal or tuberculous meningitis and leukaemic infiltrates.

Clinically, hydrocephalus in the infant is manifest as enlargement of the head, a wide, bulging anterior fontanelle and dilatation of the scalp veins. The forehead is broad and the eyes may deviate downward resulting in the sclera being visible above the iris: the 'setting sun' sign. The Dandy–Walker malformation results in a rapid increase in skull size and the skull may even transilluminate. There may be associated abnormalities and mental retardation. In the older child, deteriorating mental ability may be noted but hydrocephalus in the adult is less apparent clinically. Here it is the ventricles that enlarge rather than the cranium. Patients present with symptoms relating to the underlying cause or of chronically raised intracranial pressure.

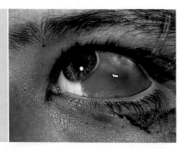

Figure 9.19.
Fracture of the anterior fossa. This has produced a subconjunctival haemorrhage.

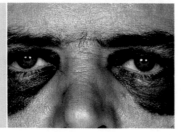

Figure 9.20.
Infratemporal bruisms from a fractured skull.

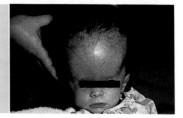

Figure 9.21.
Hydrocephalus.

Birth injuries

Intraventricular haemorrhage may occur in the premature infant due to capillary fragility and is associated with hypoxia. Ultrasound examination reveals that this is a common problem subclinically occurring in about 50% of the premature. Severe cases result in developmental delay and hydrocephalus. **Cerebral palsy** results from so-called non-progressive brain injury. This may be developmental or secondary to infection, haemorrhage or hypoxia. Developmental delay is noted. Diplegias, hemiplegias and quadriplegias may occur. Many features become more apparent as the child develops, for example dyskinetic, i.e. involuntary, movements occur which may be choreiform (jerky) or athetoid (writhing). There is spasticity with increased tone in one direction, such as flexion at the wrist. Cogwheel rigidity, toe walking and dysarthria are other features.

Intracranial abscesses

These abscesses present as chronic space-occupying lesions. They may be extradural, intradural or intracerebral. All types may arise from spread of infection from chronic otitis media or frontal sinusitis. In the case of extradural lesions there may be evidence of overlying osteomyelitis: Pott's puffy tumour. Subdural and intracerebral abscesses may result in systemic evidence of serious infection. Intracerebral abscesses may be secondary to lung abscesses, bronchiectasis or other pyaemic states. Miliary TB also affects the brain and its coverings.

Intracranial tumours
Tumour types

These may be primary or metastatic lesions. The latter account for 20% of cases, the commonest being from breast and bronchial carcinomas, although melanoma is the tumour with the greatest propensity to metastasize to the brain. In adults, 80% of tumours are supratentorial whereas in children infratentorial lesions are the most common. Primary brain tumours can arise from brain tissue, meninges, nerves, the pituitary and from various embryonic tissues and developmental abnormalities. **Gliomas** are the commonest, accounting for 45% of tumours, and of the gliomas the **astrocytoma** is the commonest.

Gliomas are malignant tumours and are graded accordingly from I to IV: **meningiomas** (15%) are slow-growing and benign; **schwannomas** (8%) most commonly arise from the eighth nerve, hence acoustic neuromas; and **pituitary tumours** are usually benign adenomas. AIDS has resulted in the appearance of rare **intracranial granulomas** and **primary lymphoma of the brain**. Tumours may present with focal features, rising intracranial pressure or epilepsy.

Focal neurological and metabolic features:

Frontal lobe tumours may result in personality changes, dementia, intellectual impairment and in speech disorders if Broca's area is involved. **Occipital lobe tumours** may cause homonymous hemianopias, e.g. loss of the right fields of both eyes for a left sided lesion. **Parietal lobe lesions** cause sensory and spatial disturbances and **temporal lobe lesions** give rise to temporal lobe epilepsy, creating mental clouding, depersonalization, feelings of *déjà vu* and hallucinations of sight, hearing, taste or smell. **Pituitary tumours** have a mass effect on the optic chiasma giving a bitemporal hemianopia, i.e. loss of both temporal fields.

Endocrine disturbances result from excessive hormonal secretion of specific hormones. Growth hormone-secreting tumours result in acromegaly in the adult, enlarging the hands and feet, and giantism in the prepubertal. Prolactin-secreting tumours cause lactation, nipple discharge and amenorrhoea; hypopituitarism may also occur. **Brain stem lesions** result in cranial nerve palsies and **cerebellar lesions** in loss of postural control, incoordination and nystagmus. **Cerebellopontine angle tumours** are usually acoustic neuromas (p.173) but, rarely, meningiomas, epidermoids and neuromas of other nerves may occur at this site.

Raised intracranial pressure

Malignant tumours grow fairly rapidly and therefore result in rising intracranial pressure. Midline tumours may obstruct the CSF pathways causing hydrocephalus.

Symptoms of rising intracranial pressure are headache and vomiting. Headache is typically worse in the morning or on bending or stooping. These phenomena are explained as follows. During sleep, pCO_2 rises causing intracranial vasodilatation and thus an increase in intracranial pressure. Dependency increases pressure in the venous sinuses as there are no valves in the great veins. In contrast to head injury, changes are gradual. Papilloedema may be observed on fundoscopy. Eventually **coning** occurs where the pressure forces the brain through the tentorium or foramen magnum. This distorts the brain stem and the oculomotor nerve resulting in coma and an ipsilateral, dilated unreactive pupil. With posterior fossa tumours the cerebellum is forced through the foramen magnum leading to pressure on the medulla. Bradycardia, rising blood pressure and slow, irregular respiration are features of medullary compression.

Epilepsy

Tumours in the posterior strip of the frontal lobe, the motor strip, may cause focal motor seizures: **Jacksonian epilepsy**.

Here the fit begins in a localized region of the contralateral half of the body but then spreads to become generalized. Temporal lobe fits are more likely to be idiopathic rather than the result of a tumour. Occipital lobe fits are rare but may produce visual hallucinations.

Severe head injury
Assessment

The principal objectives are to identify the severity of primary brain injury and to record a baseline of neurological disability. Thus subsequent deterioration from treatable causes, such as acute compressing intracranial haematomas, can be recognized.

Initial information from witnesses and from the ambulance crew, such as about the nature and velocity of the trauma and the initial state of consciousness of the patient, indicate the potential severity of the head injury. In such cases the patient is likely to have suffered other life-threatening injuries that are of more immediate relevance. The advanced trauma life support system protocol is therefore followed with airway, breathing and circulation being stabilized (p.116). The cervical spine is immobilized as there is a high incidence of associated injury. Usually a number of members of a trauma team are simultaneously involved in these tasks and so it is possible to perform an initial neurological assessment of the coma scale and pupils, as these may soon be influenced by drugs, hypoxia and endotracheal intubation. Later, a detailed neurological examination is made to look for focal neurological signs.

The **Glasgow Coma Scale** (*Table 9.1*) is a reproducible method of assessing the consciousness level. Eye opening, motor response and verbal response are quantified. When using the scale it must be remembered that factors other than cerebral injury may influence the score. Eye opening may be limited by facial trauma and periorbital oedema. Motor response is the most reliable indicator of neurological injury, and deterioration should be taken seriously. The upper limbs are most representative and it is the best motor response that is recorded. If there is no response to commands, painful stimuli are applied in the form of supraorbital or sternal pressure. A hand moving purposefully to the stimulus is regarded as localizing. Arm flexion and extension at the elbow are the lower levels of response. Verbal performance is graded as orientated conversation, confused conversation, inappropriate words, sounds (e.g. grunts) or nothing at all, but bear in mind that language difficulties, endotracheal intubation and facial trauma may greatly influence these findings.

Coma is defined as a Glasgow Coma Scale score of 8 or less. It should be noted that some versions of the scale simplify the classification of the motor response by excluding withdrawal from pain, giving a maximum score of 14 rather than 15.

Focal neurological signs may be observed in the eyes, the limbs or as the effects of medullary dysfunction on the patient's vital signs. The pupils are examined for size, inequality and reactivity to light. An acute compressing intracranial haematoma begins to compress the ipsilateral third nerve against the free edge of the tentorium as it expands. After an initial slight contraction the ipsilateral pupil begins to dilate and reaction to light becomes sluggish: the Hutchinson's pupil. Eventually, as coning supervenes, the contralateral pupil also becomes dilated and unreactive.

When observing pupillary size and response, one must allow for the effect of primary globe injury and drugs. In the Hutchinson's pupil the consensual light reflex is also lost. Thus pupillary dilatation from optic nerve injury or intraocular haematoma may be distinguished, as in these cases the consensual reflex is present. Loss of upward gaze is an important finding since this may herald imminent coning from an expanding frontal haematoma with no other localized signs (*Figure 9.22*). The development of a hemiplegia is also indicative of an acute compressing intracranial haematoma. The hemiplegia is most likely to be contralateral to the lesion.

A continued rise in intracranial pressure results in coning. Medullary compression results in **Cushing's triad** of rising blood pressure, falling pulse rate and periodic slow respiration. Pyrexia of 38°C or more may occur from damage to the thermoregulatory mechanisms.

Table 9.1. Glasgow coma scale.

Response	Details	Score
Eye opening	Spontaneous	4
	Speech	3
	Pain	2
	None	1
Verbal response	Orientated	5
	Confused	4
	Inapproproate words	3
	Incomprehensible sounds	2
	None	1
Best motor response	Obeys commands	6
	Localizes pain	5
	Withdrawal from pain	4
	Flexion to pain	3
	Extension to pain	2
	None	1

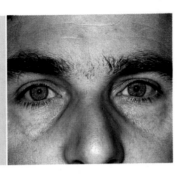

Figure 9.22.
Brain stem haemorrhage: the patient is trying to look up.

Intracranial haematomas

Acute subdural haematomas are associated with significant primary brain injury. Lacerations to the surface of the brain result in bleeding into the subdural space. The patient has suffered a severe head injury and is usually deeply unconscious on initial assessment. It is not usually associated with a lucid interval. Localizing signs may well be present. Patients presenting in this state require transfer to a neurosurgical unit for a CT scan and subsequent management. The deeply unconscious, flaccid patient with only primitive reflexes and bilateral fixed dilated pupils is likely to have suffered brain stem shearing and the situation is probably irretrievable. Primitive reflexes include:

- Glabellar tap – where tapping on the root of the nose produces persistent blinking.
- Snout reflex – stroking the upper lip produces pouting.
- Palmomental reflex – scratching the thenar eminence produces a submental twitch.

The term 'intradural haematoma' may be used to describe both subdural and intracerebral haematomas.

Acute extradural haematomas usually result from bleeding from the middle meningeal artery into the extradural space. It may occur in severe head injury but more importantly it must be recognized that the condition may arise in a more moderate injury. The classical scenario is that the patient suffers only a light blow to the side of the head but this is still sufficient to fracture the relatively thin squamous temporal bone over which the artery runs.

The patient may be only dazed initially or may have lost consciousness for a short while. Consciousness is then regained, the lucid interval after the stunning effect of the initial injury is passed. The patient gradually deteriorates over several hours as the haematoma slowly collects in the extradural space. Symptoms of rising intracranial pressure develop, i.e. worsening headache, vomiting, visual disturbances and drowsiness.

The consciousness level deteriorates and localizing signs develop such as ipsilateral pupillary dilatation, contralateral hemiparesis – with hyper-reflexia and upgoing plantar response – and Cushing's triad. The pattern of presentation of extradural haematomas is the underlying reason for admission for observation in relatively mild to moderate head injuries. Good predictive factors are skull fracture and depression of consciousness level.

Chronic subdural haematomas are not usually associated with significant head injury. These occur after a minor injury in the elderly, alcoholics or in those with clotting disorders. A small collection of blood gradually enlarges by osmosis and symptoms develop over days, weeks or even months. Headache, vomiting, mood change, irritability, incontinence and drowsiness may occur; senility may be wrongly suspected. Signs vary but pupillary inequality, long tract signs, upgoing plantars, dysphasia and fits may result.

Hypoxia and oedema

Deterioration in the patient's condition may not only be the result of intracranial haematomas. In severe brain injury, a vicious circle of oedema and hypoxia develops. Medullary compression results in respiratory depression. The fall in cerebral pO_2 causes tissue oedema and the rise in pCO_2 causes vasodilation with increase in cerebral blood volume. These changes further increase intracranial pressure and thus the cycle continues. Controlled ventilation reduces this effect. Intracranial pressure can be monitored with a probe placed via a small burr hole. Intracranial pressure greater than 20 mmHg is abnormally high.

Diffuse axonal injury

This refers to the microscopic axonal damage caused by distortion of brain tissue during the impact of the injury. A wide spectrum exists and it is used to explain the range of states seen after a head injury. It may manifest clinically as nothing more than a mild concussion or, at the other end of the spectrum, the patient may be in a profound coma. Contrary to previous thinking, such brain injury is diffuse. Macroscopic damage occurs as contusions and lacerations, these being most common on the undersurfaces of frontal and temporal lobes where the brain moves over bony ridges on impact.

Epilepsy and postconcussion syndromes

Epileptic fits may occur in the immediate period after a severe head injury though they may also occur weeks or even years later. The incidence is much higher with penetrating injuries and in those associated with an intracranial haematoma.

Postconcussion syndromes are persisting symptoms of headache, dizziness, memory impairment and lack of concentration following a head injury.

Subarachnoid haemorrhage

This results from the rupture of a vascular abnormality in the subarachnoid space; only in rare cases is trauma involved. **Berry aneurysms** occur at the junctions of the cerebral vessels in the circle of Willis. These may rupture, most commonly in the 35–60 years of age groups. **Arteriovenous malformations** account for most of these cases occurring in infancy.

Patients present with a sudden, severe, occipital **headache** and other symptoms and signs of **meningism** caused by blood in the CSF: neck stiffness, photophobia, nausea and vomiting. The differential diagnosis is meningitis. There may be signs of cerebral compression and raised intracranial pressure with papilloedema. The CSF is bloodstained and xanthochromic after centrifugation of the fresh specimen.

Brain death and the vegetative state

Brain death and the vegetative state may result following resuscitation of cardiorespiratory arrests, severe head injury and primary intracerebral catastrophe, such as subarachnoid haemorrhage. The cerebral cortex is the most vulnerable organ to hypoxic injury followed by the brain stem. Myocardium is much more resistant, thus in any of the above crises the heart and other body organs survive preferentially. Where such hypoxic injury occurs, the usual result is cortical death. The brain stem survives and thus spontaneous respiration occurs, and the heart continues to beat independently. This is the **vegetative state**.

If hypoxia is prolonged further, the brain stem also dies. The heart can still beat spontaneously but spontaneous respiration does not occur, and artificial ventilation is required. This state is **brain death**.

The Royal Colleges (in the UK) and the legal system (in the USA) have attempted to clarify the situation regarding **brain stem death**. Both decided that if the brain stem is dead, the cortex must also be dead. Death can therefore be declared when brain stem death is diagnosed rather than when the heart stops. This has important implications for the withdrawal of ventilatory support and organ donation.

Brain death results from head injury in about 50% of cases and from subarachnoid haemorrhage in about 30%. It should be noted that alcohol, neuromuscular relaxants and hypothermia may cause temporary absence of brain stem function and so must be withdrawn or corrected before the diagnosis can

be made. In brain death, the patient is apnoeic and in deep coma. Examination findings confirming brain stem death are:

- No pupillary response to light.
- No corneal reflex.
- No facial response to pain.
  No response of the larynx to movement of the endotracheal tube.
- No caloric or vestibulo-ocular response – syringeing the external auditory meatus with ice cold water normally results in vestibular nystagmus.

Once the above are established the final test is that there should be no respiratory movement after disconnection of the ventilator for sufficient time for the arterial pCO_2 to exceed 60 mmHg with 6 L min^{-1} of O_2 being applied to the endotracheal tube.

The **persistent vegetative state** is compatible with survival, sometimes even for years. It usually results from delayed resuscitation or diffuse axonal injury from a severe head injury. The patient may initially be deeply unconscious and may require ventilatory support but eventually a stable state is reached where the patient breathes spontaneously. The eyes open but there is no awareness or response. Reflex activity is present and spasticity is noted. There may be further recovery in diffuse axonal injury and it is only after 3 months that the state may be considered to be persistent.

The cranial nerves

Abnormalities detected on examination of the cranial nerves may be physical signs of intracranial problems – upper motor neurone – or pathology of the cranial nerve or its nucleus – lower motor neurone.

Olfactory nerve (**I**) function is tested for each nostril, using odour preparations. Hallucinations of the olfaction of foul odours have been reported in cases of temporal lobe tumours or abscesses. Complete loss of olfaction may result from fractures of the cribriform plate of the ethmoid.

Optic nerve (**II**) blindness is accompanied by a dilated pupil that is unresponsive to light. Lesser visual defects of each eye are mapped out by the examiner moving a finger in each quadrant, with the second eye covered. For more detailed mapping, a light spot or target disc is passed radially across the field. Multiple sclerosis (MS) is the commonest cause of optic nerve lesions. Causes of surgical importance are trauma and tumours of the orbit.

Lesions of the chiasm are usually due to pituitary tumours, these mostly being benign and potentially hormone secreting; they damage the nerve fibres of the nasal retina, resulting in bitemporal hemianopia. Damage to the optic tract, of the radiation or the visual cortex is usually due to primary or secondary malignancy; ipsilateral retinal fibres of both eyes are affected, producing a homonymous hemianopia. Cortical lesions are usually congruous, i.e. they affect the two eyes equally, whereas lesions of the optic tract and radiation are non-congruous.

The **trochlear nerve** (**IV**) supplies the superior oblique muscle, the **abducent nerve** (**VI**) the lateral rectus and the **oculomotor nerve** (**III**) the other extraocular muscles, together with the parasympathetic nerve fibres producing pupillary constriction. Injuries to the three nerves produce squint, ptosis and diplopia. Oculomotor lesions produce a dilated, unresponsive pupil, ptosis and a loss of medial, upward and downward movements. The eye is deviated laterally and downwards.

In trochlear nerve paresis, the eye is rotated and deviated laterally, and there is diplopia on looking downwards and medially. This is a particular problem when going downstairs, and the head is tilted away from the side of the lesion in an attempt to compensate. In abducent nerve paresis the eye cannot look laterally so the squint is maximum when looking in this direction.

The three nerves may be affected together in MS and vascular lesions or tumours in the region of their midbrain nuclei. They are affected to a variable extent by carotid aneurysms in the cavernous sinus, and tumours of the supraorbital fissure and orbit. The oculomotor nerve may be damaged in tentorial coning, and the long intracranial course of the delicate abducent nerve makes it susceptible to damage in raised intracranial pressure (*Figures 9.23–9.25*).

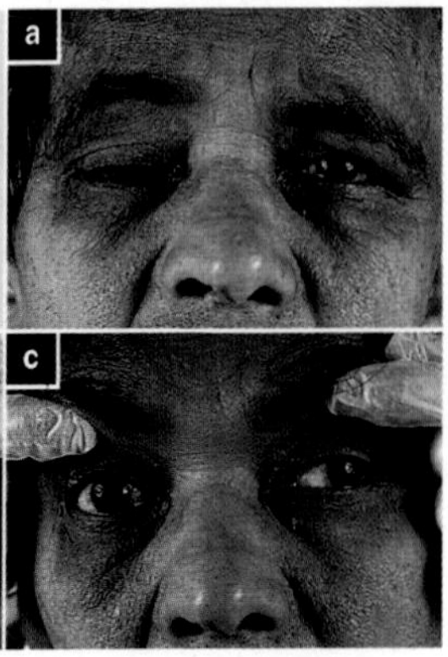

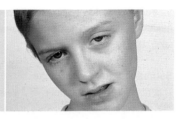

Figure 9.24. Left fourth nerve palsy.

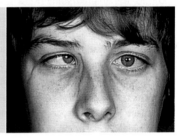

Figure 9.25. Left sixth nerve palsy. Pituitary tumour.

The **trigeminal nerve** (**V**) has four functions that may be examined:

- **Motor innervation** is to the muscles of mastication – masseter and temporalis – which are tested by palpating the muscles while the patient bites hard. If there is weakness of the pterygoid muscles, the jaw deviates to the paralysed side when the mouth is opened widely.
- **Sensation** is tested over the areas of the face supplied by the ophthalmic, maxillary and mandibular divisions. Facial bone fractures may result in sensory loss over these areas. (For trigeminal neuralgia see p.167.)
- The **corneal reflex** is elicited when stroking the cornea with cotton wool, producing blinking. The sensory component is trigeminal, the motor component is from the facial nerve. The reflex may be lost with disruption of the trigeminal or facial nerves but its clinical relevance is that its loss is also one of the features of brain stem death.
- **Taste** to the anterior two-thirds of the tongue is initially carried by the trigeminal nerve but is later taken by the chorda tympani to the facial nerve. Loss of taste has been described following divisions of the trigeminal nerve either in facial fractures or surgically in the treatment of trigeminal neuralgia.

Frey's syndrome results from inappropriate reinnervation following parotid surgery. Here parasympathetic secretomotor fibres take control of sweat glands in the skin, resulting in facial sweating to salivatory stimuli (gustatory sweating).

Figure 9.23. Acromegaly with third nerve palsy. a. At rest. b. Looking left. c. Looking straight ahead.

Facial nerve (**VII**) function is tested in the lower face by asking the patient to smile, whistle or blow out their cheeks, and in the upper face by asking the patient to 'screw up' their eyes (*Figures 9.26* and *9.27*). Weakness may also be apparent on initial inspection as a drooping of the angles of the mouth or as a loss of forehead creases. The upper face is bilaterally innervated, whereas each side of the lower face is controlled by the ipsilateral hemisphere only. Thus upper motor neurone lesions – e.g. a stroke – produce only lower facial weakness, unless they are bilateral.

Unilateral lower motor neurone facial weakness results from Bell's palsy (p.168), invasion of the nerve by malignant parotid tumours, division of branches during parotid surgery – the extent of the weakness depending upon which branches have been involved – isolated mononeuropathies, diabetes and sarcoidosis.

Bilateral facial palsy (*Figure 9.28*) is not often seen but may be the result of **Guillain–Barré syndrome** and may also occur as part of a hereditary **bulbar motor neuropathy** (p.436) where there is marked fasciculation of the tongue.

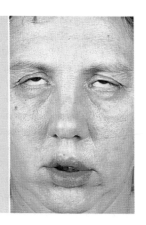

Figure 9.28.
Eyes screwed up in bilateral facial palsy.

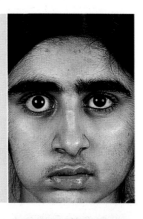

Figure 9.26. Seventh nerve palsy (at rest).

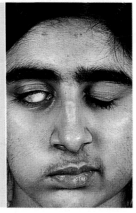

Figure 9.27. Seventh nerve palsy (eyes closed).

Unilateral or bilateral lower motor neurone damage can occur in a fracture of the base of the skull. If paralysis is of delayed onset, the injury is due to secondary oedema and eventually recovery usually occurs. The mandibular branch may be damaged in block dissections of the neck and in surgery of the submandibular salivary glands. This results in ipsilateral paralysis of the lower lip.

For the **vestibulocochlear nerve** (**VIII**) see p.173.

The **glossopharyngeal nerve** (**IX**) supplies taste to the posterior third of the tongue and also sensation to the tonsil and anterior pillar of the fauces. Its function is tested as the 'gag reflex', touching the anterior pillar with a spatula results in sudden glottic closure. It is primarily used to assess the preservation of the ability to safely swallow food or fluid in the stroke patient.

The **vagus nerve** (**X**) has many functions. Its motor innervation of the soft palate is routinely tested by observing the uvula while the patient says 'aah'. Loss of function on one side results in deviation of the uvula away from that side. Damage to the recurrent laryngeal nerve, or its fibres on the surface of the vagus as it descends in the neck, paralyses the ipsilateral vocal cord, resulting in hoarseness and inability to produce high-pitched sounds (ask the patient to say a high-pitched 'ee') and a bovine cough as the vocal cords cannot approximate to produce the explosive element of the cough. The nerves can be damaged by malignant infiltration and surgery of the thyroid gland, and structures in and around the carotid sheath.

The **spinal accessory nerve** (**XI**) innervates the sternomastoid and trapezius. Sternomastoid function is tested by asking patients to turn their heads against resistance. Turning to the right tests the left sternomastoid and vice versa. Asking patients to shrug their shoulders tests the trapezii.

The **hypoglossal nerve (XII)** innervates the tongue musculature. Paralysis of one side results in wasting and fasciculation. The tongue deviates to the affected side (*Figure 9.29*).

The ninth to twelfth cranial nerve nuclei may be collectively described as the bulbar nuclei. **Bulbar palsy** describes the lower motor neurone lesion affecting the regions supplied by these nerves, and **pseudobulbar palsy** describes the corresponding bilateral upper motor neurone lesion.

Bulbar palsy arises as part of an X-linked motor neuropathy affecting only males, with symptoms typically appearing in the over 40s. The neuropathy usually commences as lower limb weakness, which slowly spreads to the upper limbs and face. In the final stages there is a bulbar palsy, characterized by dysphagia and dysarthria, and an associated lower motor neurone facial weakness. There may be characteristic fasciculation of the tongue and lower face.

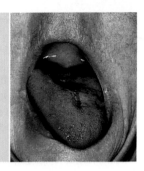

Figure 9.29.
Left hypoglossal paralysis.

Pseudobulbar palsy occurs in motor neurone disease, MS and cerebrovascular disease. There is dysarthria, with a 'gravelly voice', the jaw jerk is exaggerated but the gag reflex is preserved. The tongue moves slowly but is not wasted.

10 The face and jaws

Congenital abnormalities

In **Pierre Robin syndrome** (*Figure 10.1*) the horizontal ramus of the mandible is congenitally shortened. Facial abnormalities occur with cranial deformities in **Crouzon's** and **Apert's syndromes** (p.153).

Fibrous dysplasia of the maxilla and ethmoid occurs as part of **Albright's syndrome** (p.125). This is a combination of polyostotic fibrous dysplasia, skin pigmentation and endocrine abnormalities. Endocrine disorders may include precocious puberty, thyrotoxicosis, acromegaly and Cushing's syndrome. The distribution is usually such that the bone and skin changes occur on the same side of the body, and the most common bony deformity is of the femoral neck. The condition is more common in girls, usually presenting with secondary sexual characteristics and menstruation in infancy.

The characteristic facies of **congenital syphilis** and **cretinism** are described on pp.45 and 38, respectively.

Sinusitis

Acute sinusitis (*Figure 10.2*) is usually the result of infection secondary to one of a number of possible precipitating factors. The commonest of these are 'colds' and influenza. Dental infections, diving, barotrauma, fractures involving the sinuses, and tonsillar and adenoidal infections are also implicated.

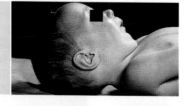

Figure 10.1.
Pierre Robin syndrome.

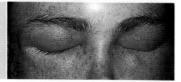

Figure 10.2.
Frontal sinusitis.

Immunodeficiency, mucociliary disorders and atmospheric irritants may also be predisposing factors.

Likely infective organisms are pneumococcus, streptococcus, staphylococcus, *Haemophilus influenzae* and *Klebsiella pneumoniae*. The maxillary sinuses are most commonly involved, sinusitis presenting with pain in the cheek or upper teeth, which may be referred to the frontal or temporal regions, with tenderness over the cheek. Most cases are secondary to nasal viral infections but about 10% arise either following a dental extraction or in relation to a dental abscess of the upper molars or premolars. The frontal sinuses and ethmoidal sinuses are usually involved secondarily to maxillary sinus infection. Involvement of the sphenoidal sinuses is very rare.

Chronic sinusitis may simply represent residual infection following recurrent acute sinusitis. Mixed organisms are usually responsible, usually streptococci and anaerobes. The symptomatology is similar to acute episodes but of a lower intensity. Other cases, however, may represent infection occurring secondary to obstruction of the sinus osteum.

Tuberculosis and **syphilis** (p.69) may rarely give rise to sinus infections and represent spread of the disease from its primary site elsewhere. **Fungal infection of the sinuses** from aspergilli may occur in the immunocompromised.

Sinusitis may result in a variety of complications by the spread of infection through bone, veins, lymphatics and perineural spaces.

Osteomyelitis usually occurs in relation to frontal sinusitis. It presents with headache and toxaemia. An oedematous area may develop on the forehead: **Pott's puffy tumour** (p.154). The risk of spread of infection to the meninges and brain is high.

All the sinuses have walls that are involved in the boundaries of the orbit. These walls may become eroded and so infection can spread to the orbit resulting in an **orbital cellulitis** and possibly a **subperiosteal abscess**. The eye becomes painful and swollen, the pain being aggravated by movement. There may be diplopia and proptosis with chemosis of the conjunctiva. Again, as with osteomyelitis, there is a risk of **intracranial infection** which may take the form of thrombophlebitis of the cavernous or sagittal sinuses, meningitis or cerebral abscess formation.

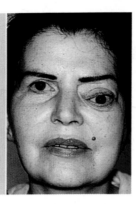

Figure 10.3.
Mucocele of the left frontal sinus, displacing the eye left.

Tumours

Cysts

Cysts associated with fusion of embryological elements forming the maxilla and cysts of dental origin tend to present as problems in the oral cavity (p.194).

Dermoid cysts (p.138) arise at the surface lines of embryological fusion. They may occur in the midline of the nose and even extend into the septum. Dermoids may also occur at the orbital margins.

Mucoceles of the paranasal sinuses (*Figure 10.3*) may result from obstruction of the sinus by a polyp, atresia of the sinus osteum or from mucous gland obstruction. Most commonly they occur in the frontal sinus and may bulge into the orbit.

Haemorrhagic bone cysts occur in the mandible, probably arising secondary to trauma occurring several years earlier. They expand painlessly, producing a radiolucent localized deformity.

Benign tumours

Osteomas arising in these regions take two forms. Localized compact osteomas occur in the frontal sinuses of young adults. They present either by displacing the eye or by giving rise to a mucocele of the sinus from frontonasal duct obstruction. Localized cancellous osteomas occur in the maxillary and ethmoidal sinuses.

Exostoses may occur in the midline of the hard palate as a **torus palatinus**. The overlying mucosa may become eroded.

Chordomas arise from notochord remnants in the nasopharynx and may result in extensive bone erosion. **Craniopharyngiomas** arising from Rathke's pouch remnants may have extracranial portions occupying the sphenoidal sinus and eroding the surrounding bone.

Malignant tumours

Squamous carcinomas (p.140) are the commonest malignant tumours of the upper airway. They may occur in the paranasal air sinuses and nasal passages, and in so doing they must be considered when looking at tumours affecting the face. In these regions most tumours arise in the maxillary antrum although the nasal passages and ethmoidal air cells are also recognized sites. They may present subtly with an involved cervical lymph node. Others may cause epistaxis or produce symptoms from local invasion.

Burkitt's lymphoma is a malignant lymphoma strongly associated with the Epstein–Barr virus. It occurs in the tropical regions of Africa, mainly affecting children in the 4–8 year age range. It may affect the maxilla alone or sometimes may simultaneously involve the maxilla and mandible on the same side. It grows very rapidly, producing a massive swelling of the face and palate within a matter of days.

Stewart's lethal midline granuloma (*Figure 10.4*) – originally thought to be a granulomatous condition – is now considered to be a T cell lymphoma. It results in a slow progressive destruction of the midface.

Other malignant tumours arising in these regions are uncommon and so are worthy of only a brief note. **Adenocarcinomas** may arise in the maxillary antrum in relation to industrial exposure to hardwood dusts. **Adenoid cystic carcinomas** may occur on the alveolus and hard palate, and olfactory neuroblastomas as nasal or ethmoidal lesions. **Malignant melanomas** (*Figure 10.5*) may arise as dark or pale polypoid masses on the septum or lateral walls of the nose. **Metastases** from other tumours may rarely occur in these regions.

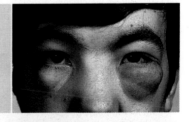

Figure 10.4.
Destructive granuloma.

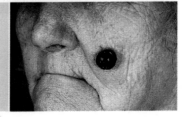

Figure 10.5.
Malignant melanoma on the cheek.

In general these tumours may produce a variety of clinical features. Unilateral nasal obstruction and unilateral persistent bleeding or discharge from the nose are suspicious symptoms. There may be swelling of the cheek, alveolar margin or nasal bridge, which is particularly rapid and pronounced in the case of Burkitt's lymphoma. Loosening of the teeth, ulceration of the palate or facial skin involvement may occur in advanced cases. Unilateral proptosis may arise at an early stage from orbital vein compression or, later and more commonly, from direct invasion through the orbital wall. Invasion of the maxillary division of the trigeminal nerve may result in facial pain or facial sensory loss. Later, severe headache may occur from invasion of the dura mater. Nasolachrymal and frontonasal duct obstruction, diplopia, optic atrophy, jaw limitation, loss of palate sensation and loss of the sense of smell may all occur.

Trauma

Maxillary fractures

Fractures of the maxilla (*Figure 10.6*) are described according to **Le Fort lines**. These lines define the level above which the midfacial skeleton is intact:

- Line I runs transversely, just above the floor of the nose through the lower third of the nasal septum.
- Line II runs through the bridge of the nose and medial orbital walls via the lachrymal bones, then crosses the inferior orbital rim at the junction of its medial one-third and lateral two-thirds. It passes through the infraorbital foramen and runs beneath the zygomaticomaxillary suture to extend backwards through the lateral pterygoid plates. The zygomatic arches remain intact.
- Line III runs parallel to the base of the skull. The fracture line runs through the nasal bone and continues posteriorly through the ethmoid, crosses the lesser wing of the sphenoid and then runs laterally upwards to the frontozygomatic suture. It normally passes below the optic foramen, but rarely may run through it.

Generally, the level of impact to the face determines the level of the fracture. Thus low level anterior and lateral impacts produce the **Le Fort I** (Guérin) fracture, the separated segment consisting of the palate, maxillary alveolar processes and the lower thirds of the pterygoid plates. Mid-

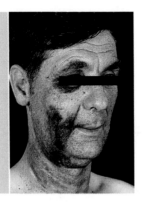

Figure 10.6.
Fracture of the right side of the maxilla.

level impacts and inferior trauma, when the mouth is open, result in the **Le Fort II**, the separated fragment being pyramidal in shape. High level impacts and superior impacts result in the **Le Fort III** where the whole midface separates from the skull. These fractures may occur symmetrically across the whole maxilla or may be in unilateral combinations, for example a Le Fort I on the left with a Le Fort II on the right. All these fractures are open to either the nose, the paranasal sinuses or the mouth. Le Fort II fractures involve the cribriform plate and should therefore be regarded as communicating with the subarachnoid space. Le Fort II and III types affect the attachments of the orbital contents.

General features of all three fracture types are **bilateral periorbital bruising**, **bilateral gross facial oedema** and **lengthening of the middle third of the face**. There may be malocclusion in the molar region and the nose is filled with blood.

Sensory loss can result if the fracture lines run through nerve canals. **Infraorbital nerve** injury gives rise to anaesthesia in the area between the inferior orbital margin and the upper lip, the side of the nose being spared. **Inferior alveolar nerve** injury results in anaesthesia of the mental region and **supraorbital nerves** may be divided by lacerations above the eyebrow giving anaesthesia above the eye.

Facial palsy is relatively rare but if present usually results from neuropraxia of the peripheral branches or less commonly from basilar skull fractures (p.154).

Surgical emphysema may be indicative of an upper airway injury.

Examination for instability of the maxilla may be possible in the unconscious or anaesthetized patient. When steadying the frontonasal junction with one hand, it may be possible to illustrate mobility in a Le Fort II and III by lifting the premaxillary region upward with the other hand. It may also be possible to spring the two maxillae apart. In the mouth the mandibular, maxillary and lingual sulci should be palpated for bony contour abnormality, but maxillary fractures are not often compound to the mouth. Percussion of the maxillary teeth may illustrate a change in the normal resonance to a 'cracked cup' sound. There is frequently gagging of the occlusion in one or both molar regions.

Zygomatic fractures

Zygoma may be part of Le Fort fractures or isolated injuries. They may go unrecognized from the initial swelling (*Figure 10.7*) but become obvious once the swelling has subsided (*Figure 10.8*). The injury may involve the temporomandibular joint, the infraorbital canal and the zygomatico-frontal suture with resultant painful mastication, numbness of the cheek and diplopia.

Mandibular fractures

Mandibular fractures are usually multiple. The commonest site is the condylar region, followed by the angle. For isolated fractures, however, the angle is the principal site. Fractures

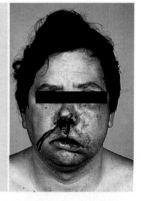

Figure 10.7.
Le Fort primary fracture of the left zygoma. In the early stages gross oedema masks the extent of the associated bony injury.

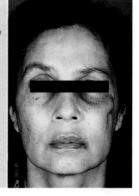

Figure 10.8.
Fracture of the zygoma. Once the swelling has subsided, bony deformity becomes evident.

of the body and opposite condyle or angle are the most likely combination but bilateral subcondylar fractures occur. Bilateral involvement of the angles or body, or three or more fracture sites are uncommon.

Condylar fractures are usually indirect, the direct result of the impact producing the body fracture. This is because the condylar region is well protected by the zygomatic arch. Most condylar fractures are actually subcondylar, running between the mandibular notch and a point above the middle of the posterior border of the ramus. Less commonly the fracture may be intracapsular, resulting in a temporomandibular joint effusion or haemarthrosis. Displacement in condylar fractures is relatively slight but the mandible tends to deviate to the side of the injury on opening the mouth, the lateral pterygoid no longer being able to influence the main fragment of the mandible. Movement at the temporomandibular joint is painful and limited by protective muscle spasm. Bilateral condylar fractures classically result when a patient loses consciousness and falls on to the chin. In combination with a parasymphyseal fracture and a characteristic laceration beneath the chin, this injury is called a **parade ground fracture**.

Temporomandibular joint dislocation is distinguished from a condylar fracture in that it produces a prominence anterior to the articular eminence and a hollow in the glenoid fossa. In unilateral cases the mandible deviates to the opposite side. There is gagging posteriorly and an inability to close the mouth. In a combined **fracture–dislocation of the condyle** the balance between the elevator muscles and lateral pterygoid is disturbed such that the jaw deviates towards the injured side. **Central dislocation of the condyle** is a rare occurrence where the condyle penetrates into the middle cranial fossa through the roof of the glenoid fossa. Fortunately the relatively weak condylar neck usually absorbs enough force to prevent this.

Fractures of the angle of the mandible tend to occur anterior to the attachment of the masseter. The elevator muscles therefore tend to pull the posterior fragment upwards, forwards and inwards, being unable to have any effect on the remainder of the mandible.

Fractures of the body of the mandible tend to occur in the region between the canine and first molar teeth. The further forward the fracture site, the more the upward pull of the elevator muscles on the posterior fragment is counteracted by the downward pull of the mylohyoid, thus reducing the degree of displacement.

In examining the mandible, the lower border can be palpated from behind and the temporomandibular joint regions inspected from the front. Movement of the condylar heads can be assessed by placing the little fingers in each external auditory meatus with the pulps pointing forwards whilst the patient attempts to move the mandible in all directions. If doubt exists as to the presence of a mandibular fracture the **compression test** may be of value. Here pain is elicited from an undisplaced fracture by applying gentle compression in two planes.

Mandibular fractures are often open to the buccal cavity, bloodstained saliva being a common finding. When this finding accompanies maxillary fractures, however, it is more likely to be due to nasopharyngeal bleeding. There may be ecchymoses of the buccal sulci near the zygomatic prominences or in the region of the greater palatine foramen: Guérin's sign. A sublingual haematoma is indicative of a fracture involving the lingual plate.

Styloid fractures are a rare accompaniment of mandibular fractures. They result either from sudden muscle spasm or from severe posterior displacement of the rami in a bilateral fracture dislocation. Dysfunction of the stylohyoid and stylomandibular ligaments, and the styloglossus and stylohyoid muscles, results in the classical symptom, a persistent difficulty in swallowing.

Soft tissue lacerations of the face are worthy of mention, in that they characteristically have a superficial and deep component. The deep injury arises from the rolling of tissues over the lower border of the mandible. A thin fascial layer separates the lacerations, hence injuries of this type should be explored to exclude a concealed foreign body.

Trigeminal neuralgia and herpes zoster

Trigeminal neuralgia is a condition of unknown aetiology that causes intense pain in the distribution of the trigeminal nerve. It affects patients over 50 years old, but it may occur in younger age groups in relation to multiple sclerosis. The condition is usually unilateral and may affect one or more divisions of the nerve. The pain very characteristically occurs in intense, knife-like paroxysms lasting only a few seconds. Touch, movement and even cold air on the face may trigger the pain, and there may be specific trigger spots. The pain seems to subside at night. Initially there may be remissions for months or even years, but in the older patient this is less likely.

Continuous pain in the trigeminal nerve distribution is not trigeminal neuralgia. In these cases malignant infiltration should be considered. Glossopharyngeal neuralgia is rare; it presents with paroxysms of agonizing pain around the oropharynx and is usually brought on by swallowing.

Herpes zoster (shingles) may also affect the trigeminal nerve, causing severe pain (*Figures 10.9–10.11*). The

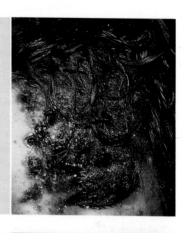

Figure 10.9.
Herpes zoster affecting the ophthalmic nerve.

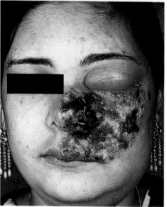

Figure 10.10.
Herpes zoster affecting the maxillary nerve.

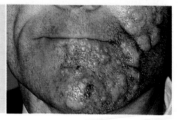

Figure 10.11.
Herpes zoster affecting the mandibular nerve.

condition is usually unilateral and may selectively involve divisions of the nerve, particularly the first. There may be initial paraesthesia over the affected dermatome. In most patients the characteristic skin eruption is preceded by the onset of shooting pains. In the young, the skin eruption may be relatively trivial but more usually the dermatome is covered with a vesicular rash. These vesicles scab over by about 7 days and settle over the following weeks. Scarring may result if the scabs are prematurely disturbed and superadded staphylococcal infection occurs. After resolution, pain may sometimes persist for years as post-herpetic neuralgia.

Bell's palsy and Ramsay Hunt syndrome

Bell's palsy is a unilateral lower motor neurone facial palsy of unknown cause. It most commonly occurs in the 20–50 year age range. It commences as aching below the ear or in the mastoid region, followed by a fairly rapid onset of facial paralysis. In severe cases there may be a loss of taste in the anterior two-thirds of the tongue, and paralysis of the stapedius makes high-pitched or loud sounds intolerable. Most cases are probably the result of segmental demyelination within the facial canal, and recovery occurs spontaneously over the following weeks. In a small proportion of cases, however, there is degeneration and subsequent reinnervation. Here function may return over several months but inappropriate reinnervation may result in twitching of the angle of the mouth on blinking.

Ramsay Hunt syndrome arises from herpes zoster infection of both the otic and genicular ganglia. Sensorineural deafness, vertigo and facial paralysis may all result. Recovery is less certain than for Bell's palsy.

11 The ear

The outer ear

Congenital abnormalities

The various congenital anomalies of the ear are accounted for by the differing embryology of the outer, middle and inner ear. The auricle develops from six auricular tubercles which appear around the margins of the first visceral cleft. The external auditory meatus develops from the ectoderm of the first visceral cleft, the malleus and incus from the mesoderm of the first pharyngeal arch and the stapes from the mesoderm of the second arch and around the membranous labyrinth. The inner ear arises from a placode of what is probably neural crest tissue.

In **microtia** *(Figure 11.1)* there is only a rudimentary pinna. In its severest form, anotia, the pinna may be absent *(Figure 11.2)*. In addition there may be **atresia of the external auditory meatus** and the inner ear may also be absent. Atresia and stenosis of the external auditory meatus may also be acquired as a result of chronic otitis externa or develop following radical mastoidectomy.

In **Collins–Franceschetti–Klein syndrome** *(Figure 11.3)* the ears are low set, the auricles have a crumpled appearance and there may be atresia of the external canal causing conductive deafness. The palpebral fissures slope downwards and laterally and the lower eyelids are notched and devoid of eyelashes. The upper lip is large, there may be a cleft palate and there is micrognathia, i.e. short horizontal rami of the mandible. The condition shows autosomal dominant inheritance with incomplete penetrance and variable expressivity.

Accessory auricles *(Figure 11.4)* may arise from abnormally sited tubercles. **Pre-auricular cysts** and **sinuses** result from incomplete fusion *(Figure 11.5)* of the tubercles and are usually found in the region of the root of the helix. Rarely there can be fistulous communications to the ear canal or middle ear.

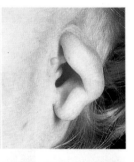

Figure 11.3.
Shell ear deformity in a child with Collins–Franceschetti–Klein syndrome.

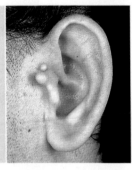

Figure 11.4.
Accessory auricles. Stenosis of the right external auditory meatus is also present.

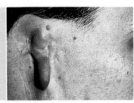

Figure 11.1.
Congenital absence of the right pinna.

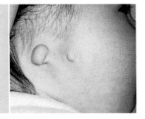

Figure 11.2.
Bilateral congenital ear deformity.

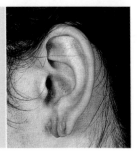

Figure 11.5.
Split ear lobes.

The commonest developmental abnormality is a prominence of the ears – '**bat ears**' *(Figure 11.6)* – which are usually bilateral.

Otitis externa

Otitis externa represents a variety of conditions that manifest as an acute or chronic reaction of the skin of the external ear, the cardinal symptom of which is irritation.

Furuncles may arise from staphylococcal infection of hair follicles in the cartilaginous portion of the external auditory meatus. Spontaneous evacuation usually occurs within a few days, relieving the irritation. Abrasion of the meatus by ear inserts, such as those used by telephonists, may encourage the condition. Diabetics are particularly susceptible and the problem may be recurrent.

Diffuse infective otitis externa *(Figure 11.7)* is a spreading dermatitis, usually starting in the external auditory canal and spreading to involve the auricle. It results in crusting and desquamation, the usual cause being streptococcal infection *(Figures 11.8 and 11.9)*.

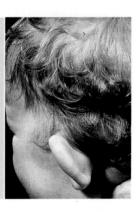

Figure 11.9.
Postauricular abscess. The associated oedema has displaced the left auricle.

In fungal infection of the external ear, **otomycosis**, the external auditory canal becomes lined with material resembling wet newspaper which has a musty odour and may be shown, on microscopic examination, to contain fungal hyphae and spores. Fungal infection usually occurs in the immuno-compromised, in association with topical antibiotic use or secondary to bacterial infection. The usual organisms are *Aspergillus niger* and *Candida albicans*.

Herpes zoster may give rise to a painful vesicular rash affecting the auricle as a component of herpes zoster oticus (see below).

Contact dermatitis may affect the ear, resulting in a localized eczematous reaction as elsewhere. For example, the posterior sulcus may be affected by nickel in the frames of glasses. **Seborrhoeic dermatitis** gives rise to greasy scaling skin; it affects the scalp, face and external ear. It may be the result of *Microbacillus cutis communis* infection.

Otitis externa malignans may rarely occur as a result of pseudomonas infection affecting the pinna in the elderly diabetic or immunocompromised patient. Infection spreads, resulting in osteomyelitis of the temporal bone. Patients have a painful discharging ear and may develop cranial nerve palsies as a number of these nerves exit the skull through foramina in the temporal bone. The seventh and last four nerves are most likely to be affected, but so may, more rarely, the fifth and sixth nerves in combination; this is **Gradenigo's syndrome**. Infection may spread to the sigmoid venous sinus and meninges with a potentially fatal outcome, cranial nerve involvement being a poor prognostic factor.

Tumours

Exostosis is the commonest benign tumour of the external ear. It refers to new bone formation projecting into the lumen of the bony canal. In its most frequent form it is bilateral but,

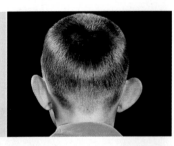

Figure 11.6.
Bat ears.

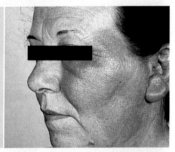

Figure 11.7.
Left otitis externa producing oedema in the adjacent face.

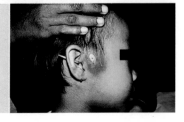

Figure 11.8.
Pre-auricular abscess.

rarely, single pedunculated tumours can occur. It may result in conductive deafness with debris and the exostosis itself covering the tympanic membrane.

Ceruminomas are firm masses under the skin of the outer meatus. They arise from ceruminous glands and are benign tumours *(Figure 11.10)*. Rarely they may give rise to adenocarcinomas.

Squamous cell carcinoma (p.140) may present as an ulcerating lesion of the meatus or auricle or simply as a serosanguineous discharge from the canal. **Basal cell carcinomas** (p.141) tend to be pre- or postauricular. They may also occur on the auricle but are relatively rare on the tragus and concha.

Trauma

Blunt trauma to the ear *(Figure 11.11)* may result in bleeding deep to the perichondrium, giving rise to a **haematoma auris** *(Figure 11.12)*. The cartilage depends on the perichondrium for its blood supply and thus, with repeated trauma, necrosis of the cartilage and resultant scarring may result in a deformed '**cauliflower ear**' *(Figure 11.13)*. Such scarring may also follow frostbite, severe infection and radiotherapy.

Miscellaneous conditions

Keloid scars may occur on the lobes. **Tophi** – subperichondrial sodium biurate deposits – may arise on the auricle in gout. **Sebaceous cysts** tend to occur on the back of the auricle and lobule *(Figure 11.14)*.

Ceruminous glands secrete cerumen (wax) into the external canal. This, together with keratin and other debris, may accumulate and form plugs of **impacted wax**. Conductive deafness, tinnitus, reflex coughing and earache may result. Such symptoms may appear suddenly when a plug is impacted against the tympanic membrane by washing, swimming or attempts at removal.

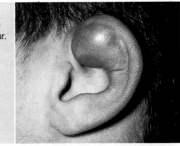

Figure 11.12. Haematoma of the pinna of the left ear.

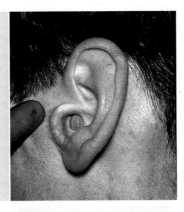

Figure 11.10. Left aural polyp.

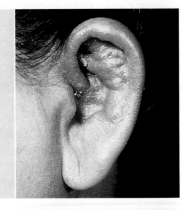

Figure 11.13. Perichondriasis in the left ear.

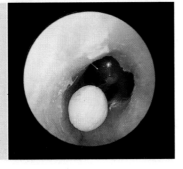

Figure 11.11. Foreign body in the external auditory meatus.

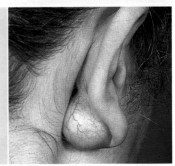

Figure 11.14. Sebaceous cyst in the right pinna.

The middle ear

Otosclerosis

This hereditary condition causes conductive deafness in the young adult, with a normal drum on otoscopy. It results from new spongy bone formation in the region of the stapes footplate, which limits its mobility. Inheritance is as an autosomal dominant condition with incomplete penetrance; about 50% of affected patients having a family history. Pregnancy may promote its development, more females being affected than males. There is an association with osteogenesis imperfecta as **van der Hoeve's syndrome**.

Acute suppurative otitis media

This common childhood infection usually arises following viral upper respiratory tract infection. Less commonly, infection may enter the middle ear via a ruptured tympanic membrane or a grommet; *Streptococcus pneumoniae* or *Haemophilus influenzae* are the usual causative organisms. Initially there is a eustachian salpingitis which then spreads to give inflammation of the tympanic membrane. There is increasing conductive deafness, earache and systemic evidence of infection. Mesenteric adenitis may cause abdominal pain. Otoscopy reveals a red, lustreless bulging drum. In the infant, acute suppurative otitis media is a common cause of pyrexia and meningeal irritation. Children may have a high temperature and febrile convulsions may result.

If untreated, the drum may perforate, relieving the pain, and **acute mastoiditis** *(Figure 11.15)* may then develop. The degree of pneumatization of the mastoid may determine the propensity to develop mastoiditis, more air cells providing a larger space for abscess formation. Clinically there is inflammation over the mastoid region and a more pronounced systemic response to infection. Rarely a similar infection may result in a pneumatization of the apex of the petrous temporal bone. Cranial nerve compression may occur causing deep pain in the distribution of the trigeminal nerve, usually retro-ocular, and paralysis of the lateral rectus muscle from abducent nerve involvement. The combination of trigeminal pain and lateral rectus palsy in conjunction with middle ear infection is **Gradenigo's triad** and, together with radiographic evidence of an abscess in the petrous temporal bone, is diagnostic of petrositis.

Recurrent otitis media may indicate a nidus of infection elsewhere, such as a sinusitis, or may occur in immune deficiency. In some recurrent cases there is a persisting effusion in the middle ear between attacks.

Chronic serous otitis media (glue ear)

Otitis media with a persisting effusion is a common problem amongst children of developed countries, with a peak incidence at 2–5 years. It may present with fluctuant hearing loss, developmental or behavioural problems (such as delayed language development), recurrent ear infections or may simply be identified on otoscopy at health screening.

Otoscopy reveals a dull, relatively immobile tympanic membrane and a fluid level is sometimes visible *(Figure 11.16)*. Many of these effusions resolve spontaneously but some cases necessitate the placement of grommets which ventilate the middle ear and prevent reaccumulation.

Chronic suppurative otitis media

This term is used to cover two unrelated conditions with markedly different outcomes. **Tubotympanic disease** refers to repeated reinfection via a perforation in the pars tensa of the tympanic membrane, or from an upper respiratory tract source, such as persisting adenoidal hyperplasia or a cleft palate. The condition does not have serious sequelae.

Atico-antral disease or **cholesteatoma** is also regarded as a form of chronic suppurative otitis media but its nature and outcome are far more serious. A cholesteatoma is effectively an epidermoid cyst arising in the middle ear. The aetiology is

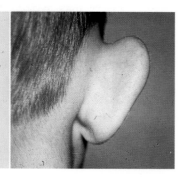

Figure 11.15.
Acute mastoiditis. The associated oedema has produced a 'bat ear' appearance.

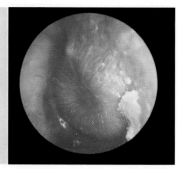

Figure 11.16.
View of the tympanic membrane in a patient with otitis media and an effusion (glue ear).

unknown but it may arise as a retraction pocket of the tympanic membrane, perhaps drawn inwards by negative pressure associated with a blocked eustachian tube. A cholesteatoma is locally destructive, resulting in perforation of the tympanic membrane and destruction of any of the structures within the temporal bone. Patients present with smelly discharge from the ear and conductive hearing loss. Otoscopy may reveal the perforations described or debris in the ear canal; the contents of the cholesteatoma itself may be visible through the perforation as a grey substance.

Complications

Serious complications are most often the result of acute exacerbations of chronic infection associated with cholesteatoma.

Localized infection and destruction of the temporal bone and its contained structures can result in **cranial nerve palsies**, particularly of the facial nerve. Erosion of the inner ear may cause **sensorineural deafness and vertigo**.

Infection spreading through the temporal bone may manifest itself externally as subperiosteal abscesses. These are usually postauricular (lying over the mastoid) but may also be preauricular (pus escaping from zygomatic air cells) or lie in the substance of the sternomastoid muscle (**von Bezold's abscess**).

Intracranial infection may result from direct spread from temporal bone osteomyelitis, by retrograde thrombophlebitis via small veins from the brain substance which communicate with Haversian canals, through the various foramina or via old basilar fractures. **Thrombophlebitis of the sigmoid sinus, meningitis** and **brain abscesses** may result.

Ear and sinus infections account for about half of all brain abscesses, most of these being otogenic. Brain abscesses arising from middle ear infection may either be in the **ipsilateral temporal lobe** or in the **ipsilateral cerebellar hemisphere**. Symptoms may be acute or insidious, with systemic evidence of sepsis, raised intracranial pressure and focal signs specific to the area involved. In the case of the temporal lobe this may take the form of temporal lobe epilepsy, dysphasia – dominant hemisphere – and upper quadrantic hemianopia for the opposite field of vision. Cerebellar abscesses may cause vertigo, nystagmus and balance problems.

Acute suppurative otitis media may result in **perforations** of the tympanic membrane. These may be marginal or central and may be closed by a thin membrane. They usually result in conductive deafness, less so in closed cases. Scarring of the tympanic membrane (**tympanosclerosis**) and adhesions between the ossicles (**adhesive otitis**) may also result in conductive deafness following infection.

Other types of middle ear infection

Tuberculous otitis media may rarely occur secondary to pulmonary disease with infection spreading via the eustachian tube. Caseous necrosis in the middle ear results in multiple painless perforations of the tympanic membrane causing otorrhoea and conductive deafness of insidious onset. In addition, aminoglycoside antibiotics used in treatment may cause sensorineural deafness and vertigo.

Syphilitic otitis media is another rare form that occurs as a combined inner and middle ear infection: otolabyrinthitis. It may occur in congenital syphilis and in the tertiary stage of acquired syphilis and appears as a painless otorrhoea with sensorineural deafness.

Traumatic rupture of the tympanic membrane

Foreign bodies, unskilled instrumentation or syringeing, sudden changes in air pressure (e.g. flying, diving or nose blowing), basal skull fractures passing through the petrous temporal bone and electrocution may all result in perforation of the tympanic membrane. There is pain, deafness, tinnitus, vertigo and blood in the meatus, the perforation being visible on auroscopy.

The inner ear and vestibulocochlear nerve

Herpes zoster oticus

Herpes zoster infection may occur in the vestibular ganglion, causing intense pain in the ear. Sensorineural deafness may result, forming part of the **Ramsay Hunt's syndrome** (p.168).

Acoustic neuroma

This is a benign tumour of the acoustic nerve that presents with sensorineural hearing loss, tinnitus and vertigo. Bilateral cases occur in **type 2 neurofibromatosis** (i.e. central neurofibromatosis) but the condition is not associated with type 1 neurofibromatosis (von Recklinghausen's disease, p.149).

The trigeminal nerve may become involved causing pain or numbness in any division and loss of the corneal reflex. In addition, the tumour may compress the fourth ventricle causing headache from rising intracranial pressure. Cerebellar symptoms, diplopia and facial nerve palsy may also later develop. Eventually death may result from the effects of further increases in intracranial pressure.

Other conditions causing sensorineural deafness or vertigo

Meniere's disease is a condition of unknown aetiology characterized by intermittent attacks of vertigo, low frequency sensorineural hearing loss and tinnitus. All three features are required for its diagnosis. It is usually unilateral and affects more females than males. Accumulation of endolymphatic fluid is thought to result in rupture of the inner ear membranes with subsequent mixing of endolymph and perilymph. The disturbance of electrolyte balance that this creates gives an abrupt vestibulocochlear failure. Most cases resolve spontaneously.

Paraganglionomas are rare benign tumours arising from non-chromaffin paraganglionic tissue in the head and neck, the best known being carotid body tumours. In the temporal bone these may be in the middle ear (glomus tympanicum), the jugular bulb (glomus jugulare) or with the vagus nerve (glomus vagale). They classically cause pulsatile tinnitus and sensorineural deafness. Palsies of the facial, glossopharyngeal and hypoglossal nerves may occur. Otoscopy may reveal a pulsatile mass behind the tympanic membrane and there may be an audible bruit over the temporal bone.

Noise-induced hearing loss may result from sudden severe noise exposure, which can recover if not too severe, or from prolonged exposure such as in industry.

Barotrauma refers to the damage caused by sudden pressure changes such as those encountered in unpressur-ized flying or diving. It may cause rupture of the inner ear membranes with endolymph fistula formation, the patients presenting with sensorineural deafness, tinnitus and vertigo. There may be a positive **fistula test** where raising and lowering the external ear pressure by a pumping action on the tragus induces nystagmus and vertigo.

Sensorineural hearing loss may also occur as a result of damage to the inner ear from transverse **basal skull fractures** and as a sudden, unexplained hearing loss following **viral infections**. Viral infections may also possibly give rise to the phenomenon of **acute vestibular failure** or **vestibular neuronitis** where there is a sudden severe vertigo that resolves spontaneously over a few days. **AIDS** (p.98) may be associated with auditory **nerve neuropathy** and resultant sensorineural hearing loss.

Presbyacusis is the name given to age-related hearing loss. It is a bilateral, symmetrical condition where high frequency sounds are most affected. As consonants tend to be high frequency sounds, these patients have difficulty in understanding speech. In addition, the cochlea loses the ability to accommodate. Shouting therefore adds nothing to their ability to understand and may decrease the resolution of sounds.

Ototoxic drugs such as aminoglycosides, high dose salicylates and some chemotherapeutic agents may produce tinnitus, sensorineural deafness and vertigo. Some are selective, for example streptomycin tends to affect the vestibular apparatus, whereas others, such as gentamicin, affect both systems.

12 The orbit

Periorbital disease

Dermoid cysts are congenital subcutaneous cystic lesions that occur mainly around the eyes. They result from the sequestration of skin along lines of embryonic closure and differ from sebaceous cysts histologically in that they are lined by an epidermis complete with appendages. The commonest site is over the external angular process of the frontal bone, the **external angular dermoid** (*Figure 12.1*). The cyst may become adherent to the periosteum of the underlying bone, which becomes hollowed. The outer eyebrow overlies the cyst, which distinguishes it from a swelling of the lachrymal gland. Less commonly, **internal angular dermoid cysts** arise that lie over the root of the nose. Sublingual dermoids are described on p.192.

    Herpes zoster ophthalmicus – shingles – results from an infection of the trigeminal ganglion with herpes zoster or chickenpox virus (p.167). It occurs mainly in the elderly and immunocompromised and takes the form of a painful vesicular skin rash over the forehead and side of the nose corresponding to the distribution of the trigeminal nerve. The vesicles become dry scabs over a few days and the lesions gradually subside over the following weeks, sometimes resulting in scarring. The pain may persist for months after the rash has subsided as post-herpetic neuralgia.

The eyelids

Congenital conditions of the eyelids include epicanthus, ptosis and coloboma. **Epicanthus** (*Figure 12.2*) is usually bilateral and takes the form of additional concave skin folds extending from the nasal aspect of the upper eyelids to the lower eyelids at the medial canthus. It may give the impression of a convergent squint but becomes less prominent with facial growth. **Ptosis** (*Figures 12.3* and *12.4*) may occur congenitally from the incomplete development of the levator palpebrae superioris. It refers to a drooping of the eyelid which may be unilateral or bilateral.

    Blepharitis (*Figure 12.5*) is a chronic inflammation of the eyelid margins from staphylococcal infection. Crusty exudates

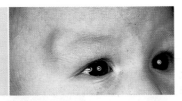
Figure 12.1.
External angular dermoid cyst.

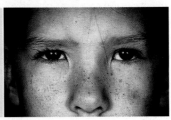
Figure 12.2.
Prominent epicanthic folds and naevi, left cheek.

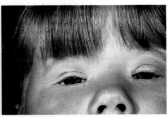
Figure 12.3.
Congenital ptosis.

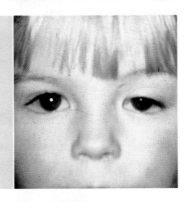
Figure 12.4.
Bilateral congenital ptosis.

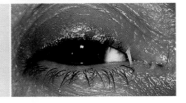
Figure 12.5.
Blepharitis.

Figure 12.6.
Trachomal infection occurs in 500 million people worldwide, resulting in blindness in over 5 million individuals.

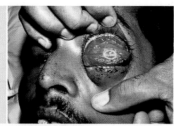

Figure 12.7.
Stye.

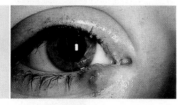

Figure 12.8.
Chalazion. Left upper lid.

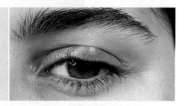

Figure 12.9.
Cysts of Zeis and Moll.

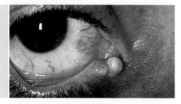

Figure 12.10.
Retention cyst.

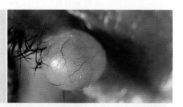

Figure 12.11.
Squamous cell carcinoma of the medial canthus.

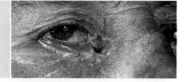

Figure 12.12.
Right entropion.

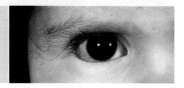

form on the inflamed lids and the eyelashes may be lost. **Acute allergic blepharitis** arises rapidly in response to a variety of common allergens such as pollens, dusts, make-up, eyedrops and seafood. Chronic inflammation of the eyelids may also result from infection with *Chlamydia trachomatis*: **trachoma** (*Figure 12.6*). Here the conjunctiva lining the inner surface of the eyelid becomes studded with follicles.

Cystic lesions include styes, meibomian cysts and cysts of Moll. **Styes** (*Figure 12.7*) result from acute staphylococcal infection of an eyelash follicle and present as red, discharging swellings of the eyelid margin. As with furuncles elsewhere, repeated affliction may raise the suspicion of diabetes. **Meibomian cysts** (chalazion, *Figure 12.8*) are painless mobile lumps in the eyelid resulting from trapped sebum in a meibomian gland. **Cysts of Moll** (*Figures 12.9* and *12.10*) are translucent swellings at the eyelid margin arising from obstructed glands of Moll.

Papillomas and vascular malformations may occur on the eyelids. **Venous malformations** appear as red or blue soft swellings of the lid and almost always regress in the first few years of life. **Capillary malformations** appear as a purple skin discoloration (port wine stain) and may be associated with meningeal and choroidal haemangiomas and juvenile glaucoma in the Sturge–Weber syndrome.

Basal cell carcinomas (p.141) are the commonest malignant tumour of the eyelids. **Squamous cell carcinomas** (p.40; *Figure 12.11*) occur less commonly, usually at the canthus. Pre-auricular and submandibular nodes are often involved from lymphatic spread.

Entropion (*Figure 12.12*) is an inturning of the lower lid which may occur without apparent cause in the elderly or less commonly may result from scarring of the tarsal conjunctiva or from spasm secondary to irritation from a foreign body. The eyelashes may abrade the conjunctiva or cornea resulting in watering and inflammation of the eye. In **ectropion** (*Figure 12.13*) the lower lid sags downward. Again it usually occurs in the elderly but may result from scarring or facial palsy.

Xanthelasma (*Figure 12.14*) are yellow lipid deposits in the skin of the eyelids. They occur in the hyperlipidaemia associated with diabetes and myxoedema and also in primary hypercholesterolaemias.

Figure 12.13.
Ectropion of the lower lid.

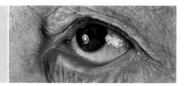

Figure 12.14.
Xanthelasma in a
patient with hyper-
cholesterolaemia.

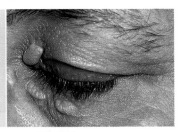

The lachrymal apparatus

Acute dacryocystitis (*Figure 12.15*) results from infection of the lachrymal sac secondary to nasolachrymal duct obstruction. There is a rapid onset of a painful, inflamed swelling just below the medial canthus at the side of the nose. **Chronic dacryocystitis** is a longstanding watering of the eyes – epiphoria – in the elderly patient associated with chronic nasolachrymal duct obstruction. This obstruction can also give rise to a **mucocele** of the lachrymal sac, presenting as a quiescent swelling of the sac. In the same way occlusion of the frontonasal duct may give rise to a **mucocele of the frontal sinus** (p.164) resulting in a swelling either in the position occupied by the lachrymal sac or lying over the bridge of the nose. As these swellings enlarge they may displace the globe. **Congenital obstruction of the nasolachrymal duct** may give rise to unilateral or bilateral sticky eyes in the infant. The duct may later open and the condition usually resolves.

Dacryoadenitis refers to inflammation of the lachrymal gland presenting as an inflamed swelling at the lateral aspect of the upper eyelid. It may result from acute infection, TB, mumps and sarcoidosis.

Neoplasms of the lachrymal gland present as hard, irregular swellings, enlarging over several months. They are relatively rare and usually occur in midlife. Mixed tumours are the commonest but adenoid cystic carcinomas, lymphomas and lymphosarcomas also occur. Involvement of the gland with lymphoma is usually associated with widespread reticulosis.

The eye

Red eye

The conditions that may result in a **red eye** are summarized in *Table 12.1*.

Conjunctivitis (*Figure 12.16*) may result from bacterial infection (staphylococcus; *Haemophilus influenzae*; streptococcus), viral infection (*Figure 12.17*; herpes simplex; adenovirus), *Chlamydia trachomatis* infection, trauma, chemical irritation, exposure to UV light and from inadequate tear secretion (conjunctivitis sicca). Pre-auricular lymphadenopathy and conjunctival follicles are additional features of adenoviral,

Table 12.1. The red eye.

Condition	Symptoms	Signs
Conjunctivitis	Bilateral red eyes 'gritty' eyes 'sticky' eyes	Conjunctival hyperaemia Oedematous eyelids Mucoid discharge
Iritis/uveitis	Unilateral red eye Lachrymation Photophobia Blurred vision Pain	Reduced acuity Ciliary injection Constricted pupil Anterior chamber flare Keratic precipitates Oedematous eyelid
Keratitis	Unilateral red eye Lachrymation Photophobia Blurred vision Pain	Reduced acuity Ciliary injection Localized corneal opacification (Dendritic ulcer)
Acute glaucoma	Unilateral red eye Lachrymation Photophobia Blurred vision Pain Haloes	Reduced acuity Ciliary injection Corneal oedema Half-dilated, oval pupil Raised ocular tension

Figure 12.16.
Bacterial conjunctivitis.

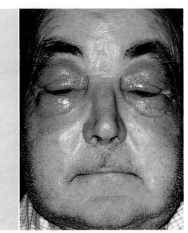

Figure 12.15.
Acute dacrocystitis.

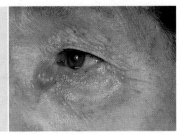

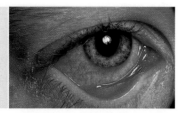

Figure 12.17.
Viral conjunctivitis.

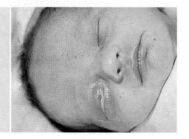

Figure 12.18.
Gonococcal
ophthalmia
neonatorum.

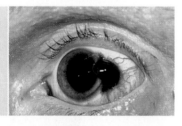

Figure 12.19.
Chlamydial
conjunctivitis.

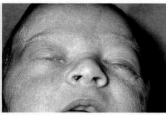

Figure 12.20.
Pterygium of the
right eye.

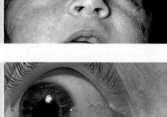

Figure 12.21.
Conjunctival
malignant
melanoma.

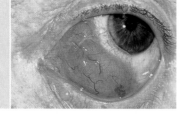

Figure 12.22.
Conjunctival
lymphoma.

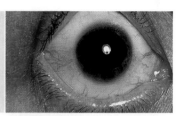

Figure 12.23.
Iritis of the right eye.

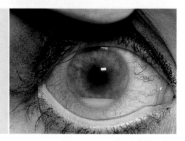

Figure 12.24.
Hypopyon.

herpes simplex and chlamydial conjunctivitis. Lymphoid follicles appear as rounded nodules in the inferior conjunctival
fornix. **Neonatal conjunctivitis**, from *Neisseria gonorrhoeae*
(*Figure 12.18*) or chlamydial infection (*Figure 12.19*), results
from contact with an infected birth canal. **Pterygium** (*Figure
12.20*) is a form of chronic conjunctivitis occurring in hot, dry
dusty countries, characterized by an ingrowth of the palpebral
conjunctiva on to the cornea. The conjunctiva may be the site
of malignant deposits (*Figures 12.21* and *12.22*).

Iritis (*Figure 12.23*) is an autoimmune condition associated with the seronegative arthritic and chronic inflammatory
disorders listed below. Inflammation may involve any part of
the uveal tract but the clinical distinction between iritis, cycli-
tis, anterior uveitis and uveitis is not clear. Deposition of inflammatory cells in the anterior chamber produce a hypopyon
(*Figure 12.24*). It is a common feature of Behçet's disease.
Conditions associated with iritis are:

- Sarcoidosis.
- Reiter's disease.
- Ankylosing spondylitis.
- Still's disease.
- Behçet's disease.
- TB.
- Syphilis.
- Leprosy.

Keratitis describes inflammation of the cornea, which may
result from bacterial (staphylococci; streptococci), viral
(herpes simplex; adenovirus; herpes zoster) or chlamydial

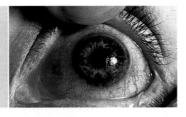

Figure 12.25.
Corneal (dendritic)
ulcer.

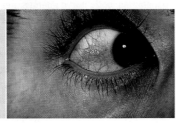

Figure 12.26.
Bilateral scleritis.

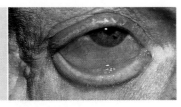

Figure 12.27.
Scleritis due to
Crohn's disease.

infection. A localized corneal opacity results from an oede-matous area of the cornea, which becomes infiltrated with inflammatory cells. In the case of **herpes simplex** infection, the corneal lesion forms a characteristic **dendritic ulcer** (*Figure 12.25*) that may be more apparent on staining with fluorescein or Bengal rose. **Adenovirus keratitis** occurs in epidemics and can easily be spread by the clinician's unwashed hands. **Trachoma keratitis** gives rise to a char-acteristic vascularized opacity called **panus**, which com-mences in the upper cornea but may extend to involve the whole cornea. Scarring from associated conjunctivitis may result in entropion and trichiasis, i.e. ingrowing eyelashes.

Scleritis (*Figure 12.26*) occurs in association with rheuma-toid arthritis, selected collagen disorders and inflammatory bowel disease (*Figure 12.27*). There is a dull aching pain and ciliary hyperaemia over part of the eye, which may continue for up to a year. In contrast, **episcleritis** is a relatively minor con-dition of unknown aetiology where there is hyperaemia of the episcleral vessels close to the corneal margin.

Glaucoma

Glaucoma is a condition where rising intraocular pressure damages the optic nerve, resulting in visual field loss. Glaucoma may be primary or secondary.

The primary glaucomas are:

- Congenital glaucoma.
- Acute (closed angle) glaucoma.
- Chronic simple (open angle) glaucoma.

Secondary glaucomas may occur with:

- Iritis.
- Injury.
- Central retinal vein thrombosis.
- Steroid eyedrops.
- Pseudoexfoliation of the lens capsule.

Congenital glaucoma is usually bilateral and occurs mainly in males. It may be noticed at birth or become appar-ent during the first few months of life. There is a huge enlargement of the eyes (called buphthalmos which means ox eyes), photophobia, clouding of the corneas and exces-sive lachrymation.

Acute glaucoma (*Figures 12.28* and *12.29*, closed angle glaucoma) is an ophthalmic emergency where there is a rapid rise in intraocular pressure which may result in permanent visual loss without immediate intervention. A narrow anterior chamber predisposes to the condition which usually affects one eye at a time. Days or weeks before, the patient may notice haloes, i.e. coloured rings, around artificial light sources, caused by diffraction by an oedematous cornea. There is then a rapid loss of vision, over several hours, with severe orbital aching pain, photophobia and nausea. The eye is red and watery with circumcorneal hyperaemia; the oedematous

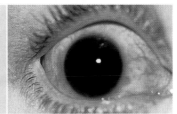

Figure 12.28.
Acute (rubeotic)
glaucoma with fresh
blood in the anterior
chamber.

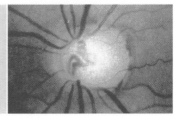

Figure 12.29.
Optic atrophy. Acute
glaucoma.

cornea appears cloudy. The pupil may be oval in shape, partly dilated and unreactive to light. The high intraocular pressure is apparent on digital palpation of the globe.

Chronic simple glaucoma – open angle glaucoma – results from a gradual rise in intraocular pressure, usually bilaterally, which tends to affect the over-40s. A partial visual field loss develops, which may be demonstrated by perimetry, and there is a deterioration of close vision. Fundoscopy reveals a cup-to-disc ratio of more than 0.5 and increased intraocular pressure is revealed by tonometry. This condition is a common cause of blindness worldwide.

Proptosis and exophthalmos

Proptosis refers to a protrusion of the entire orbital contents whereas **exophthalmos** is a protrusion of the globe alone, but this distinction is rarely made and so the terms are often used synonymously. Congenital abnormalities, infection, orbital masses, arteriovenous fistulae and thyrotoxicosis can all lead to such a protrusion.

Congenital proptosis occurs in craniofacial deformities such as Apert's and Crouzon's syndromes (p.153).

Orbital cellulitis (*Figure 12.30*) can result from the spread of infection from the frontal and ethmoidal sinuses, and from the lachrymal gland. The ethmoidal sinus is particularly implicated as it is only separated from the orbital contents by the thin lamina papyracea. Clinically it presents with a painful inflammatory oedema of the periorbital tissues, protrusion of the globe and a purulent conjunctival discharge. There is a risk of optic nerve damage, meningitis and cavernous sinus thrombosis. **Thrombophlebitis of the cavernous sinus** results from the spread of infection from the face along the angular ophthalmic vein, the middle ear along the lateral and petrosal venous sinuses, peritonsillar abscesses through the pterygoid venous plexus and from orbital cellulitis via the ophthalmic vein. Symptoms progress rapidly from severe headache and rigors to delirium. There is proptosis, chemosis (*Figure 12.31*, oedema of the ocular conjunctiva) and later ophthalmoplegia and loss of pupil reactivity. Blindness and death may ensue.

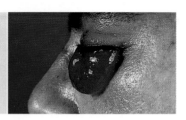

Figure 12.31. Conjunctival chemosis.

Retro-ocular and **ocular neoplasms** may displace the globe causing proptosis (*Figures 12.32–12.34*), strabismus and diplopia from interference with the extraocular musculature and decreased visual acuity from optic nerve compression. **Primary retro-ocular tumours** include **haemangiomas**, **optic nerve gliomas**, **neurofibromas**, **meningiomas**, **lymphomas** and **osteogenic sarcomas**. In addition, dermoid cysts, lachrymal gland tumours and swellings of the lachrymal sac may displace the globe. Secondary tumours include direct intraorbital extension of nasopharyngeal malignancies and metastatic deposits from breast and lung carcinomas.

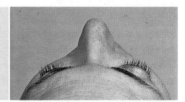

Figure 12.32. Retro-orbital tumour producing proptosis of the right eye.

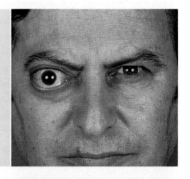

Figure 12.33. Carcinoma of the ethmoidal air sinus producing proptosis of the right eye.

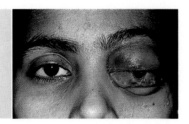

Figure 12.30. Orbital cellulitis.

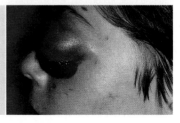

Figure 12.34. Rhabdomyosarcoma of the orbit.

Tumours of the fundus present with visual field changes or may be found on routine fundoscopy. Only rarely may they progress sufficiently to result in proptosis. **Malignant melanomas of the choroid** (*Figure 12.35*) may be seen on fundoscopy as a raised brown area near the posterior pole of the fundus. A gradually increasing shadow may be noted in the visual field but more rapid deterioration of vision may occur with secondary retinal detachment. Benign choroidal melanomas occur as flat, pigmented areas on the fundus near the posterior pole. Here there is no field defect and the lesion is usually simply a finding on fundoscopy.

Retinoblastoma (*Figure 12.36*) is the only primary malignant tumour of the retina and presents in the first two years of life. A raised white area is noted on fundoscopy. Sometimes the parents notice the appearance of a white pupil due to reflected light from the tumour. More advanced cases progress to strabismus, proptosis and ultimately a fungating mass. The tumour may spread along the optic nerve to the brain and haematogenous metastases may also arise. It is now believed that the condition is inherited in a recessive manner. A point mutation on chromosome 13 gives this predisposition but the tumour only appears in homozygotes. Most cases arise when the child is homozygous for the affected gene as a result of a second mutational event. One quarter of cases are bilateral and there is also an associated risk of the subsequent development of osteogenic sarcoma.

Carotid cavernous fistulae (*Figure 12.37*) arise when an aneurysm of the intracranial carotid artery ruptures into the cavernous sinus. This may occur spontaneously or as a result of trauma. There is a rapid onset of throbbing orbital pain, a buzzing noise in the head and blurred vision. Examination reveals a pulsating proptosis with a loud orbital bruit, the pulsation ceasing on occluding the ipsilateral carotid artery in the neck. Pulsating proptosis may also be a feature of a highly vascular orbital neoplasm or an ophthalmic artery aneurysm.

Primary thyrotoxicosis may result in ophthalmopathy. **Non-infiltrative ophthalmopathy** results from increased sympathetic activity, leading to upper eyelid retraction. This gives the appearance of bulging, staring eyes from the widening of the palpebral fissures. This can be accentuated by von Graefe's sign in which, when the patient follows the examiner's finger up and down, the upper lid is seen to lag behind the corneoscleral limbus ('lid lag'). **Infiltrative ophthalmopathy** is a process of cellular infiltration and mucopolysaccharide deposition resulting in oedema of the orbital and periorbital tissues. There is proptosis – actual protrusion of the globes (*Figure 12.38*) – which is usually, but not always, bilateral. Proptosis is demonstrated by examining the patient from behind while tipping the head backwards. Ophthalmoplegias (*Figure 12.39*) develop, particularly of the superior rectus and inferior oblique muscles, causing diplopia which is most marked on an upward and outward gaze. There is weakness of convergence and loss of co-ordinated eye movements. There is a reduced blink

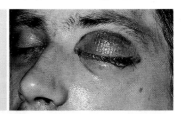

Figure 12.37.
Carotid cavernous fistula.

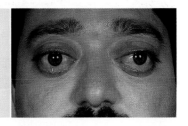

Figure 12.38.
Malignant exophthalmos.

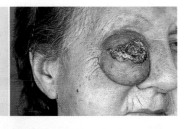

Figure 12.35.
Malignant melanoma.

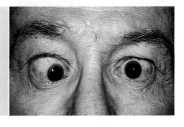

Figure 12.39.
Exophthalmic ophthalmoplegia.

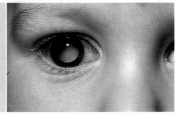

Figure 12.36.
Retinoblastoma of the right eye.

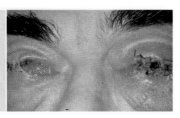

Figure 12.40.
Thyrotropic exoph-
thalmos with
chemosis.

reflex, which, with the increased area of eye exposure, can lead to corneal irritation, chemosis (*Figure 12.40*) and corneal ulceration. Visual acuity deteriorates with the development of papilloedema, retinal oedema, haemorrhages and optic nerve damage. Severe cases – malignant exophthalmos – progress to blindness.

Eye injury

Small, high velocity bodies, such as metal fragments from engineering processes, may result in intraocular foreign bodies (*Figure 12.41*). More usually such fragments are of lower velocity and tend to become corneal foreign bodies.

Trivial injury to the conjunctiva may result in a **conjunctival haemorrhage** (*Figure 12.42*). This is distinguished from subconjunctival haemorrhage in that it moves with the conjunctiva on moving the eyelid. Glancing blows from a fingernail or twig may result in a **corneal abrasion**. There is inflammation and watering of the eye which may recur over

a period of weeks from later breakdown of the healing epithelium. **Hyphaema** is the name given to haemorrhage into the anterior chamber. On sitting or standing, a fluid level of blood is seen between the cornea and the iris. There is a danger of subsequent haemorrhage for about 10 days after the injury and glaucoma may later develop in some of these patients. Injuries resulting in hyphaema may also tear the iris at its periphery: **iridodialysis**. Retinal tears and retinal haemorrhage occurring at the time of injury may give rise to a **retinal detachment** (*Figure 12.43*) developing over the following days. These are all manifest as a sudden loss of vision, impending retinal detachment being heralded by the perception of flashes of light. **Choroidal rupture** and **complete rupture of the globe** may also occur.

Lens abnormalities

Cataracts (*Figures 12.44* and *12.45*) are opacities of the crystalline lens. The types of cataract are summarized in *Table 12.2*.

Lens displacement results from defects of the suspensory fibres or lens capsule and is associated with Marfan's syndrome, homocystinuria, ocular injury and ageing. The iris may appear to wobble and the displaced edge of the lens may be apparent in the pupil; displacement may be complete (dislocation) or partial (subluxation). Rapid changes in visual acuity occur as the lens moves.

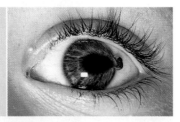

Figure 12.41.
Foreign body.

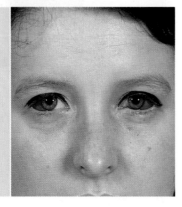

Figure 12.42.
Subconjunctival
haemorrhage
following severe
vomiting.

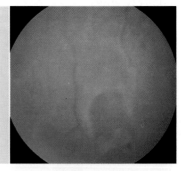

Figure 12.43.
Retinal detachment
and hole.

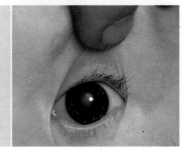

Figure 12.44.
Cataract in the left
eye.

Figure 12.45.
Cataract.

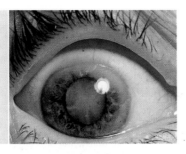

Table 12.2. Types of cataract.

Type	Features
Developmental	Minor 'blue dot opacities', which do not affect vision
Congenital (bilateral)	Severe opacities resulting from intra-uterine infection (rubella), drugs or congenital syndromes (Down's; syphilis; galactosaemia; diabetes mellitus)
Congenital (unilateral)	Associated with retinoblastoma, toxoplasmosis and microphthalmos
Age associated ('senile')	Progressive, usually bilateral, loss of acuity over years (almost all people over 65 years old have some minor degree of cataract)
Secondary to ocular disease	Iritis; injury; radiation; keratitis
Associated with systemic disease	Hypoparathyroidism; dystrophia myotonica; systemic steroids; Down's; galactosaemia

Table 12.3. Common refractive errors.

Error	Acuity	Cause
Hypermetropia	Blurring of close objects	Axial length of eye too short Age-related accomodation failure (presbyopia)
Myopia	Blurring of distant objects	Axial length of eye too long
Astigmatism	Focus varies in different meridians	Irregular cornea

Table 12.4. Reasons for rapid changes in refraction.

Age-related cataract
Diabetes mellitus
Eyelid lumps
Lens subluxation
Miotic eye drops (pilocarpine): artificial myopia
Mydriatic eye drops (cyclopentholate): artificial hypermetropia
Keratoconus (rapid onset of conical cornea in adolescents)

Figure 12.46.
Keratoconus and normal eyes.

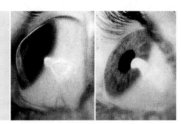

Figure 12.47.
Congenital squint.

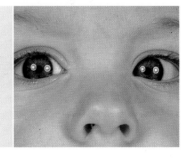

Refractive errors

Table 12.3 summarizes common refractive errors and *Table 12.4* lists the causes of rapid changes in refraction (*Figure 12.46*).

Strabismus

Normal eye movements are co-ordinated so that both eyes move together in parallel, the gaze only converging to view near objects or diverging in sleep or anaesthesia. Strabismus is the loss of this normal conformity of eye movements. It may be nonparalytic (concomitant) or paralytic (incomitant).

In **non-paralytic strabismus** (*Figure 12.47*) the angle of deviation of the affected eye remains constant in all directions of gaze. The extraocular muscles are intact and the range of ocular movements is not restricted, the squint probably being the result of a failure in the development of binocular reflexes. The affected eye may turn in any direction but the commonest configuration is the convergent squint where the eye turns inward. The image from the affected eye is suppressed by the visual cortex and, with time, vision may be permanently reduced: **strabismic amblyopia**. Conversely a refractive error may be the precipitating factor.

Nonparalytic strabismus most commonly develops at 1–3years old. The child may be noted to have a squint by the parents or amblyopia may be found at a routine school eye examination. On examination it is important to exclude an abnormality of the affected eye such as a cataract or retinoblastoma. The angle of the squint may be estimated from the appearance of the corneal reflections. In the cover test, each eye is covered in turn whilst the child looks at a pen torch. If the uncovered eye moves to take up fixation on the torch then a squint is present. There is a familial tendency to nonparalytic strabismus.

Paralytic strabismus results from extraocular muscle paralysis. The angle of the squint varies with the direction of the gaze and the squint is maximal on looking in the direction of action of the affected muscle.

Congenital cases result from birth trauma or developmental abnormalities in the cranial nerve nuclei. The lateral rectus is most commonly involved resulting in a convergent squint and limitation of abduction of the affected eye. Such a squint occurs in **Möbius' syndrome** where there are combined congenital palsies of the abducent and facial nerves. Developmental abnormalities of the extraocular muscles may also give rise to a congenital paralytic strabismus. In **Duane's retraction** (*Figure 12.48*) there is fibrosis of the lateral rectus which results in retraction of the globe and limitation of abduction. Similarly, tethering of the superior oblique limits elevation of the eye in abduction.

The majority of paralytic squints are acquired in later life from head or orbital injury, meningoencephalitis, multiple sclerosis (MS), intracranial neoplasms, myasthenia gravis and thyrotoxicosis. Third nerve palsies result in a divergent squint with limited elevation, abduction and depression of the eye. In addition there may be ptosis (drooping of the upper eyelid) and pupillary dilatation. With fourth nerve palsy (superior oblique paralysis) there is a vertical squint, i.e. the eye deviates upward, with limitation of depression of the eye in abduction. Sixth nerve palsy (lateral rectus paralysis) gives a convergent squint with limitation of abduction. Diplopia is common in all cases.

Nystagmus

Nystagmus describes rhythmic, involuntary eye movements that may be congenital, voluntary, physiological or a localizing sign of CNS disease. As a localizing sign, nystagmus is most often described in relation to vestibular and cerebellopontine angle disease.

Eye movements are controlled by the paired vestibular nuclei. Each nucleus drives the eye towards the opposite side, and hence the opposing forces of the pair keep the eyes in a stable position. If a pathological process affects one side, the remaining nucleus drives the eye slowly to the opposite side (the slow phase of nystagmus). This is then rapidly corrected (the fast phase of nystagmus). The direction of nystagmus is defined by the fast phase.

Horizontal nystagmus results from disease processes affecting the semicircular canals, vestibulocochlear nerve or vestibular nuclei. The fast phase is away from the side of the lesion and the nystagmus is accentuated by deviating the eyes in the direction of the fast phase; this is Alexander's Law.

Vertical nystagmus – where the abnormal movements occur in the vertical plane – occurs in fourth ventricle lesions (fast phase upwards) and in tonsillar herniation through the foramen magnum (fast phase downwards).

Cerebellopontine angle tumours initially result in vestibular horizontal nystagmus where the fast phase is away from the tumour. In the later stages, however, the fast phase is directed towards the lesion and is evoked by turning the gaze in that direction.

Pupillary abnormalities

Abnormalities of the shape of the pupil may result from **colobomata** (*Figure 12.49*), congenital notches in the iris or may be secondary to globe injury or glaucoma.

Abnormal pupillary responses (*Figure 12.50*) may be a sign of CNS disease but may also result from disease of the optic and oculomotor nerve, and from the effects of disease and drugs on the eye itself.

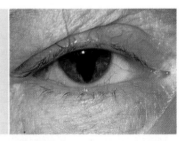

Figure 12.49.
Iris coloboma of the right eye.

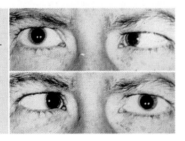

Figure 12.48.
Squint. Duane's retraction syndrome.

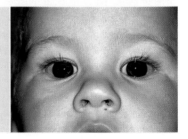

Figure 12.50.
Congenital asymmetry of the pupils (in subdued light).

An **acute compressing intracranial haematoma** compresses the ipsilateral oculomotor nerve against the edge of the tentorium, resulting in dilatation of the ipsilateral pupil: **Hutchinson's pupil**. The pupil is poorly reactive in both direct (light in the affected eye) and consensual (light in the other eye) light reflexes. **Coning** results in bilateral pupillary dilatation.

Globe injury may result in a dilated, unreactive pupil (to light in both the affected and unaffected eye).

Optic nerve injury or disease (*Figure 12.51*) results in a dilated pupil that is unreactive to direct light but reacts a little to light in the unaffected eye. The unaffected eye has a diminished response to stimulation of the affected eye by light.

Optic tract disease does not affect resting pupillary size but gives absent pupillary reflexes of the eye on the opposite side to the lesion, to light stimulation of either eye.

Injury or disease affecting the **oculomotor nerve** gives a dilated pupil, unreactive to light stimulation of either eye, with a divergent paralytic squint (p. 160; *Figure 9.23*).

The **Argyll Robertson pupil**, which is a feature of neurosyphilis, is small and unreactive to light but reacts to convergence.

The **Holmes–Adie pupil** shows no normal reactions to light or convergence but may slowly dilate in a darkened room. It results from myotonia, occurring in association with depressed tendon reflexes and limb anhidrosis.

Horner's syndrome (*Figure 12.52*) results from damage to the cervical sympathetic chain, and is characterized by miosis (pupillary constriction), ptosis (drooping of the eyelid) and vasodilatation and anhidrosis of the face, all occurring on the same side as the causal lesion. The causes of Horner's syndrome are summarized in *Table 12.5*. Eye signs may occur in isolation with interruption of the intracranial sympathetic plexus around the carotid artery. The combination of Horner's syndrome and loss of the first division of the trigeminal nerve, **Raeder's syndrome**, may result from tumour invasion at the skull base.

Drug-induced pupillary constriction occurs with miotic eyedrops, such as pilocarpine, and opiates. Drug-induced pupillary dilatation occurs with anticholinergic drugs, including mydriatic eyedrops, such as atropine, and cocaine.

Visual field loss and blindness

Visual loss, both temporary and permanent, may be a feature of disease processes and injuries affecting the globe (including the retina), optic nerve, visual pathways and visual cortex. Distinctive patterns of visual loss identify the site of disease, as shown in *Table 12.6*.

Conditions affecting the globe, such as **glaucoma**, **injuries** and **ocular tumours**, have already been discussed (p.180).

Table 12.5. Causes of Horner's syndrome.

Congenital
Idiopathic
Trauma (particularly cervical sympathectomy)
Brain stem vascular and demyelinating diseases
Aneurysms of aortic arch, subclavian artery and carotid bifurcation
Malignancy:
    lymph node metastasis
    anaplastic thyroid cancer
    chemodectomas
    Pancoast tumour (upper lobe apical bronchogenic carcinoma)
    tumours of the skull base

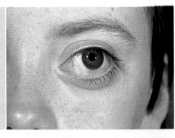

Figure 12.51.
Optic nerve glioma producing proptosis: the pupil reacted poorly to light.

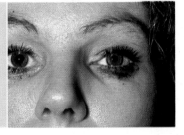

Figure 12.52.
Horner's syndrome of the left eye demonstrating ptosis and pupillary constriction.

Table 12.6. Patterns of visual loss.

Globe	Field defect or complete visual loss for affected eye only
Retina	Focal field defect
Optic nerve	Dilated unresponsive pupil with field loss varying from focal to blindness
Chiasma	Bitemporal (heteronymous) hemianopia, a field defect in the temporal field for each eye
Optic tract	Homonymous hemianopia, a field defect in the nasal field of the eye on the side of the lesion and the temporal field of the other eye
Visual cortex	As for optic tract

Central retinal artery occlusion (*Figure 12.53*) may result in sudden loss of vision in one eye. The usual cause is embolism from carotid atheroma or from the heart. On general examination there may be atrial fibrillation, evidence of generalized atheromatous disease and a carotid bruit may be present in the case of carotid atheroma. The eye shows perception of light only with a decreased or absent direct light reflex. With the ophthalmoscope, the fundus is pale but the macula appears relatively bright as a 'cherry red spot'. As the central retinal artery is an end artery recovery is unlikely. As a precursor to this dramatic event the patient may experience transient blurring of vision or visual loss lasting for minutes or even hours caused by smaller emboli that do not cause a complete occlusion of the central retinal artery. This phenomenon is called **amaurosis fugax**.

Retinal detachment (p. 182) is most common in the over-50s and is associated with myopia. Visual loss occurs suddenly, a dark shadow descending across the visual field of the eye. Sometimes specks or flashes of light in the visual field may be noticed the same day, or sometimes days beforehand. On fundoscopy, the detached portion of the retina appears grey. Detachment often commences on the temporal side of the retina and a tear may be seen at the periphery. Trauma may be involved in some cases.

Macular degeneration is a common cause of blindness in western countries, where there is an age-related, gradual deterioration in vision over many years. Fundoscopy reveals speckled pigmentation of the macular region.

Diabetic retinopathy and **hypertensive retinopathy** give characteristic appearances on fundoscopy but their discussion is beyond the scope of this text.

Optic nerve disease is summarized in *Table 12.7*.

Papilloedema (*Figure 12.54*) is the term used to describe swelling of the optic disc, where there is raised intraocular pressure. The disc is reddened with loss of its concavity and has blurred margins. The eye shows a decreased direct light reflex and there is an increased blind spot on visual field testing. True papilloedema results from **raised**

intracranial pressure** but disc swelling may also occur in **ischaemia** such as **central retinal artery occlusion** or **cranial arteritis**, and **inflammatory processes** such as the **optic neuritis** of MS.

The **optic chiasma** may be compressed by **pituitary adenomas, craniopharyngiomas, meningiomas, intracranial aneurysms** and **optic nerve gliomas**. **Ischaemic damage** to the chiasma may occur in severe head injury.

The **optic radiation** has lower fibres – upper visual fields – which loop forwards from the geniculate body into the temporal lobe and then back up to join the fibres from the upper part of the radiation – lower visual fields – which pass through the parietal lobe. Temporal lobe tumours or infarction may therefore produce an upper quadrantic homonymous field defect on the opposite side. Parietal lobe tumours or infarction may produce a lower quadrantic homonymous hemianopia on the opposite side to the lesion. The optic radiation is susceptible to ischaemia, being supplied by a single deep penetrating branch of the middle cerebral artery.

Table 12.7. Conditions affecting the optic nerve.

Developmental dysplasia

Hereditary atrophy

Nutritional neuropathies: thiamine (alcoholism)) and B_{12} (pernicious anaemia) deficiencies

Toxic neuropathies: ethambutol; streptomycin; chlomycetin; digitalis; chloroquine

Optic neuritis (aetiology unknown): MS; viral (measles; mumps; chickenpox; infectious mononucleosis; herpes zoster); post viral; granulomatous inflammation (syphilis; TB; cryptoccocus; sarcoidosis)

Optic nerve infarction

Intrinsic tumours

Extrinsic tumours

Papilloedema

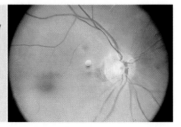

Figure 12.53. Central retinal artery occlusion. Note the paucity of vessels radiating from the optic disc.

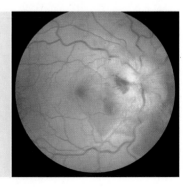

Figure 12.54. Papilloedema. Note the pale, swollen optic disc.

The **visual cortex** is arranged so that the posterior cortex receives fibres representing central vision whereas the medial occipital lobes receive fibres representing peripheral vision. The lower fields are represented above the calcarine fissure and the upper fields in the area below the fissure. The blood supply to these cortical regions differs, the posterior cortex being supplied by a branch of the middle cerebral artery and the medial cortex by the posterior cerebral artery. Ischaemia of the visual cortex may produce homonymous hemianopias, but it is possible for central vision to be spared if it is the posterior cerebral artery that is occluded.

The orbit

Orbital fractures

Depressed fractures of the zygomatic bone result from a direct blow to the zygoma. Fracture separations occur at the infraorbital rim, the zygomaticofrontal suture and in the zygomatic arch. The wall of the related maxillary sinus may be shattered. There may be unilateral epistaxis from tearing of the mucous membrane of the maxillary sinus, a black eye with subconjunctival haemorrhage from the orbital floor injury and flattening of the contour of the cheek, although this may be masked by oedema.

Additional physical signs may be present that assist in the clinical diagnosis. The fracture may be palpable as a notch or irregularity of the lateral orbital margin at the zygomatic suture line or tenderness may be noted at this point. If the fracture extends through the orbital floor across the path of the infraorbital foramen there may be anaesthesia or even hyperaesthesia over the upper lip from damage to the infraorbital nerve. These sensory changes may be temporary in the case of a neuropraxia or permanent if there is complete shearing of the nerve. There may be diplopia from entrapment or displacement of the attachments of the extraocular muscles and displacement of the lateral attachment of the suspensory ligament of the eyeball to the zygoma. Air may enter the overlying tissues from the maxillary sinus resulting in surgical emphysema.

Zygomatic fractures are not always easily seen on radiography, but if the orbital floor is involved blood may obliterate the normal radiolucency of the maxillary sinus. This is particularly evident on an occipitomental view: Waters projection.

Orbital blow-out fractures classically result from a relatively focused but blunt impact with the globe, such as from a squash ball. Whilst the globe itself is damaged, a significant proportion of the impact is dissipated by the globe and extraocular tissues being displaced through one of the surrounding orbital walls. This may occur through the lamina papyracea, the roof of the orbit, the greater wing of the sphenoid or, most commonly, through the orbital floor. Most orbital floor fractures occur in the area medial to the infraorbital canal but anterior to the inferior orbital fissure as the orbital floor here is relatively weak. Periorbital fat and the inferior rectus and inferior oblique muscles may remain depressed into the maxillary antrum.

On initial clinical examination there may be bruising of the periorbital tissues but the globe is probably relatively undisplaced, the pupils being level, as a result of tissue oedema compensating for the orbital floor deficit. Weeks later, when the oedema has subsided, the globe may be inferiorly displaced and there may be enophthalmos from atrophy of the retro-ocular tissues. In contrast to zygomatic fractures involving the orbit, the infraorbital nerve is rarely damaged as the fracture zone avoids the infraorbital canal. Diplopia may subsequently develop secondary to globe displacement and entrapment or fibrosis of the inferior ocular musculature.

13 The mouth

The teeth and gums

Congenital and developmental abnormalities

Congenital and developmental abnormalities are listed in *Table 13.1*. Additional teeth are not uncommon and may be **supernumerary**, where they are of an abnormal conical appearance, or **supplementary**, having the appearance of a normal tooth.

Absent teeth usually represent failure of eruption, which may result from any cause of reduced space, from early loss of deciduous teeth, an abnormal position, additional teeth, dentigerous cysts or the retention of a deciduous tooth. The commonest causes world-wide, however, are rickets and cretinism.

Congenital syphilis

Congenital syphilis may give rise to characteristic dental deformities. **Hutchinson's incisors** (*Figure 13.1*) are small and tapered, and may have a cresenteric incisal ridge. Upper central incisors are most often affected. **Moon's molars** (*Figure 13.2*) are dome-shaped, first upper molars.

Odontomes

Odontomes are hamartomas of the dental tissues, tumours of developmental origin. They range in appearance from enamel pearls on an otherwise normal tooth, to larger rounded masses. These may erupt from beneath the gums, and, once exposed, are prone to infection.

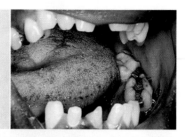

Figure 13.1.
Hutchinson's teeth in congenital syphilis.

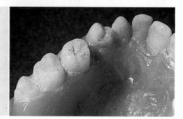

Figure 13.2.
Moon's molars in congenital syphilis.

Caries, pulpitis and periapical periodontitis (toothache)

Dental caries

Dental caries is the process of progressive, irreversible bacterial damage to the teeth. This damage allows bacteria to penetrate to the dentine, resulting in pulpitis which leads to the death of the pulp. Infection may then spread through the apical foramina to the periapical tissues, called periapical periodontitis. This succession of processes is the commonest cause of toothache and loss of teeth in young people. (Gingivitis is the commonest cause of loss of teeth in older age groups.)

Caries (*Figures 13.3* and *13.4*) develop in the presence of three factors: bacterial plaque, bacterial substrate (sugar) and a susceptible tooth surface. Plaque is a matrix of organic debris containing bacteria that forms in the absence of tooth brushing, giving the dental surface a ground-glass appearance. *Streptococcus mutans* is the principal cariogenic organism.

The earliest sign of caries is a 'sticky fissure' on the crown of the tooth. A sharp probe does not normally 'stick' in an occlusal fissure but early decalcification in these areas allows it to do so. There may be a chalky appearance to the surrounding enamel, which softens and later collapses to form

Table 13.1. Chronology of dentition.

Teeth	Deciduous (months)	Permanent (years)
Lower incisors	6–9	6–8
Upper incisors	6–9	7–9
Lower canines	16–18	9–10
Upper canines	16–18	11–12
Premolars	Absent	10–12
1st molars	12–14	6–7
2nd molars	20–30	11–13
3rd molars	Absent	17–21

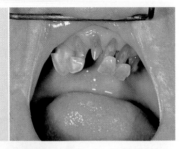

Figure 13.3.
Gross dental attrition.

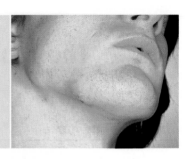

Figure 13.5.
Apical abscess of the lower right canine pointing externally.

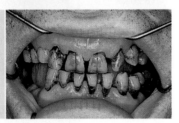

Figure 13.4.
Dental caries following local radio-therapy.

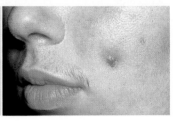

Figure 13.6.
Facial sinus of dental origin.

a visible cavity. Interstitial caries are difficult to detect clinically and at an early stage may only be identified as lucencies on dental radiographs. Later, a dark grey discoloration develops at the edge of the tooth, where it is in contact with its neighbour.

Pulpitis

Pulpitis results from infection of the dental pulp secondary to caries. It is the commonest cause of pain from the teeth, jaw or surrounding area and is recognized principally by this symptom. The presence of a carious cavity may suggest, but does not confirm, the responsible tooth. Application of hot or cold to the tooth elicits the pain and there may be tenderness on percussion with a dental instrument. Toothache originating in a tooth that has undergone a restorative procedure, however, is more likely to be the result of exposure of the pulp.

Periapical periodontitis

Periapical periodontitis is inflammation of the periodontal membrane surrounding the apex of the tooth and follows death of the pulp as a result of pulpitis. Initially the tooth is described as uncomfortable rather than acutely painful; this is because the oedematous periodontal membrane lifts the tooth slightly so that the bite falls more heavily upon it. As the process continues, an abscess forms (*Figure 13.5*) and throbbing pain develops, which continues for several days until it is relieved by the pus penetrating the bone. There may be a low grade fever and regional lymphadenopathy. If an upper canine is affected, the eyelid

may become oedematous. The responsible tooth either has a large carious cavity or is discoloured from death of the pulp. The typical sign is tenderness on dental percussion with the absence of pain on application of hot or cold. Chronic abscesses may remain without symptoms and only be discovered as a lucency on radiographs, or they may form dentigerous cysts (p. 191). An abscess may discharge externally, with sinus formation (*Figure 13.6*).

Gingivitis
Acute ulcerative gingivitis

Acute ulcerative gingivitis (*Figure 13.7*) – Vincent's angina – is a rare condition associated with poor oral hygiene, smoking, upper respiratory infection and general debilitation. As one of the many afflictions of troops in the First World War, it was also known as 'trench mouth'. The exact pathology is unknown but Vincent's organisms, *Spirochaeta denticola*, are associated. A rapid progressive ulceration begins at the tips of the interdental papillae and spreads along the gingival margins, destroying the periodontal tissues. There is an offensive halitosis.

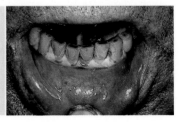

Figure 13.7.
Vincent's angina.

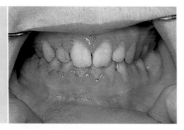

Figure 13.8.
Chronic gingivitis.

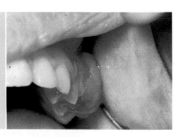

Figure 13.9.
Fibrous epulis.

Chronic gingivitis

Chronic gingivitis (*Figure 13.8*) is a common condition result-ing from the accumulation of plaque around the necks of the teeth. The alveolar margin resorbs and the gum forms redun-dant tissue around the necks of the teeth, allowing debris to collect and thus establishing a cycle of progressive damage. The condition begins in young people and progresses over years to be the main cause of loss of teeth in older age groups. It can be prevented by careful brushing of the teeth and the use of dental sticks.

Gingivitis may also occur in **uraemia**, **pregnancy**, **acute leukaemias** and **scurvy**. In acute leukaemias of childhood, it may be the earliest sign. The phenomenon arises because of abnormal white cell function. The region requires defence from infection but the only response the cells can mount is to infiltrate the gums in large numbers.

Dental and gingival tumours
Cysts

Periodontal cysts

Periodontal cysts are the commonest cause of a major swelling of the jaw and may present at any time in adult life. They form secondary to infection of a dental root and appear as a rounded, hard, painful swelling of the alveolus. The swelling later softens as the surrounding bony walls are pen-etrated, thus relieving the pressure.

Dentigerous cysts

Dentigerous cysts are attached to the neck of a developing tooth, surrounding the crown and preventing eruption. They may be found at any time in adult life and are often noticed in the search for a non-erupted tooth or if they become symp-tomatic through infection.

Benign tumours
Epulis

An epulis (*Figure 13.9*) is a fibrous, granulomatous or bony swelling that arises from the alveolar margin.

Ameloblastoma

Ameloblastoma is a rare odontogenic tumour, which forms a hard, slow-growing mass, usually in the mandible.

Malignant tumours

There are no commonly occurring malignant tumours of dental tissue. Squamous carcinomas of the gums and tumours of the mandible are considered in the section on oral tumours (p. 195).

Dental impaction and wisdom teeth

A tooth that is prevented from erupting because of lack of space is said to be impacted. Although already mentioned as a cause of absence of a tooth, impaction may give rise to other symptoms. The lower third molar – the wisdom tooth – is most frequently affected, the upper canines and upper third molars taking second and third places. Wisdom teeth are the most commonly symptomatic impacted teeth, not only because they are the commonest tooth to be impacted but because they are often partially erupted. Young adults are most often affected but problems may also arise in the elderly, where alveolar atro-phy uncovers a previously buried tooth. The partially erupted tooth is covered with a flap of gum, the operculum, which acts as a stagnation area encouraging caries of the crown or of the second molar at their point of contact. A pericoronal abscess may form and the spread of infection may lead to osteomyelitis of the mandible, a submandibular abscess or Ludwig's angina.

A non-infected impacted wisdom tooth may cause local soreness, referred otalgia and swelling of the cheek, and is the most common cause of trismus. The operculum may be missed on clinical examination if not specifically searched for.

Miscellaneous conditions
Hereditary gingival hyperplasia

Hereditary gingival hyperplasia (*Figure 13.10*) occurs as an autosomal dominant condition, in association with hypertri-chosis (hairiness), epilepsy and mental retardation. The gums may be so grossly enlarged as to bury the teeth.

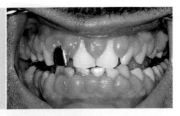

Figure 13.10.
Gingival hyperplasia.

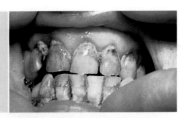

Figure 13.12.
Discoloured lines of
the teeth following
lead poisoning.

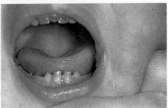

Figure 13.11.
Discoloured teeth
following a course of
tetracycline.

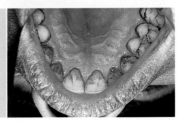

Figure 13.13.
Discoloration of the
teeth of a betel nut
chewer.

Pigmentation

Pigmentation of the teeth results from exposure to causal agents during dental development. **Tetracyclines** (*Figure 13.11*) are taken up by calcifying tissues, initially causing bright yellow discoloration, which later turns to brown or grey. **Fluoride** may give a mottled appearance to the enamel.

Lead line

Lead line (*Figure 13.12*) refers to a black–purple line around the gingival margin which results from lead accumulation in these tissues, from exposure through industry. Similar appearances may result from excessive exposure to gold, bismuth, mercury and certain drugs. New cases are less likely to be encountered since the introduction of improved health and safety controls and changes in drug therapy for syphilis. In tropical areas it is common to chew the betel nut – the nut is mixed with quicklime and rolled in a vine leaf. There is purple staining of the mouth, brown staining of the teeth (*Figure 13.13*) and, long-term, an increased incidence of oral cancer.

Phenytoin-induced gingival hyperplasia

Phenytoin-induced gingival hyperplasia occurs in some patients taking the drug. There is an overgrowth of the interdental papillae, which become bulbous and overlap the teeth; the gums may take on an orange-peel appearance.

Receding gums

Receding gums result from normal ageing and wear. The roots of the teeth become exposed, but the gingival margins are healthy and there is no great increased risk of dental loss if dental hygiene is maintained.

Lips and oral cavity

Congenital abnormalities
Sublingual dermoid cysts

Sublingual dermoid cysts arise when ectodermal tissues become trapped in the deeper tissues during embryological midline fusion. Although congenital, the cyst is most often noticed in early adult life as a swelling under the tongue or at the point of the chin. The lump is visible at these sites, and is firm and fluctuant but does not transilluminate.

Cleft lip is described with cleft palate on p. 198.

Stomatitis

The causes of stomatitis – inflammation and ulceration of the oral mucosa – are summarized in *Table 13.2*.

Herpes simplex and varicella-zoster viruses

Herpes simplex (*Figure 13.14*) – cold sores; type 1 herpesvirus – produces oral infections, whereas varicella-zoster (chickenpox) – type 2 herpesvirus – is the cause of genital and neonatal infection. Transmission of herpes simplex is by mucosal contact, usually kissing. Primary infection commences with a sore throat and influenza-like symptoms; there may be cervical adenopathy and splenomegaly. After several days vesicular lesions appear on the lips, palate and gums. These break down to form shallow painful ulcers, healing over 10–14 days. After primary infection has passed, the virus lies dormant in the sensory ganglia of the trigeminal nerve. Recurrences may occur, which are usually trivial in comparison with the primary infection. Trigger factors for recurrence include febrile illness, UV light and trauma.

Table 13.2. Causes of stomatitis and ulceration.

Acute bacterial infection	Poor oral hygiene; Vincent's stomatitis; cancrum oris
Acute viral infection	Koplik's spots; herpes simplex; hand-foot-and-mouth disease
Chronic bacterial infection	TB; syphilis
Fungal infection	Candidiasis; actinomycosis; blastomycosis; histoplasmosis
Trauma	Toothbrush; dentures; damaged tooth
Allergy	Cosmetics
Metals	Lead; gold; bismuth; mercury
Drugs	Phenytoin
Miscellaneous conditions	Aphthous ulceration; Behçet's syndrome; lichen planus; pemphigus; pemphigoid; hyperkeratosis; leukoplakia; erythroplakia; AIDS; pernicious anaemia; agranulocytosis; leukaemia; scurvy; pellagra

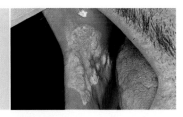

Figure 13.15. Chronic candidal infection of the mouth.

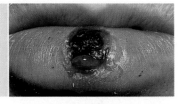

Figure 13.16. Primary chancre of the lower lip.

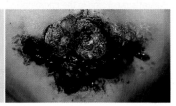

Figure 13.17. Cancrum oris.

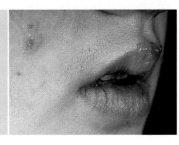

Figure 13.14. Herpes simplex vesicular lesion of the lip.

Recurrent lesions occur in the cutaneous distributions of the maxillary and mandibular branches of the trigeminal nerve, usually on the lips or around the nostrils. Typically, there is itching and tingling, followed, after hours or days, by the eruption of a cluster of small blisters filled with clear fluid. Lesions heal by crusting over the following 10 days but may become secondarily infected. Recurrences do not normally produce significant systemic upset, but in the immunocompromised there may be severe generalized infection with hepatitis, pneumonitis or encephalitis. In patients with skin conditions such as eczema, the virus may spread to produce an extensive vesicular rash. Steroid treatment may facilitate the spread of the virus. Parents who have children afflicted with eczema should be warned that they must prevent close contact with those who have active cold sores.

Candida albicans

Candida albicans (*Figure 13.15*) causes oral infections in children, the debilitated and immunocompromised, and as a com-

plication of antibiotic therapy. It appears initially as small red patches on the buccal mucosa and tongue but later as raised white lesions. The mouth is painful, and salivation excessive. Painful swallowing may be indicative of pharyngeal involvement.

Syphilis

Syphilis (*Figure 13.16*) may affect the mouth in any of its stages. Primary disease may result in a chancre of the lips or tongue. In the secondary stage, mucous patches may appear on the oral mucosa as 'snail track ulcers'. A **gumma** may occur in the palate or tongue, usually in the midline. Destruction of the tissues may result in a hole in the palate.

Cancrum oris

Cancrum oris (*Figure 13.17*) is a rare and fatal disease beginning as ulceration of the buccal mucosa and progressing to a rapidly spreading gangrene which destroys the cheek. It is associated with severe malnutrition; Vincent's organisms may be responsible.

Acquired immunodeficiency syndrome (AIDS) – these oral manifestations are described on p. 88.

Aphthous ulceration

Aphthous ulceration (*Figure 13.18*) is a condition of unknown cause, characterized by the appearance of recurring painful

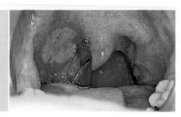

Figure 13.18.
Bilateral aphthous ulcers of the faucial pillars.

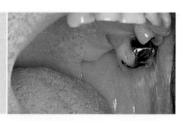

Figure 13.19.
Lichen planus of the mucosa of the left side of the cheek.

ulcers anywhere on the oral mucosa, which last for days or even weeks. The ulcers have a sloughing base, with a surrounding ring of hyperaemia, and typically, as one heals, the next one appears.

Behçet's syndrome

Behçet's syndrome is the combination of oropharyngeal and genital ulceration, with iritis and hypopyon, i.e. pus in the anterior chamber of the eye. The ulcers have a punched-out appearance with a surrounding red halo. The cause is unknown and males are mainly affected. Rarely, acute encephalitis and blindness may follow after several years.

Pemphigus

Pemphigus is a rare and sometimes fatal condition of unknown cause, characterized by the formation of large bullae on the skin and other mucosal surfaces, which rupture to leave ulcers. Lesions in the mouth are painful and are the first to appear. **Pemphigoid** is a non-fatal condition with otherwise similar characteristics. **Lichen planus** (*Figure 13.19*) manifests in the mouth as glistening white papules, which, in large numbers, give a lace-like appearance. It cannot be removed by scratching and may persist for over a year.

Oral tumours

The range of tumours encountered in the oral cavity is shown in *Tables 13.3* and *13.4*. Tumours arising from dental tissues are described on p. 189.

Cysts

Cysts (*Figures 13.20* and *13.21*) may be inflammatory, developmental or neoplastic (*Table 13.3*). Regardless of their origin, however, most present as slowly enlarging tumours of the jaws. The **ranula** (*Figure 13.22*) is a retention cyst of the sublingual salivary gland (p. 194).

Benign tumours

Osteomas

Osteomas are common, localized overgrowths of bone – exostoses – which appear as hard, rounded swellings. As a

Table 13.3. Oral soft tissue tumours.

Cysts	Sublingual dermoid*; thyroglossal*; ranula*; mucocele*; lymphoepithelial*
Benign	Papilloma; adenoma; fibroma; lipoma; myxoma; haemangioma; neurilemmoma; teratoma; chordoma; salivary tumours; lingual thyroid*
Malignant	Carcinoma; salivary tumours; melanoma; sarcomas; lymphomas; Kaposi's sarcoma

* non-neoplastic lesions

Table 13.4. Tumours of the teeth and jaws.

Cysts	Periodontal*; dentigerous*; eruption*; primordial*; nasopalatine*; solitary bone*; neoplastic (ameloblastoma)
Benign	Teeth – ameloblastoma; odontomes; dentinoma; cementoma; composite odontoma Jaw – fibroma; osteoma; giant cell granuloma
Malignant	Osteogenic sarcoma; fibrosarcoma; chondrosarcoma; secondary carcinoma

* non-neoplastic lesions

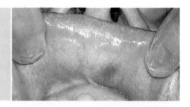

Figure 13.20.
Cysts of the lip.

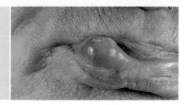

Figure 13.21.
Angioma of the lower lip.

torus palatinus (*Figure 13.23*), the osteoma appears in the midline of the hard palate, and as a **torus mandibularis** (*Figure 13.24*), it lies on the lingual aspect of the mandible, opposite the mental foramen.

Figure 13.22.
Ranula.

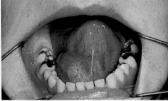

Figure 13.23.
Palatal torus.

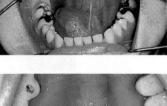

Figure 13.24.
Mandibular torus.

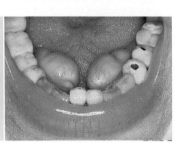

Figure 13.25.
Oral leukoplakia.

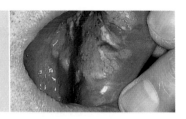

Figure 13.26.
Carcinoma of the
lower lip.

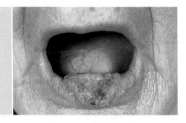

Figure 13.27.
Carcinoma of the
inside of the cheek.

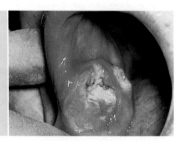

Figure 13.28.
Carcinoma over the
mandible.

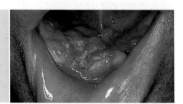

Figure 13.29.
Squamous
carcinoma on the
floor of the mouth.

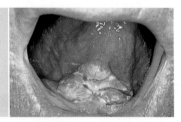

Oral carcinoma

Leukoplakia and erythroplakia

Leukoplakia (*Figure 13.25*) and erythroplakia, which appear as white or raised red areas of the mucosa, are premalignant lesions. Approximately 3% of areas of leukoplakia undergo malignant change over 5 years. These lesions may be found in a separate site to an oral carcinoma, supporting the theory of field change in response to carcinogens.

Squamous carcinoma

Squamous carcinoma (*Figures 13.26–13.29*) may arise from the mucosal surfaces of all areas of the oral cavity and present as bleeding, ulcerated lesions with everted edges. The underlying tumour mass may be fixed by invasion of adjacent tissues. Symptoms of local invasion are summarized in *Table 13.5*. Cervical lymph node metastases are common and contralateral nodes may be involved in advanced cases.

Pipe smoking, chewing tobacco and, to a lesser extent, cigarette smoking are the principal aetiological factors; alcohol may act as a facilitator. In the Far East, chewing of betel nuts and reverse smoking of chuttas are additional risk factors, with the result that in these regions oral cancers account for half of all malignancies.

Table 13.5. Features of local invasion by oral carcinoma.

Structure	Feature
Muscles of mastication	Trismus
Inferior alveolar nerve	Mandibular anaesthesia
IX and X cranial nerves	Referred otalgia
XII cranial nerve	Ipsilateral tongue weakness/wasting
Base of tongue	Deviation to the affected side on protrusion

Carcinoma of the lip

Carcinoma of the lip most commonly appears as a bleeding, ulcerating lesion on the lower lip, and is associated with excessive exposure to UV light. Tumours of the upper lip grow more quickly and metastasize early.

Carcinomas of the hard palate

Carcinomas of the hard palate are particularly rare except where reverse smoking is practised. A tumour of the hard palate is equally likely to be a tumour of a minor salivary gland.

Malignant tumours of the jaw

Malignant tumours of the jaw are rare but two clinical pictures are worth mentioning. **Osteogenic sarcoma** (*Figure 13.30*) is a highly malignant tumour and is the main malignant neoplasm of bone. It is rare but primarily occurs in the jaw and is seen in adolescents, patients with Paget's disease and secondary to radiation. Presenting as a rapidly growing, painful swelling of the jaw, it quickly metastasizes to the lungs. **Secondary deposits of carcinoma** from tumours that commonly metastasize to bone may occasionally occur in the jaw. Severe pain, swelling and paraesthesia of the lip, from invasion of the mental nerve, are the features.

Miscellaneous conditions

Peutz–Jeghers syndrome

Peutz–Jeghers syndrome (p. 290; *Figure 23.25*) is an autosomal dominant condition characterized by melanotic macular pigmentation of the lips and oral mucosa. The associated polyposis of the small intestine may rarely give rise to malignancy.

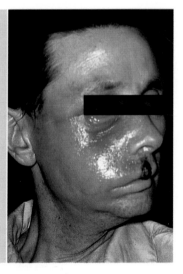

Figure 13.30. Osteogenic sarcoma on the floor of the mouth.

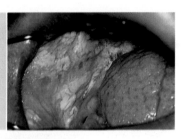

Figure 13.31. White spongy naevus of the mouth.

White sponge naevus

A white sponge naevus (*Figure 13.31*) takes the form of a 'shaggy white patch' on the buccal surfaces, which can be peeled away to reveal normal mucosa but is fairly rapidly re-established. The condition, which has autosomal dominant inheritance, appears in childhood and is of little consequence.

Multiple endocrine neoplasia syndrome

Multiple endocrine neoplasia syndrome, type 2B – phaeochromocytoma and medullary thyroid carcinoma – is associated with multiple nodules (neuromas) of the oral mucosa and eyelids.

Fordyce's spots

Fordyce's spots are yellow or white nodules from the presence of heterotopic sebaceous glands in the oral mucosa. They are of no clinical significance.

Leukoedema

In leukoedema, the buccal mucosa is thrown into folds which have a milky-white opalescence. The condition is of no significance.

The tongue

Congenital abnormalities

Congenital abnormalities of the tongue are listed in *Table 13.6*. **Macroglossia** (p. 14; *Figure 1.48*) occurs in cretinism, Down's syndrome ('mongolism') and acromegaly. **Ankyloglossia** (*Figures 13.32* and *13.33*) – tongue-tie – results from the tethering of the tongue by a short frenulum linguae and can cause speech difficulties if the frenulum is not surgically divided. A **lingual thyroid** (*Figure 13.34*) appears as a purple-red swelling at the back of the tongue; it may enlarge and bleed in pregnancy, it may represent the only functioning thyroid tissue and its removal may render the patient hypothyroid.

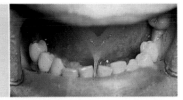

Figure 13.32.
Tongue tie.

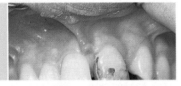

Figure 13.33.
Congenitally short upper lip frenulum.

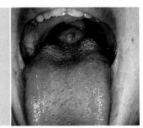

Figure 13.34.
Lingual thyroid.

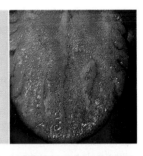

Figure 13.35.
Congenital fissuring of the tongue.

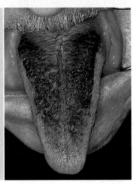

Figure 13.36.
Black, hairy tongue.

Glossitis

Many causes of glossitis (*Table 13.6*) are those of stomatitis. This section covers those conditions more specific to the tongue. Candidiasis typically produces lesions on the tongue (p. 202).

Geographic tongue

Geographic tongue is a clinically characteristic condition of unknown aetiology. Red patches with yellow borders form a pattern on the dorsum of the tongue, which changes in configuration from day to day. The condition starts in childhood and continues throughout life, although some cases remit spontaneously.

Hairy tongue

Hairy tongue (*Figures 13.35* and *13.36*) refers only to the appearance of the tongue and does not involve the development of actual hairs. **Black, hairy tongue** occurs in response to some antibiotics and antiseptics. There is an overgrowth of filiform papillae which become stained black by bacteria, medication or tobacco. **Hairy leukoplakia** is a white, friable lesion of the tongue seen in AIDS.

Pernicious anaemia

Pernicious anaemia causes a smooth inflamed tongue known as **Hunter's glossitis**. There may be pallor of the lips and oral mucosa, and an angular cheilitis.

Pellagra

Pellagra – a deficiency of the B$_2$ complex of vitamins – results in an inflamed, fissured tongue and angular cheilitis. It was commonly seen in prisoner of war camps during the Second World War.

Agranulocytosis

Agranulocytosis is a fatal state that may be induced by drugs containing the benzene ring. It presents with a sudden onset of sore throat, ulceration and false membrane formation on the tongue and other oropharyngeal mucosal surfaces.

Table 13.6. Disorders of the tongue.

Congenital abnormalities	Glossitis
Aglossia (absent t.)	Geographic t.
Microglossia (small t.)	'Hairy' t.
Macroglossia (large t.)	Pernicious anaemia
Glossoptosis (abnormally mobile t.)	Pellagra
Ankyloglossia (tongue tie)	Agranulocytosis
Bifid t.	Causes of stomatitis
Fissured t.	Median rhomboid glossitis
Lingual thyroid	
Accessory thyroid	
Thyroglossal cysts	

Median rhomboid glossitis

Median rhomboid glossitis (*Figure 13.37*) is characterized by the appearance of a rhomboid or oval mass in the midline of the tongue, immediately in front of the foramen caecum. The mass is slightly raised and smooth, being devoid of papillae. It probably results from candidal infection.

Carcinoma of the tongue

Carcinoma of the tongue usually occurs on the lateral border of the middle third of the tongue, but occasionally on the dorsum. There is often a prior history of leukoplakia (*Figure 13.38*). Deviation of the tongue to the side of the lesion, on protrusion, is a sign of deep tumour fixation. A classical picture (*Figure 13.39*) is that of the hardy, middle-aged, male smoker, with a high alcohol intake, who has ignored the local lesion, presenting instead with earache (referred otalgia) that he has treated himself with a cotton wool pad in the ear. Cirrhosis and the Plummer–Vinson syndrome are also associated with this carcinoma.

Wasting and deviation of the tongue

There may be unilateral wasting of the tongue in hypoglossal nerve lesions. The tongue deviates to the affected side, other causes of deviation include tumour fixation. Bilateral weakness of the tongue occurs in bulbar and pseudobulbar palsy (p. 162, *Figure 9.29*) and is associated with fasciculation in the former.

The palate

Cleft lip and palate

Cleft lip and palate (*Figures 13.40–13.43*) are congenital deformities that occur in approximately 1 in 800 births and result from failure of the mesenchyme to penetrate the junctions between the primary processes that fuse to form the nose, lips and palate. Clefts begin at the vermilion border of the lip or at the uvula and extend to a varying degree from these points. They occur on either side or both sides of the midline, the least degree of deformity being the bifid uvula. Patterns of deformity are such that a quarter have a cleft lip alone, a quarter have a cleft palate alone and half have both a cleft lip and palate.

Cleft lip is primarily a cosmetic problem but a cleft palate may cause feeding problems, interfere with the development of normal speech and result in an increased risk of respiratory infections and deafness.

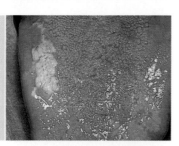

Figure 13.37. Median rhomboid glossitis.

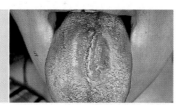

Figure 13.38. Leukoplakia of the tongue.

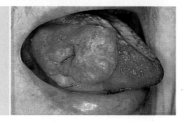

Figure 13.39. Carcinoma of the tongue.

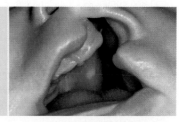

Figure 13.40. Left-sided cleft lip.

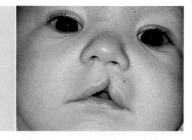

Figure 13.41. Left-sided cleft lip and palate.

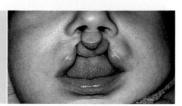

Figure 13.42. Bilateral cleft lip and palate.

There is a strong genetic tendency to cleft lip with a 1 in 25 incidence in the child of an affected parent. The relationships are not so clear for cleft palate.

Cleft palate occurs in association with micrognathia – 'shrew-like' facies – and glossoptosis, a poorly anchored tongue that is easily displaced backwards, as in **Pierre Robin syndrome** (p. 163; *Figure 10.1*).

Syphilitic gumma

A hole in the middle of the soft palate may be evidence of a previous syphilitic gumma (*Figure 13.44*; pp. 45 and 69). As syphilis is now uncommon in the west, a hole in the palate is more likely to result from attempts at operative closure of a cleft, radiotherapy or from erosion by carcinoma.

Inflammatory conditions

Inflammatory conditions (*Figure 13.45*) affecting the mucosa of the palate are those causing stomatitis (p. 192).

Carcinoma

Carcinoma (*Figure 13.46*) presents as painful ulceration or as the inability to wear an upper denture. Tumours are divided equally into those arising from the oral mucosa and adenocarcinomas of the ectopic salivary glands (p. 211).

Paralysis

Paralysis of the soft palate – shown by the absence of movement on saying 'Aah' – may result unilaterally from a lesion of the vagus nerve or bilaterally in bulbar poliomyelitis.

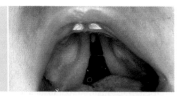
Figure 13.43.
Cleft palate.

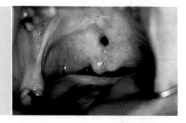
Figure 13.44.
Palatal fistula.

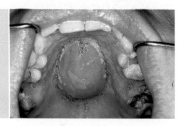
Figure 13.45.
Palatal abscess.

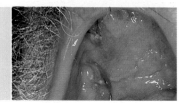
Figure 13.46.
Carcinoma of the palate.

14 Nose and throat

The nose

Congenital abnormalities

Defects of embryological midline fusion may rarely give rise to a **bifid nose**. **Dermoid cysts** are also thought to be related to this process, and may occur on the bridge of the nose.

Atresia or stenosis of the anterior nares

These abnormalities are very rare but **atresia of the posterior nares** may result from persistence of the primitive bucconasal membrane. This extends between the base of the sphenoid, the medial pterygoid plates, the vomer and the hard palate. It may be bony or membranous and its persistence is commoner in females than males. If the problem occurs unilaterally it may go unnoticed, the only symptom being a persisting nasal discharge. Bilateral cases, however, should be evident at or soon after birth. Usually there is intermittent asphyxia or asphyxia during feeding. A few cases may present later with nasal discharge and failure to develop taste and smell. If the condition is suspected in the infant, the diagnosis is supported by a number of simple examination findings. A mirror placed beneath the nostrils does not develop any condensation and it is impossible to pass a soft plastic tube through the nose.

Rhinitis

Acute and chronic rhinitis

Acute rhinitis presents with rhinorrhoea, nasal obstruction and constitutional disturbances. The usual cause is the common cold and, in more pronounced cases, influenza. It may also arise in diphtheria, secondary to disease in the throat.

In its simplest form, chronic rhinitis may represent nothing more than relapsing attacks of acute rhinitis. In other cases, the nasal mucosa may hypertrophy and fibrose, or atrophy and degenerate. Dusty environmental surroundings may be responsible or the rhinitis may be secondary to sinusitis.

Wegener's granulomatosis

Wegener's granulomatosis (*Figure 14.1*) is an autoimmune disorder that represents a rare cause of rhinitis. The condition may involve the lungs, kidney, sclera, subglottic region,

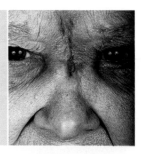

Figure 14.1.
Wegener's granuloma.

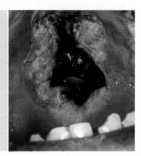

Figure 14.2.
Midline granuloma.

nasal cavity and ears. It takes the form of a periarteritis nodosa and diagnosis may be difficult. Subtle features including splinter haemorrhages in the nails, a flitting arthritis and granulomatous, punched-out skin lesions.

Stewart's midline granuloma

Stewart's midline granuloma (*Figure 14.2*) causes rapid destruction of the nose and midface region. It was once thought to be an inflammatory condition and is hence worthy of mention when considering chronic rhinitis. It is now regarded as a T-cell lymphoma.

Syphilis

Syphilis (*Figures 14.3* and *14.4*) may cause nasal symptoms in both congenital and acquired forms. Congenital syphilis most commonly causes a purulent rhinitis in infants up to about 3 months old; it may also present later at puberty with deformities similar to those of tertiary disease. In the acquired form it may cause a chancre at about 3–6 weeks and, later, a persistent rhinorrhoea at about 6–9 weeks. The commonest nasal

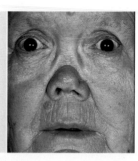

Figure 14.3.
Congenital syphilis.

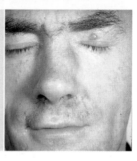

Figure 14.4.
Gumma of the nose.

manifestation of syphilis, however, is a gumma of the nose. This occurs in the tertiary stage of the disease as a result of systemic spread, about 1–5 years after the initial infection. The gumma starts to develop in the periosteum of the septum, leading to perforation. The bridge of the nose then sinks, resulting in the characteristic saddle deformity. **Yaws** (or framboesia) is a tropical condition that may affect the nose; the condition is clinically indistinguishable from syphilis.

Tuberculosis

Tuberculosis (TB, *Figure 14.5*) may affect the nose as **lupus vulgaris**. The source is frequently another family member with TB. Low virulence bacilli are thought to be inoculated as a result of nose picking. There is a chronic unilateral rhinitis, which may result in ulceration of the nose or pharynx. More typically, lupus vulgaris is identified as a cutaneous

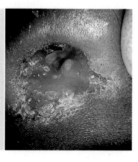

Figure 14.5.
Tuberculosis of the vestibule.

infection, which has a characteristic 'apple jelly' appearance when a glass slide is pressed against it. More virulent forms of TB affecting the nose may give rise to a **tuberculoma** of the cartilaginous septum, which becomes eroded and perforates. Here the infection may be the result of miliary spread from the lungs.

Sarcoidosis

Sarcoidosis is a granulomatous condition clinically similar to TB; histologically, however, there is no caseation. In the nose it may give rise to nodules on the septum or in the vestibule. **Leprosy** may be conveyed to the nose, giving rise to a nodular, ulcerated area on the septum. **Diphtheria** may cause rhinitis, secondary to pharyngeal involvement.

Scleroma

Scleroma is a chronic inflammatory condition of unknown cause. It affects young adults, causing nasal obstruction as a result of the soft, red masses that it produces on the nasal mucosa. The condition is seen in central and Eastern Europe and in Central and South America.

Rhinosporidiosis

Rhinosporidiosis gives rise to a bleeding, raspberry-like polyp on the nasal mucosa, and results from a sporozoal infection. India, Sri Lanka and Africa are the geographical regions of occurrence.

Leishmaniasis

Nasopharyngeal leishmaniasis causes ulceration of the mucosa and may recur years after the primary infection, destroying the facial tissues. The parasite is transferred by the sandfly and the condition is most prevalent in South America, although other regions are affected.

Fungal infections

Fungal infections tend to occur in the debilitated or immuno-compromised. **Aspergillosis** gives rise to grey areas on the mucosa with a musty discharge, but it occurs in the nose much less commonly than in the ear. **Candidiasis** occurs as white plaques and tends to be secondary to antibiotic use; in this site it is much rarer than in the mouth.

Vasomotor rhinitis

Vasomotor rhinitis is the name given to a chronic combination of sneezing, watery rhinorrhoea and nasal obstruction of unknown aetiology. Atmospheric conditions and dusty environments trigger paroxysmal symptomatology. Hereditary and psychological factors may have a role.

Allergic rhinitis

Allergic rhinitis usually occurs in response to inhaled stimuli such as dust and pollen but can arise less commonly from exposure to allergens through other routes. It tends to first manifest in children of school age, and there is a common progression from eczema in the infant to rhinitis and later asthma. Clinically the condition is identifiable as a profuse, watery rhinorrhoea with paroxysms of sneezing. The responsible allergen may be recognizable from the history, such as pollen in seasonally related cases of hay fever.

Nasal tumours
Rhinophyma

A rhinophyma (*Figure 14.6*) is a benign swelling of the whole of the tip of the nose. It results from hyperplasia and fibrosis of sebaceous glands in the skin, and occurs in relation to acne rosacea.

Capillary haemangiomas

Capillary haemangiomas (p. 389) may occur on the external surface of the nose as a strawberry naevus or may occur on the septum, causing epistaxis. The strawberry naevus usually spontaneously resolves at puberty. Venous and capillary malformations (p. 390) may also occur.

Nasal polypi

Nasal polypi (*Figures 14.7* and *14.8*) may take many histopathological forms. They may occur in isolation or be associated with other conditions such as vasomotor rhinitis or rhinosporidiosis. **Malignant polyps** may be polypoid forms of squamous carcinoma, melanoma, lymphoma or sarcoma.

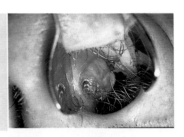

Figure 14.7.
Bleeding polypus in the septum.

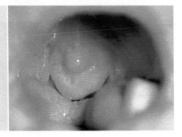

Figure 14.8.
Posterior nasal polyp presenting in the choana.

Most polyps arise in the ethmoidal air cells. The middle turbinates are the next commonest site, and the antrum the least common. Regardless of their site of origin, most polyps tend to grow into the anterior nares where large polyps may be visible. Adult males are most commonly affected, the principal symptom being a gradual onset of nasal obstruction. Anosmia, speech defects and snoring may result from this obstruction. Rhinorrhoea and bleeding may accompany inflammatory and neoplastic variants.

Nasal trauma
Fractures

Fractures (*Figure 14.9*) may take three forms:

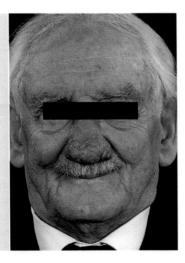

Figure 14.6.
Rhinophyma.

- Type 1 – the thin distal portion of the nasal bone is displaced and the nasal septum is fractured vertically. It results from frontal trauma and may be known as the Chevallet fracture.
- Type 2 – lateral trauma produces a C-shaped fracture of the perpendicular plate of the ethmoid and quadrilateral cartilage.
- Type 3 – caused by a more significant blow than that which causes types 1 and 2. Here there is marked depression, the perpendicular plate of the ethmoid rotating backwards and the septum collapsing inwards. The tip of the nose turns upwards.

Figure 14.9.
Compound nasal fracture.

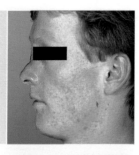

Figure 14.10.
Deviated nasal septum.

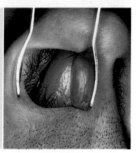

In all fracture types the deformity may initially be concealed by external swelling and there may be periorbital bruising. There is often epistaxis, and nasal obstruction may be indicative of a septal injury.

Haematoma of the septum

A haematoma of the septum may arise in response to injury, as a collection of blood beneath the mucoperichondrium or mucoperiosteum. Haematomas are usually bilateral and appear as soft, red, septal swellings on nasal examination; there is often complete nasal obstruction. To test for septal deviation (*Figure 14.10*) or haematoma, the patient may be asked to exhale through the nose whilst each nostril is occluded in turn with finger pressure. Limited egress of air is suggestive of such a problem. A septal abscess may occasionally complicate a haematoma.

Perforation of the septum

Perforation of the septum may occur directly as a result of injury or operative trauma, or may arise from a variety of other causes. Erosion may result from acid fumes in chromium platers, cocaine abuse and secondary to nasal foreign bodies. Chronic inflammatory conditions such as syphilis, TB and Wegener's granulomatosis, and pressure from haematomas or polyps, may also cause perforation. The perforation may manifest as irritation, crusting in the nostrils, epistaxis or may cause whistling noises on nasal breathing.

Foreign bodies

A foreign body in the nose should be suspected if a child is brought in with unilateral, purulent nasal discharge. Inspection with a nasal speculum is usually diagnostic.

Miscellaneous conditions
Epistaxis

Epistaxis is bleeding from the nose. It most commonly arises at Little's area, a vascular region of the anterior inferior septum containing Kiesselbach's plexus. Bleeding may solely pass into the pharynx and may present as apparent haematemesis, haemoptysis or even melaena. Hypertension does not in itself cause epistaxis but increases the severity and prolongs spontaneous bleeding. The lower atmospheric pressure and dry air associated with high altitude may predispose to spontaneous bleeding. Local trauma may result in epistaxis, usually when a fingernail scratches the septum. Fractures involving the nasal cavity, sinuses and the base of the skull are more severe examples. Bleeding may be associated with inflammatory and neoplastic conditions and may follow nasal operations.

A number of systemic disorders may indirectly result in epistaxis. The raised venous pressure of cardiac and pulmonary disease may give rise to such bleeding, as do conditions where normal blood clotting is disturbed (p. 23).

Snoring

Snoring may be a sign of partial obstruction of the upper airway during sleep; often this is simply due to laxity of the palate or pharynx. Snoring may be associated with sleep apnoea where there is a cessation of airflow for more than 10 seconds. In these cases there may be a more identifiable cause of nasal obstruction such as a polyp or septal deviation.

The pharynx

Congenital abnormalities

A **bifid uvula** is the commonest malformation in this area, probably constituting a minor degree of cleft palate. **Congenital strictures** of the pharynx may cause speech difficulties or dysphagia, but they are rare.

Pharyngitis

Acute pharyngitis tends to occur in the nasopharynx as part of a rhinitis, and in the laryngopharynx as part of a laryngitis. Symptomatology and causative organisms reflect these associated conditions. Less commonly, a number of more specific forms may be identified.

Vincent's angina

Vincent's angina or acute membranous pharyngitis is an acute ulcerative infection of the tonsils, spreading to the oropharynx. It occurs in overcrowded conditions in debilitated, malnourished people. There may be a high fever and a grey, membranous slough over the affected areas. A number of organisms have been implicated, including a spirochaete.

Diphtheria

Diphtheria tends to affect children in the 2–5 year age group, and results from *Corynebacterium diphtheriae* infection. Rare now in the developed world, the condition presents with a mild pyrexia and sore throat. There is a characteristic grey–white pseudomembrane covering the tonsils, faucial pillars, soft palate and posterior pharyngeal wall. The pharyngeal wall bleeds on separation of the membrane. There may be cervical lymphadenopathy.

Candida

Candida may cause painless, white patches on the pharynx as part of an oral candidiasis.

Herpes simplex

Herpes simplex may cause painful ulceration in association with lesions on the lips and face.

Chronic pharyngitis

Chronic pharyngitis is the name sometimes given to chronic irritation and clearing of the throat. It may be a result of smoking or dusty working environments, and is more common in patients who have had a tonsillectomy.

Ulceration and obstruction

Tuberculosis and **syphilis** may result in painless chronic ulceration. Tuberculous involvement is secondary to pulmonary infection and syphilis is usually the tertiary stage. Syphilitic ulcers are serpiginous in shape. Syphilitic gumma formation results in a firm, red swelling of the posterior pharyngeal wall or palate. Tissue destruction may result in a perforation of the soft palate. This may give rise to vocal changes and regurgitation of fluids into the nose.

   Leprosy, **sarcoidosis** and **Wegener's granulomatosis** are other rare causes of painless pharyngeal ulceration. Leprous ulcers are characteristically stellate.

   The inflammatory masses produced in **scleroma** may also involve the nasopharynx and palate, producing nasal obstruction.

Tonsillitis and adenoidal hypertrophy
Acute tonsillitis

Acute tonsillitis (*Figures 14.11* and *14.12*) results from group A haemolytic streptococcal infection and may occur in epidemics. Sore throat, earache and difficulty in swallowing are common complaints. Most cases resolve spontaneously but some give rise to peritonsillar abscesses, rheumatic fever, otitis media and chronic tonsillitis.

Peritonsillar abscess

A peritonsillar abscess (*Figure 14.13*) or quinsy is an abscess lying between the capsule of the tonsil and the lateral pharyngeal wall. The condition causes a high pyrexia and severe pain in the throat. The abscess may be visible in the soft palate above the tonsil. Rarely it may extend parapharyngeally to produce a swelling in the neck.

Rheumatic fever

Rheumatic fever is a condition that may follow acute infection of the tonsil or throat with group A β-haemolytic streptococcus; it is rare in the western world. Typically affecting children in the 6–15 year age groups, in most cases it presents 1–3

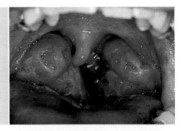

Figure 14.11. Tonsillitis.

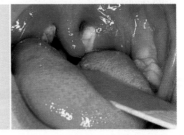

Figure 14.12. Tonsillar ulceration in glandular fever.

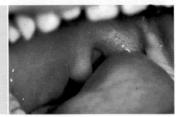

Figure 14.13. Tonsillar abscess (quinsy).

weeks after a sore throat with a number of possible features. There may be an **arthritis** which moves from joint to joint, and may affect the wrists, elbows, ankles and knees.

Carditis is its most important manifestation and, in developing countries, about half of the cases present in this way. Valvulitis results in mitral regurgitation – apical systolic murmur – and sometimes later aortic regurgitation – early diastolic murmur; residual valve damage may result though the tricuspid and pulmonary valves are rarely involved. Myocarditis may impair cardiac function and the accompanying pericarditis may cause chest pain and a pericardial rub.

Sydenham's chorea may occur as a late manifestation, up to 6 months after the acute illness. It takes the form of jerky body movements, exaggerated by tension. These may be tested for as finger movements within a sustained hand grip. **Erythema marginatum** may occur as red macules, which spread outward, whilst the originally red central region fades to the normal skin colour. **Rheumatoid nodules** may appear as firm, painless subcutaneous nodules lying over bony prominences.

Chronic tonsillitis

Chronic tonsillitis represents a chronic inflammatory hypertrophy causing a persistent sore throat, difficulty in swallowing and a chronic cough. There may be cervical node enlargement and problems from obstruction of the eustachian tubes. It usually affects children and adolescents. Calcification of chronically infected material within the tonsillar follicles may result in **tonsiloliths**. The presence of surrounding infection may lead to intratonsillar abscesses.

Tuberculosis

Tuberculosis of the tonsil may give rise to painless cervical lymphadenitis.

Adenoids

Adenoids are hypertrophied, nasopharyngeal tonsils. Spontaneous regression usually occurs during adolescence. If these areas are sufficiently enlarged they may cause obstructive symptoms. Nasal obstruction may result in breathing through the mouth, a toneless voice and nostrils with a pinched appearance. Eustachian tube obstruction causes conductive deafness. An egg-white plug of mucus visible behind the uvula is diagnostic.

Retropharyngeal abscess

Such an abscess lies in the potential space between the buccopharyngeal and prevertebral fascia. It may arise from two different disease processes.

Acutely, the condition may be caused by suppuration of the retropharyngeal lymph nodes, which become infected secondary to nasopharyngeal or oropharyngeal infections. This usually occurs in the infant and is manifested as breathing and suckling difficulties. There is toxaemia and the abscess may cause death by aspiration if it ruptures spontaneously. The abscess may be palpable on palpation of the posterior pharyngeal wall.

Tuberculosis of retropharyngeal nodes, or spread from tuberculous involvement of cervical vertebrae, may give rise to a chronic retropharyngeal abscess; this is more likely to occur in older children and adults. The collection is effectively a 'cold abscess' and presents with dysphagia or cervical adenitis.

Pharyngeal tumours
Squamous carcinoma

This is the commonest tumour arising in the pharynx. Its aetiology and presentation differ between the regions of the pharynx.

Carcinoma of the nasopharynx

Carcinoma of the nasopharynx occurs particularly in the Chinese, and there is an association with the Epstein–Barr virus. It often presents simply as a cervical lymph node metastasis but may cause symptoms from local invasion. A combination of such features comprises **Trotter's triad**: conductive deafness; pain in the side of the head; and elevation and fixity of the soft palate unilaterally. The conductive deafness results from eustachian tube invasion, and the pain from invasion of the trigeminal nerve at the foramen lacerum. Invasion of the orbit and paralysis of the second, fourth and sixth cranial nerves may occur. Jugular foramen syndrome, with paralysis of the ninth, tenth and eleventh cranial nerves is also a possibility, as is nasal obstruction and epistaxis.

Carcinoma of the oropharynx

This is most common in elderly males and is associated with smoking and alcohol. Sore throat, dysphagia, blood in the saliva, cervical nodes and referred otalgia may be presenting symptoms.

Carcinoma of the laryngopharynx

This arises in a number of areas, the largest group being those in the piriform fossa. These may cause a 'catch in the throat', pain on swallowing referred to the ear and dysphagia. In this case, hard masses in the neck are more likely to represent direct extension than nodes. Dysphagia is the main symptom of carcinomas arising on the posterior pharyngeal wall and in the cervical oesophagus.

Figure 14.14.
Lymphoepithelioma
of the tonsil.

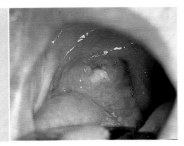

Figure 14.15.
Barium swallow
showing a large
pharyngeal pouch.

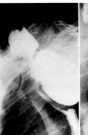
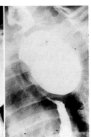

Post-cricoid carcinoma

Post-cricoid carcinoma arises between the upper border of the cricoid cartilage and the oesophageal opening. It presents with dysphagia but is distinct from the other squamous malignancies of these regions in that it almost exclusively affects females.

Paterson–Kelly (Plummer–Vinson) syndrome

This syndrome predisposes to the development of post-cricoid carcinoma. Again, females are almost exclusively affected and there is a relationship with iron deficiency. Pyridoxine deficiency, abnormal tryptophan metabolism and gastrectomy are associated. Dysphagia for solids and later liquids develops as a result of a chronic, atrophic inflammation of the cricopharyngeal region. There is concentric stenosis and a web may be present. Features of iron deficiency are pallor, angular stomatitis (fissures at the angle of the mouth), glossitis and koilonychia (spoon-like nails).

Other malignant tumours

Malignant tumours, other than squamous carcinoma, are extremely uncommon though some do occur, mainly in the oropharynx. **Lymphoepitheliomas** (*Figure 14.14*) are probably highly anaplastic, squamous carcinomas; **lymphomas** may also occur. **Adenocarcinomas** may arise from the minor salivary glands.

Benign tumours

Benign tumours are also uncommon. **Papillomas** may arise on the palate and tonsil. **Angiomas** of the nasopharynx may cause epistaxis or nasal obstruction. **Neurilemmomas** may occur behind the tonsil and removal may result in damage to the vagus nerve and carotid arteries.

Pharyngeal pouch

This arises as a herniation of the pharyngeal mucosa through Killian's dehiscence (between the thyro- and cricopharyngeal part of the inferior constrictor muscle). The pouch sags behind the oesophagus and so may obstruct it. Patients are usually elderly and complain of longstanding dysphagia and regurgitation of undigested food; there is a danger of aspiration. There may be a swelling in the neck, usually on the left. This may gurgle and empty on pressure (*Figure 14.15*).

The larynx

Congenital abnormalities

Complete occlusion of the larynx by a **laryngeal web** results in a stillbirth; lesser obstruction presents with stridor at or soon after birth. **Laryngeal cysts, subglottic haemangiomas** and **laryngomalacia** – where the laryngeal inlet is reduced by an abnormal shape – all produce such symptoms. In addition, **subglottic stenosis** – resulting from intubation trauma in premature infants – is included in this group.

Laryngitis

Acute laryngitis causes hoarseness, a sore throat and a dry cough; general malaise and fever precede and accompany these symptoms. In adults, the condition is usually viral in origin and resolves uneventfully over a few days. In other upper respiratory tract infections, smoking and alcohol are associated.

In children, upper respiratory tract infections produce a more pronounced obstruction of the upper airway as a result of the greater quantity of surrounding lymphoid tissue. These conditions present with acute stridor, the commonest being **acute laryngotracheobronchitis**. This usually occurs in the 1–2 year age group and is the result of infection from the parainfluenza virus, respiratory syncytial virus or rhinovirus. There is little constitutional disturbance, with cold-like symptoms followed by a cough and hoarseness, settling over a few days. The condition is commonly known as viral 'croup'. A small group of children, however, have the much more serious condition of **acute**

epiglottitis. The causative organism here is *Haemophilus influenzae* and the condition tends to affect the 2–3 year age group. The child is unwell with a high fever and acute onset of stridor. They are anxious and swallowing is painful, resulting in drooling of saliva. There is a danger of life-threatening upper airway obstruction, which may be precipitated by inspecting the throat. Hence, in cases of stridor in children, the throat should only be inspected by those capable of performing a rapid intubation.

Chronic laryngitis

Chronic laryngitis gives a persisting hoarseness and cough and is usually the result of chronic exposure to irritants such as cigarette smoke and alcohol. Dusty atmospheres, industrial fumes and chronic sinus infection are also implicated.

Diphtheria

Diphtheria may affect the larynx as an extension of pharyngeal involvement. If the characteristic grey–white inflammatory pseudomembrane involves the vocal chords, progressive stridor and croup may develop. This is particularly dangerous in young children, for whom emergency trachotomy may be required. Although the immunization programme in the UK has eradicated diphtheria, it is still endemic in many areas worldwide.

Tuberculous laryngitis

Tuberculous laryngitis usually results from infected sputum, secondary to pulmonary infection. The posterior portion of the larynx tends to be involved, having a nodular ulcerated appearance, and it may be noted that there is impaired adduction of the cords.

Syphilis

Syphilis may affect the larynx, usually in the tertiary stage. The commonest laryngeal finding is a gumma of the epiglottis but diffuse infiltration may occur.

Leprosy

Leprosy affects the larynx in about 10% of cases; it is always associated with disease elsewhere. In common with TB and syphilis, this condition may result in cartilaginous destruction, leading to scarring and stenosis with residual stridor and vocal weakness.

Mycotic infection

Mycotic infection of the larynx is very rare, only occurring in the immunocompromised.

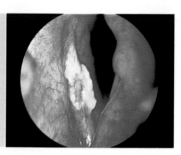

Figure 14.16. Carcinoma of the vocal cord.

Laryngeal tumours

Leukoplakia

Leukoplakia, or hyperkeratosis of the larynx, is a premalignant condition appearing as raised, white patches on the cords.

Benign neoplasms

Benign neoplasms of the larynx are most likely to be papillomas, but fibromas, chondromas and angiomas also occur. Hoarseness is the usual symptom.

Squamous carcinoma

This is the only common malignant tumour of the larynx. The vocal cords, hence glottic carcinoma (*Figure 14.16*), are the commonest site. Carcinoma of the undersurface of the cords – subglottic – is viewed as a separate locational type, and is the next most common. Supraglottic growths are the least common, occurring in the anterior half of the vestibule or on the ventricular band and in the underlying vestibular sac. The condition tends to affect males in the 40–60 year age group.

The presentation of laryngeal carcinoma varies with its site.Glottic carcinoma invades locally but does not show early metastases because of the paucity of lymphatics in the area. Thus, cases tend to present with hoarseness and stridor. Subglottic forms are also mainly locally invasive but tend to present late. In these cases, hoarseness may result from recurrent laryngeal nerve palsy. The tumour may initially be concealed when the cords are viewed on indirect laryngoscopy. Supraglottic forms may cause laryngeal pain before hoarseness. Cervical lymph node metastases are much more likely as a result of the better lymphatic drainage of the upper larynx.

Referred otalgia

In laryngeal pain it is important to consider referred otalgia. This phenomenon may arise in neoplastic and inflammatory conditions of the larynx. As the larynx is innervated by the vagus nerve, pain may be referred to the auricular branch of the vagus. This branch supplies the concavity of the concha of the ear. Hence, otherwise unexplained pain occurring at this site must always raise the suspicion of laryngeal conditions.

Laryngeal trauma
Blunt trauma

Blunt trauma from a blow or strangulation may result in hoarseness, dyspnoea and dysphagia. There may be external bruising and swelling, and, in severe cases, surgical emphysema of the neck or upper body. If laryngeal cartilages are fractured there may be a rapidly fatal subglottic swelling that obstructs the airway.

Penetrating injuries

Penetrating injuries are often associated with fatal injuries of the great vessels or cervical spine. Isolated cases from stabbing or cutting type injuries are usually apparent in the emergency room, functioning as a surgical airway. There may be dyspnoea from anxiety and associated haemorrhage and oedema. Surgical emphysema of the neck or mediastinal emphysema may accompany the injury.

Burns

Thermal burns may result in association with facial and other burns from flame inhalation. Chemical burns may result from the inhalation or swallowing of corrosive liquids. The larynx becomes oedematous and upper airway obstruction may supervene.

Intubation injury

Intubation injury may later result in scarring and laryngeal stenosis. The problem occurs in those requiring prolonged intubation in the intensive care unit. Also, the use of too large a tube, or a cuffed tube in the child, may lead to the condition.

'Singer's nodes'

These nodes (*Figure 14.17*) may result from excessive use and straining of the voice, hence singers, actors and teachers are most often affected. The condition presents with hoarseness, which may arise insidiously over a period of months, or suddenly after an episode of vocal straining. On indirect laryngoscopy, the nodes appear as small nodules occurring at a fairly constant site: the junction of the anterior third and posterior two-thirds of the cord. **Contact ulcers** may occur in the same groups but are relatively uncommon. They take the form of depressions over the vocal processes and are thought to be the result of hammering of one vocal process of the arytenoid cartilage against the other. **Acute submucosal haemorrhages** may occur on the cords, as a result of forceful approximation in coughing or shouting.

Laryngocele

A laryngocele (*Figures 14.18* and *14.19*) is an elongation or protrusion of the laryngeal vestibule. They tend to occur in males in the 50–70 year age group, and the condition is related to occupations involving forced expiration, such as glassblowers and trumpet players. An internal laryngocele is confined to the framework of the larynx, whereas an external laryngocele passes through the thyrohyoid membrane, probably via the points of entry of the superior laryngeal nerve and artery. The external laryngocele is apparent externally on coughing as an expanding swelling in the neck. It transmits a cough impulse, can be filled by a Valsalva manouevre, and can be emptied by digital pressure.

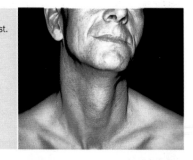

Figure 14.18.
Laryngocele at rest.

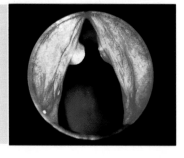

Figure 14.17.
'Singer's nodes'.

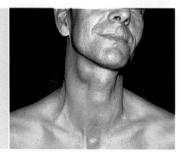

Figure 14.19.
Laryngocele becoming evident when the patient performs a Valsalva manoeuvre.

Miscellaneous conditions

Oedema

Oedema of the larynx can result in dyspnoea and stridor; **angioneurotic oedema** may occur suddenly in response to drug or food allergy. Excitement and psychological overlay may have a role. Inflammatory and neoplastic conditions, and myxoedema, may also cause laryngeal swelling.

Paralysis of the larynx

Paralysis of the larynx may occur in a variety of forms and degrees of severity. In the CNS the larynx is represented bilaterally, thus upper motor neurone lesions are unlikely. However, lesions of the vagus and of the superior or recurrent laryngeal nerves may result in such paralysis. In many cases the cause is unknown but common malignancies of the cervical structures and surgical injury, for example at thyroidectomy, are likely causes. Peripheral neuritis from chemical and bacterial toxins is also recognized.

Laryngeal nerve palsy

In **unilateral recurrent laryngeal nerve palsy** the patient may be asymptomatic if the active cord compensates, otherwise hoarseness may result. In **bilateral recurrent laryngeal nerve palsy** there may still be some compensation but dyspnoea may result on exertion or with laryngitis. **Superior laryngeal nerve palsy** results in a voice that tires easily. In combined lesions the voice may be very weak and food aspiration may be a problem. On laryngoscopy the cords are in the 'cadaveric' position, lying midway between their midline phonatory position and their abducted inspirational position. In an **isolated recurrent laryngeal nerve palsy** the affected cord lies near to the midline.

Functional paralysis

Functional paralysis gives rise to a hysterical aphonia. The condition mainly affects young women, reducing the voice to a whisper. **Myasthenia gravis** may rarely give rise to laryngeal paralysis.

Crico-arytenoid arthritis

Crico-arytenoid arthritis is a rare cause of hoarseness. It results from rheumatic fever, gonococcal infection, injury, chronic inflammatory conditions and, rarely, in rheumatoid arthritis.

15 Salivary glands

Introduction

The spectrum of salivary gland pathology is shown in *Table 15.1*. Salivary tumours are most often encountered in the parotid gland, whereas sialolithiasis more commonly affects the submandibular gland. The probability of a salivary tumour being malignant, however, is far greater in the submandibular (35–60%), sublingual (35–90%) and minor (35–90%) salivary glands than in the parotid gland (10–35%). The inferior lingual glands of Blandin and Nuhn may undergo cystic degeneration, and ectopic glands may give rise to adenocarcinomas of the palate.

Sialadenitis

Mumps (*Figure 15.1*) is the commonest cause of acute parotitis. A highly contagious paramyxovirus causes epidemics in non-immunized children, usually in the 4–12 year age group. After an incubation period of 21 days there is general malaise followed by a bilateral or unilateral painful parotid swelling, with fever and arthralgia. The swelling spreads down the neck, giving a double chin appearance. Rarely there may be associated orchitis, meningoencephalitis, pancreatitis, thyroiditis or sensorineural hearing loss. In most cases, however, the condition subsides uneventfully.

Acute bacterial sialadenitis (*Figures 15.2* and *15.3*) is seen postoperatively in the elderly and neonates. Dehydration, general debilitation, poor oral hygiene and stricturing or stones in Stensen's duct are factors. Typically there is sudden, painful swelling of one parotid gland, trismus, dysphagia and fever. Less commonly, the submandibular gland is affected.

Chronic sialadenitis – from obstruction or narrowing of Stensen's or Wharton's ducts by a calculus or stricture – may cause recurrent swelling and aching of the parotid or submandibular glands, particularly before eating. On examination, the affected gland is enlarged and rubbery hard. Stricturing of the duct results from repeated infection (associated with poor oral hygiene and ill-fitting dentures), congenital abnormality or trauma.

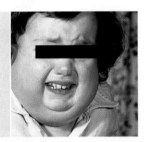

Figure 15.1.
Mumps giving rise to bilateral facial oedema over the infected parotid glands.

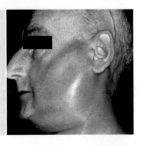

Figure 15.2.
Parotid abscess in an ageing patient.

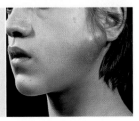

Figure 15.3.
Parotid abscess in a young girl.

Table 15.1. Salivary gland pathology.

Salivary gland tumours		Other salivary conditions
Benign	*Malignant*	Sialolithiasis (stones)
Pleomorphic adenoma	Mucoepidermoid carcinoma	Stricture of ducts
Warthin's tumour	Adenocystic carcinoma	Sialadenitis – mumps; acute bacterial sialadenitis; TB; actinomycosis; cat-scratch disease; Mikulicz's syndrome
Monomorphic adenoma	Malignant mixed tumour	Autoimmune conditions – Sjögren's syndrome
Oncocytoma	Acinic cell carcinoma	
	Adenocarcinoma	
	Squamous cell carcinoma	
	Undifferentiated carcinoma	

Mikulicz's syndrome is the combination of bilateral salivary and lachrymal gland enlargement. There may be many causes, likely examples being sarcoidosis, leukaemia/lymphoma and Sjögren's syndrome.

Sjögren's syndrome (*Figures 15.4* and *15.5*) is a rare autoimmune condition affecting the salivary glands and can occur in combination with other autoimmune connective tissue disorders. It may take many forms, as shown in *Table 15.2*.

Radiotherapy for head and neck malignancy may result in **salivary gland atrophy**, decreased salivary secretion and increased risk of caries.

Salivary gland tumours

The **pleomorphic adenoma** (*Figures 15.6–15.8*) – mixed salivary tumour – is a benign tumour, the commonest salivary tumour and the commonest tumour of the parotid gland. Typically it forms a mass in the lateral lobe, which slowly enlarges over many years, women in their forties most often being affected. On palpation the tumour is firm, non-tender and smooth or lobulated in texture. Initially spherical and encapsulated, it may eventually spread more deeply, with the result that recurrence after resection is common. Facial nerve palsy does not usually occur and is suggestive of a malignant tumour. On oral examination, the deep part of the gland may have pushed the tonsil and pillar of the fauces towards the midline. The key differential diagnosis is that of an enlarged pre-auricular lymph node. A useful feature in their distinction is mobility – the parotid gland, and tumours arising from it, are relatively fixed, whereas the pre-auricular node usually occurs outside the capsule of the gland and so is very mobile.

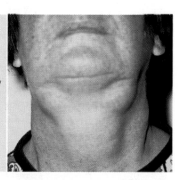

Figure 15.4.
Submandibular enlargement of allergic adenitis. The causative agent can be difficult to identify – drugs, pollen and foodstuffs have been implicated.

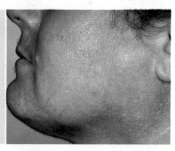

Figure 15.5.
Sjögren's syndrome.

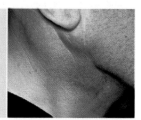

Figure 15.6.
Parotid swelling. These often begin behind the angle of the mandible.

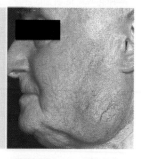

Figure 15.7.
Parotid swelling. Diagnosis is frequently not established until cytological evidence is available.

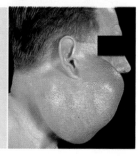

Figure 15.8.
Large, mixed parotid tumour.

Table 15.2. Manifestations of Sjögren's syndrome.

Condition	Manifestation
Keratoconjunctivitis sicca	Deficient tear film
Xerostomia	Deficient salivation and gland enlargement
Primary glandular sicca syndrome	Both of the above
Primary extraglandular sicca syndrome	The above with hyperglobulinaemic purpura, vasculitis, or Raynaud's phenomenon or B cell lymphoma
Secondary Sjögren's syndrome	Any of the above occurring together with rheumatoid arthritis, systemic lupus erythematosus or other recognizable connective tissue disorders

The **adenolymphoma** – Warthin's tumour – is a benign tumour, the second commonest salivary tumour, and is found exclusively in the parotid gland. It affects males in their fifties, forming a slow-growing, painless swelling over the angle of the jaw; there is a high incidence of bilateral disease. The tumour arises just beneath the capsule of the gland, usually at the level of the lower border of the mandible (lower than a pleo-morphic adenoma). It is smooth, soft and often fluctuant, its superficial nature and slight mobility sometimes giving the appearance that it is separate from the gland. The site, con-sistency and sometimes the bilateral involvement may allow this type of tumour to be suspected on clinical grounds.

Less common benign tumours include the **monomorphic adenoma** and **oncocytoma**.

Adenocystic carcinoma (*Figures 15.9* and *15.10*) is the commonest malignant salivary tumour and occurs in the sub-mandibular, sublingual and minor glands. In contrast, **mucoepidermoid carcinoma** predominantly occurs in the parotid. Other malignant tumour types are **adenocarcinoma**, **squamous carcinoma**, **undifferentiated carcinoma**, **acinic cell carcinoma** and **malignant mixed tumours**.

Typically, malignant tumours produce indistinct, rapidly growing masses and malignant cervical lymphadenopathy. For the submandibular gland, numbness of the anterior two-thirds of the tongue from lingual nerve infiltration is diagnostic, whereas sublingual tumours may cause deviation of the tongue from invasion and fixation.

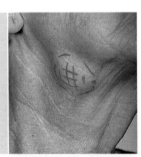

Figure 15.9.
Adenocystic carcinoma of the submandibular gland.

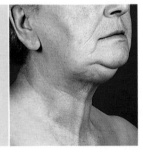

Figure 15.10.
The presentation of the right submandibular malignancy in this woman was with the more obvious metabolic lymph node lower in the neck.

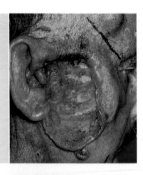

Figure 15.11.
Squamous carcinomas of the parotid region may be due to invasion from cutaneous lesions as here, or to metastatic spread from other sites.

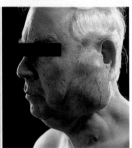

Figure 15.12.
Arteriovenous malformation of parotid region. The differential diagnosis from other parotid swellings is made by the pulsatile nature of the lesion and the associated bruit.

Malignant parotid tumours tend to occur in older age groups and most take the form of solitary, hard nodules with deep fixation. There may be local pain, exacerbated by open-ing the mouth, referred otalgia and varying degrees of facial nerve palsy. Undifferentiated carcinoma forms a large, rapidly growing mass. Squamous carcinoma should be considered to be metastatic, until proved otherwise, and a primary tumour sought (*Figures 15.11* and *15.12*).

Sialolithiasis

Salivary calculi (*Figures 15.13* and *15.14*) most commonly occur in the submandibular – Wharton's – duct. They may occasionally occur in relation to the parotid but a number of features of the submandibular gland predispose to stone for-mation. The opening of Wharton's duct lies above the level of the gland, encouraging stasis. Saliva from the submandibular gland contains more mucus and calcium and is more alkaline. Submandibular calculi tend to occur in young to middle-aged patients, causing a dull aching pain and swelling in the sub-mandibular region which worsens just before and during eating. Symptoms may be relieved by pressing the gland but this releases foul-tasting, purulent saliva. There is often a pat-tern of remission and relapse over days or weeks, as the stone moves in the duct; eventually the stone may pass.

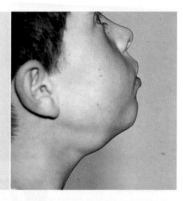

Figure 15.13. This unilateral submandibular swelling proved to be due to a submandibular calculus.

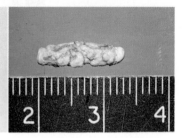

Figure 15.14. Submandibular calculus.

Inspecting the floor of the mouth with a torch may reveal an inflamed duct ampulla, exuding pus or occasionally a stone in the duct orifice. There may be an asymmetry of the floor or a bulge from the swollen gland. A dry swab may be placed beneath the tongue and gland secretion stimulated with lemon juice on the dorsum of the tongue. Normally, when the swab is removed, saliva is seen flowing or being ejected from the ducts. With calculus obstruction, there is little or no secretion from the affected side.

The submandibular duct may be palpated with the index finger. The patient's head should be flexed and tilted to the affected side to relax the musculature, and any dentures removed. The alveolar margin is followed back to its posterior extremity and the finger then rotated so its pulp faces downward. The duct can then be palpated along its course, from behind forwards, the other hand providing support from below the jaw. The gland itself may be palpated bimanually. It may be evident on inspection of the neck as a swelling just beneath and in front of the angle of the jaw. Stimulation of salivation with lemon juice may induce swelling in a patient with suggestive symptoms.

16 The neck

Lumps in the neck

A lump is the most likely clinical problem to be encountered in the neck. Symptoms and signs to be elicited are those to be considered in describing any lump (p. 60). Lumps may be classified in relation to the 'triangles of the neck' (*Figure 16.1, Tables 16.1* and *16.2*) or according to their structure of origin.

Skin and subcutaneous tissue

Sebaceous cysts (p. 138), lipomas (*Figure 16.2*; p. 148), neurofibromas (p. 149), capillary malformations (p. 390) and a variety of common skin conditions (p. 129) and tumours (Chapter 8) may occur on the neck.

Sternomastoid muscle

The sternomastoid tumour of infancy is either an organizing haematoma or an area of fibrosis secondary to ischaemia in the middle third of the sternomastoid muscle. Associated with breech presentation, it is uncertain whether the problem represents a birth injury or is the result of an intrauterine phenomenon.

The condition may be discovered soon after birth as a smooth, fusiform swelling in the middle third of the sternomastoid, or may present 3–6 weeks later with torticollis. Torticollis results from fibrotic shortening of the muscle, turning the child's head away from the affected side and slightly

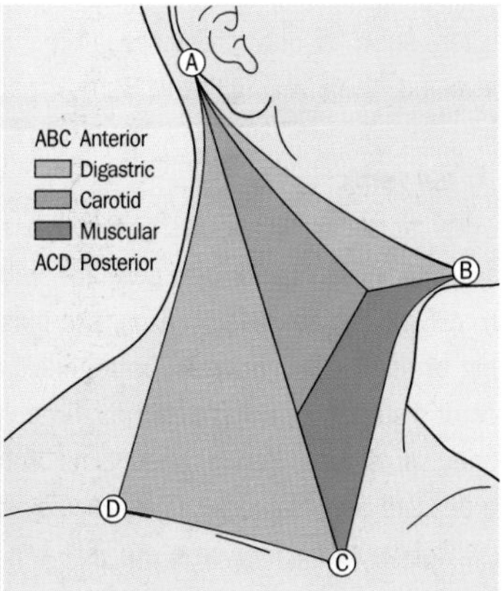

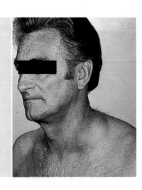

Figure 16.2. Subcutaneous lipoma in the roof of the neck.

Figure 16.1. Figure of triangles of the neck.

ABC Anterior
- ▢ Digastric
- ▢ Carotid
- ▢ Muscular

ACD Posterior

Table 16.1. Anatomical regions of the neck.

Triangle	Anatomical boundaries	Contents
Anterior	Midline	May be subdivided into the digastric, carotid and muscular triangles as described below
	Anterior border of sternomastoid	
	Inferior border of the ramus of the mandible	
Digastric	Inferior border of the ramus of the mandible	Submandibular gland
		Facial artery
	Anterior and posterior portions of the digastric muscle, slung to the hyoid bone	Lymph nodes
Carotid	Omohyoid	Common carotid artery, dividing at the level of the hyoid bone into the internal and external carotid arteries
	Anterior border of sternomastoid	
	Posterior portion of digastric	Internal jugular vein
		Vagus nerve
		Lymph nodes
Muscular	Omohyoid	Laryngeal structures
	Midline	Thyroid: goitres extend beyond this area, beneath the sternomastoid and may extend into the posterior triangle
	Anterior portion of digastric	
Posterior	Posterior border of sternomastoid	Lymph nodes
	Anterior border of trapezius	Scalenus anterior muscle
	Upper border of the middle third of the clavicle	Accessory nerve

Table 16.2. Lumps in the neck.

Region	Type or cause of lump
All regions	Skin and subcutaneous tissues: sebaceous cyst; lipoma; neurofibroma
	Lymphadenopathy: acute infective; chronic infective (TB); primary malignant (lymphoma); secondary malignant (nodal metastases)
	Superior vena caval obstruction (generalized swelling of the head and neck with venous dilatation)
Midline	Sublingual dermoid
	Thyroglossal cyst, sinus or fistula
	(Pharyngocele)
	(Laryngocele)
	(Ranula)

The ranula lies just to one side of the midline but does not arise from a unilateral midline structure. The pharyngocele and laryngocele do not lie in the midline but arise from the midline structures

Digastric triangle	Submandibular gland tumours
	Ranula
Carotid triangle	Carotid tortuosity
	Carotid aneurysm
	Carotid body tumour
	Pharyngocele
	Branchial cyst, sinus or fistula
Muscular triangle	Thyroid swellings (these extend beneath the sternomastoid and may enter the posterior triangle)
	Laryngocele
	Innominate tortuosity
	Innominate aneurysm
Posterior triangle	Thyroid swellings
	Subclavian aneurysm
	Cystic hygroma

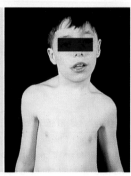

Figure 16.3.
Sternomastoid tumour in a child.

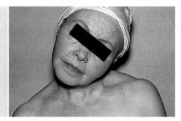

Figure 16.4.
Sternomastoid tumour producing torticollis in an adult.

or under the muscle. Attachment to the muscle may be demonstrated as a loss of mobility of the lump when the sternomastoid is contracted. Here it is important to remember that to tense the left sternomastoid, you must ask the patient to turn their head to the right and vice versa.

Other neck-related conditions can be found as follows: pharyngeal pouch (p. 207); laryngocele (p. 209); and thyroid lesions (Chapter 17).

Arteries

The commonest cause of a pulsatile swelling in the neck is prominence and tortuosity of the right common carotid, subclavian or innominate arteries; this tortuosity and lengthening results from hypertension and atherosclerosis, and is most often seen in older females. If the innominate artery is involved, the swelling lies in Burns' space.

Aneurysms

Extracranial carotid aneurysms may present as a pulsatile neck swelling, neck pain or with cerebral embolic symptomatology (p. 364). They exhibit an expansile pulsation with an overlying bruit. The majority are iatrogenic, arising in relation to carotid surgery or trauma, although rarely true atherosclerotic aneurysms occur. Tender aneurysms of the extracranial carotid artery are associated with Takayasu's arteriopathy.

Subclavian aneurysms are rare but may occur as poststenotic aneurysms in thoracic outlet syndrome (p. 366). They

upwards (*Figure 16.3*), forced movements to correct the deformity being resisted.

An adult patient (*Figure 16.4*) may be encountered who had the condition as a child. Here, the signs to be elicited are those of shortening of the affected sternomastoid. Shortening of the left muscle turns the' head to the right and tilt the head to the left. In the rare case of an adult patient presenting *de novo* with a tumour of the sternomastoid, a rhabdomyosarcoma should be considered. The differential diagnosis includes traumatic swellings of the muscle, and neck lesions lying over may appear as a pulsatile mass in the supraclavicular fossa with an overlying bruit or give rise to embolic phenomena (p. 367).

Innominate aneurysms have been reported in syphilitic aortitis.

For more on arteries, see also Chapter 28.

Veins

Superior vena caval syndrome (p. 246) results from extrinsic compression of the vena cava by mediastinal masses or, less commonly, from fibrosis, thrombosis or invasion of the vein. The patient may notice a feeling of 'fullness' in the ears or nose which is accentuated by lying down. In addition, symptoms may arise from compression of the airway and recurrent laryngeal nerve by the causal mass. There is venous engorgement and oedema of the face, neck and arms. There may be periorbital oedema and chemosis, which is accentuated by leaning forwards.

Venous malformations (*Figures 16.5a, b*) are described on p. 391.

Lymphatics

The cystic hygroma (*Figure 16.6*) is described on p. 147.

Lymph nodes

An enlarged cervical lymph node is the commonest cause of a lump in the neck. It is usually secondary to acute infection but when due to malignant spread, the primary lesion is sited in the head and neck in 90% of cases. The distribution of

cervical node groups, and the areas they drain are shown in (*Figure 16.7*). Cervical lymph nodes may become enlarged as a result of inflammatory or neoplastic processes; these are summarized in *Table 16.3*.

Figure 16.7. The distribution of nodes in the neck. The numbers indicate a possible sequence for examination.

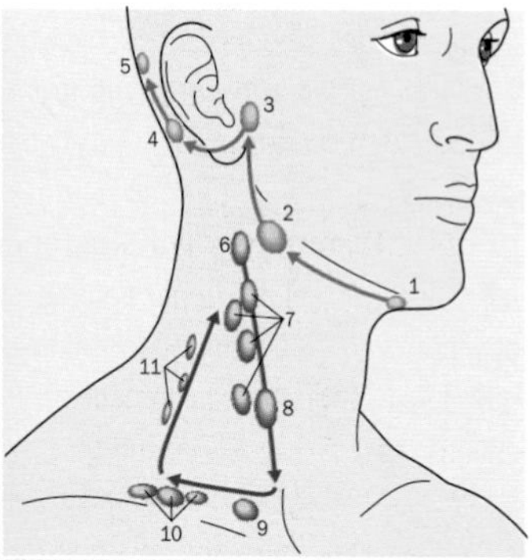

1 Mental
2 Submandibular
3 Preauricular
4 Postauricular
5 Occipital
6 Jugulodigastric
7 Internal jugular (deep cervical)
8 Jugulo-omohyoid
9 Scalene
10 Supraclavicular
11 External jugular (superficial cervical)

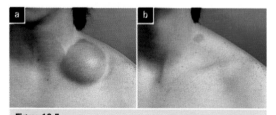

Figure 16.5.
a. Venous malformation in the root of the neck. The patient has undertaken a Valsalva manoeuvre. b. The patient breathing normally.

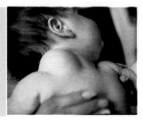

Figure 16.6.
Cystic hygroma.

Table 16.3. Causes of lymphadenopathy

Condition	Cause
Acute inflammation	Common infections of the upper aerodigestive tract: tonsillitis; pharyngitis/laryngitis; parotitis; dental abscess
	Common superficial infections of the head and neck: acne; furuncle/abscess; infected wounds; infected skin malignancies
	Infectious mononucleosis: glandular fever; Epstein–Barr virus infection
	Toxoplasmosis
	Cytomegalovirus
	Actinomycosis
	Cat-scratch disease
Chronic inflammation	TB
	Sarcoidosis
	Histiocytosis X
Lymphomas	Hodgkin's
	Non-Hodgkin's
Metastatic carcinoma	Carcinomas of the upper aerodigestive tract
	Skin tumours of the head and neck: squamous cell carcinoma; basal cell carcinoma; melanoma
	Rarely, carcinoma at other body sites

In general, acute suppurative conditions result in firm, tender nodes, about 1–2 cm in diameter. The features of the underlying condition may well be more marked than those of the lymphadenopathy. Tuberculous adenopathy presents more subtly with a variety of possible appearances depending upon the stage of the disease. Lymphomas result in large, rubbery nodes whereas those involved with secondary carcinoma are small and hard; the greater cornu of the hyoid bone may be mistaken for such a node.

Acute inflammatory lymphadenopathy

Acute infection of the upper aerodigestive tract may result in cervical lymphadenopathy. Tonsillitis – usually from group A haemolytic streptococcal infection – most commonly affects children, producing a sore throat, tonsillar swelling and systemic upset. Associated lymphadenopathy usually affects the upper cervical chain and it is common to find an enlarged node at the angle of the mandible, which is thus often called the tonsillar node. Infectious mononucleosis – glandular fever – affects young adults, resulting in general malaise, sore throat and cervical lymphadenopathy. The causative agent, the Epstein–Barr virus, is spread by mucosal contact or as an aerosol, and infects B-lymphocytes. The condition is self-limiting but general weakness may persist for weeks or even months. Cytomegalovirus infection occasionally results in a glandular fever- like condition. The virus is spread by transfusion and is common in transplant recipients either as primary infection or reactivation by immunosuppression.

Toxoplasmosis

Toxoplasmosis is a protozoal infection that occurs world-wide. Cats are the definitive hosts, humans becoming infected by ingesting oocysts – which reach food preparation surfaces from cat faeces – or by eating infected meat. Infection is often subclinical but in some cases cervical lymphadenopathy, malaise and fever may be noted. When acquired in pregnancy, or by the immunocompromised, the infection may result in more serious sequelae. Congenital infection may result in abortion or congenital syndromes whereas in AIDS cerebral toxoplasmosis may occur.

Actinomycosis

Actinomycosis may result in a painful intraoral swelling of the jaw, cheek or submandibular region with associated lymphadenopathy. Although uncommon, the condition usually arises following a dental extraction, the causative organism – *Actinomyces israelii* – being a mouth commensal, occurring particularly in association with dental caries. Rarely, sinus formation to the overlying skin may result, the exudate classically containing sulphur granules.

Chronic inflammatory lymphadenopathy

Tuberculous cervical adenitis (*Figures 16.8–16.10*) may result from tonsillar infection from contaminated milk, in areas where bovine TB is common. Where milk is pasteurized, cases are relatively rare but may occur in association with pulmonary TB and in immigrants from high prevalence areas.

The condition insidiously results in caseous necrosis of the upper and middle deep cervical nodes. Classically, four stages are identified, which may progress over weeks or months:

- Stage I – initially there are fairly solid, moderately enlarged nodes.
- Stage II – the lymph nodes break down and liquefy, pus collecting beneath the deep fascia. A fluctuant mass is palpated that, unlike an acute abscess, has little or no overlying inflammation.
- Stage III – eventually the deep cervical fascia is eroded, resulting in a release of pus beneath the superficial fascia. This dumb-bell like arrangement is termed a collar stud abscess.
- Stage IV – following spontaneous discharge or surgical drainage of the abscess, a chronic discharging sinus results.

Surprisingly, pus or biopsies obtained from these abscesses or sinuses have a low isolation rate for tubercle bacilli. It is possible that such lymphadenopathy represents a reactive hyperplasia rather than tuberculous nodal involvement.

Sarcoidosis

Sarcoidosis is a condition characterized pathologically by the presence of non-caseating tuberculoid granulomas, in the absence of an identifiable infective agent. It affects young

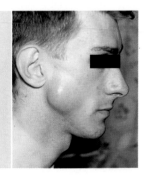

Figure 16.8.
Tuberculous abscess developed from a preauricular lymph node.

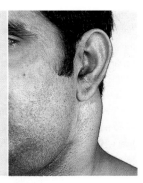

Figure 16.9.
Tuberculous abscess from
deep cervical lymph chain.

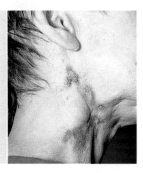

Figure 16.10.
Chronic scarring following
tuberculous infection with
sinus formation.

adults, often those of African descent, causing erythema nodosum, arthropathy, uveitis, fever and hilar lymphadenopathy on chest radiography. It is a rare cause of cervical lymphadenopathy, which is present in only 3–4% of cases.

Histiocytosis X

Histiocytosis X may cause numerous and varied clinical pictures, the only common diagnostic factor being a uniform histological picture in which histiocytes predominate. The condition may result in massive, painless, cervical node enlargement in small children. Most of these cases form part of a generalized syndrome but if the condition affects the neck in isolation it may be termed sinus histiocytosis or Rosai–Dorfman syndrome.

Cat-scratch disease

This is characterized by a regional lymphadenitis occurring 2–3 weeks after a skin injury in the area drained by the nodes. After the initial injury there is a localized, crusted pustule that disappears just before the lymphadenitis develops. No causative organism has been identified.

Neoplastic lymphadenopathy

Lymphoma describes primary malignant tumours of the reticuloendothelial system, which may be grouped into Hodgkin's and non-Hodgkin's types. A Hodgkin's lymphoma is defined

Table 16.4. Classification of lymphoma.

Hodgkin's lymphoma

Characterized by the binucleate Reed–Sternberg cell which does not carry B or T cell identity

Non-Hodgkin's lymphoma

Low grade lymphomas	Lymphocytic lymphoma	
	Immunocytic lymphomas	Waldenström's macroglobulinaemia
		Myeloma
Follicular cell lymphomas		
High grade lymphomas	Centroblastic lymphomas	
	Immunoblastic lymphomas (associated with immunosuppression)	
	Adult T cell leukaemia/lymphoma syndrome (associated with HIV)	
	Burkitt's lymphoma (associated with Epstein–Barr virus infection and chromosomal defect)	

Ann Arbor staging of Hodgkin's lymphoma

I. Single node region or extralymphatic site

II. Two or more node regions on the same side of the diaphragm, or single node region and one extra lymphatic site on one side of the diaphragm

III. Node regions on both sides of the diaphragm

IV. Diffuse involvement of one or more extralymphatic sites

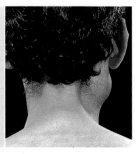

Figure 16.11.
Lymph node enlargement in
Hodgkin's disease.

by the histological finding of Reed–Sternberg cells – binucleate cells lacking the markers that normally identify the cells as T- or B- lymphocytes. A variety of conditions thus fall into each category, as shown in *Table 16.4*.

Hodgkin's lymphoma

Hodgkin's lymphoma (*Figure 16.11*) occurs in young adults and may be associated with chromosomal abnormalities and Epstein–Barr virus infection. Typically, they cause large, painless, rubbery cervical or axillary lymphadenopathy. In approximately a quarter of cases there are constitutional symptoms of malaise, weight loss and a pyrexia of unknown origin, often characterized by night sweats. The condition may be staged with the Ann Arbor classification shown in *Table 16.4*. Occasionally, upper mediastinal lymphadenopathy may result in superior vena caval obstruction (p. 246).

Non-Hodgkin's lymphoma

Non-Hodgkin's lymphoma (*Figures 16.12* and *16.13*) usually occurs in the 60–80 year age group. Lymphadenopathy is a common presenting feature although unlike Hodgkin's types there is no clear anatomical pattern and extra-lymphoidal tissue is frequently involved. About a third of cases present as extranodal disease.

Secondary carcinoma

Secondary carcinoma (*Figures 16.14–16.17*) is the most likely cause of a malignant cervical node. The primary tumour is nearly always situated in or on the head or neck, most commonly in the upper aerodigestive tract. Thus male patients in their fifties, who are heavy smokers or have a heavy alcohol intake, are most likely to be affected. On finding a suspicious node, examination should be directed towards identification of the primary tumour. A full inspection of the skin of the head and neck excludes common malignant skin tumours. The thyroid should be examined, papillary and medullary thyroid carcinomas being noted for their ability to produce cervical node metastases. A careful examination of the oral cavity and salivary glands should be made, remembering that tumours are often missed at the lateral border or base of the tongue. The nasopharynx, piriform fossae and larynx require evaluation with indirect laryngoscopy and flexible nasopharyngeal endoscopy.

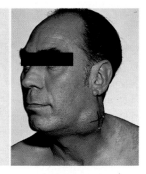

Figure 16.15.
Nodal metastasis in a patient with carcinoma of the tongue treated with radiotherapy.

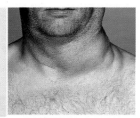

Figure 16.12.
Lymph node enlargement in a patient with a low grade lymphoma.

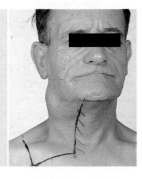

Figure 16.16.
Secondary malignant lymph nodes from melanoma of the leg.

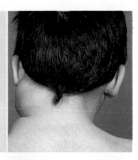

Figure 16.13.
Follicular lymphoma.

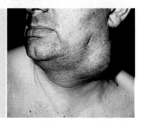

Figure 16.14.
Nodal metastases from a retropharyngeal malignancy.

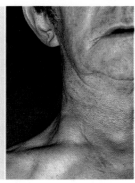

Figure 16.17.
Supraclavicular malignant lymph nodes secondary to carcinoma of the lung. An enlarged scalene node, commonly from a lung or breast malignancy, lies deep to the lower end of the sternomastoid muscle which must be relaxed during palpation.

Carcinomas arising outside the head and neck area (below the clavicle) may produce cervical node secondaries but should be considered only when a head and neck primary has been excluded or if there is other supportive evidence. The great exception to this rule is the supraclavicular fossa where three quarters of the associated primary tumours are infraclavicular in origin: bronchogenic, breast, gastrointestinal or genitourinary malignancy. In particular, isolated left supraclavicular lymphadenopathy may result from spread along the thoracic duct from gastric or pancreatic carcinomas (Troisier's sign).

For salivary glands see Chapter 15.

Embryological remnants or defects

In embryological development, the mandibular region and neck are formed from the six paired branchial arches. Abnormalities in this developmental process give rise to the branchial cyst, sinus and fistula. Branchial cysts are thought to arise from remnants of ectodermal placodes from the first, second or fourth branchial clefts. Hence they are usually lined by stratified squamous epithelium. Those lined by columnar epithelium are thought to represent pharyngeal pouch remnants. The branchial sinus and fistula may be remnants of the cervical sinus. Alternatively a sinus may result from the drainage of a cyst, either surgically, or spontaneously following infection.

Although a congenital abnormality, a branchial cyst (*Figure 16.18*) commonly presents in young adults. The theory behind this is that initially the cyst is an empty sac of embryological tissue. Over subsequent years epithelial debris accumulates and infection may occur, the cyst thus becoming more apparent. Cysts usually lie between the carotid sheath and the sternomastoid muscle, bulging into the carotid triangle from beneath the anterior border of the muscle. Typically ovoid in shape, the cyst may be as large as 5–10 cm across. It is usually painless, soft and fluctuant but infected cysts are hard

and tender with overlying inflammation. Cysts contain a yellow fluid, which on microscopy is rich in cholesterol crystals, hence they do not usually transilluminate.

Branchial fistulae (*Figure 16.19*) present at or soon after birth as a discharging orifice on the anterior aspect of the neck. The site of the orifice is much lower than that of a branchial cyst, usually lying at the anterior border of the lower part of the sternomastoid muscle. The fistulous tract passes from the skin, between the internal and external carotid arteries, superior to the hypoglossal nerve, inferior to the glossopharyngeal nerve, to open into the tonsillar fossa. Untreated, the fistula intermittently becomes infected and discharge.

A congenital branchial sinus may resemble a fistula but has only an external opening. A branchial sinus, arising from surgical or spontaneous drainage of an infected branchial cyst, however, has an external opening at a higher position in the neck than a fistula.

The thyroglossal cyst, sinus and fistula are described on p. 225 and the sublingual dermoid and ranula are described on p. 194.

Neuroendocrine tissue

Carotid body tumours (*Figure 16.20*) are chemodectomas and arise from the chemoreceptor cells of the carotid body. They form part of a group of tumours arising from glomus tissue, paraganglionomas, which include tumours of the vagus body, the glomus jugulare and phaeochromocytomas. Carotid body tumours are slow growing and, in most cases, do not invade or metastasize. They occur more often in

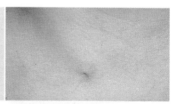

Figure 16.19.
Opening of a branchial fistula.

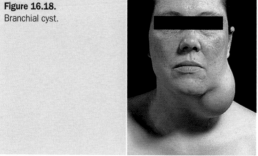

Figure 16.18.
Branchial cyst.

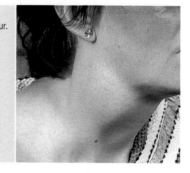

Figure 16.20.
Carotid body tumour.

people and cattle living at high altitude, where carotid body hyperplasia results from longstanding hypoxaemia. There is an autosomal dominant genetic tendency, which may account for bilateral cases.

The tumour presents as a painless lump in the neck in the 40–50 year age group. In about 10% of cases there may be localized nerve damage resulting in palsies of the seventh, ninth, tenth, eleventh or twelfth cranial nerves. On examination, the tumour is a hard, regular mass at the carotid bifurcation – the level of the hyoid bone – and exhibits a transmitted pulsation. It may be moved horizontally but has little vertical mobility. If very vascular it may be expansile.

Thoracic outlet syndromes and cervical vertebral pathology are considered on p. 366 and in Chapter 30, respectively.

17 The thyroid and parathyroids

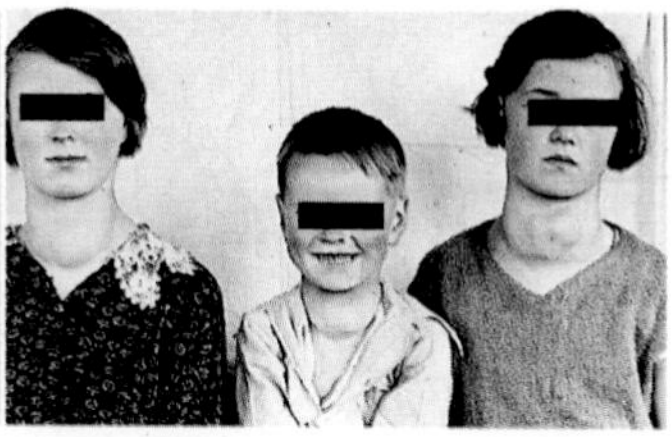

The thyroid

Goitre in the euthyroid

A goitre is an enlargement of the thyroid gland. The euthyroid patient with a goitre may notice a swelling in the lower anterior neck or may be unaware of their condition. Large goitres, compressing the trachea by more than 75%, may cause stridor. Dysphagia is usually the result of anxiety but a posterior nodule may compress the oesophagus sufficiently to cause this symptom. Pain and hoarseness usually indicate malignant involvement of the recurrent laryngeal nerve, but occasionally these symptoms result from haemorrhage into a cyst, which expands suddenly stretching the nerve, or from thyroiditis.

The isthmus of the normal gland may be visible. In the obese, inspection is facilitated by the patient pressing their occiput back on to their clasped hands. A goitre appears as a swelling in the lower anterior neck, which may be asymmetric, and rises on swallowing because of its attachment to the larynx. Palpation is traditionally performed from behind with the chin lowered to relax the musculature. A normal thyroid may be palpable in a thin individual. A goitre may be smooth or nodular. Any localized swelling arising from the gland may be re-examined and delineated from the front. Retrosternal extension is manifest either as a gland that rises out of the superior mediastinum on swallowing or as superior vena caval obstruction. Percussion over the manubrium may detect such extension but in practice is of limited value. Tracheal deviation may be noted and latent tracheal impingement is demonstrated by stridor on compression of the lateral lobes.

A **smooth euthyroid goitre** – simple goitre – is a compensatory hypertrophy of the gland in response to dietary iodine deficiency, or a congenital defect of thyroxine synthesis, goitrogens and increased physiological demand. Physiological goitres occur at puberty or pregnancy. Defects of hormone synthesis may be hereditary although this group of conditions is rare and familial goitre may be related to dietary iodine deficiency (*Figure 17.1*). **Pendred's syndrome** is the association of congenital deafness with juvenile goitre.

Multinodular goitres (*Figure 17.2*) result from a disordered thyroid metabolism, where some areas of the gland

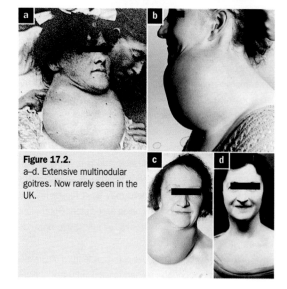

Figure 17.1.
Three siblings with deficiency goitres.

Figure 17.2.
a–d. Extensive multinodular goitres. Now rarely seen in the UK.

become hyperplastic and form nodules, which later degenerate, fibrose and calcify. Multinodular goitres either arise primarily or develop from a pre-existing smooth goitre. They are larger and are more likely to produce mechanical problems. Haemorrhage into a cyst can cause pain, sudden enlargement and tracheal compression. Malignant change occurs in 5% of cases.

Thyrotoxicosis

Thyrotoxicosis is described in the section on clinical states (p. 36). The clinical features and the causes are summarised on p. 224, *Table 17.1*.

Table 17.1. Thyrotoxicosis.

Clinical features	Causes
Weight loss	Graves' disease
Diarrhoea	Toxic nodular goitre
Irregular menstruation (amenorrhoea)	Plummer's disease (toxic adenoma)
	Iatrogenic (excessive thyroxine)
Heat intolerance	Thyroiditis
Sweating	Metastatic thyroid carcinoma
Tremor	Struma ovarii
Weakness	TSH-secreting pituitary tumour
Myopathy	Choriocarcinoma and hydatidiform mole
Palpitations; tachycardia; arrhythmias	Neonatal thyrotoxicosis
Ophthalmic signs	

Grave's disease – primary thyrotoxicosis – is manifest as a diffuse toxic goitre with ophthalmic signs. It results from hypertrophy in response to thyroid stimulating antibodies of the IgG type which are probably produced in the thyroid gland, cervical nodes or bone marrow. Associated autoimmune diseases include vitiligo, myasthenia gravis and pernicious anaemia.

The gland is hypervascular and a bruit is heard in 70% of cases. The goitre is seldom massive and is unlikely to produce pressure symptoms; it tends to arise in women in the 20–40 year age group and there may be a family history, HLA-B8 and HLA-DW3 antigens being associated. Ophthalmic signs may be due to non-infiltrative or infiltrative ophthalmopathy (p. 181).

Pre-tibial myxoedema is a less common feature of Grave's disease, where mucopolysaccharide skin infiltration gives symmetrically distributed, non-pitting plaques over the shins. Thyroid acropachy is the association of finger clubbing and osteoarthropathy.

Toxic nodular goitre – secondary thyrotoxicosis – results when thyrotoxicosis develops in a pre-existing, multinodular goitre. The condition mostly affects older females; cardiac signs are common (p. 37).

Thyroid crisis is an acute, life-threatening exacerbation of hyperthyroidism. Fortunately it is rare. It occurs in the first 24 hours after thyroidectomy when thyrotoxic patients have been inadequately prepared with antithyroid drugs. Gland manipulation during surgery results in the release of large quantities of thyroid hormones. The patient becomes distressed, restless and dyspnoeic and may have vomiting and diarrhoea. There is a tachycardia and hyperpyrexia, which my progress to delirium and coma.

Malignant goitre

A malignant goitre is more likely to be painful and may invade nerves, resulting in hoarseness in the case of the recurrent laryngeal nerve and Horner's syndrome (p. 185) in the case of the cervical sympathetic chain. The goitre is hard and enlarges rapidly, invading the surrounding tissues and losing its upward mobility on swallowing. The carotid arteries may be displaced backwards: Berry's sign.

Cervical lymphadenopathy supports the diagnosis and occasionally thyroid malignancy may present primarily as an enlarged cervical node.

Papillary carcinoma accounts for 70% of cases. Patients are more likely to be female and in their third or fourth decades. Therapeutic irradiation of the neck in childhood is associated, the latency period being up to 35 years. Lymphadenopathy is common but haematogenous spread is rare.

Follicular carcinoma accounts for only 15% of cases. Again, more females than males are affected but the age groups involved are older. Incidence is increased in endemic goitre areas, and thyroid-stimulating hormone (TSH) may have a role. Haematogenous spread to the lungs and bone is more common than lymphatic spread.

Anaplastic carcinoma (*Figure 17.3*) is most common in the elderly. It spreads locally invading the trachea and oesophagus, and commonly produces recurrent laryngeal nerve damage. The disease has a poor prognosis.

Malignant lymphoma is a rare cause of a rapidly enlarging goitre in the elderly. Many cases occur in longstanding Hashimoto's thyroiditis.

Medullary carcinoma arises from the parafollicular C cells. It accounts for 5–10% of cases and has equal sex incidence; 20% of cases are familial and occur as part of the multiple endocrine neoplasia (MEN) syndromes type II. The familial form tends to be bilateral whereas sporadic cases are unilateral. Lymphadenopathy is common – 50% at presentation. The tumour synthesizes prostaglandins, serotonin and vasoactive intestinal polypeptide, which may cause diarrhoea.

Multiple endocrine neoplasia type II takes two forms: MEN IIa is the combination of primary hyperthyroidism, phaeochromocytoma and medullary thyroid carcinoma; MEN

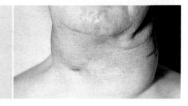

Figure 17.3. Anaplastic carcinoma of the thyroid.

IIb patients have phaeochromocytoma and medullary thyroid carcinoma but do not develop hyperparathyroidism. They may develop marfanoid features or ganglioneuromas. Ganglioneuromas of the gastrointestinal tract may result in constipation, diarrhoea or megacolon.

Rare goitres and thyroiditis

Hashimoto's thyroiditis is an autoimmune disorder resulting in the destruction of follicles with lymphoid infiltration and fibrous replacement of the gland. Antibodies to thyroglobulin and to the microsomes of thyroid acinar cells may be found but there is no evidence that they are the cause of the condition. Typically it presents with a firm goitre, which may be diffuse or localized, in a postmenopausal female. The patients are usually hypothyroid but may be euthyroid.

Reidel's thyroiditis is very rare. It takes the form of fibrous replacement of the gland, presenting as a firm goitre causing mechanical problems. Retroperitoneal fibrosis may also occur in these patients. There is an equal sex incidence.

De Quervain's thyroiditis presents with a 'flu-like' illness and a tender goitre. The patient may become hypothyroid if the condition persists but eventually returns to the euthyroid state.

Thyroid amyloidosis is a rare condition that presents as a rapidly enlarging smooth goitre.

Solitary nodules

At surgery about 50% of solitary nodules (*Figures 17.4* and *17.5*) are found to be part of a multinodular goitre. Consideration of the solitary nodule is important, however, because others represent carcinomas or adenomas. About

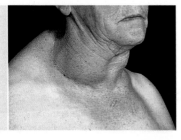

Figure 17.4.
Non-toxic solitary nodule that proved to be benign.

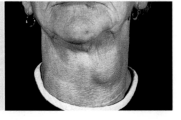

Figure 17.5.
Non-toxic solitary nodule that proved to be follicular carcinoma.

10% of solitary nodules are carcinomas but this proportion is higher in children and the elderly, and 5% of those forming part of a multinodular goitre are malignant.

The clinical assessment of a solitary nodule must therefore include a search for evidence of malignancy and determination of thyroid status. Thyrotoxicosis may suggest that the nodule is a toxic adenoma.

Hypothyroidism

Most spontaneous cases of hypothyroidism – underactive thyroid – arise as the end stage of autoimmune thyroiditis. Many of the cases encountered in surgical practice, however, are iatrogenic. Hypothyroidism can develop weeks, months or years after thyroid surgery, but the long half life of thyroxine prevents this occurring in the immediate postoperative period. Radio-iodine used to treat thyrotoxicosis results in a greater incidence. Overtreatment with antithyroid drugs – propylthiouracil and carbimazole – may also render a patient hypothyroid.

In addition to primary failure of the gland, hypothyroidism may be secondary to pituitary disorders – resulting in decreased TSH production – such as craniopharyngiomas, pituitary tumours and pituitary infarction (Sheehan's syndrome).

Neonatal hypothyroidism may result from agenesis of the thyroid or from genetic defects of thyroid hormone synthesis associated with goitres.

The clinical states resulting from hypothyroidism are myxoedema (p. 38) and cretinism (p. 38).

The thyroglossal tract

The thyroid gland develops from a cell mass arising at the base of the tongue and descends along the midline of the neck to lie anterior to the third and fourth tracheal rings. This line of descent, the thyroglossal tract, therefore extends from the foramen caecum of the tongue to the isthmus of the thyroid gland and should atrophy completely. Abnormalities of these embryological processes give rise to a number of physical signs.

Ectopic thyroid tissue arises if all or part of the developing gland fails to descend. This can lie anywhere along the tract, even at the foramen caecum of the tongue.

Thyroglossal cysts (*Figures 17.6–17.8*) result from failure of part of the tract to atrophy. Again they lie along the line of the tract: 90% in front of the hyoid, 8% below and 2% lingually. Although they are developmental abnormalities, they are not often apparent in the infant. Most present later in childhood or in early adult life. The cyst not only moves upwards on swallowing but also on protrusion of the tongue, as it is attached by the tract remnant to the foramen caecum. Thus it can be differentiated from a nodule arising from the isthmus of the thyroid.

A **thyroglossal sinus** (*Figure 17.9*) arises when a cyst becomes infected and drains spontaneously or when a cyst is incompletely excised.

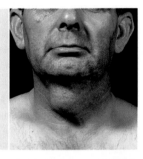

Figure 17.6.
Infrahyoid thyroglossal remnant.

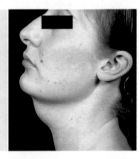

Figure 17.7.
Suprahyoid thyroglossal cyst.

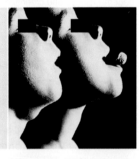

Figure 17.8.
Views of a thyroglossal cyst demonstrating elevation on protrusion of the tongue.

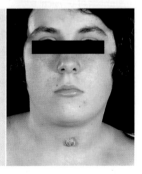

Figure 17.9.
Sinus following the incomplete removal of a thyroglossal cyst.

The parathyroids

Parathyroid disease presents as disturbed endocrine function, never as a swelling in the neck. It may take the form of hyper- or hypoparathyroidism.

Primary hyperparathyroidism results in hypercalcaemia from increased secretion of parathyroid hormone, which mobilizes calcium from bone and increases calcium uptake and phosphate loss from renal tubules. Primary overactivity can result from an adenoma (90% of cases), hyperplasia (9%) or carcinoma (1%). Hyperplasia may occur as part of the MEN IIa syndrome (p. 289). Patients may present with symptoms of hypercalcaemia or may have asymptomatic hypercalcaemia on routine serum analysis. A traditional mnemonic describes the features of hypercalcaemia as 'bones, stones, moans and abdominal groans'.

Calcium-containing renal calculi – the stones – are the commonest presenting feature. Gastrointestinal symptoms – the abdominal groans – occur from peptic ulceration as a result of hypercalcaemia-induced gastrin secretion. Acute and chronic pancreatitis are also associated. Bone disease is common histologically but is not often clinically overt. Radiological appearances resembling rickets may occur in children from the resorption of metaphyseal bone. Osteitis fibrosa cystica – brown tumours – arises from a process of subperiosteal bone resorption with patchy fibrous replace-ment. Radiologically these resemble giant cell tumours but occur in sites not typical for these, such as the mandible or skull. Mental disturbances include behavioural changes, psy-chosis and dementia. Calcification can occur in other tissues such as cartilage, resulting in pseudogout, and in the cornea as band keratopathy (*Figure 17.10*). Other features of hyper-calcaemia include hypertension and myopathy.

Differential diagnosis is from other causes of hypercalcaemia such as disseminated malignancy, myeloma, sarcoidosis, milk–alkali syndrome and excessive vitamin D ingestion.

Secondary hyperparathyroidism is a reactive hyper-plasia of the glands in response to chronic calcium-losing states such as malabsorption or chronic renal failure. Calcium levels may be normal and there is unlikely to be an identifiable clinical state.

Tertiary hyperparathyroidism arises after renal trans-plantation, when the overactivity of the parathyroids, associ-ated with chronic calcium loss, becomes autonomous.

Hypoparathyroidism usually results from surgery to the thyroid. The parathyroids may be contused, rendered ischaemic or inadvertently excised. The incidence follow-ing thyroidectomy is about 1%. Low calcium levels in the

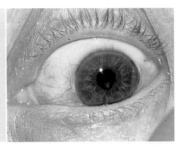

Figure 17.10.
Calcific corneal band in a patient with hypercalcaemia.

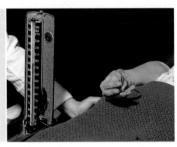

Figure 17.11.
Positive Trousseau's sign in a patient with hypercalcaemia.

immediate postoperative period are usually due to changes in calcium distribution and do not represent hypoparathyroidism, which may be latent for years until there is an increased calcium demand such as in pregnancy or lactation. Hypocalcaemia results in paraesthesia of the face, fingers or toes and in abdominal cramps. Carpopedal spasm – tetany – may result; latent tetany may be detected by:

- Chvostek's sign – facial muscle contraction in response to tapping with a tendon hammer over the facial nerve as it emerges in front of the auditory meatus.
- Trousseau's sign (*Figure 17.11*) – carpal spasm induced by arterial occlusion of the forearm with a sphygmomanometer cuff at 200 mmHg for 5 minutes. The fingers are noted to be extended at the interphalangeal joints and flexed at the metacarpophalangeal joints, the thumb being strongly adducted.

18 Breast and axilla

Introduction

Breast problems make up to 20% of the workload of a surgical outpatient department in the UK. Patients, mostly female, commonly present complaining of a lump in the breast, pain or nipple discharge. Although the commonest cause of symptoms is benign breast disease, carcinoma of the breast is one of the commonest cancers affecting women. In many countries, increasing numbers of women now undergo screening for malignant breast disease and require further management of their asymptomatic breast disease.

Anatomy

The mammary glands are modified sweat glands and arise form a cord of tissue that runs from the axilla to the groin on each side. The glands develop *in utero* as a rudimentary duct system and may become prominent due to high levels of maternal hormones. Although some development of the duct system occurs in childhood, the main growth and development of the breast in the female takes place at puberty. After development of large numbers of acini and the deposition of fat, the breast has a variable and usually asymmetric size and shape. It normally overlies the second to sixth ribs, on each side extending down from the axilla along the anterior axillary line and across to near the midline with its tail passing into the axilla.

Further development of the female breast occurs at pregnancy when hormonal changes cause enlargement and development of the duct and acinar systems to allow lactation, and the nipples become darker and the Montgomery tubercles enlarged. After pregnancy, the breast reduces in size but the areolar changes remain. After the menopause the breast usually further reduces in size and becomes less protuberant as the interlobular fibrous tissue atrophies and the glandular epithelium involutes.

The male breast does not normally develop past the childhood stage although slight temporary enlargement may occur at puberty.

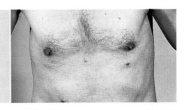

Figure 18.1.
Accessory nipples.

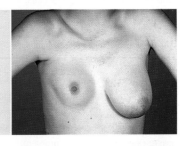

Figure 18.2.
Hypoplasia of the right breast.

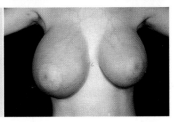

Figure 18.3.
Mammary hyperplasia in a 13-year-old child.

Anomalies

Occasionally one or both breasts fail to develop giving rise to amastia (amazia). It is also possible for accessory breasts to develop in both men and women, which may be rudimentary or complete, usually occurring along the milk line (*Figure 18.1*) from the axilla to the groin. Truly symmetrical breasts are rare. Most women have breasts that are slightly different in both size and shape and occasionally these differences are significant enough to be obvious (*Figures 18.2* and *18.3*).

Pathophysiology

The breast is a specialized organ of the skin and is subject to any condition that affects the skin and subcutaneous tissues, such as basal cell and squamous cell carcinomas, melanomas, lipomata and haemangiomata. The development and activity of the breast are under the control of the hypothalamus and pituitary via hormones produced by the pituitary and ovaries during growth and development, normal menstrual cyclical activity, pregnancy and in response to suckling. Any imbalance in the levels of the circulating hormones may lead to increased secretory or proliferative activity within the breast and therefore to an alteration of function, symptoms and to changes in appearance. As the acinar and ductal cells undergo proliferation during development and reproductive activity, it is not surprising that the regulation of this process may become deranged and lead to neoplastic growth of both the acinar and ductal cells.

History

The duration, variation in size and associated pain or discomfort of a breast lump, or breast thickening or enlargement, should be noted. The rate of enlargement of malignant lumps is usually progressive and not related to the menstrual cycle. Conversely, benign lumps often arise and disappear rapidly and repeatedly if they are cysts, and benign breast problems are often cyclical. Pain without a lump is a recognized presenting symptom of carcinoma of the breast and, characteristically, the pain is fairly well localized and constant, in contrast to the cyclical diffuse discomfort of benign breast disease. Pain, however, may be referred from the chest wall and thoracic organs to the breast.

Nipple discharge may be from one or more ducts. Bloody nipple discharge usually indicates a benign or malignant neoplasm of the duct system. Bright red blood is characteristic of a duct papilloma. Green, yellow or sometimes a clear discharge occurs in benign breast disease. Pus may arise from a breast abscess. Milk can appear in pregnancy or secondary to a pituitary prolactinoma.

Other features of note in the history include previous history of breast disease, its course and management, the menstrual history, including the age of menarche and menopause, and the obstetric history, especially pertaining to breast feeding and its complications. A drug history should be obtained with special regard to oral or parenteral contraceptives and hormone replacement therapy. A family history is important as there is an increased incidence of carcinoma of the breast in first degree relatives of those with carcinoma of the breast. Family history of carcinoma and carcinoma of the colon is also associated with breast cancer.

Examination

Seclusion, warmth and privacy are particularly important in examination of the breast, to avoid discomfort and embarrassment to the – usually and understandably – very anxious patient. Good lighting is essential to detect minor abnormalities. The patient should be asked to undress to the waist and initially be sitting comfortably upright.

The first stage is **inspection**. The size and shape of the breasts are noted. There is marked variation in the appearance of women's breasts and the size of an individual woman's breast may change during development, the normal menstrual cycle, pregnancy, lactation and ageing. Breasts are rarely symmetrical but any recent changes in symmetry should be ascertained and noted. The nipple usually points forward, more noticeably so when erect. Unilateral or bilateral nipple retraction (*Figure 18.4*) may be congenital or occur during development but recent change may be a manifestation of underlying disease. The nipple darkens with age and during pregnancy. Discharge or eczema of the nipple is noted and compared with the other side.

Lumps that are large in comparison to the size of the breast or situated near the surface of the breast may be evident on first inspection (*Figure 18.5*). Further abnormalities may be evident if the arms are moved. The patient is first

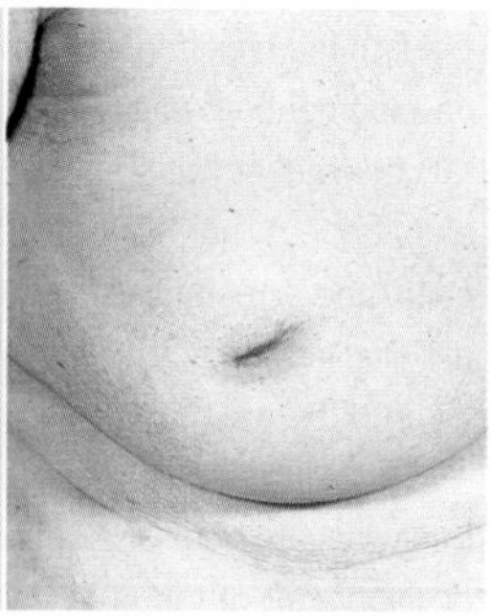

Figure 18.4.
Nipple retraction due to underlying breast neoplasia.

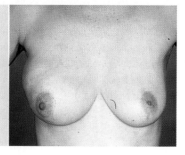

Figure 18.5.
Benign fibroadenoma of right breast.

asked to lift their arms above their head (*Figures 18.6 and 18.7*) and then – when inspection in this position is complete – the arms are brought down to the hips and the patient presses her hands into her hips to contract the pectoral group of muscles (*Figure 18.8*). Abnormalities in large pendulous breasts may become more evident if the patient leans forward so that the breasts fall away from the body. During these movements the breast is inspected, with special note made of any differences in the freedom of movement. Pathology may be revealed by the presence of any redness, oedema, *peau d'orange*, ulceration, skin nodularity and abnormal venous patterns (*Figure 18.9*).

Redness and erythema may arise from inflammatory or neoplastic diseases of the underlying breast. *Peau d'orange* (*Figure 18.10*) – French for orange peel – is a characteristic appearance of underlying neoplastic disease: infiltration of the lymphatic drainage of the breast gives rise to cutaneous oedema; the appearance of the tiny pits of orange peel is produced by deep tethering of the sweat glands. Nodularity of the skin may arise from neoplastic infiltration; ulceration (*Figure 18.11*) is a late change where the underlying neoplasm give rises to necrosis of the overlying skin.

A few veins are normally visible on the skin of the normal breast and these venous patterns enlarge and become more apparent during pregnancy. Arising outside pregnancy they may be a manifestation of underlying malignancy. Neoplasms may interfere with the supporting fibrous architecture of the breast and give rise to skin dimpling or puckering and retraction or deviation of the nipple. Eczema of the nipple and areola

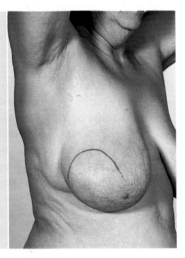

Figure 18.6.
Carcinoma of right breast on elevation to test for cutaneous and deep fixity.

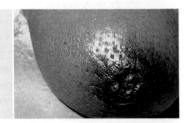

Figure 18.9.
Mondor's disease. The superficial phlebitis is self-limiting, the pain subsiding within a few weeks. The condition does not signify any underlying malignancy nor have the sinister links with malignancy that superficial phlebitis carries at other sites.

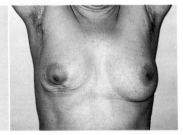

Figure 18.7.
Arm elevation showing skin puckering from an underlying neoplasm.

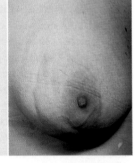

Figure 18.10.
Peau d'orange.

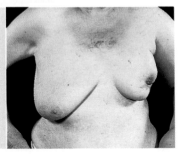

Figure 18.8.
Hands pressing down on hips tenses the pictoralis major muscle and demonstrates fixity of the overlying left breast cancer.

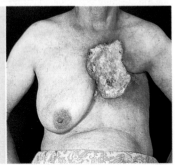

Figure 18.11.
Extensive, neglected, malignant ulcer replacing the left breast.

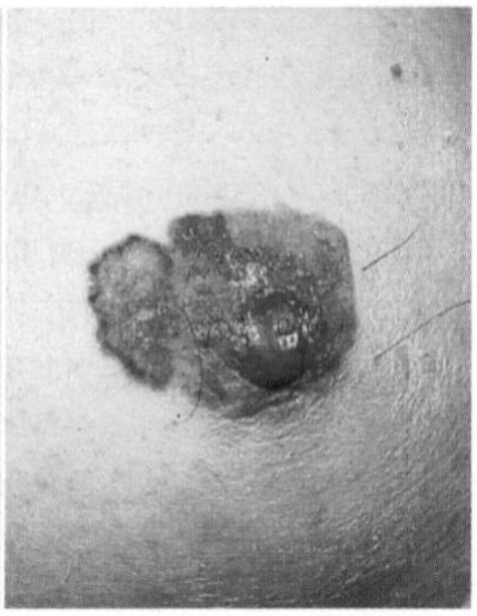

Figure 18.12.
Paget's disease of the nipple.

may be due to dermatitis or eczema but when it is unilateral, may be due to neoplastic spread through the duct system to the nipple – this is known as Paget's disease of the breast (*Figure 18.12*). During early lactation the nipple is prone to inflammation, cracking and infection.

In **palpation** it is usual to examine the normal breast first. The patient is asked to lie flat and then to put the hand of the side to be examined behind her head and then roll slightly to the opposite side, so that the breast lies flat on the chest wall and becomes more easily palpable. The breast is palpated with the flat of the hand quadrant by quadrant, including beneath the nipple, finally examining the axillary tail. Any lump in the breast is noted and examined for site, size, shape, consistency, fluctuation, tenderness, characteristics of the overlying skin, fixity of the lump to the skin and to the underlying chest wall, and the attendant lymphatic drainage.

The fixity of a breast mass to the pectoral muscles is determined by palpating the mass while the patient contracts her pectoral muscles, by asking her to push her hand into her hip (*Figure 18.8*). The fixity of a breast mass to the serratus anterior is determined by palpating the mass while the patient contracts her serratus anterior, by asking her to push her hand forwards into your shoulder. Skin fixation has serious prognostic implications. It is carefully looked for by gently squeezing the overlying skin to demonstrate mobility or puckering. The presence of fixity to the skin of retroareolar lumps is of less concern as even benign masses demonstrate this property due to the proximity of many ducts leading to the nipple.

Where the presenting complaint is mastalgia, ask the patient to show where the pain originates from and then to gently palpate this area to elicit tenderness of the underlying pectoral muscles, ribs and costal cartilages, as all of these structures can give rise to inflammation leading to mastalgia.

Examination of the nipple and retroareolar areas is essential. The nipple is palpated between the thumb and

fingers for tissue nodularity. If there is a history of nipple discharge, an attempt should be made to produce this discharge by firm palpation of the retroareolar area and then each quadrant of the breast. The patient may be able to express the discharge themselves. In each case palpation should proceed in a systematic fashion – such as a 'round the clock' pattern – so as to identify the individual duct(s) responsible for the discharge. The location and number of ducts which produce the discharge should be noted as well as the character of the discharge.

If the breasts are very large or pendulous it may be impossible to examine adequately the breast against the chest wall. It may therefore be necessary to use bimanual palpation to increase the ability to palpate the entire mass of breast tissue. This is facilitated by asking the patient to lean slightly forward so the breasts hang away from the chest wall. Where the breasts are very large and adequate examination is not possible, mammography should be undertaken.

Examination of the lymphatic drainage of the breast should never be omitted; this usually starts with the axillae. If the patient's left axilla is to be examined, the left arm is taken and supported by the left hand of the examiner, so that the muscles of the shoulder girdle are relaxed to allow easy access to the axilla. The examiner's right hand palpates the anterior part of the axilla and the nodes between the pectoral muscles. The hand is then introduced gently into the apex of the axilla to palpate the apical group of lymph nodes and passed down to palpate the medial group before the posterior group, around the serratus anterior and latissimus dorsi, and the lateral group, around the neck and shaft of the humerus. The posterior and lateral groups can more easily be felt from behind. The presence of axillary lymph nodes is normal but they are usually quite small and either impalpable or barely so. The size, number, consistency and mobility of the nodes must be fully documented. Obstruction of the axillary lymphatics – for instance from neoplastic invasion or damage secondary to radiation – gives rise to oedema of the arm.

The right axilla is examined in a similar fashion except that the arm is supported by the right hand and examined with the left hand. Other groups of nodes that must be examined are the supraclavicular and the infraclavicular nodes found in the infraclavicular and supraclavicular fossae. Note particularly the presence and characteristics of the scalene node, behind the insertion of the sternocleidomastoid. The other lymphatic organ examined is the liver, a common site for metastatic disease; other sites for such disease include the lungs and pleura, giving rise to pleural effusions, and the skeleton, most notably the spine, giving rise to tenderness and pathological fractures.

Malignant disease of the breast

Breast cancer vies with lung cancer as the commonest type of cancer in women in the western world today. The incidence is in the order of 5–15% of women, 1–2% are synchronous and after developing one cancer, women are five times more likely to develop another (*Figure 18.13*). It is 50 times more common in women than in men.

Hormonal activity or sensitivity are likely aetiological factors because of the associations with female sex, nulliparity, early menarche, late menopause and late age of first birth. There are also links with high social class, smoking and obesity which may be interrelated. There is a strong genetic component as the risk is significantly greater in those whose first degree relatives have been affected, especially in premenopausal disease.

The size of a breast tumour at diagnosis and treatment is inversely proportional to survival, so attention has been directed at the earlier detection of tumours by self examination and screening programmes using mammography and/or clinical examination. However, breast cancer still presents with metastatic disease, and the presence of micrometastases at the time of early diagnosis has been demonstrated. The prognosis at diagnosis is also determined by the presence of involved lymph nodes; the involvement of four or more nodes confers a decrease in survival of 20–30%. Invasion of local structures – e.g. the skin and chest wall – also carries a poor prognosis. Most of this information can be drawn by eliciting the relevant clinical signs, although where possible it should be confirmed by imaging techniques and the histological examination of diseased, or potentially diseased, tissue. As well as answering important questions of prognosis, these factors have considerable bearing on the management of the disease.

Malignant breast lumps tend to enlarge progressively and have a more insidious onset. There is less variation of symptoms with the course of the menstrual cycle. Pain is a relatively common symptom of malignant disease and is usually deep-set and constant; it may not occur in relation to a lump. Nipple discharge if present is usually serous or serosanguineous. The location of the duct or ducts from which the discharge issues is related to the location of the tumour. Eczema or Paget's disease of the nipple (*Figure 18.12*) – which is caused by infiltration of the nipple with Paget or foam cells from an underlying tumour – is another manifestation of malignant disease. Skin changes may be present from previous radiotherapy (*Figure 18.14*).

Like many neoplasms, the prognosis and further behaviour of the disease, and therefore its further management, can in part be predicted by the extent to which the disease has already progressed at the time of diagnosis. This is known as the stage of the disease. Although further investigations – and in some cases the operative and pathological findings – may allow more accurate staging of the disease, some idea of the stage may be evident from the clinical examination. Two staging methods are in common use, the simpler International Classification and the more precise but complex TNM system, where the T refers to the tumour, N to the regional lymph nodes and M to the metastases.

International Classification

I A lump or Paget's disease demonstrating no fixity to skin or chest wall, no lymph node involvement and no distant metastasis.

II Where there is ipsilateral axillary mobile lymphadenopathy, nipple retraction or skin tethering.

III Where there is extensive skin tethering (including *peau d'orange*), fixity to the chest wall, skin ulceration or fixed ipsilateral lymph nodes.

IV The presence of distant metastases (liver; bone; lung; pleura; skin), contralateral or supraclavicular lymphadenopathy or a lump in the other breast.

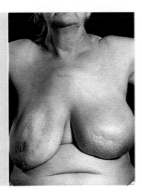

Figure 18.13.
Bilateral carcinoma of the breast with external protrusion from secondary bone deposits.

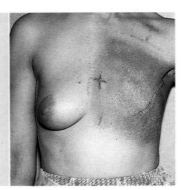

Figure 18.14.
Secondary cutaneous changes following radiotherapy to the left breast.

TNM classification

T1   Less than 2 cm – or Paget's disease – with no fixation or nipple retraction.

T2   2–5 cm, or less than 2 cm with skin tethering or nipple retraction.

T3   5–10 cm, or less than 5 cm with infiltration or ulceration of the skin or *peau d'orange* over tumour or fixation to muscle.

T4   Larger than 10 cm, infiltration, ulceration or *peau d'orange* wide of tumour or chest wall fixation.

N0   No palpable lymph nodes.

N1   Axillary lymph nodes palpable but mobile.

N2   Axillary lymph nodes fixed (to each other or related structures).

N3   Supraclavicular lymph nodes – either fixed or unfixed – or arm oedema.

M0   No evidence of distant metastasis.

M1   Distant metastasis (including liver, bone, skin, lung, plura, brain), contralateral breast or lymph node involvement.

Sarcoma

The commonest sarcoma is the cystosarcoma phyllodes tumour (Brodie's disease; *Figure 18.15*). These often large, rapidly growing masses account for approximately 1% of breast tumours. They occur in slightly older women than carcinoma and present as a progressive enlargement of either a lump or the whole breast; they are often painful. They characteristically have an uneven consistency and a bosselated surface. The breast may be tense and firm with thin skin and enlarged veins. Occasionally the skin becomes ulcerated over the tumour, the healthy, sensitive, skin edges appearing punched out and the base of the ulcer revealing the tumour,

which may present as a fungating mass. Usually it is not fixed to skin or deep structures and there is rarely spread to lymph nodes or distant metastasis. The tumour is thought to arise in a large fibroadenoma that undergoes cystic degeneration and sarcomatous change.

Other types of sarcoma that occasionally arise in the breast include fibrosarcomas, leiomyomasarcomas, and rhabdomyosarcomas.

Nipple discharge

Discharges may be evident on the clothing or on palpation of the breast. The properties of the discharge may point to the underlying diagnosis but in every case careful examination of the breasts, together with further investigations including cytological examination of the discharge, are required.

The types of discharge are as follows:

- Bright red blood – The most frequent cause is a benign duct papilloma. Other causes include a duct carcinoma and, rarely, carcinoma in a lactating breast. The diagnosis therefore depends on the further examination of the breast and of cytological examination of the fluid. Papillomas and cysts may also present as a painless nipple swelling (*Figure 18.16*).
- Dark, altered blood – This can occur as a result of a papilloma obstructing a duct so that the discharge of blood is delayed.
- Slightly bloodstained fluid – Together with the presence of a sizeable cystic swelling, this discharge strongly suggests an intracystic papilliferous carcinoma (rare: Disease of Reclus).
- Clear, yellow, serous fluid – With a lumpy breast, this discharge is often due to benign breast disease with retention cysts but can occur in women taking the oral contraceptive pill.
- Thick, green discharge – Duct ectasia is the common cause of this discharge. In this condition the ductal tissue is hyperproliferative producing a cellular discharge. Duct ectasia is associated with nipple retraction and an increased incidence of developing carcinoma.
- Milky discharge (*Figure 18.17*) – Usually due to insufficient suppression of lactation after weaning but may rarely be the manifestation of a secreting prolactinoma of the pituitary gland.

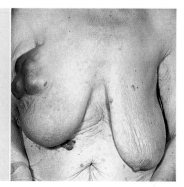

Figure 18.15.
Brodie's cystosarcoma phyllodes of the right breast.

Figure 18.16.
Benign cystic lesion
of the nipple.

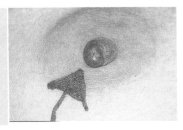

Figure 18.17.
Galactorrhoea in a
patient with a
prolactinoma.

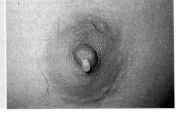

Nipple retraction

Nipple retraction may be congenital where the nipple may evert at any time as the breast develops or changes, at times such as pregnancy, or when the breast undergoes involution. Not only may the appearance of nipple retraction cause women to request correction but it tends to make breast feeding difficult and leads to increased incidence of infective complications. The causes of acquired nipple retraction are duct ectasia and periductal mastitis, previous surgery and biopsy, infections notably tuberculosis, and most importantly malignancy. Where the symptom occurs then careful examination and radiological and cytological investigation must be undertaken to rule out any serious underlying condition.

Benign breast disease

Benign breast disease is a very common condition, especially in women of age 20–40 years. The incidence falls after the menopause, in contrast to malignant breast disease. Over the years it has had a variety of synonyms such as fibroadenosis, chronic mastitis, fibrocystic disease, cystic or benign mammary dysplasia, cystic mastopathy and benign breast condition. One of the newer terms – aberration of normal growth and development – is more general and descriptive of the current proposed aetiology of the condition. This aetiology is poorly understood but is likely to involve the action of cyclical circulating hormone levels on breast tissue. The breast is functioning optimally when lactating but at other

times breast tissue is subject to cyclical changes in the hormonal environment, influenced by the menstrual cycle, pregnancy, oral contraceptives, hormone replacement therapy and probably factors such as diet and smoking. The exaggeration of normal physiological responses may give rise to overgrowth or over-activity of one or more of the lobular, duct or fibrous tissue elements of the gland. Just as normal cyclical changes may give rise to discomfort, these exaggerated changes may give rise to pain, known as cyclical mastalgia, a common condition in younger women. This condition needs extensive investigation to exclude a carcinoma although, in the majority of cases, no abnormality is found.

Microscopic changes include adenosis, cyst formation, papillomatosis, epithelial hyperplasia, fibrosis and lymphatic infiltration. These in turn may be accompanied by pain, tenderness, nodularity and occasionally larger cyst formation. The symptoms tend to occur over a large time span and may change. A common characteristic of these symptoms from benign conditions is that they change during the patient's normal menstrual cycle. Changes in the woman's perception of the characteristics of her breast tissue not surprisingly give rise to alarm and lead her to seek medical advice. As the characteristics of breast tissue vary from woman to woman and progressively and cyclically with time, the woman herself is often the best judge of any significant change.

Often there is a change in the nodularity of the breast tissue which can be diffuse or focal, unilateral or bilateral. When diffuse, the whole of a large proportion of the breast(s) may change considerably in their consistency and the whole breast may feel replaced by a mass. When focal, it can be perceived as a discrete breast lump. The commonest site for lumps or changes in nodularity is the upper outer quadrant and axillary tail (*Figure 18.18*). Lumps can be single or multiple and characteristically are sudden in onset, enlarge rapidly and are tender. They can also regress spontaneously and are subject to variation with the menstrual cycle, usually being larger and more tender premenstrually. The changes in the secretory activity of the breast tissue commonly give rise to a

Figure 18.18.
Large benign lesion
of the upper outer
quadrant of the right
breast.

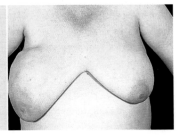

cyst; such cysts may be single or multiple and vary from barely palpable to very large. Defined cysts are usually smooth, round and of variable consistency; they are not tethered to deep structures or skin. Fluctuation of the lump can be elicited if the lump is relatively superficial and is often best elicited from behind. Very tense cysts feel hard and are not fluctuant.

The distinction between a benign lump or cyst and that caused by a malignancy is not always easy to make; it is usual to apply further diagnostic tests to obtain a definitive diagnosis. One of the easiest methods of doing this in the outpatient setting is to attempt to aspirate a suspected cyst with a needle and syringe. The fluid obtained from a benign cyst is typically turbid yellow-green but may be clear, white, brown or black and should contain no blood. The aspirate can be sent for cytological examination to exclude the presence of malignant cells as can the cellular material obtained from lesions that prove to be solid lumps. Following successful aspiration, there should be no residual mass and the breast should be re-examined several weeks later to ensure it has not reaccumulated.

Fibroadenoma of the breast

These common benign breast lumps – usually occurring in women under the age of 30 – are not strictly speaking neoplasms as they do not arise from a single cell and are classified as aberrations of development; they are commoner in black women. They are hormonally dependant and therefore commonly arise after puberty, in young adulthood or pregnancy and undergo involution around the menopause.

Fibroadenomata are characteristically small firm or hard lumps, usually spherical or ovoid, possibly with an undulating surface, usually very mobile and may disappear from between the fingers on palpation (hence the term 'breast mouse'). They are commonly multiple and bilateral. Fibroadenomata may be mistaken for a carcinoma and are biopsied or removed to exclude this diagnosis. Occasionally they may become very large, usually arising in adolescence and are then known as giant fibromata if exceeding 5 cm in diameter. These are common in Africa and may contain areas of atypical epithelial hyperplasia which nonetheless are managed in the same way as ordinary fibromata. Removal may involve considerable destruction of breast tissue leading to marked asymmetry. Very occasionally (approximately. 1 in 1000) a carcinoma may arise in a fibroadenoma but where this is confined to the fibroadenoma the prognosis is excellent.

Fibromatosis

Fibromatosis – a benign proliferation of myofibroblasts – can occur in the breast and is similar to desmoid tumours – extraperitoneal fibromatosis. It is managed by wide local excision and frequently recurs.

Fat necrosis

This usually occurs as a painless lump in the breast, arising as a result of trauma to the breast though, in many cases, no instance of trauma can be recalled. It is usually indistinguishable from early carcinoma and therefore further investigations or excision should be undertaken to exclude a carcinoma.

Galactocele

These usually arise in a lactating or recently lactating breast, usually resulting from a blockage in the duct system causing a build up of milk from the proximal branches of the lactiferous tubules. In cases of pituitary prolactinomas, which secrete prolactin, galactocele formation may be the only symptom. A cystic swelling is identified without evidence of any infection. Aspiration yields milk and the mass should disappear.

Acute inflammation of the breast

In addition to eczema of the nipple, the inflammation arising from ulcerating carcinomas and Paget's disease of the breast, inflammation of the breast can be due to infection or trauma. In infants, both male and female, mastitis may arise due to the stimulation of the neonatal breast tissue by maternal hormones. The infant breast secretes a milk-like substance. Occasionally this leads to retrograde infection of the breast tissue that usually resolves spontaneously. A similar condition may occur at puberty. Certain viral infections – e.g. mumps – can lead to a mastitis.

Most infections of the breast follow trauma, the commonest cause of which is breast feeding. The nipple can become cracked and painful and local infection commences around the crack. The infection can lead to cellulitis, around the crack, and from there a deep-seated infection and then abscess formation may occur.

Breast abscesses (*Figure 18.19*) present with a history of recent trauma and painful swelling that starts as a dull ache and develops into a throbbing pain. Where the infection is widespread or severe, systemic effects of infection such as malaise, anorexia, pyrexia and sweating may occur. There is usually oedema and erythema around the swelling and cracking or cellulitis may be present at the nipple. There may be demonstrable fluctuation if the abscess is not too painful or too tense. Although aspiration demonstrates the presence of pus, further management usually requires surgical drainage. When the history is prolonged, the tenderness is not marked and there is generalized induration and mastitis carcinomatosa; a rapidly advancing carcinoma should be excluded.

Where an abscess discharges spontaneously near the nipple, where the adjacent ducts are large, the resulting tract may epithelialize to form a mammary fistula (*Figure 18.20*) which discharges clear or occasionally bloodstained fluid from an opening near the nipple

Infections can also occur in the glands of Montgomery, giving rise to subareolar mastitis (*Figure 18.21*). Blocked glands of Montgomery give rise to periareolar lumps usually full of inspissated secretions.

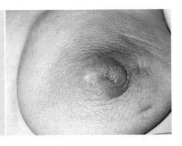

Figure 18.19.
Oedema and inflammation of the right breast from an underlying abscess.

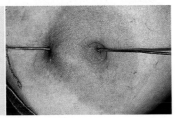

Figure 18.20.
Mammary fistula.

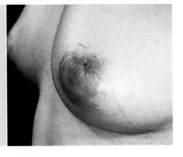

Figure 18.21.
Periductal mastitis.

Other common causes of trauma to the breast arise as a result of abrasion, usually during exercise in the previously unexercised where stiff abrasive clothing is worn ('jogger's nipple' or traumatic mastitis).

Chronic inflammation of the breast

Chronic inflammation may arise as a result of inadequately treated acute infections. Where they are common, chronic infective agents such as tuberculosis or actinomycosis can give rise to chronic breast abscesses, presenting as a mass or sinus with a purulent discharge. In tuberculosis there may be regional lymph node involvement as well as a primary focus in the lung, gut or other organ. Chronic intramammary abscesses present as breast lumps, usually with skin induration, *peau d'orange* and even skin tethering, and may be clinically indistinguishable from carcinoma.

Chronic submammary abscesses are associated with nipple retraction and are recurrent if the nipple remains retracted. When an abscess involving the duct system, with or without duct ectasia or nipple retraction, a mammary fistula may result. This presents as recurrent abscess and purulent discharge and usually persists until surgical excision.

Syphilis of the breast is now rare and used to be contracted from nursing an infected child or kissing by an infected person and gave rise to a primary chancre and then numerous ulcers all centred around the nipple. Occasionally – in tertiary syphilis – gummata can arise in the breast tissue itself.

Breast augmentation

Women may be dissatisfied with the appearance of their breasts and seek surgical improvement in order to change the shape, or enlarge or diminish the size of their breasts. Previously this was attempted by the injection of paraffin liquid or liquid silicon into the submammary space. These injections can lead to a chronic inflammatory response that may be mistaken for a carcinoma years later. Migration of the material may lead to further confusion. Nowadays the augmentation is effected by the placement of silicone gel enclosed in a silastic bag placed in the submammary space, but this bag can also provoke an inflammatory response leading to it being enclosed in a hard or tense capsule. A breast that has an implant can be examined in the normal fashion and can also be subjected to radiological investigation in the usual fashion. Needle aspiration has the added risk of perforation of the silastic envelope. Recently there has been much alarm over the possibility that these silicone implants may give rise to a connective tissue disorder, giving rise to a number of systemic symptoms. At the present time no definite link has been proven.

Breast screening programmes

Although a careful history and examination form the cornerstone of the management of symptomatic breast disease, the fact that many cancers are thought to metastasize before they either cause symptoms or are palpable on routine or self-examination, the efficacy of radiological screening has been evaluated. In a number of studies in Scandinavia, USA and the UK, the ability of mammography to detect significant numbers of asymptomatic carcinomas has been demonstrated, although benefit in terms of increased life expectancy has not always been demonstrated. Despite the use of guided cytological sampling and examination of equivocal mammographic lesions, it is not uncommon for many potentially harmless lesions to be removed surgically after wire localization. Of further interest is the fact that many palpable lesions are first detected by mammography.

The male breast

Although rudimentary, the male breast occasionally becomes the source of disease. Mastitis may arise in the male infant and the pubertal male as it does in the female. Trauma from abrasion may occur as may infections such as mumps, all causing painful breasts.

Breast lumps may arise in the male breast and are caused by the same pathological processes as in the female. Carcinoma of the male breast (*Figure 18.22*) – although much

less common at 1% of all breast carcinoma – presents at a much later stage due to the small size of the male breast relative to the tumour, but is readily palpated for the same reason.

Gynaecomastia (*Figure 18.23*) – enlargement of the male breast – is the commonest complaint arising from the male breast. It is usually due to elevated levels of oestrogen or oestrogen-like compounds. It is also commoner in Klinefelter's syndrome, a chromosomal abnormality with the genotype XXY.

The causes are:

- Physiological – Neonatal, due to circulating maternal and placental hormones; puberty, which may be uni- or bilateral and usually resolves spontaneously; and old age.
- Hypogonadism – As a result of gonadotrophin insufficiency, decreased Leydig cell function, or androgen resistance.
- Tumours –Producing sex hormones such as testicular tumours, adrenal tumours and others producing ectopic hormones such as bronchogenic carcinoma.
- Hepatic – The liver is the site of oestrogen breakdown; in hepatic dysfunction of any cause, elevated levels of circulating oestrogen may lead to breast enlargement.
- Hyperthyroidism – As a result of excessive sex hormone binding globulin and increased sex hormone production.
- Iatrogenic – Through the administration of oestrogens or oestrogen-like compounds such as stilboestrol, for prostatic carcinoma, or steroids. Cimetidine affects the hepatic metabolism of oestrogens; neurotransmitter agonists such as methyldopa, phenothiazines, and tricyclic anti-depressants cause gynaecomastia probably by affecting prolactin secretion. Other drugs include spironolactone and digitalis.

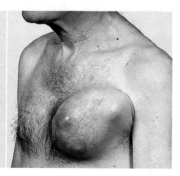

Figure 18.22. Carcinoma of the male breast.

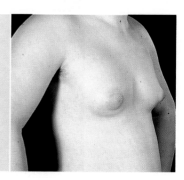

Figure 18.23. Gynaecomastia.

19 The thorax (including the oesophagus)

Examination of the respiratory system and the thorax

General examination

The presence of shortness of breath, cyanosis, clubbing and cough must always be determined when examining the respiratory system. If the patient is short of breath particular attention must be paid to the respiratory rate, depth, regularity, the use of accessory muscles, stridor and the presence or absence of a wheeze.

Laryngeal or tracheal obstruction

Stridor is a harsh noise produced as inspiratory and expiratory air passes through a partially obstructed main airway. Dyspnoea, cyanosis and restlessness are observed as a result of fighting for breath and are cardinal signs of obstruction of the major air passage. The larynx moves forcibly up and down with respiration and, particularly in adults, the accessory muscles of respiration are used with each inspiratory effort. Simultaneously, the distended jugular veins become empty and indrawn, refilling when inspiration is replaced with expiration. This is indicative of the pronounced negative intrathoracic pressure brought about by the increased inspiratory drive. On examining the thorax, the lower end of the sternum together with the adjacent rib interspaces, the supraclavicular fossae and epigastrium, are drawn-in during inspiration. This is especially noticeable in thin adults and young children.

If the patient has a **productive cough** the sputum should be examined:

- Mucoid sputum suggests acute or chronic bronchitis.
- White or pink and frothy sputum suggests pulmonary oedema.
- Yellow or green sputum suggests bacterial infection or eosinophilic sputum in asthma.
- Rust-coloured sputum suggests pneumococcal pneumonia.
- Blood-stained sputum suggests tumour, pulmonary embolus, tuberculosis (TB) or infection.

Clubbing

The causes of clubbing (p. 7; *Figure 1.14*) in the respiratory system include bronchial carcinoma, chronic suppurative lung disease, bronchiectasis, lung abscess, empyema, pulmonary fibrosis, and pleural and mediastinal tumours.

Examination of the chest

This should be examined with the patient laying at 45° and then sitting upright so that the front and back of the chest may be viewed.

Inspection

The symmetry and shape of the chest should be inspected together with any thoracic spinal curvature.

An exaggerated anteroposterior curvature of the spine is known as a **kyphosis** and a lateral curvature as a **scoliosis**. Sternal depression is known as **pectus excavatum** and a protuberant sternum as **pectus carinatum**.

The symmetry and extent of the movements of the chest on deep inspiration and expiration should be determined. In the absence of any spinal deformity, diminished movement on one side usually indicates disease on that side. The adequacy of chest movements can be tested by measuring (by tape measure) the inspiratory to expiratory difference of chest circumference at nipple level, which is normally greater than 5 cm.

Rib counting

It is often necessary to know which rib is injured or diseased. Running the finger downwards from the suprasternal notch, a transverse ridge can be felt and often seen – the angle of Louis (or sternal angle). The finger, moved to the side along this ridge, passes directly on to the second rib. Ribs are counted from this point.

Note abnormal dilated veins on the chest wall and the presence of any operation scars.

Centralization of the trachea is checked by noting the position of the trachea relative to the tip of a finger placed in the suprasternal notch. The trachea may be displaced by tumours in the neck or upper mediastinum, or by a shift of the mediastinum due to lung collapse, massive pleural effusion or a pneumothorax.

Such findings may be confirmed by examining the movements of the two sides of the chest and the position of the apex beat.

Compare the **tactile vocal fremitus** on the two sides of the chest at two or three levels by placing the hand lightly on the chest and asking the patient to repeat a resonant word (e.g. 99). It is increased over consolidated lung and diminished when air, liquid or if a thickened pleura separates the lung from the chest wall, or when a major bronchus is obstructed.

Percussion

The chest is percussed at four or five different levels comparing one side with the other. The note elicited on percussion is determined by the thickness of the chest wall, by the aeration of the lungs and by any structures intervening between the lung and the chest wall. The lower limits of pulmonary resonance on each side are determined. On the right side, lung resonance gives way to liver dullness and on the left side, lung resonance gives way to tympany of the stomach and large bowel. Over normal lung it is resonant; over liquid or solid (e.g. pneumonic consolidation) it is dull; over gas under tension (e.g. pneumothorax) it is tympanitic.

Auscultation

The **breath sounds** on the two sides of the chest at three or four levels are compared. The sound generated by air passing through the large airways during breathing is modified by conduction through the normal lung and chest wall, thus the sound heard over the thorax is softer and less harsh than that heard over the larynx. In health, the inspiratory noise is heard clearly throughout inspiration whereas the expiratory noise is quieter, less harsh and usually only heard for the first half or two-thirds of expiration. Such normal sounds are known as **vesicular breath sounds**.

The breath sounds are **diminished** when thickened pleura, air or liquid separates the lung from the chest wall and in muscular or obese individuals. They are also diminished when the respiratory flow rate is considerably reduced (e.g. in severe asthma) and occasionally when there is bronchial obstruction.

When the sound heard over the thorax is similar to the sound heard over the larynx – i.e. it is unmodified by passage through aerated lung – the breath sounds are called **bronchial breath sounds**. These are best heard over consolidated lung.

Added sounds

Crackles, **wheezes** and the sound caused by the two layers of the pleura rubbing together (**pleural rub**) may be heard. The sound of crackles are largely derived from the opening and closing of airways and does not necessarily imply intraluminal fluid. As the airways are normally narrower during expiration, wheezes are particularly pronounced during expiration.

Fine crackles may be heard in pulmonary oedema, fibrosing alveolitis and during the early stages of pneumonic consolidation.

Medium and **coarse crackles** are characteristically associated with bronchiectasis and pneumonia but may be heard in severe pulmonary oedema, at the lung bases in emphysema and over bronchi containing secretions.

Wheezes imply airway narrowing and are usually multiple and of varying pitch. A solitary localized wheeze, not abolished by coughing, indicates a localized airway narrowing and is suggestive of a tumour, foreign body or inspissated mucus.

Pleural rubs indicate pleural inflammation but do not differentiate the cause.

Physical signs
Thoracic injuries
Fractured rib

Pain is experienced in the region of the fracture upon inspiration. Palpation along each rib in this region may reveal local tenderness and it is possible that the fracture may be felt. Signs of concomitant injury of the pleura and lung, and on the left splenic rupture, should be sought.

Sternal fracture

The patient is commonly bent forward and in great pain. The accessibility of this bone means that such a fracture is easily detected. The patient must be assessed with particular regard to myocardial contusion and the possibility of an associated spinal injury.

Lung injury

Two important early signs of lung injury are haemoptysis and subcutaneous emphysema.

Haemoptysis indicates that contusion or laceration of the lung parenchyma has occurred, with release of blood into the alveoli or bronchioles.

Subcutaneous emphysema is the result of the extravasation of air into the subcutaneous tissue, most commonly the result of a rib fracture. In severe cases the emphysema may spread widely from the face to the perineum (including the scrotum in the male) and upper thigh. Such a situation may develop after a wound or rupture of the trachea or large bronchus, or following laceration of the adjacent lung by a fractured rib or stab wound (*Figure 19.1*). Minor degrees of subcutaneous emphysema are common after thoracic operations.

Figure 19.1.
Subcutaneous emphysema of the right axillary region. The gas shadows are obscuring the normal muscle contours.

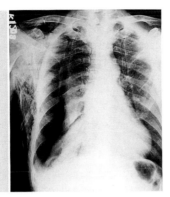

Figure 19.2.
Flail section of the posterolateral aspect of the left chest. a. At rest there is slight asymmetry of the two sides of the chest. b. On inspiration the asymmetry is increased due to drawing-in of the flail chest segment.

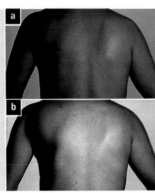

Lung contusion may lead to the signs of consolidation as a result of bleeding within the lung substance.

Lung laceration may produce a communicating or a tension pneumothorax.

Haemothorax and **haemopneumothorax** may follow thoracic fractures. The diagnosis, though suspected clinically, is easily confirmed radiologically.

A **bronchial tear** following major trauma produces a tension pneumothorax which must be treated by tube drainage. A continuing massive leak of air indicates that a main bronchus has been torn and that urgent thoracotomy is essential. Many patients present with massive subcutaneous emphysema.

Flail chest is the result of a crushing injury producing comminuted fractures of a number of ribs, each with a fracture posteriorly at or near the costochondral junction. A more serious variant is when a number of ribs or costal cartilages are fractured on either side near the sternum, rendering the sternum flail. In either case the flail segment is sucked in during inspiration and driven out during expiration; the breathing is therefore **paradoxical** (*Figure 19.2a, b*). The injured side of the thorax moves in while the uninjured side moves out; this results in air being shunted from the injured to the uninjured side and back again, rather than being exhaled. There is therefore a progressive accumulation of carbon dioxide (CO_2) which, together with loss of effective cough and resulting accumulation of tracheobronchial secretions, produces respiratory embarrassment. The increasing anoxia and CO_2 retention result in increased dyspnoea and more pronounced paradoxical movement with worsening respiratory failure – a vicious cycle that can be broken only by mechanical ventilation.

Pneumothorax occurs when air has collected between the two layers of the pleura. Normally the intrapleural pressure is negative but this is lost once a communication is made with atmospheric pressure. If the communication between the

airways and the pleura remains open a bronchopleural fistula is created. Once the communication between the lung and the pleural space is obliterated, air is eventually reabsorbed. In older patients a pneumothorax may be associated with asthma or chronic bronchitis and, rarely, with a peripheral bronchial carcinoma. A **spontaneous pneumothorax** tends to occur in tall, asthenic young men and women (*Figure 19.3*). It is liable to recur and the condition is frequently bilateral. A small bleb may occasionally be seen on the lung surface; the patient complains of unilateral chest pain and slight dyspnoea. Other causes of pneumothorax include trauma, placement of a central venous line, oesophagoscopy, surgical operations (thyroid; trachea; kidney) and mechanical ventilation.

Traumatic pneumothorax due to rib fracture or stab injury commonly results in a tear in both the parietal and visceral pleura. Such a pneumothorax may result in a sucking wound in which air is drawn in and out at each respiration. In such a case a **tension pneumothorax** can develop where air enters the pleural cavity from the lung during inspiration but does not escape during expiration, hence the term 'valvular' is often applied. Subcutaneous emphysema (*Figure 19.1*) may be present.

Figure 19.3.
Right spontaneous tension pneumothorax with complete collapse of the right lung. The right pleural cavity is more lucent than the left and there is absence of any lung markings.

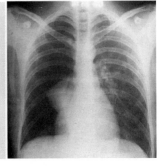

Increasing dyspnoea and cyanosis are predominant features of a pneumothorax. Absence of breath sounds, hyperresonance, cardiac displacement, pallor, poor pulse and hypotension are cardinal signs. As the air accumulates in the pleural cavity, the mediastinum and trachea become more and more displaced, resulting in a decrease in blood returned to the heart with circulatory embarrassment. Urgent chest tube drainage and plugging of the wound are the essential resuscitative measures.

Deformities of the thoracic cage
Pectus excavatum (funnel chest; *Figure 19.4*) and **pectus carinatum** (pigeon chest; *Figure 19.5*) are both the result of a congenital elongation of the costal cartilages so that the sternum is pushed backwards or forwards. In pectus excavatum the lower sternum forms a fixed irreversible deformity which, if severe, may cause the patient to suffer from dyspnoea on exertion. Pressure upon the heart may also embarrass the contractile function of the myocardium leading to circulatory inadequacy.

Solid swellings of the thoracic cage
The normal guidelines for the examination of a lump apply. All lumps that can be found on the skin can occur on the thorax but the following section deals with swellings specific to the thorax.

Non-specific costochondritis – Tietze's syndrome – is a varyingly painful swelling of the chest wall. The most common cartilage to be affected is the second. On palpation the swelling is due to an expansion of the cartilage as it joins the rib.

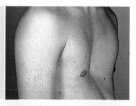

Figure 19.4.
Pectus excavatum.

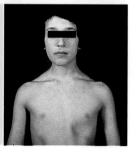

Figure 19.5.
Pectus carinatum.

Neoplasms of the rib commonly lie in the long axis and expands the rib. In this position the swelling is unlikely to be caused by excessive callus around a fracture but may be due to a primary or secondary neoplasm, most commonly the latter. Should such a tumour be situated within a rib beneath the breast it may cause an apparent swelling of that structure. Chondrosarcoma is the most common *primary* rib neoplasm. In the case of *secondary* carcinoma of a rib, pain and local tenderness are marked and may be present long before a swelling is manifest. Spontaneous fracture of the rib may also occur. Neoplasms of the sternum are considerably less frequent than those of the ribs. Secondary tumours of this structure are, however, more likely.

Cold abscess arising in the thoracic wall
Anterior swelling (with no underlying pleural effusion)
The abscess has either originated in a tuberculous rib or costal cartilage, or the site of origin of the abscess is a tuberculous internal mammary lymph node. In the latter, the related ribs and costal cartilages look and feel normal. A cold abscess of the lateral thoracic wall is uncommon.

Posterior swelling
This may arise from a tuberculous rib, a tuberculous dorsal vertebra or a perinephric abscess.

Empyema necessitans
The swelling normally appears on the anterior or lateral aspects of the thorax somewhere between the third and sixth intercostal spaces. Fluctuation is obtained readily. If the flat of the hand is laid over the swelling and the patient is asked to cough, a fluid thrill can usually be felt.

Discharging sinuses of the thoracic wall
Chronic empyema sinus
If a sinus continues to discharge following drainage of an empyema, possible causes are inadequate drainage, underlying suppurative lung disease, osteomyelitis of the ribs, TB and actinomycosis.

Aortic aneurysm
A syphilitic aneurysm of the ascending aorta may give rise to a pulsatile swelling near the sternum. It is very rare.

Pulmonary infection
Surgical patients, like the rest of the population, are subject to chronic bronchitis, emphysema and pneumonic infection (*Figure 19.6*). Some surgical groups – such as patients with

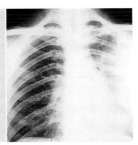

Figure 19.6.
Pneumonic consolidation of the mid-zone of the left lung.

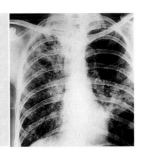

Figure 19.7.
Pulmonary TB. Patchy consolidation is present in both lung fields.

cardiovascular disease and bronchial carcinoma – may be aged and heavy smokers, and are particularly susceptible to these problems. In addition, patients undergoing surgical procedures – particularly under general anaesthesia and with assisted ventilation or in whom the level of consciousness is diminished – are prone to pulmonary infection, pulmonary consolidation and atelectasis.

These problems are due to deficient ventilation of the whole lung and to aspiration of saliva and gastric secretions. Infection can also arise from pre-existing disease in the nasal air sinuses, tonsils, teeth or general sepsis, and chronic infection such as TB. The organisms are commonly *Streptococcus pneumoniae*, *Staphylococcus aureus*, *Haemophilus influenzae* and *Klebsiella pneumoniae*. TB (*Figure 19.7*) is common in developing countries and is also increasing elsewhere, due to the ease of travel, increased migration and susceptibility of patients who have HIV infections. Atypical pneumonia occurs in hospital-acquired infections as well as in patients with an altered immune response.

Clinical symptoms are a productive cough with purulent sputum, pyrexia, tachycardia, tachypnoea, dyspnoea, and scattered crackles and wheezes. Consolidation is dull to percussion with bronchial breath sounds; a sympathetic effusion is dull to percussion with reduced breath sounds. In chronic disease there may also be haemoptysis, night sweats and weight loss.

Complications of pulmonary infection include lung abscess and bronchiectasis. Postoperative pneumonia occurs most commonly around the third or fourth day, often in elderly patients, when it can be accompanied by a degree of confusion. Another postoperative syndrome – which must be considered in a patient with respiratory distress – is the inhalation of vomited gastric juices: Mendelson's syndrome. A chemical inflammatory process is induced by the gastric acidity and is accompanied by bronchospasm, pulmonary oedema and, in severe cases, circulatory collapse.

Atelectasis (*Figure 19.8a, b, c*) is the collapse of part or the whole of a lung following an occlusion in the bronchial tree. The block may be due to a bronchial neoplasm but atelectasis is also common postoperatively. The latter may occur during anaesthesia, or pain may inhibit normal expansion, allowing the retention of secretions and the development of a plug of inspissated mucus. There is continued blood flow through the collapsed segment producing interpulmonary shunting and hypoxia.

On clinical examination the patient may be dyspnoeic and cyanosed and there is often a spike of pyrexia. Movement and air entry are reduced over the collapsed segment and, if this is large, there is tracheal shift and movement of the apex beat towards the side of the lesion.

Atelectasis may also follow inhalation of a **foreign body**. Young children are at particular risk as are adults with a diminished level of consciousness, such as in inebriation, a

Figure 19.8.
Atelectasis. a. Right apical lower lobe. b. Right lower lobe. c. Left lung.

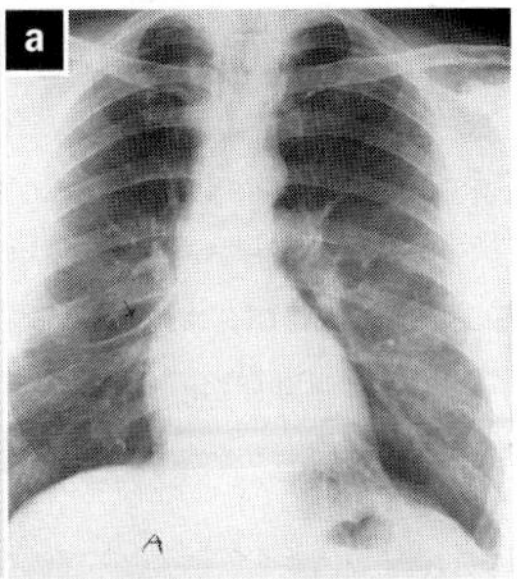

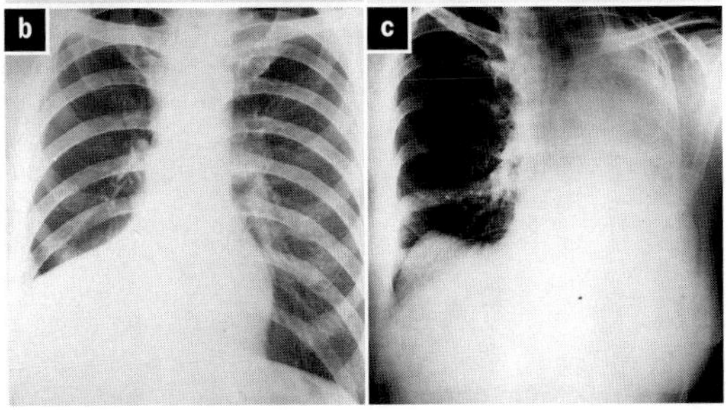

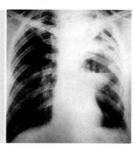

Figure 19.9.
Lung abscess in the left mid-zone. Note the horizontal line at the pus/air interface.

head injury and during an epileptic fit or anaesthesia. The anatomy of the bronchi is such that 80% of foreign bodies pass into the right lung. Symptoms may be minimal after the initial paroxysm of coughing. Chest radiography shows a radiopaque object and there may be atelectasis or obstructive emphysema present. Radiolucent bodies, however, may go unnoticed. Metal objects are surprisingly well tolerated but organic material, notably a peanut, can excite a marked inflammatory response with secondary infection and possibly abscess formation and, later, bronchiectasis.

A **lung abscess** (*Figure 19.9*) may follow a virulent infection accompanied by bronchial obstruction such as in atelectasis, tumours, foreign bodies, inadequate treatment of pneumonia and in TB. It may also follow penetrating pulmonary injuries. Abscesses less commonly encountered in the UK include an infected hydatid cyst and abscesses spreading from abdominal amoebiasis. The clinical picture is similar to that of the underlying pulmonary infection (see above) together with cachexia, swinging pyrexia and anorexia, due to the purulent collection. Chest radiography reveals the air fluid level of the abscess cavity. Rupture of the abscess may be into the pleural cavity or into the bronchial tree; in the latter there is a risk of spilling the contents into the opposite lung.

Bronchiectasis (*Figure 19.10*) is irreversible damage, dilatation and chronic infection of the medium-sized bronchi.

It follows severe infection accompanied by some degree of obstruction. It usually starts in childhood when the supporting cartilage is soft and easily damaged by both bronchiolitis and external damage from the inflammatory changes of adjacent lymph nodes. It is particularly seen after whooping cough and measles; TB must also be excluded. Focal bronchiectasis may occur after damage from a foreign body. Bronchiectasis may be associated with the deposition of systemic amyloid.

The clinical picture is of recurrent chest infections, with copious sputum, often foul-smelling, and accompanied by cachexia and weight loss. Haematemesis may be massive as is seen in inflammation at other sites (e.g. peptic ulceration; diverticulitis) rather than the chronic haemorrhage from malignant lesions. Physical signs may be minimal but wheezing is usually present as is clubbing in long-standing disease.

Pulmonary embolism

This is the passage of detached thrombus from peripheral veins, through the right side of the heart into the lungs (*Figure 19.11*). A paradoxical embolus is the passage of the embolus through a congenital cardiac defect into the systemic circulation. The thrombus usually comes from the lower limbs. Calf vein thrombosis commencing around the valves of the soleal venous sinuses is very common, occurring in more than 50% of hospital surgical patients.

The causes of thrombosis fall into Virchow's triad of stasis, damage to the vessel wall and increased hypercoagulability. Bed rest, immobility, calf pressure on the operating table and surgical procedures stimulate all these factors. Other patients at risk are those with coagulopathies and a history of previous thrombosis, women taking oestrogen contraception, and during pregnancy and the puerperium, patients with malignancy, generalized sepsis or nutritional abnormalities, and after major trauma. Uncommon causes of embolism are dislodgement of renal carcinoma that has grown into the renal vein and inferior vena cava, and amniotic fluid from the pregnant uterus.

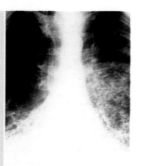

Figure 19.10.
Bilateral basal bronchiectasis. Bronchial markings are increased due to thickening of the walls, retained sputum and infected debris.

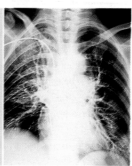

Figure 19.11.
Pulmonary embolism. The catheter injecting the contrast medium can be seen passing above the body of the right scapula and descending into the right atrium. The left pulmonary artery is deficient over many of its branches in the upper and middle lobes, and there are also scattered areas of non-filling on the right side.

The vast majority of leg thrombi remain asymptomatic and gradually recanalize. However, calf venous thrombosis can propagate into the popliteal, femoral and iliac systems or thrombus can arise *de novo* across the pelvic veins producing increased venous pressure in the limb. The clinical features of this pressure increase are those of a white or blue leg, as considered on p. 385. The increased pressure within the limb may dislodge a small or larger length of thrombus. The symptoms of these pulmonary emboli fall into four categories:

- Small emboli can be asymptomatic although recurrent showers can give rise to the late sequelae of pulmonary hypertension.
- Larger emboli give rise to pleuritic pain and haemoptysis. There may be a pleural rub associated with the pain and scattered crackles and wheezes on auscultation.
- Longer lengths of vein can pass into one or both lungs and produce systemic circulatory collapse, increased respiratory rate, tachycardia, pyrexia, sweating and marked dyspnoea. The patient is pale and cyanosed. The diagnosis of myocardial infarction may be considered but the electrocardiogram in major pulmonary emboli shows S waves in lead 1, and Q waves and inverted T waves in lead 3 (S1; Q3; T3). Chest radiographs may be normal but a ventilation–perfusion (VQ) scan demonstrates the differential of normal air entry, with reduced or absent blood flow through affected areas of lung.
- Massive pulmonary emboli produce a powerful vagal stimulus – the patient characteristically urgently calls for a bedpan but has died by the time it arrives. The large quantities of thrombus coil in the heart giving rise to ventricular fibrillation and obstructing the pulmonary outflow tract, producing lethal pulmonary hypertension. This high mortality is reflected in the 20 000 deaths per annum in the UK and hence the search for routine prophylaxis in all surgical patients over the age of 45, and in other high risk groups or situations.

Carcinoma of the bronchus

Carcinoma of the bronchus (*Figure 19.12*) is the commonest malignancy in the male and second only to the breast in the female. It is a disease primarily affecting the older male smoker but pollution and radiation have also been implicated. The commonest lesion is a **squamous carcinoma**

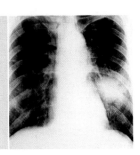

Figure 19.12.
Carcinoma of the left lung. The large lesion in the mid-zone is accompanied by increasing distal markings due to consolidation and collapse.

(60%) followed by an **anaplastic lesion** (20–30%), a small-cell, highly malignant lesion often associated with endocrine syndromes such as Cushing's and atopic ADH secretion. **Adenocarcinoma** (10%) is a slow-growing, more peripherally sited lesion. Equally common in the female, it metastasizes late to the liver, brain, bone, and adrenal and lymph nodes. **Alveolar cell carcinomas** are usually distally situated, solitary lesions and curable by resection, but multicentric carcinomas have a poor prognosis. They may be associated with a myopathy.

The symptoms of carcinoma of the bronchus may initially be indistinguishable from a chest infection. There is a persistent cough with non-specific chest pain and dyspnoea. An important symptom, however, is haemoptysis, bloodstained sputum being present in approximately half the patients (*Figure 19.13a, b*).

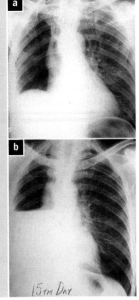

Figure 19.13.
Right pneumonectomy undertaken for a carcinoma of the bronchus. a. First day post operation showing the air-filled right chest with no pulmonary markings. b. Fifteenth day radiograph showing a pleural effusion with an air/fluid horizontal interface and mediastinal shift to the right.

The more frequent manifestations of the disease – which should arouse suspicion – are tobacco staining, clubbing of the fingers and signs of obvious weight loss.

Bone metastases

These occur in the ribs, long bones or spine. Pain is the predominant feature in the majority of patients, with a swelling possibly appearing as a late sign. **Pathological fractures** (*Figure 19.14*) are not infrequent, particularly in the long bones or vertebrae. **Hypertrophic pulmonary osteoarthropathy** (*Figure 19.15*) – a subperiosteal new bone formation occurring around the end of long bones, particularly of the wrists and ankles – also occurs in some benign and malignant pleural lesions.

Enlarged lymph nodes

When in the neck or axillae these are typically stony hard in consistency. It is also not unknown for enlargement of other nodes, e.g. the groin, to be the first sign.

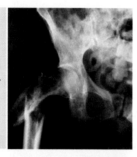

Figure 19.14.
Pathological transverse fracture of the upper end of the shaft of the right femur through secondary metastatic disease from carcinoma of the bronchus.

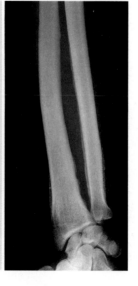

Figure 19.15.
Hypertrophic osteoarthropathy of the distal right radius and ulna in a patient with carcinoma of the bronchus.

Recurrent laryngeal nerve paralysis

This results in hoarseness. It may be due to carcinomatous infiltration originating in a bronchus. Local invasion may also extend into adjacent structures such as the aorta and oesophagus (*Figure 19.16*).

Liver enlargement

Malignant enlargement of the liver or **ascites** are occasional presentations, as are pleural effusions.

Secondary carcinomatous deposits

These deposits in the skin may be single or multiple; they are rarely the first sign. They are of a hard consistency and vary in size from 2 cm in diameter down to minute swellings which can only be detected by running the pulp of the index finger over them. The history is usually that they have appeared in a matter of days or weeks.

Superior vena caval obstruction

Visible engorgement of the veins of the neck is usually an indication of metastases in the posterior mediastinum pressing upon the superior vena cava (p. 386; *Figure 29.8*). It can be due to other causes such as a primary neoplasm or a cyst pressing upon this vein.

Pancoast syndrome

Pancoast syndrome results from a growth in the apex of the lung that is usually silent for a long period. It may feature some of the following manifestations: distension of the veins of the neck (the result of pressure on the superior vena cava); swelling of the face from the same cause; Horner's syndrome (from pressure on the sympathetic chain) and pains that radiate down the arm as a result of tumour infiltration of the lower brachial plexus.

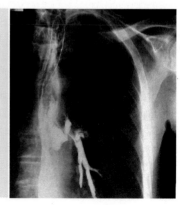

Figure 19.16.
Invasion of carcinoma of the bronchus into the oesophagus. A barium swallow has demonstrated an oesophagobronchial fistula.

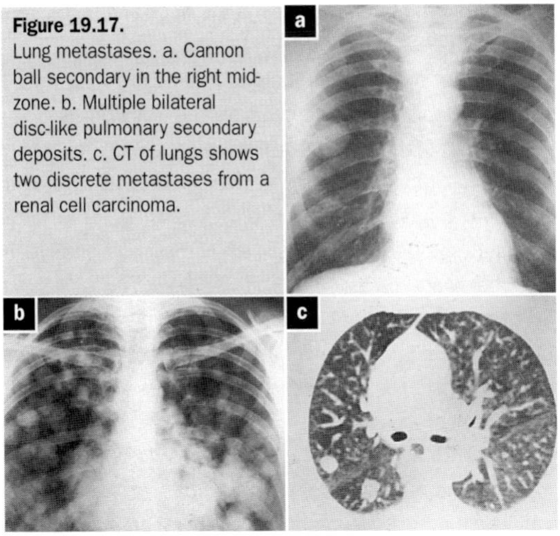

Figure 19.17.
Lung metastases. a. Cannon ball secondary in the right mid-zone. b. Multiple bilateral disc-like pulmonary secondary deposits. c. CT of lungs shows two discrete metastases from a renal cell carcinoma.

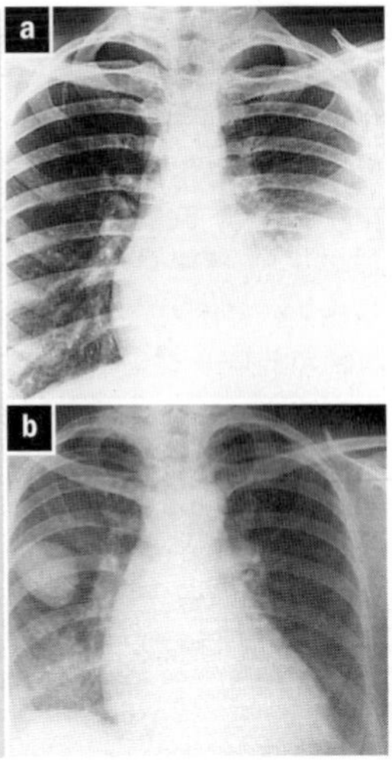

Figure 19.18.
Left pleural effusion. a. The dense opacity extends over the lateral chest wall obliterating the lung markings and the outlines of the chest wall and diaphragm. b. Interlobar right pleural effusion; note its similarity to the appearance of the pulmonary metastasis in Figure 19.17a.

Paraneoplastic syndromes

Paraneoplastic syndromes associated with carcinoma of the bronchus include atopic ADH production, Cushing's syndrome and hypercalcaemia.

Other bronchial neoplasms

Non-carcinomatous lesions of the bronchial tree are uncommon. Carcinoid tumours of varying malignancy occur and may present with carcinoid syndrome (p. 306), adenoid cystic carcinomas (cylindromas) are malignant, mainly locally invasive tumours, while benign lesions include fibromas, hamartomas and epitheliomas, the lesion being usually identified when investigating persistent or recurrent pulmonary infections, atelectasis or abnormal shadowing on a chest radiograph. Pulmonary metastases (*Figure 19.17a, b, c*) are not uncommon and are often cannon ball in appearance on a chest radiograph. They originate from a wide range of carcinomas and sarcomas, including bone sarcomas and gut, renal and breast carcinomas.

Pleura

The lung develops as an outpouching from the primitive foregut into the pleural cavity. The mesothelial lining of the cavity is thus divided into visceral pleura covering the lung, and parietal pleura lining the chest wall and the mediastinum. The parietal pleura is innervated by the intercostal nerves, and pain is well localized. Sensation from the visceral pleura, however, is vague and less well defined. In health, the visceral and parietal pleura move over each other, lubricated by 10–15 mL of pleural fluid.

If pulmonary infection spreads to the pleura, the inflamed surfaces rub on each other, producing pleuritic pain during respiratory excursions. A pleural rub may be heard over these areas. In disease, the amount of pleural fluid can increase dramatically (effusion; *Figure 19.18a, b*). Separation of diseased pleural layers can eradicate the pleural pain and the rub. The signs of an effusion are dullness to percussion and reduction of breath sounds. When the lung is compromised, there is associated dyspnoea and cyanosis, progressive collapse and secondary infection. Effusions can occur in trauma, when they may be haemorrhagic from a lacerated intercostal artery or a major mediastinal vessel, while damage of the thoracic duct can produce a chylous collection. Sterile effusions occur in collagen diseases, congestive cardiac failure and Meigs' syndrome (p. 298).

Malignant effusions are most commonly due to metastatic infiltration, particularly from primary disease of the lung, breast, ovary or lymphomas. The fluid is often bloodstained. **Mesothelioma** is a primary malignancy of the pleura and peritoneum; in about half the cases, prior exposure to asbestos can be identified (*Figure 19.19*). Although the disease may

Figure 19.19.
Thickening of the right lower mediastinal and diaphragmatic pleura in an individual previously exposed to asbestos.

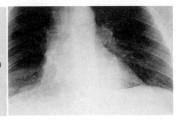

take 10–20 years to develop it is highly malignant, with pleural pain, effusion, pyrexia, night sweats and progressive dyspnoea and weight loss.

Infection of an effusion gives rise to an **empyema.** This may occur from contaminated traumatic wounds or spread from bony infection of the ribs or vertebrae. Purulent infection can spread from acute lung infections, abscesses, bronchiectasis and chronic infective processes such as TB, fungal infections, hydatid and amoebiasis. Malignant lung masses may also break down and undergo suppuration. Oesophageal rupture into the mediastinum (p. 249) usually spreads into an adjacent pleural cavity, and subphrenic and liver abscesses can spread through the diaphragm or its openings to involve the pleural cavity.

The mediastinum

The mediastinum lies between the pleural cavities and contains the heart and great vessels. For descriptive purposes it is divided into the superior mediastinum (above a horizontal line from the sternal angle) and below this into the anterior, middle and posterior mediastinum, the middle containing the heart. The mediastinum is well protected from the exterior but is subject to a number of cysts and tumours (*Figure 19.20a–d*), air can enter it through surgery or other trauma, and rupture of the oesophagus (p. 249) and bronchus pro-

duces surgical emphysema round the neck and sometimes the whole of the body ('Michelin man').

Superior mediastinal lesions include low-lying thyroid lesions, ectopic parathyroid tumours and lymphomas.

Lesions of the **anterior mediastinum** include tumours of the thymus, lymphomas, and germ cell remnants that fail to complete migration from the urogenital ridge. The latter include teratomas, desmoids, seminomas, and embryonal and choriocarcinomas.

Middle mediastinal lesions are usually congenital cysts, due to aberrant development of the pericardium, sequestration of bronchogenic remnants or enterogenous cysts from duplication of the gut.

Posterior mediastinal lesions are a wide variety of neurogenic tumours and include neurofibromas, neurilemmomas, ganglioneuromas, neuroblastomas, chemodectomas and phaeochromocytomas.

Diaphragmatic hernias

The diaphragm is subject to herniation through two congenital defects – Bochdalek and Morgagni – through the oesophageal hiatus (hiatus hernia, p. 250) and through a traumatic rupture. Denervation or atrophy of one or both hemidiaphragms produces elevation (**eventration**; *Figure 19.21a, b*) compromising pulmonary expansion and occasionally producing paradoxical movement, i.e. elevation rather than descent on inspiration, and descent on expiration.

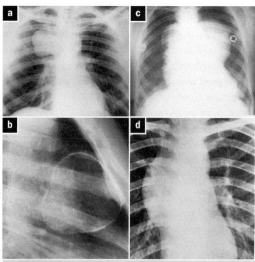

Figure 19.20.
a–d. Mediastinal tumours. These are often incidental radiological findings.

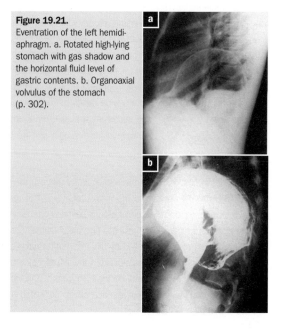

Figure 19.21.
Eventration of the left hemidiaphragm. a. Rotated high-lying stomach with gas shadow and the horizontal fluid level of gastric contents. b. Organoaxial volvulus of the stomach (p. 302).

Figure 19.22.
Bochdalek's hernia. The left chest is filled with abdominal contents, with mediastinal shift to the right.

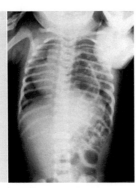

A **Bochdalek hernia** (*Figure 19.22*) is through a posterolateral defect, there being free communication between the pleural and peritoneal cavities; it is on the left side in 90% of cases, and commoner in males. Breath sounds are replaced by gut sounds, and the heart is shifted to the right (giving apparent dextrocardia), the trachea being similarly deviated. The abdomen is drawn in (scaphoid). Obstruction and strangulation of the bowel is rare but, as the contents of the thoracic bowel increase, there is progressive respiratory distress.

Hernia of Morgagni is anteriorly situated and small. It is asymptomatic at birth, symptoms developing in middle age. Omentum and colon pass into the defect, promoted by obesity, trauma and pregnancy. The condition is usually an incidental radiological finding but the neck of the sac is narrow and obstruction can occur.

Traumatic rupture (*Figure 19.23*) may be due to a penetrating subcostal injury but, more commonly, is from a rapid abdominal blow against a closed glottis. In some cases it may be herniation into a pre-existing congenital sac. The liver acts as a protective cushion on the right, and left sided ruptures are more common. Symptoms may be minor and the diagnosis missed on chest radiography. The traumatic incident may, therefore, have been forgotten when the patient presents later with emaciation and strangulation of the contents of the sac.

The oesophagus

The oesophagus is inaccessible to physical examination. Nonetheless, by the application of indirect physical signs a great deal of information can be ascertained. In some instances a diagnosis may be made by their aid alone. This should be confirmed by contrast radiology, endoscopy and functional studies. Congenital anomalies of the oesophagus are considered on p. 232.

Spontaneous rupture of the oesophagus

An early diagnosis followed by immediate resuscitation and operation may avoid death. Dyspnoea, cyanosis and rapidly increasing circulatory failure are commonly observed. The majority of patients are males with a history of alcoholism. Following a heavy meal there is vomiting, and during one of these expulsive episodes the oesophagus ruptures in its lower third. Extreme pain is experienced usually in the left side of the lower thorax which radiates to the back. Generally vomiting ceases with the onset of the rupture but if it continues the vomitus is commonly streaked with bright red blood. In many instances subcutaneous emphysema may be apparent around the neck (*Figure 19.24*). A hydropneumothorax may result from the extravasated gas and fluid bursting through the parietal pleura.

Rupture may also be **iatrogenic** in origin, the wall being penetrated during oesophagoscopy, possibly through a diseased segment, such as a carcinoma. The symptoms are much less than those seen in spontaneous rupture and may be minimal or even overlooked. This is because oesophageal fluid rather than gastric acid is released into the mediastinum, and the small volume, and the absence of the pressure effects of vomiting reduce the likelihood of subsequent mediastinitis.

Vomiting may produce mucosal tears around the oesophagogastric junction. These may produce minor symptoms but occasionally can produce major haemorrhage and are termed **Mallory–Weiss tears**.

Figure 19.23.
Ruptured left hemidiaphragm. The stomach and other viscera are sited in the left pleural cavity and there is mediastinal shift to the right.

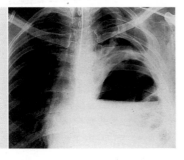

Figure 19.24.
Ruptured oesophagus. This shows extensive subcutaneous emphysema and a left pleural effusion.

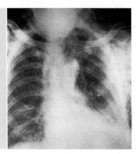

The oesophagogastric junction is one of the sites of portosystemic anastamoses that develop in portal vein obstruction and portal hypertension. Other sites are retroperitoneal veins and between the superior and inferior rectal plexuses. The **oesophageal varices** (*Figure 19.25*) are the most likely source of haemorrhage, producing haematemesis and melaena. The deposition of large quantities of blood in the gut is equivalent to a protein meal and further accentuates the symptoms of liver failure (p. 285).

Hiatus hernia

There are two primary types of hiatus hernia: sliding (85%) and rolling (5%). Types III and IV are respectively when the lesions occur together (10%) and when organs other than the stomach, e.g. the colon, are also situated within the hernial sac.

In a **sliding hiatus hernia** (*Figure 19.26*) the oesophagogastric junction is sited in the chest. The condition is usually asymptomatic until there is associated incompetence of the oesophogastric sphincter; **oesophageal reflux** is present (p. 252).

In a **rolling** (**paraoesophageal**) **hiatus hernia** there is a peritoneal-lined hernial sac passing through the oesophageal hiatus alongside the oesophagus, and a variable amount of stomach rolls into this space. The sac is usually sited anterior to and to the left of the oesophagus. There is progressive increase in the size of the hernia as the pleural pressure is less than that of the abdominal cavity; the whole stomach may end up in the chest.

Dysphagia and heartburn – the predominant symptoms in a sliding hiatus hernia – may be present but are much less prominent as the oesophagogastric junction is usually competent. Postprandial discomfort is prominent, together with nausea and a substernal pressure sensation. The latter may be relieved by belching and regurgitation of food. The presence of a large amount of stomach in the chest can cause breathlessness and suffocation. The stomach in the hernial sac is subject to the complications of volvulus, obstruction, gangrene and perforation. The severe retrosternal pain in these lesions can be mistaken for myocardial infarction. Chronic symptoms include marked anaemia due to chronic blood loss from inflamed gastric mucosa within the sac.

Dysphagia

A large variety of lesions give rise to dysphagia, as shown in *Table 19.1*. They can be divided into external, within the wall and intrinsic lesions. The diagnosis must be determined

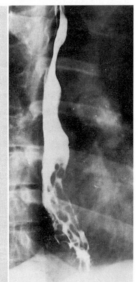

Figure 19.25.
Oesophageal varices. The barium is indented by the diffuse pattern of bulging varicosities at the lower end of the oesophagus.

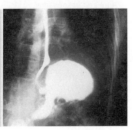

Figure 19.26.
Paraoesophageal hiatus hernia. The cardiac end of the stomach has passed through the oesophageal hiatus alongside the oesophagus and is sited above the diaphragm.

Table 19.1. Oesophageal obstruction.

Extrinsic pressure	Abnormalities of the wall		Abnormalities within the lumen
	Stricture	*Abnormalities of oesophageal contraction*	
Thyroid	Post traumatic	Achalasia	Foreign bodies
Pharyngeal pouch	Benign & malignant neoplasms	Failure of relaxation of the crico-pharyngeus	Webs
Aortic aneurysm	Acute & chronic oesophagitis	Cerebrovascular accidents	Schatski's rings
Abnormal aortic arch	Corrosives	Diffuse oesoph-geal spasm	
Mediastinal tumours	Crohn's disease		
	Post radiotherapy		
Paraoes-ophageal hiatus hernia	Oesophageal diverticulum		
	Scleroderma		

radiologically and by oesophagoscopy; nevertheless, there are certain key points which should be sought during the clinical examination.

A general examination should pay particular attention to whether the patient is anaemic or has signs of weight loss. The patient should be asked to indicate the point where the food is arrested, the mouth should be examined and the neck palpated for enlarged lymph nodes particularly in the supra-clavicular fossae. The abdomen should be examined for hepatomegaly and ascites.

Extrinsic oesophageal compression

Large thyroid lesions can compress both the trachea and oesophagus, producing dyspnoea and dysphagia; the symptoms can also be marked with infiltrating anaplastic lesions of the gland. A pharyngeal pouch (*Figure 19.27*; p. 207) can compress the upper oesophagus, and a paraoesophageal hernia the lower end, while vascular compression is usually at the mid-oesophagus. The latter include aortic aneurysms (*Figure 19.28*) and congenital anomalies of the arch. Mediastinal tumours causing dysphagia are usually primary malignancies or secondary nodal metastases.

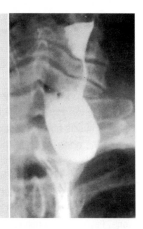

Figure 19.27.
Pharyngeal pouch.

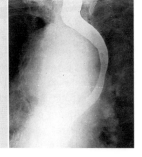

Figure 19.28.
Aneurysm of the aortic arch displacing the upper thoracic oesophagus.

Dysphagia lusoria (vascular ring)

Anomalous development of the primitive aortic arches can leave a vascular ring containing the trachea and oesophagus. This does not usually produce obstructive symptoms at birth but, as these structures grow more rapidly than the arteries, dysphagia and stridor may appear within a matter of months. A baby thus affected commonly lies with its neck extended. In this position, pressure on the trachea and oesophagus is reduced; flexion of the neck brings on stridor and dysphagia.

Abnormalities within the oesophageal wall

Cancer of the oesophagus is the commonest cause of dysphagia but strictures also occur in a number of benign lesions, particularly oesophagitis associated with a sliding hiatus hernia. Traumatic strictures may follow perforation of the oesophagus or the inflammation resulting from the ingestion of corrosives or the prolonged use of oesophageal tubes. The E of the CREST syndrome denotes the 'esophagus' (from the American coining of the term) due to vasculitic changes of the vessel wall in scleroderma. Abnormalities of motility include local disease such as achalasia and diffuse spasm.

Carcinoma of the oesophagus (*Figure 19.29*) accounts for 5% of malignancies in the UK. It is twice as common in males and usually occurs in the fifth and sixth decades. It is a common lesion in the Far East and has a high incidence in the Bantu tribe in Africa. The latter is thought to be due to a high intake of nitrosamines in the diet. Other risk factors include smoking, high alcohol intake, lye strictures, achalasia and Plummer–Vinson syndrome. The majority of lesions are squamous in origin but a few adenocarcinomas occur at the lower end of the oesophagus.

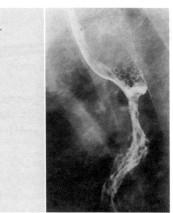

Figure 19.29.
Carcinoma of the mid-oesophagus.

Figure 19.30.
Hamartomatous polyp of the upper oesophagus indenting the barium column from the right side.

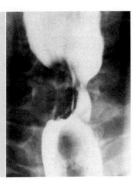

Figure 19.31.
Post-corrosive stricture.

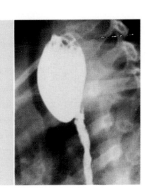

Clinically, presentation is usually within 3 to 6 months of origin, the prime symptom being dysphagia. Any individual over the age of 45 with a recent history of dysphagia must, therefore, be considered as having oesophageal cancer until proven otherwise. Dysphagia is usually to solids but rapidly progresses to include fluids, and the starvation is accompanied by anorexia, cachexia and weight loss, while occult bleeding causes anaemia. Saliva cannot be swallowed and the overspill into the larynx can give rise to chest infection.

Pain is a late feature and is usually non-specific, poorly localized and retrosternal discomfort. Invasion through the oesophageal wall may involve the trachea and the recurrent laryngeal nerves. A postcricoid lesion in the Plummer–Vinson syndrome usually presents while still in the benign state but local invasion of the larynx and its innervation may require pharyngolaryngectomy if surgical excision is being considered.

Benign tumours of the oesophagus make up approximately 5% of neoplasms. Leiomyoma is the commonest lesion. It is submucosal and, therefore, mucosal bleeding is uncommon and dysphagia is not prominent. Vague, poorly localized discomfort may be present but the lesion is usually an incidental radiological finding. Other tumours include papillomas, fibromas and lipomas (*Figure 19.30*).

Oesophagitis

Oesophagitis may be acute or chronic. **Acute oesophagitis** occurs in response to burns, scalds, ingestion of corrosives, the trauma of a long-standing oesophageal tube and, less frequently, to the effects of gastric acidity. Acute infective lesions are uncommon and, when present, are usually an extension of pharyngitis.

Corrosive strictures (*Figure 19.31*) are usually in children but may be the result of attempted suicide. The lesions are more common in Asia and Africa, where home industry is more prevalent, as are the many strong alkalis and acids associated

with these ventures. Cleaning agents and bleach are, however, common world wide. The burn involves the mouth and pharynx and may also produce laryngeal injury. The agent is diluted in the stomach where the gastric mucosa is more resistant to damage than the oesophagus. The oesophageal burn is usually full thickness and, after the initial acute inflammatory phase, there is extensive and progressive fibrosis producing dysphagia and lifelong management problems.

Chronic oesophagitis is usually associated with reflux from a sliding hiatus hernia. Some degree of sliding hiatus hernia can be demonstrated radiologically in a large number of patients, with appropriate positioning and abdominal pressure. However, a number of factors are normally involved with maintaining competency at the gastro-oesophageal junction. The gastric mucosal folds form a rosette around the sphincter, and the acute angle at which the oesophagus enters the stomach serves as a flap valve. This angle is partly maintained by the arrangement of spiral gastric muscle fibres. The lower 2 cm of oesophagus are within the abdomen, and the abdominal pressure has a valvular effect, while the encircling fibres of the right crus serve as a pinchcock mechanism. Competency of this mechanism is reduced in the aged and obese, when the elasticity of tissues is reduced, as is the normal muscle tone. Factors giving rise to increased abdominal pressure, such as pregnancy or ascites, increase reflux; the symptoms in pregnancy usually subside immediately post partum.

The symptoms of a **sliding hiatus hernia** (*Figure 19.32*) are primarily **heartburn** and **dysphagia**. Heartburn is retrosternal burning, accompanying regurgitation of gastric juice; there is a bitter, sour taste. It is brought on by stooping and lying, being particularly noted when first going to bed and relieved by sleeping propped up on a number of pillows. This early nocturnal pain differs from duodenal pain, which awakes an individual one or two hours later.

Figure 19.32. Sliding hiatus hernia. The upper narrowing is at the oesophagogastric junction and the lower at the level of the diaphragm.

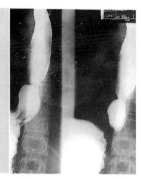

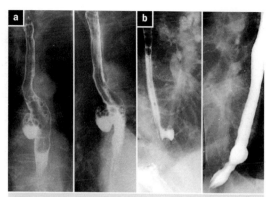

Figure 19.33.
Oesophageal diverticula. a. In the mid-oesophagus. b. Sited near the diaphragm.

Figure 19.34.
Achalasia of the oesophagus. There is gross dilatation of the oesophagus with smooth tapering at the lower end. The barium column is mixed with food residue.

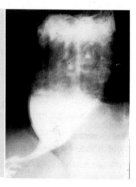

Dysphagia is an early symptom and sited behind the lower sternum. It commences with fluids, particularly cold fluids, possibly due to local oedema. Initially solids do not produce symptoms, and this is in contrast to the dysphagia of a malignant neoplasm. There is early fullness at meal times, and occasional vomiting. Larger hernias produce pulmonary symptoms, there being gurgling in the chest with pressure producing dyspnoea. Regurgitation may be accompanied by aspiration, possibly during sleep, giving rise to a persistent cough; this can progress to bronchitis, pneumonia and lung abscess formation. Of note is the absence of any epigastric or subcostal tenderness.

Once oesophagitis intervenes, retrosternal pain is more prominent. It may be postprandial; this is not necessarily so but it can be precipitated by hot food, hot fluids and alcohol. As the condition progresses, pain radiates into the epigastrium, the neck and the shoulders, and may be mistaken for myocardial infarction.

The history is usually of recurrent exacerbations of symptoms but inflammatory changes later become irreversible; dysphagia is to fluids as well as solids as the fibrosis progresses. Occult bleeding, with anaemia, is common. Haematemesis is unusual unless gastric mucosa is present in the oesophagus. This can occur through mucosa being drawn up by the fibrous response. Previously, the presence of such mucosa – termed 'short oesophagus' or 'Barret's oesophagus' – was considered to be due to congenital rests but it is now thought to result from chronic oesophagitis.

Oesophageal diverticula (*Figure 19.33a, b*) may be congenital, pulsion, traction or pseudodiverticula. **Congenital diverticula** are probably incomplete versions of tracheo-oesophageal fistulae or enterogenous cysts, which are found along the length of the alimentary canal and represent various stages of duplication of the gut. **Pulsion diverticula** are due to high intraluminal pressures produced in motility dis-

orders. The term **traction diverticula** was applied to many of these abnormalities and was considered to be due to adhesions from tuberculous mediastinal nodes: this aetiology, however, is probably very rare. **Pseudodiverticula** are radiologically demonstrated, rigid-walled ulcers, penetrating the full thickness of the mucosa.

Achalasia (**cardiospasm**; *Figure 19.34*) is an aganglionic defect in Auerbach's plexus, that gives rise to a failure of relaxation of the gastro-oesophageal junction, and dysphagia. It occurs primarily in the third and fourth decade and is equally distributed in the sexes. The oesophagus progressively dilates, producing a **megaoesophagus**. In the UK the condition is probably congenital in origin but an indistinguishable lesion is found in South America, due to infection from American trypanosomiasis: Chagas' disease. This infection can also produce megaduodenum and megacolon.

Clinically, presentation is usually with dysphagia but this is insidious and may progress over many years, thus differing from the acute presentation of carcinoma of the oesophagus. The patient often complains of vomiting but on detailed

Figure 19.35.
Corkscrew oesophagus.

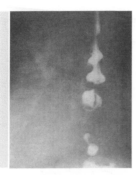

questioning, this is found to be regurgitation of copious amounts of foul-smelling, partly digested food and frothy sputum. An associated oesophagitis can produce retrosternal discomfort.

As the dysphagia progresses and the stenosis becomes complete, there is weight loss, malnutrition and cachexia. Aspiration of the regurgitated oesophageal contents produces respiratory infection. There is an increased incidence of malignancy, these changes usually occurring in the mid-oesophagus. Radiological studies usually demonstrate the megaoesophagus, the stenosed segment and the absence of a stomach air bubble.

Failure of relaxation of the cricopharyngeus muscle can occur in cerebrovascular disease. Spasm of this muscle produces the sensation of a lump in the throat: globus hystericus. Although this used to be considered hysterical in origin, it is probably spasm in response to oesophageal reflux.

Diffuse oesophageal spasm, **corkscrew oesophagus** (*Figure 19.35*) and **tertiary contractures** are some terms applied to entities that were diagnosed initially radiologically and later from abnormal motility studies. Patients usually present with episodic chest pain and dysphagia, the former often having features of angina, which has to be differentiated. In some of these conditions, pathological abnormalities are discovered, e.g. in approximately half the patients with diffuse spasm there is marked thickening of the oesophageal smooth muscle along its length.

Abnormalities within the lumen

Foreign bodies (*Figure 19.36a–d*) blocking the oesophagus include fish bones, coins, pins and dentures. The history is usually available, the lesions may be shown radiographically and are identified and removed endoscopically. The web in Plummer–Vinson syndrome is situated in the postcricoid region (*Figure 19.37*) whereas the thin web of Schatski's rings occurs in, and encircles, the lower oesophagus.

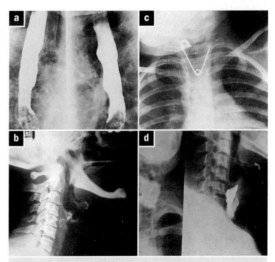

Figure 19.36.
Foreign bodies in the oesophagus. a. Meat bolus. b. Chicken bone sited between the trachea and the C7 and T1 vertebral bodies. c. Open safety pin. d. Denture.

Figure 19.37.
Post-cricoid oesophageal web.

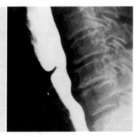

Sideropenic dysphagia (Plummer–Vinson syndrome)

In this the patient is usually a middle-aged woman. Typically the patient complains of choking and the delayed swallowing of food, localized at the level of the cricoid cartilage. Not all the physical signs are necessarily present. The lips and corners of the mouth are commonly cracked, known as **angular stomatitis** or **cheilosis**.

The tongue is usually devoid of papillae, smooth and pale. The finger nails may be brittle and tend to be spoon shaped: **koilonychia**. The spleen is occasionally enlarged as in other iron deficiency anaemias. Koilonychia, an inflamed tongue and cheilosis are not unusual in sideropenia *per se*, and therefore the syndrome can only be set apart by the presence of the associated characteristic dysphagia. Endoscopic examination of the laryngopharynx and the oesophagus is necessary as the condition is premalignant and a postcricoid carcinoma may have supervened. Achlorhydria is sometimes present.

20 Evaluation of the cardiac surgical patient

Introduction

Heart disease may be classified as acquired or congenital. This chapter deals with acquired lesions of the coronary arteries, heart valves, major blood vessels, the myocardium and the endocardium. (A brief comment on congenital heart disease has been included at the end of the chapter.)

Despite the development of sophisticated invasive and non-invasive techniques for cardiac investigation, the clinical history and examination retain a key role in pre- and postoperative evaluation. For example, deterioration in the clinical symptoms of dyspnoea and fatigue in a patient with a known lesion of a heart valve may encourage earlier operative intervention, even if there has been no deterioration of echocardiographic contractile ability. Similarly, if echocardiographic data and/or information gained from cardiac catheterization is at variance with the clinical history and physical signs, the investigation needs repetition. In contrast to eliciting a thorough history, it should be remembered that these investigations demonstrate the patient's haemodynamics at only one point in time, often extending to no more than a few heart beats.

Clinical assessment

History
Risk factors for coronary artery disease are:

- Family history of coronary artery disease.
- Diabetes, diet controlled, oral therapy or requiring insulin.
- Hypercholesterolaemia (>6.5 mmol/L or treated).
- Hypertension (>140/90 mmHg or treated).
- Hypothyroidism.
- Smoking, calculated as the number of 'pack years'.
- Advancing age.
- Previous myocardial infarction.

Further aspects of the cardiovascular history are:

- History of rheumatic fever.
- History of bacterial endocarditis.
- Known congenital valve abnormality.
- Ankylosing spondylitis, Marfan's syndrome, osteogenesis imperfecta or Ehlers–Danlos syndrome, all of which may lead to heart valve abnormalities.
- Previous cardiac or thoracic surgery.
- Lower limb intermittent claudication or rest pain.
- Cerebrovascular symptoms.

Symptoms
In the assessment of a patient whose predominant features are angina or dyspnoea, a system of grading by severity of symptom occurrence has been instituted by the New York Heart Association (NYHA). It represents a means by which subsequent improvement or deterioration may be measured:

- NYHA 1 – No limitation of ordinary physical activity.
- NYHA 2 – Ordinary physical activity causes discomfort.
- NYHA 3 – Moderate to great limitation of ordinary physical activity.
- NYHA 4 – Unable to perform any physical activity without discomfort.

The following symptoms should be sought together with their duration and whether they have recently deteriorated.

Chest pain
Chest pain is a common feature of cardiac surgical disease. **Angina pectoris** is pain derived from the heart itself when the oxygen demand of the myocardium exceeds supply. This may be the result of coronary artery stenosis as a result of arterial narrowing due to atheroma (*Figure 20.1*). Angina is not only a feature of coronary artery disease, it may also occur when the oxygen supply is insufficient to meet the

Figure 20.1.
Left coronary arteriogram showing a bifurcation stenosis.

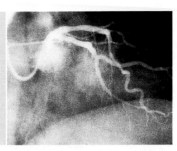

demands of an increase in cardiac muscle mass as a result of aortic stenosis or systemic hypertension. In these cases the increased bulk of the myocardium is due to left ventricular hypertrophy. A low cardiac output – which may occur from ischaemic damage or a cardiomyopathy – may also cause angina. It is not uncommon for these factors to coexist.

Angina is a strangulating pain felt substernally that may radiate to the arm, jaw or neck. It is commonly exacerbated by exercise and cold weather, and relieved by rest and sublingual nitrates. It may occur at night and wake the patient from sleep, and it may occur after eating. Angina may be atypical, e.g. presenting as epigastric pain and thus mimic the pain of a peptic ulcer. An episode of pain lasting longer than a few minutes and associated with nausea or vomiting may signify that the angina has become 'unstable' or that the patient has sustained a myocardial infarction.

Severe pain felt in the anterior chest with radiation through to the back is characteristic of an acute dissection of the thoracic aorta.

Pleuritic pain may be felt on either side of the chest. It is sharp and synchronous with respiration, and is indicative of infarction of part of the lung as may occur with a pulmonary embolism. It is characteristically associated with a pleural rub.

Dyspnoea

Dyspnoea encountered in the cardiac surgical patient is the result of loss of elasticity of the lungs, as a result of passive congestion. This may be due to left ventricular failure or valvular obstruction. In these cases congestion is said to be passive, contrasting with active congestion which occurs due to increased pulmonary blood flow as occurs with a left-to-right shunt in congenital heart malformations. The lungs in congestion become turgid and consequently require increased work of breathing to inflate.

Orthopnoea is breathlessness on lying flat and is the result of increased venous return to the heart when the patient is in a recumbent position. This increased blood flow cannot be adequately dealt with by a failing or obstructed heart. Also, when the patient is supine, there is 'splinting' of the diaphragm by the abdominal viscera and the volume of lung expansion reduced. It is useful to enquire how many pillows a patient sleeps with as more help to reduce the splinting effect.

Paroxysmal nocturnal dyspnoea is breathlessness occurring during sleep that awakes the patient, who is gasping for air. The mechanism is similar to orthopnoea but because sensory awareness is reduced during sleep severe interstitial and alveolar oedema can accumulate.

Wheezing may occur, in association with the above conditions, due to bronchial endothelial oedema (cardiac asthma) and the sputum may be tinged with blood.

Syncope

Syncope of cardiac origin is of sudden onset and of brief duration. It occurs in patients suffering from aortic stenosis when they exert themselves. It may be due to a decrease in cerebral blood flow as peripheral resistance falls secondary to exercise, or to high intraventricular pressures generated within the left ventricle. Pulmonary valve stenosis and mitral valve stenosis – when associated with pulmonary hypertension – may also cause syncope when associated with exercise. The fixed low cardiac output which results from these conditions is unable to increase to accommodate the demands of exercise. In the evaluation of syncope it should be noted that other causes should also be considered in the cardiac surgical patient, e.g. arrhythmias and atrioventricular block, themselves caused by ischaemic heart disease. Rarely, tumour or clot within the left atrium may cause a low cardiac output due to diminished ventricular filling.

Palpitations

A palpitation is an increased awareness of the normal heart beat. It may be the result of extrasystoles or tachyarrhythmia, an example of the latter being atrial fibrillation which often occurs in patients with mitral stenosis due to enlargement of the left atrium; atrial fibrillation may also be due to ischaemic heart disease. Palpitations may also be due to an increased force of contraction, as occurs in aortic regurgitation, due to volume loading of the left ventricle.

Fatigue

Fatigue is tiredness and lethargy. This symptom is of little use as an indicator of heart disease. However, in patients with severe heart failure, fatigue is commonly experienced as a result of a poor cardiac output, leading to reduced cerebral and peripheral perfusion. Beta-blockers used in the treatment of hypertension or angina may also cause fatigue.

Haemoptysis

A variety of pathological processes may cause haemoptysis. Mitral stenosis is a common cardiac cause. It may be due to the rupture of congested bronchial capillaries or pulmonary hypertension causing pulmonary congestion. Pulmonary apoplexy is the effortless sudden coughing of a large volume of bright red blood. It occurs in cases of pulmonary venous hypertension, the event acting as a physiological venesection.

The pink, bloodstained, frothy sputum of pulmonary oedema has a sinister significance. Pulmonary infarction – which may occur as a result of pulmonary embolism – is another cause of haemoptysis. Pulmonary venous or arterial thrombosis as a result of a large left-to-right shunt is a rarer cause.

Oedema

The oedema of heart failure (*Figures 20.2* and *20.3*) is the result of salt and water retention. Retained fluid accumulates in the feet and ankles of ambulant patients, and over the sacrum in bedridden patients. It generally worsens during the day and may be absent on initial rising as the fluid is resorbed on lying down. In severe cases pulmonary oedema, ascites, pleural effusions and leg and thigh oedema (*Figure 20.4*) may occur.

Additional medical history/identification of risk factors

Routine cardiac surgery is now commonplace and the mortality for operations such as coronary artery bypass grafts is around 1–4%. Nevertheless it is still a major undertaking and the low mortality is a reflection of improved surgical techniques, technological advances in cardiopulmonary bypass, myocardial preservation techniques and, at least in part, the

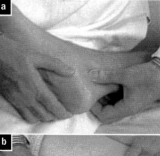
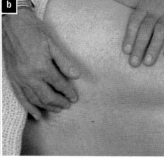

Figure 20.4. Oedema is demonstrated by digital pressure, leaving skin dents (pitting). Small amounts are first identified around the ankles, over the shin and on either side of the tendo Achilles and, after recumbency, over the sacrum.

identification of risk factors for morbidity and mortality. The latter is of paramount importance if complications are to be avoided, and if adequate prophylaxis and the early institution of therapy are to be carried out.

Related areas that should be considered in the cardiac history are shown in *Table 20.1*.

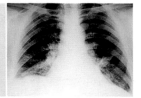

Figure 20.2. Radiograph of a patient in cardiac failure. This shows an enlarged heart, enlargement of the pulmonary conus (left hilar marking between the aortic knuckle and the left ventricle) and increased pulmonary vascular markings.

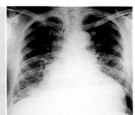

Figure 20.3. Radiograph of patient with pulmonary oedema. This is most marked at the lung bases.

Table 20.1. Related areas in the cardiac history.

GI tract	Peptic ulcer	Diverticular disease
	Hiatus hernia	Inflammatory bowel
	Gallstones	disease
	Alcoholism (men > 15,	Previous abdominal
	women > 12 units/week)	surgery
Renal	Functioning transplant	Acute renal failure:
	Creatinine ≥ 200 µmol/L	dialysis
		Chronic renal failure:
		dialysis
Respiratory	Chronic airflow limitation	Tuberculosis
	Asthma	
Valvular	Rheumatic/scarlet fever	Active endocarditis
	Previously treated	
	bacterial endocarditis	
Vascular	Carotid bruit	Peripheral vascular
	Transient ischaemic attack/	disease
	cerebrovascular accident	
	Deep venous thrombosis/	
	pulmonary embolus	
	Varicose veins	

Physical examination

General examination

The initial general assessment should determine whether the patient is well, unwell, ill or very ill, and whether the patient is anaemic, jaundiced, obese or cachectic. Examination of a patient's teeth is of particular importance when implanting a new heart valve as poor dental hygiene is a common source of valve infection.

Examination of the cardiovascular system

Clubbing

The common cardiac causes are subacute infective endocarditis and cyanotic congenital heart disease (p. 6; *Figure 1.8*). It takes many months to develop and is therefore not seen in infants, neonates or in acute endocarditis. The mechanism remains obscure – it might be due to hepatic impairment or as part of the condition of hypertrophic pulmonary osteoarthropathy. Another likely mechanism is the production of a blood-borne factor produced in the lungs or elsewhere and which has failed to be removed by the lungs. This latter cause would explain its occurrence in conditions of right to left shunts where a portion of the blood effectively bypasses the pulmonary circulation. Clubbing appears first in the thumb and in the great toe.

Cyanosis

The dusky blue discoloration of the skin and mucous membranes is due to the presence of unoxygenated haemoglobin (at least 5 g/dL). It is uncommon in the anaemic patient and is more common in the polycythaemic patient. Cyanosis may be central or peripheral. **Central cyanosis** (p. 11; *Figure 1.37*) occurs when the tongue, lips and conjunctivae are cyanosed, indicating the mixing of venous and arterial blood; it is improved by breathing oxygen. **Peripheral cyanosis** is observed in the extremities and is due to vasoconstriction and stasis of blood in these areas with a concomitant increased oxygen extraction. It will occur when there is an inadequate peripheral circulation as in shock, exposure to cold and in severe low cardiac output as in cardiac failure.

The arterial pulse should be examined with respect to:

- Rate.
- Rhythm.
- Character.
- Volume.
- Vessel wall.

The radial pulse should be examined for not less than 30 seconds. In cases of atrial fibrillation the **rate** counted at the wrist does not indicate the true rate of ventricular contraction. In this case the heart rate should be counted by auscultation at the apex, and the difference between this and the rate at the wrist is recorded as the pulse deficit. This phenomenon is the result of a varying length of diastole in patients with atrial fibrillation. When diastole is short, the heart barely fills and consequently the stroke volume is small and as such is not felt at the wrist although the heart has contracted.

The examiner should decide whether the **rhythm** is regular or irregular. If it is irregular the next decision is whether it is regularly irregular (usually the result of ectopic beats) or irregularly irregular (atrial fibrillation). In normal patients the pulse may be felt to slightly quicken in inspiration, and to slightly slow down in expiration, so-called **sinus arrhythmia**.

The **character** is best determined by palpation of the carotid pulse (*Figure 20.5*). The normal pulse has a moderately rapid upstroke coinciding with left ventricular ejection. As the left ventricular pressure falls, the aortic and ventricular pressures fall to their different diastolic levels. **Corrigan's sign** is when a large volume carotid pulse is visible in the neck. It may occur in states of high cardiac output and in aortic regurgitation.

In certain situations the character and volume of the pulse is detectably abnormal.

Slow rising 'plateau' pulse

This is typically found in aortic stenosis. It is small in volume and slow in rising to a peak as a result of the prolonged ejection phase of the left ventricle.

Collapsing 'water hammer' pulse

This is typically found in aortic regurgitation. It is characterized by a rapid upstroke and rapid descent of the arterial pressure wave. The rapid upstroke is due to an increased stroke

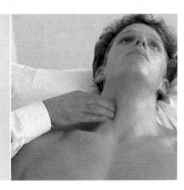

Figure 20.5.
Assessment of the character of the carotid pulse.

volume consequent upon a leaking or regurgitant valve. The rapid decline in pressure is due to the leak back into the left ventricle and also to a reduced systemic vascular resistance.

Pulsus bisferiens

This is a combination of a slow rising and collapsing pulse found in mixed aortic valve disease and hypertrophic obstructive cardiomyopathy. This is in fact a 'double pulse'. When the left ventricle is obstructed or empties slowly, the elastic recoil of peripheral vascular bed – which normally occurs in diastole and produces the dicrotic notch – occurs in late systole and is felt as a double pulse. In the case of mixed aortic valve disease it is the increased volume loading produced by a regurgitant aortic valve that causes prolonged emptying, and it is this together with an obstructed aortic valve that cause a double wave form.

Bigeminal pulse ('pulsus bigeminus')

This is the result of a premature ectopic beat following a sinus beat. There is a compensatory pause following the extra systole which makes the sinus beat larger than normal.

Pulsus paradoxus

This is an exaggeration of the normal response. During inspiration there is a fall in the systolic pressure and the pulse pressure (systolic pressure–diastolic pressure). It is normally less than 10 mmHg. Deep inspiration causes a reduction in intrathoracic pressure. This has a twofold effect – right ventricular volume increases and pooling of blood occurs within the pulmonary circulation. The overall result is that with inspiration the left ventricular volume falls, resulting in a lower **stroke volume**. It is an important sign in patients with cardiac tamponade. In these patients the fluid within the pericardium exerts its own pressure and the normal physiological response is exaggerated by further compromising the volume of the left ventricle. It is also an important sign in patients with severe asthma – in this situation severe air flow limitation produces a sudden and increased negative intrathoracic pressure which exacerbates the normal physiological response.

The paradox is that the heart may still be auscultated although there may be no pulse palpable at the wrist.

Pulsus alternans

This is when, in successive beats, the ventricle beats strongly and then weakly; there is an indication that there is severe damage to the left ventricular muscle mass.

The **arterial vessel wall** can be conveniently assessed in the radial artery at the wrist. The normal artery is easily com-

pressed on the radius. A rigid artery, e.g. in atherosclerosis, diabetes and renal disease, retains its cylindrical shape and may be incompressible. For this reason calcified vessels can give a falsely high blood pressure reading when measured with a sphygmomanometer cuff.

The jugular venous pulse

A measure of right atrial pressure may be attained from the jugular venous pulse (JVP). It does not measure volume but its level may give the observer an indication of the level of 'filling' of the cardiovascular system. It is an indicator of the competence of the right heart to accept and deliver blood.

The JVP is defined by three waves (a, c, v) and two negative descents (x, y):

- **a wave** – Produced by atrial systole.
- **x descent** – Occurs when atrial contraction finishes.
- **c wave** – Interrupts the x descent. It is a small positive deflection caused by a displacement of the tricuspid annulus into the right atrium as the right ventricular pressure rises. It is synchronous with ventricular systole.
- **v wave** – Results from the passive rise in pressure that occurs as venous return continues to the right atrium during ventricular systole.
- **y descent** – Represents the fall in right atrial pressure when the tricuspid valve opens and blood enters the right ventricle.

The **a wave** is distinguished from the **v wave** by palpation of the carotid artery. The a wave occurs immediately before the carotid pulsation.

Measurement of the jugular venous pressure

The patient should recline at an angle of 45° with the neck supported and the neck muscles relaxed. In this position, in the normal subject, the peaks of the JVP waves are just visible in the internal jugular vein. The distance between the right atrium and the sternal angle is constant whatever the position of the patient, however, with the patient sitting upright, the JVP in the normal subject is hidden from the observer's view by part of the thoracic cage.

Without distinguishing the three separate waves, there is a mean level which is the perpendicular height of the blood column above the right atrium. In healthy subjects this is the same level as the sternal angle: its value is 6–8 cm of water and this is the central venous pressure. In practice the jugular pressure is measured as the vertical distance between the manubriosternal angle and the top of the venous column, using the reclining position. It is usually less than 3 cm of water.

Variations in the jugular venous pressure

A **low JVP** occurs in hypovolaemic states. It cannot be measured clinically but the central venous pressure can by pressure transduction of the internal jugular vein.

A **high JVP** occurs in:

- Heart failure.
- Cardiac tamponade.
- Fluid retention including fluid overload.
- Constrictive pericarditis.
- Superior vena caval obstruction.

In cardiac tamponade or constrictive pericarditis, ventricular filling is impeded. During inspiration, when venous return is increased, the JVP is seen to elevate. This is known as **Kussmaul's sign**.

Absent a waves are waves that do not occur in atrial fibrillation as there is no atrial contraction. **Frequent a waves** occur in atrial flutter.

Large a waves occur when there is increased resistance to ventricular filling, e.g. tricuspid stenosis, pulmonary stenosis and pulmonary hypertension, all of which result in right ventricular hypertrophy. Commonly in tricuspid stenosis the patient is in atrial fibrillation and therefore the waves are not noticed. **Cannon waves** occur when the right atrium contracts against a closed tricuspid valve in complete heart block.

Large v waves result from tricuspid regurgitation as the ventricular contraction is transmitted directly to the internal jugular veins.

Examination of the precordium

The surface anatomy of the precordium is shown in *Figure 20.6*.

Inspection

Deformities of the chest wall should be noted, for example, pectus excavatum (funnel chest) or pectus carinatum (pigeon chest). Attention should also be paid to the spinal curvature, e.g. kyphoscoliosis. Gross thoracic skeletal deformities may produce functional embarrassment of the heart as well as making surgery and anaesthesia more difficult.

Palpation

The **apex beat** is the most lateral and inferior point of cardiac pulsation. It is usually felt in the mid-clavicular line at the level

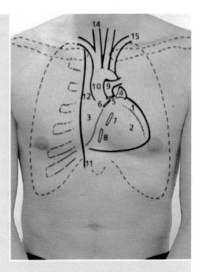

Figure 20.6. Surface markings of the heart and great vessels.

1	Left ventricle	
2	Right ventricle	9 Pulmonary trunk
3	Right atrium	10 Ascending aorta
4	Left auricular appendage	11 Inferior vena cava
5	Pulmonary valve	12 Superior vena cava
6	Aortic valve	13 Left innominate vein
7	Mitral valve	14 Right common carotid artery
8	Tricuspid valve	15 Left subclavian artery

of the left fifth intercostal space but is subject to great variation as a result of thoracic cage deformities and underlying lung disease, which push or pull it from its usual site.

In many cases palpation of the left and right ventricular impulses may be of greater value. They yield information as to which ventricle is under strain and whether the load is due to an increased stroke volume or is obstructive in nature.

Left ventricular impulse

The examiner's palm locates the apex beat. The nature of this impulse is of greater value than its position. In aortic stenosis the left ventricle is obstructed and hence the myocardium hypertrophies. This is felt as a powerful heaving impulse. In aortic regurgitation the ventricle deals with increased volumes of blood, the resulting impulse being turbulent and hyperdynamic. The left ventricular enlargement produces a rather more diffuse impulse.

Right ventricular impulse

This is palpable to the left of the sternum. Similar observations may be made when it is hypertrophied as, for example, in atrial septal defect and pulmonary stenosis when a definite 'lift' may be felt.

Thrills

These are palpable murmurs felt with the flat of the hand. They are caused by turbulent flow produced by blood flowing through stenosed valves or large volumes of blood passing through normal valves. Thrills indicate a definite abnormality. Systolic thrills in the aortic area are commonly due to aortic stenosis and, at the apex, are due to mitral regurgitation. A diastolic thrill at the apex is usually due to mitral stenosis. A thrill from aortic regurgitation is uncommon.

Auscultation

By the time the examiner uses a stethoscope there should be a well founded clinical suspicion of the diagnosis. It should thus be regarded as a confirmatory diagnostic tool. However, once the mechanics underlying the heart sound are understood, further information may be elicited.

There are four areas where the heart sounds and murmurs are most easily heard:

- **Aortic area** – Second right intercostal space just to right of the sternum.
- **Pulmonary area** – Second left intercostal space just to left of sternum.
- **Tricuspid area** – Fourth intercostal space, to the left of the sternum (left sternal edge).
- **Mitral area** – Point at which the apex beat is heard.

Heart sounds

First heart sound is caused by the closure of mitral (M1) and tricuspid (T1) valves. The cessation of mitral valve flow might also contribute to the sound. Electrical and mechanical events on the left side of the heart slightly precede those on the right. Therefore mitral valve closure slightly precedes tricuspid closure. The split is best heard over the mitral and tricuspid areas, but may be inaudible.

Second heart sound is due to the closure of aortic and pulmonary valves. The second sound is also normally split and is best heard in the corresponding aortic and pulmonary areas. The presence of two distinct components indicates that both valves are present and working. The aortic (A2) component slightly precedes the pulmonary (P2) component.

The gap between the first and second heart sounds represents the systolic phase of the cardiac cycle.

Third heart sound is due to the rapid expansion of the left ventricle. It is due to ventricular filling and is caused by the rapid filling of the left ventricle in early diastole; it therefore closely follows the second sound. It is a normal finding in patients with hyperdynamic states and in individuals under 30 years old. Later in life a dilated left ventricle, and mitral and aortic regurgitation, give rise to a third heart sound.

Fourth heart sound is, like the third sound, due to ventricular filling and results from atrial contraction, hence it immediately precedes the first heart sound. It occurs when the ventricle is non-compliant as in cardiac hypertrophy, as observed in systemic hypertension or aortic stenosis. It has been observed as a normal finding in young athletes but is much more commonly associated with an underlying pathology.

Additional sounds

An **opening snap** of the mitral valve strongly suggests that the valve is thickened and fibrotic. It is heard just after the second sound and indicates mitral stenosis. It is heard best just medial to the apex beat. In surgical terms it signifies pliability of the valve which may be suitable for a valve conservation procedure known as valvotomy, i.e. the division of fused leaflets. This does not occur with a heavily calcified valve.

Friction rubs are scratching/crunching noises produced by the movement of the inflamed pericardium. As they are high pitched they are best heard with the diaphragm of a stethoscope in systole although they may also be recognized in diastole.

Cardiac murmurs

Cardiac murmurs are shown in *Figure 20.7*. The heart sound and any murmurs should always be timed with the carotid pulse. The heart should be listened to in all four areas (aortic; pulmonary; mitral; left sternal edge) together with the neck and axilla. The patient is turned on to the left side to listen for mitral stenosis and asked to sit forward on expiration to listen for aortic regurgitation.

Listen first for sounds, then added sounds and finally murmurs. The bell of the stethoscope picks up low pitched sounds, e.g. third and fourth sounds and the murmur of mitral stenosis. The diaphragm picks up high-pitched sounds, e.g. first and second heart sounds and most murmurs.

Turbulent flow causes heart murmurs; it may be produced when there is high flow through a normal valve or normal blood flow through an abnormal valve.

Features of murmurs
Loudness and length

Loudness and length are proportional to the pressure gradient, along which the blood passes but they are not good indi-

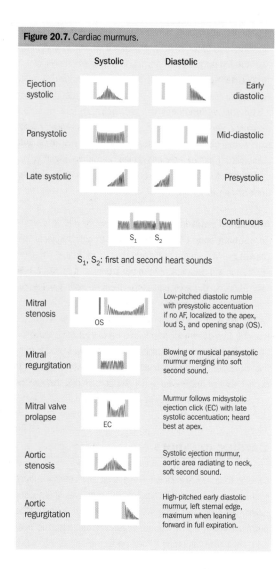

Figure 20.7. Cardiac murmurs.

Ejection systolic murmurs

- Aortic stenosis.
- Aortic sclerosis.
- Pulmonary stenosis.
- Atrial septal defect (ASD).

Aortic stenotic murmurs are harsh and radiate to the neck. They are best heard over the aortic area. Pulmonary stenosis and ASD are best heard at the left sternal edge on inspiration.

Pansystolic regurgitant murmurs

- Mitral regurgitation.
- Tricuspid regurgitation.
- Ventricular septal defect (VSD).

Mitral regurgitation is best heard at the apex and radiates to the axilla. Tricuspid regurgitation and VSD are best heard at the left sternal edge.

Mid-diastolic murmurs

- Mitral stenosis.
- Tricuspid stenosis.
- Austin Flint murmur.

Mitral stenosis is best heard at the apex. There is a loud mitral first sound, opening snap and low-pitched, rumbling, diastolic murmur. The patient should be rolled to the left side; the murmur is accentuated on exertion. A presystolic murmur may also be heard. The latter is caused by the cusps almost closing together at the end of diastole. Tricuspid stenosis is best heard at the left sternal edge. The Austin Flint murmur is sometimes heard in aortic regurgitation; it is produced where the flow of blood back into the left ventricle partially closes and obstructs the mitral valve.

Early diastolic murmur

- Aortic regurgitation.
- Pulmonary regurgitation.
- Graham Steell's murmur.

Aortic regurgitation is best heard at the left sternal edge and apex with the patient sitting forward and in expiration. Pulmonary regurgitation is best heard to the right of the sternum and is louder on inspiration. Graham Steell's murmur is

cators of the severity of the lesion. This is because, with a severely stenotic valve, the blood flow is so little that no murmur is present.

Character

- Mitral/tricuspid diastolic – Low pitched and rumbling.
- Aortic/pulmonary diastolic – High frequency, decrescendo.
- Mitral/tricuspid systolic – Blowing quality.
- Aortic/pulmonary systolic – Harsher, rushing.

heard in pulmonary hypertension, when it is due to mitral stenosis; this leads to pulmonary regurgitation.

Examination of other areas

- **Liver** – Should be palpated to see if it is enlarged, tender and, in the case of tricuspid regurgitation, pulsatile.
- **Ascites.**
- **Spine and limbs** – Check for pitting oedema of the sacrum and ankle.
- **Lung bases** – Listen for crackles after the patient has coughed.

Heart valves

Heart valves maintain the forward flow of blood through the heart. Pathology may affect the valve by making the valve orifice smaller, i.e. a stenosis, or by producing reverse backflow or regurgitation through the valve. Both stenosis and incompetence may coexist.

Stenosis produces a pressure load on the cardiac chamber immediately proximal to it. This chamber responds by becoming hypertrophied. Back pressure on other chambers and vessels may follow.

Regurgitation produces a volume load which has an effect both up- and downstream of the valve. The heart chamber enlarges predominately by dilatation but also to some extent by hypertrophy.

Pathophysiology of heart valve disease
Aortic valve
The haemodynamic effects of aortic valve disease are seen mainly on the left ventricle.

Aortic stenosis
A pressure overload is directed on to the left ventricle which responds by hypertrophy. With increasing size of the left ventricle there is an increased oxygen demand by the myocardium. When supply exceeds demand, the patient experiences angina in the absence of coronary artery disease *per se*. Syncopal attacks may also be a presenting feature particularly on exertion; these are due to the normal vasodilatation that occurs on exercise but the heart is unable to keep pace. Hypertrophy represents a compensatory feature for the progressive reduction in the valve aperture creating a gradient across the valve. As the aperture becomes smaller, so the compensatory mechanisms begin to fail and

progressive ventricular dilatation occurs. This leads to heart failure. Surgery is used to improve prognosis and to relieve symptoms, particularly if the aortic valve gradient is in excess of 60 mmHg.

Aortic regurgitation
A volume load is produced on the left ventricle, which responds primarily by dilatation. It is usually better tolerated then aortic stenosis but progressively leads to myocardial failure.

Mitral valve
Mitral stenosis
An immediate pressure load is placed on the left atrium. This is transmitted to the pulmonary circulation, which responds by progressive pulmonary hypertension. The left atrium is not usually dilated. As the pulmonary arterial pressure increases so there is an increasing load on the right ventricle. In due course the tricuspid valve, right atrium and liver suffer the effects of back pressure (congestive cardiac failure). In the early stages of mitral stenosis acute pulmonary oedema may occur, often as paroxysmal nocturnal dyspnoea. This occurs when the left atrial pressure exceeds the oncotic pressure in the pulmonary circulation. In some cases this is precipitated by the development of an atrial arrhythmia, characteristically atrial fibrillation. In long-established cases, pulmonary oedema occurs less frequently. Surgery is performed for symptomatic deterioration, particularly NYHA classes 3 or 4. A valve area of less than 1.0 cm is a further indication. The left atrium may contain thrombus, making systemic embolization particularly likely, especially if atrial fibrillation has developed – this constitutes a further reason for operation.

Mitral regurgitation
A volume load is produced on the left atrium and is also associated with dilatation of the left ventricle. When this occurs slowly, large increases in cardiac chamber size may occur before any increase in pulmonary artery pressure develops. In the situation where regurgitation develops suddenly due to rupture of a papillary muscle or chorda, the left atrial volume is small, the pulmonary vascular pressure rises abruptly and pulmonary oedema ensues with severe hypoxia. In the acute situation surgery may be lifesaving. The case is more complex for the patient with chronic mitral regurgitation. Valve replacement in this situation does not affect the damaged and dilated ventricle, which continues to require a high filling pressure. Overall the timing of surgery should be judged on the basis of left ventricular function as well as the symptoms.

Tricuspid valve disease

The majority of cases are due to secondary tricuspid regurgitation. This is due to right ventricular failure with long-term dilatation of the tricuspid valve annulus. This may occur, for example, with mitral valve disease. The clinical signs are those of congestive cardiac failure, prominent jugular venous pulsations, liver congestion, ascites and peripheral oedema. In a small number of cases the pathological process is rheumatic fever. Operations for these conditions are uncommon in the UK and are frequently performed in association with other valve replacements.

Pulmonary valve disease

This condition is almost always a paediatric condition and as such it will not be discussed further.

An atrial myxoma (*Figure 20.8*) is a rare tumor of the interatrial septum. It may interfere with cardiac function, and embolization of parts of the tumour may give rise to peripheral ischaemic symptoms.

Congenital heart disease (CHD)

Abnormalities of cardiac development include incomplete division into right and left sides (ASDs and VSDs), anomalies of the valves between the cardiac chambers, venous anomalies and combinations of these lesions (e.g. Fallot's tetralogy and patent ductus arteriosus – *Figure 20.9*). In addition, abnormalities of the aorta include aberrant aortic vessels and aortic coarctation (*Figure 20.10*). Coronary heart disease occurs in about 10/1000 live births. Although many lesions are incompatible with life, an ASD, for example, may be asymptomatic. Within these possible extremes, presentation in childhood is very variable, and a defect can go undetected. About 50% of such patients need medical or surgical help during infancy.

The most helpful clinical classification of CHD is into cyanotic and acyanotic varieties. Cyanosis most commonly indicates a right-to-left cardiac shunt with blood bypassing the lungs. It may also be due to mixing of the systemic and pulmonary circulations, abnormal communication through anomalous vessels or pulmonary AV fistulae. High degrees of central cyanosis are accompanied by polycythaemia and clubbing of fingers and toes. There is dyspnoea and exertional incapacity. The child is undersized, which eases the burden on the heart.

Fallot's tetralogy is an example of a complex anomaly. The primary defect is obstruction to the pulmonary outflow tract. The aorta overrides both ventricles, there is an associated VSD and consequent hypertrophy of the right ventricle. A characteristic feature of Fallot's is that the child takes up the squatting position when tired. Cyanosis may not be present in the early months in Fallot's patients. It may also occur much later in other conditions, for example, in a patient with an isolated pulmonary stenosis and a septal defect; cyanosis may be delayed until the shunt is reversed in the third or fourth decade.

Cardiac examination demonstrates palpable thrills, abnormal heart sounds and murmurs characteristic of each lesion.

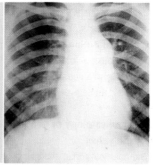

Figure 20.9.
Patent ductus arteriosus. The pulmonary conus is enlarged, the aortic knuckle reduced and there are prominent vascular markings.

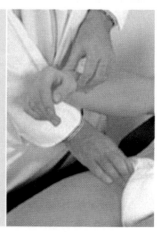

Figure 20.10.
In aortic coarctation the narrow segment is usually at the site of the primitive ductus arteriosus. Hypertension develops and the collateral channels are particularly noted in the intercostal arteries, notching of the ribs being present on radiographs. Radiofemoral delay is detected by the simultaneous palpation of radial and femoral arteries, the latter being attenuated.

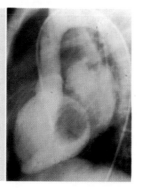

Figure 20.8.
Atrial myxoma.

Pericardium

The serous internal layer of pericardium, like the peritoneum and pleura, can become inflamed, producing pain. It may also develop an effusion. A further complication is calcification of the pericardium and this can interfere with cardiac function.

Pericarditis may be produced by viruses, bacteria such as TB, and inflammatory disorders such as rheumatic fever, scleroderma and polyarteritis nodosa. It follows 15% of myocardial infarcts and trauma such as cardiac surgery. These conditions may have an associated pericardial effusion as may chronic renal failure and malignant invasion such as with mesothelioma or sarcomatous lesions.

Pericardial pain is a retrosternal ache and can be aggravated by movement. It has to be differentiated from angina and the pain of myocardial infarction: it may also mimic upper alimentary symptoms.

A **pericardial effusion** (*Figure 20.11*) may produce **cardiac tamponade** when the amount of fluid reaches 1–2 L and interferes with ventricular function. Cardiac output is reduced and a pulsus paradoxus (an accentuation of the normal fall of cardiac output during inspiration) and cardiac arrhythmias may be present.

Constrictive pericarditis, due to fibrosis and calcification (*Figure 20.12*), interferes particularly with right ventricular filling, producing cardiac failure with a raised JVP, a large liver, jaundice, ascites and peripheral oedema. Another sign of pericardial disease is a pericardial rub. The sound may have atrial and ventricular components and be increased in certain postures and in inspiration. Electrocardiographic changes include reduced voltage, ST elevation and changes in the T wave. Chest radiographs show a globular, enlarged heart shadow with normal lung fields: calcification may be present in the pericardium.

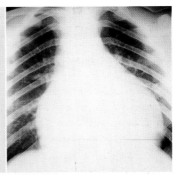

Figure 20.11.
Pericardial effusion. There is a globular enlarged cardiac shadow with loss of the normal cardiac contour.

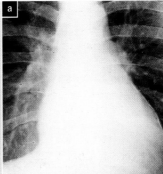

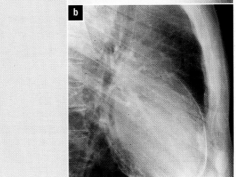

Figure 20.12.
a, b. Calcified pericardium.

21 The abdominal wall, umbilicus and the groin

The abdominal wall

The abdominal wall consists of the skin, subcutaneous fat and fascia, the three mammalian layers of muscles, transversalis fascia and peritoneum. It is important to determine whether a lump is intra- or extraperitoneal; a lump deep to the abdominal wall may be palpable in relaxed patients but impalpable when patients raise their extended legs off the bed – this is **Carnett's sign**. The skin and subcutaneous tissues of the abdomen may be subject to the same pathologies as those seen anywhere on the body. **Campbell de Morgan's spots** (p. 147; *Figure 8.59*) are common in the elderly and are of no significance.

Divarication of the **rectus abdomini muscles**, with bulging of the intervening tissues on straining or tensing of the abdominal wall, is usually seen in the two extremes of life. In babies the separation is above the umbilicus and resolves spontaneously. In the elderly, the subject is usually a multiparous female. The tensed recti can be palpated along the lines of separation, and the fingertips inserted into the defect on relaxation. The condition can give rise to cosmetic problems but is otherwise asymptomatic.

Spreading infection across the abdominal wall may be a grave sentinel sign of intestinal leakage and warrants emergency treatment.

Gas gangrene of the abdominal wall (*Figure 21.1*) occasionally follows spreading faecal contamination. It is accompanied by severe sepsis, malodorous pus, gas bubbles and a severe systemic disturbance. It is important to remember that air can be trapped in the abdominal wall at operation and so crepitus may be demonstrable for a few days. This is of no clinical consequence.

Haematomas of the rectus sheath are produced by tears of the rectus muscles or rupture of the inferior or superior epigastric arteries. The condition usually occurs in fit, young adults but may also be seen in the late stages of pregnancy or in the elderly. The onset of pain is acute and usually follows strenuous exercise. It may be associated with trauma or bouts of coughing and straining, and occasionally occurs spontaneously. It should be considered in patients on anticoagulants.

The haematoma is very tender, the commonest site being below the arcuate line where the posterior sheath is deficient. The superficial mass disappears on tensing of the recti but pain may prevent the elicitation of this sign. Bruising appears lateral to the recti but is slow to develop and may be absent. The condition may be misdiagnosed as appendicitis, an appendix mass or torsion of an ovarian cyst. A strangulated spigelian hernia is particularly difficult to differentiate. A tear of the right superior epigastric artery can mimic acute cholecystitis.

Skin discoloration is seen after applications of hot water bottles (**erythema ab igne**; *Figure 21.2*) in a patient's attempts to relieve unremitting pain. Haemorrhagic pancreatitis may be associated with discoloration of the flanks (**Grey Turner's sign**; *Figure 21.3*) or around the umbilicus (**Cullen's**

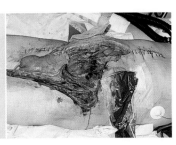

Figure 21.1.
Gas gangrene of the abdominal wall following large bowel infarction.

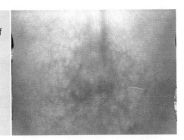

Figure 21.2.
Erythema ab igne of the lower back following the application of a hot water bottle to relieve pain in this area.

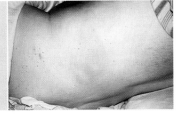

Figure 21.3.
Discoloration of the flanks in a patient with haemorrhagic pancreatitis: Grey Turner's sign.

sign; *Figure 21.4*) and leakage from aortic or iliac artery aneurysms may be associated with flank bruising (*Figure 21.5*).

Abdominal striae are stretch marks. They are most commonly seen in pregnancy where they are termed striae gravidarum (*Figure 21.6a, b*) and are pink, fading to thin white marks with time. The striae of Cushing's disease (p. 40; *Figure 2.33*) are typically purplish in colour.

The abdominal wall is subjected to innumerable **surgical incisions** world-wide and the majority heal without complications. There is an 8% incidence of wound infection but this is usually limited to mild erythema. Severe sepsis, as considered above, is uncommon and associated with pre-existing abdominal sepsis or faecal contamination.

A **burst abdomen** occurs in 1% of incisions. It may be related to poor closure techniques or materials but is usually due to underlying disease processes such as sepsis, the enzymes of acute pancreatitis, jaundice, hypoproteinaemia, malignancy, anaemia and obesity. Violent coughing, vomiting and abdominal distension may also contribute, as does pregnancy. The condition occurs 5 to 8 days after operation, usually commencing with a pinkish, serous discharge from the wound. This indicates that the deep layers have given way and that the skin is likely to follow if the wound is not resutured. The presentation of the gut through the wound after a bout of straining usually receives prompt attention. Minor degrees of disruption probably go unnoticed but may present later as incisional hernias (p. 275).

A fatty apron (*Figure 21.7*) may cover unsuspected and possibly symptomatic incisional, inguinal or femoral hernias and other groin pathology. Fibrosarcomata and desmoid tumours may arise deeper in the abdominal wall in relation to the muscles (*Figure 21.8a, b*). Mesotheliomas arising from the anterior parietal peritoneum have the clinical signs of an intraperitoneal mass.

Figure 21.4.
Periumbilical staining in a patient with acute pancreatitis: Cullen's sign.

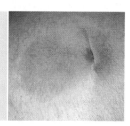

Figure 21.5.
Flank bruising following rupture from an abdominal aortic aneurysm.

Figure 21.7.
A fatty apron may cover unsuspected groin pathology.

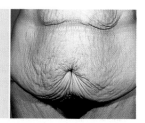

Figure 21.8a, b.
Tumours of the abdominal wall may be from skin subcutaneous tissue or the muscular layers. They may reach large proportions. a. Lipoma of the left side of the lower abdomen. b. Benign leiomyoma.

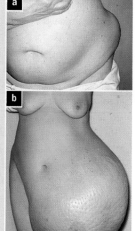

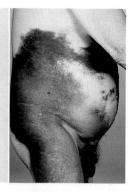

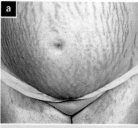

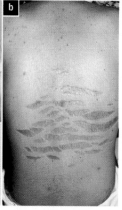

Figure 21.6.
Cutaneous stretch marks.
a. Striae gravidarum.
b. Skin marks following acute pancreatitis.

The umbilicus

The umbilicus is normally situated almost equidistant along a line joining the tip of the xiphisternum with the superior border of the symphysis pubis. It is displaced upwards by a swelling arising from the pelvis (p. 345; *Figure 27.14*) or downwards by ascites (**Tanyol's sign**; *Figure 21.9a, b*). When the abdomen becomes distended the umbilicus tends to partly unfold. This is a helpful sign in early cases of intestinal obstruction or if there is doubt about the presence of ascites. Unfolding also occurs in late pregnancy. The umbilicus is subject to a wide range of congenital and acquired lesions (see *Table 21.1*).

Umbilical infection

This may be secondary to congenital or acquired fistulae or may occur primarily due to poor hygiene, particularly in the obese, dermatitis, intertrigo and bacterial or fungal invasion. On rare occasions, infection can spread from the peritoneal cavity such as in a tuberculous peritonitis.

The following conditions are discussed elsewhere: **umbilical hernia** (p. 275); **exomphalos** (p. 331); **omphalitis** (p. 331); and **congenital umbilical fistula** (p. 331).

Acquired umbilical fistula

The umbilicus is a creek into which nature may divert a variety of fistulous pathologies. For instance gallstones have been discharged through the umbilicus and a discharging umbilicus has led to the discovery of a retained swab (inadvertently left in the peritoneal cavity at previous surgery); colonic diverticulitis and malignancy may rarely be associated with a faecal umbilical discharge.

Table 21.1. Abnormalities of the umbilicus.

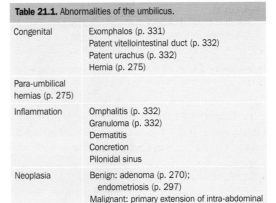

Congenital	Exomphalos (p. 331) Patent vitellointestinal duct (p. 332) Patent urachus (p. 332) Hernia (p. 275)
Para-umbilical hernias (p. 275)	
Inflammation	Omphalitis (p. 332) Granuloma (p. 332) Dermatitis Concretion Pilonidal sinus

Neoplasia	Benign: adenoma (p. 270);
	    endometriosis (p. 297)
	Malignant: primary extension of intra-abdominal
	    pathology; secondary (Sister Joseph's) nodule

Venous dilatation	

Umbilical concretion

Concretions within the umbilicus are surprisingly common, especially in the elderly. They are usually black and composed of dirt and desquamated skin. They are usually asymptomatic and often have never been noticed by the patient but they may cause local inflammation and a bloodstained discharge.

Pilonidal sinus of the umbilicus

This is diagnosed by the hairs protruding from the orifice; it is subject, like these lesions elsewhere, to recurrent infection.

Umbilical tumours are rare but incorporate a wide variety of benign (*Figures 21.10* and *21.11*), primary (*Figure 21.12*) and secondary malignancies.

Endometriosis of the umbilicus

In this unusual condition the umbilicus becomes the focus of a deposit of endometrial tissue. The principal signs and symptoms of this disorder are pain, swelling and bloody discharge of the umbilicus that usually, but not always, follows the pattern of the patient's menstrual cycle. Treatment is by surgical excision. This condition has also been described following surgical abdominal incisions involving the umbilicus such as Caesarean section and laparoscopy.

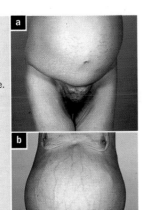

Figure 21.9.
The umbilicus is usually displaced upwards by pelvic swellings and downwards by ascites, but ovarian masses can sometimes modify this rule. a. Ascites in a patient with advanced breast neoplasia. b. Large ovarian mass.

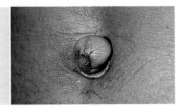

Figure 21.10.
Umbilical fibroma.

Figure 21.11.
a. Adenoma of the umbilicus.
b. Excised specimen demonstrates a remnant of vitello-intestinal duct attached to nodule.

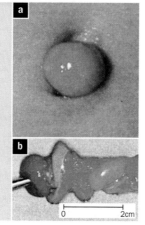

Figure 21.13a, b.
Demonstrating blood flow. The direction of flow within a vein can be demonstrated by pressure at a point (right side in a) and expressing blood first in one direction, controlling the pressure and releasing the original pressure point (right side in b). If the segment fills, blood is flowing in the direction of the expressed segment.

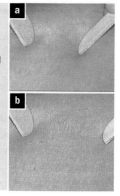

Figure 21.12.
Carcinoma of the urachus.

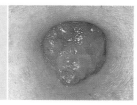

It should be borne in mind as a differential diagnosis in cases of umbilical swellings in women.

Secondary umbilical deposit

Widespread intra-abdominal malignancy, especially advanced adenocarcinoma of the stomach, may seed to the umbilicus where it grows as a nodule, known as **Sister Joseph's nodule**.

Venous engorgement around the umbilicus

This is shown on p. 386; *Figure 29.7*. Normal venous flow in the abdominal wall below the umbilicus is downward. In **portal obstruction** the direction of flow is unchanged whereas in **inferior vena caval obstruction** the flow below the umbilicus is reversed because some of the blood is shunted through the superficial veins to the superior vena cava. Determination of the direction of flow along a vein (*Figure 21.13a, b*) was initially and well described by Harvey in the 17th century (*De motu cordis*).

Lymph nodes in the groin

The superficial inguinal lymph nodes are, for clinical purposes, divided into a horizontal group, lying beneath and parallel to the inguinal ligament, and a vertical group, overlying the

femoral vessels. An enlarged lymph node, or nodes, may be the result of a primary source of **inflammation** from where lymph drainage is to the groin, or may be part of a generalized lymphadenopathy. Clinical examination must therefore include a thorough examination of the head, neck and axillae – sites of palpable lymphadenopathy – as well as those sites that drain to the inguinal nodes. Do not forget to examine between the toes, the anus and natal cleft, and the external genitalia (including the coronal sulcus in males). If no primary focus is evident on clinical examination, it is wise to consider:

- Cat-scratch disease.
- HIV infection. '
- Tuberculous lymphadenitis.
- Venereal diseases, especially syphilis, chancroid, lymphogranuloma venereum and granuloma inguinale.

Continued suppuration in infected inguinal lymph nodes may result in abscess formation. A careful history and examination should allow an accurate distinction of primary suppurative lymphadenitis from a psoas abscess pointing in the groin (p. 65; *Figure 4.6*) and a retroperitoneal enterocutaneous fistula arising in malignant or other inflammatory enteric disease.

Malignant nodes may be primary lymphomas or metastatic deposits from sites considered under inflammation – occasionally, the primary lesion may be widely separated or not identified (*Figure 21.14*).

Figure 21.14.
Malignant groin lymph nodes from unknown primary.

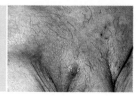

22 Abdominal hernias

General details and classification

A hernia is a protrusion of a viscus, in part or in whole, through a normal or an abnormal – congenital or acquired – defect in the wall that contains it. Abdominal hernias are common in both sexes and are an important cause of morbidity and mortality. Most are easily detected on clinical examination but a minority may be missed if the examination is not thorough. In abdominal hernias there may be a history of straining or heavy lifting, and obesity is common in hernias of late onset.

Groin hernias – inguinal and femoral – are the commonest forms (at approximately 80% and 10% respectively) except in early life and in black people, in whom congenital umbilical hernias are more common. Hernias may be found incidentally on examination, they may present with a lump or local discomfort and may be the presenting complaint of patients with increased abdominal pressure, particularly ascites. Patients with hernias most commonly present electively to the surgical outpatient clinic, but they also commonly present as surgical emergencies with life-threatening obstruction and strangulation.

A useful clinical classification is into reducible, irreducible, obstructed and strangulated hernias. In **reducible hernias** the contents of the sac can be completely returned to their original cavity. This may involve lying down or applying external pressure, or both. Although **irreducibility** may be due to adhesions of the gut or omentum in a long-standing sac, and may be asymptomatic, it can predispose to, and may indicate the onset of, obstruction and strangulation. The term 'incarcerated' is also applied to irreducible hernias, but as some authors also include 'obstruction' in this form it is best avoided.

Obstruction indicates blocking to the passage of gut contents, leading to the onset of colicky abdominal pain, constipation, vomiting and abdominal distension. It also predisposes to strangulation. In **strangulation** the blood supply to the sac contents is impaired, initially the venous and later the arterial supply dies – after which the gut becomes atonic – and perforates. The gangrene is accompanied by local inflammatory signs as well as accompanying toxaemia and systemic disturbance. Occasionally the contents of a sac may become infected, e.g. in appendicitis or from an ill-fitting truss. The signs are local to the hernia and the sac is not tense, although surgery may be required to differentiate this from strangulation.

Another diagnostic pitfall is a **Richter's hernia**, in which only one side of a loop of gut gets trapped in the sac. This knuckle, however, can strangulate without obstruction of the lumen. This occurs when the neck of the sac is small, such as in a femoral hernia, and the local signs are easily missed. The consequences are serious as perforation of the knuckle decompresses the sac, allowing the release of gut and septic contents back into the peritoneal cavity.

Abdominal hernias have three important physical signs:

- They occur at well-recognized congenital or acquired places of weakness in the abdominal wall.
- Most can be reduced.
- Most have a visible and palpable expansile cough impulse.

An impulse is often better seen than felt. If the patient is already lying on a couch, first ask them to cough and then raise their head and shoulders off the bed without the use of their hands. Visible hernias become more apparent and other lumps may appear during these manoeuvres. If the bulges are indistinct, ask the patient to stand erect with their head turned away from the examiner and to cough, while you observe the abdominal wall closely. With groin hernias, compare one side with the other while the patient is coughing. A palpable cough impulse is also examined for when lying and standing (*Figure 22.1a, b, c*).

After examining a groin it should be possible to say if a hernia is present, whether it is bilateral, whether it is indirect or direct inguinal, or femoral, whether it descends into the scrotum, whether it is reducible and what it contains.

Inguinal hernias

Inguinal hernias present above and medial to the pubic tubercle as they emerge through the superficial inguinal ring. They may be **indirect** (*Figure 22.2*) – starting at the deep inguinal

Figure 22.1.
Palpation of the superficial ring, above and medial to the pubic tubercle. a. Lying. b. Standing. c. A finger can be inserted into the superficial inguinal ring if passed along the course of the spermatic cord, by invagination of the scrotum. The invagination must be gentle and pass deep to the subcutaneous tissues of the groin. A cough impulse, coming through the ring, is then easily palpable. This manoeuvre is only required when a hernia is suspected but not identified by direct palpation for a lump and a cough impulse.

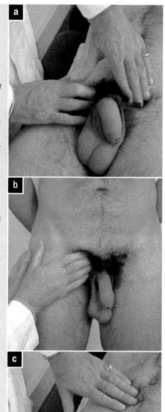

Figure 22.2.
Indirect inguinal hernia. It is not possible to palpate above the scrotal mass. This is filled with abdominal contents, passing through the superficial inguinal ring into an indirect inguinal hernial sac. The testis is sited posteroinferior to the hernia. It is possible to palpate above the scrotal pathology on the right side, which is a collection of spermatoceles above the testis.

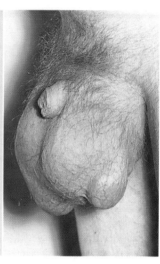

Figure 22.3. Diagram of Hesselbach's triangle.

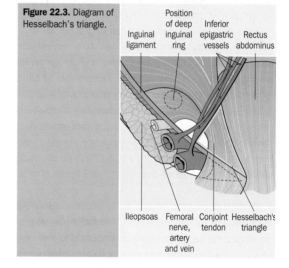

ring and passing obliquely down the inguinal canal within the three fascial layers of the spermatic cord (or round ligament) towards the scrotum (or labium majora) – or **direct**, starting in the weaker medial posterior wall of the inguinal canal medial to the inferior epigastric artery, through Hesselbach's triangle (Figure 22.3).

A clinical distinction between the two varieties of inguinal hernia is difficult: direct hernias rarely descend into the scrotum, reduce more easily when the patient lies down and emerge directly forwards rather than obliquely. Both forms are commonly bilateral but direct hernias appear later in life, are rare in women, do not occur in children and rarely strangulate.

A **sliding hernia** is an uncommon form of inguinal hernia, in which an extraperitoneal structure, such as the rectosigmoid junction, slides into the hernia alongside the peritoneal sac.

Recurrent hernias, following surgery on the direct or indirect variety, can occur throughout the length of the canal. They can be recognized by the overlying scar and are termed recurrent rather than their original form. In some thin subjects there can be an oval-shaped longitudinal bulge produced on straining, above and parallel to the medial half of the inguinal ligament. This is **Malgaigne's bulge**. It is a normal finding and not necessarily associated with a concomitant inguinal hernia. The key to the diagnosis of the latter is the protrusion of hernial contents through the superficial inguinal ring.

Examination of an inguinal hernia

Exposure should include the whole abdomen and down to the knees.

- Inspection – Look carefully at both groins. Inguinal hernias lie above the groin crease whereas femoral hernias lie below the groin crease. Look to see whether the lump extends into the scrotum or whether there are any other scrotal swellings.
- Palpation – Before starting, ask the patient if and where there is any tenderness and examine with this in mind. Feel the scrotal contents from the front as coincidental scrotal pathology is common (*Figures 22.2, 22.4*). If you can get above a scrotal mass, it cannot be a hernia. In women, an irreducible inguinal hernia must be distinguished from a hydrocele of the canal of Nuck (smooth; fixed; fluctuant; translucent; and a cyst of Bartholin's glands (confined to the labium majora and therefore one can get above it; p. 328). A lipoma of the cord often accompanies an indirect hernia and may occur independently.

Feel the groin from the side to determine the following characteristics of the lump:

- Position.
- Colour of the overlying skin.
- Temperature.
- Tenderness.
- Size.
- Shape.
- Composition.
- Cough impulse.
- Reducibility.

Inguinal hernias in babies and children are indirect, with a 25:1 male predominance. If the diagnosis is difficult to confirm, encourage descent of the hernia by holding a baby across the mid-abdomen with the legs dangling and gently swinging. Encourage infants to jump up and down, and children to run around. Remember that 15% of these hernias are bilateral.

Reduction should not be attempted in the presence of intestinal obstruction, or redness and oedema over a mass, since these factors suggest the possibility of dead bowel within a hernial sac, and this must not be returned to the abdominal cavity. First ask the patient if the hernia usually reduces and, if so, ask them to reduce it themselves. If this is not possible, the examiner should try. Pressure on the

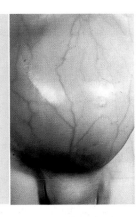

Figure 22.4.
Ascitic fluid has passed into a right indirect inguinal hernial sac.

fundus of the sac just pushes the contents over the top of the neck rather than through it. The thumb and finger of the examiner's hand lateral to the hernia is, therefore, used to squeeze and narrow the sac contents adjacent to the neck. Alternating this pressure with fundal pressure with the other hand usually reduces the contents of the hernia.

If the sac is full of gut loops the first part of the reduction may be difficult but, once started, the remainder reduces easily. In long-standing, large hernias, the omentum may become stuck within the sac. Initial expulsion of gut loops is easy but total reduction is difficult and may be impossible.

- Percussion – To determine the composition; usually tympanic gas but may be ascitic fluid.
- Auscultation – Listen for bowel sounds; absent in an omentocele and strangulation.

Don't forget to examine the other side (*Figure 22.5*). Examine the abdomen completely. If the patient's description is of a hernia yet no lump is found, re-examine them standing after they have walked up and down stairs and remained standing until the examination. If an abnormality is still not detected, re-examine after a month and then less frequently until an abnormality is found or until the symptoms disappear.

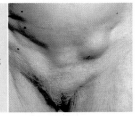

Figure 22.5.
Left inguinal hernia sited above the pubic tubercle. On further inspection a second cough impulse and bulge were present below and lateral to the right pubic tubercle, there being an associated right femoral hernia.

Differential diagnosis of inguinal hernias

- Femoral hernia.
- Communicating hydrocele.
- Hydrocele of the cord or the canal of Nuck.
- Undescended testis.
- Lipoma of the cord.

A **hydrocele of the cord** may be difficult to diagnose but if, on palpation, the lump can be grasped and brought down, towards the scrotum, and one can then get above it, the diagnosis should be entertained. Communicating hydroceles transilluminate and, if large, cannot be reduced; they may obscure palpation of the testis on that side.

Femoral hernias

Femoral hernias (*Figure 22.6*) are much less common than inguinal hernias (with a ratio of 1:8) and are rare before puberty. They are more common in women than men (4:1) although in women inguinal hernias are more common than femoral; 20% are bilateral. The neck of the femoral hernia lies between the lacunar ligament medially and the femoral vein laterally, and the inguinal and pectineal ligaments anteroposteriorly. The sac descends in the femoral sheath and becomes superficial by passing through the saphenous opening.

Femoral hernias may cause intestinal obstruction without the patient noticing a lump, and indeed, unless examination – especially of the obese female – is thorough, may not be noticed by the clinician. Femoral hernias arise below and lateral to the pubic tubercle, passing into the femoral triangle. Further expansion downwards is prevented by the blending of fascias and so expansion proceeds upwards to overlie the inguinal canal. Irreducibility is encountered ten times more frequently with a femoral hernia than with an inguinal hernia because of the narrowness of the neck of the hernia (within the femoral canal) so any attempts at reduction by the clinician must be extremely careful.

A much rarer form of femoral hernia – the prevascular femoral hernia – arises in the thigh anterior to the femoral vessels in the femoral sheath. It has a wide neck and a flattened wide sac; it is therefore usually reducible and rarely strangulates, although surgical repair is difficult.

Differential diagnosis of femoral hernias

- Inguinal hernia.
- Enlarged lymph nodes.
- Saphena varix.
- Ectopic testis.
- Psoas abscess.
- Psoas bursa.
- Femoral aneurysm.
- Lipoma.
- Hydrocele of a femoral hernial sac.

Differentiation from an inguinal hernia may be made by placing the little finger gently into the inguinal canal from below. If the lump is still present, or if it appears when the patient is asked to cough, it cannot be an inguinal hernia. A saphena varix may be visible as a lump with a blue discoloration in thin subjects (p. 388; *Figure 29.15*). It feels softer than a hernia, has a fluid thrill when the patient coughs – Cruveilhier's sign – and, if associated as it usually is, with pronounced varicosity of the long saphenous vein, there is a positive percussion or tap sign (p. 388).

Differentiation from a solitary enlarged lymph node (*Figure 22.7*) – especially when the enlarged node is in the femoral canal (Cloquet's node) – can be difficult, and the finding of a lump in the groin means that all areas from which lymph drainage passes to the groin must be examined: the lower limbs, buttocks, perineum, anus and genitalia. Femoral hernias in old, thin patients may cause visible distension of the superficial epigastric and/or circumflex iliac veins.

If the lump is an ectopic testis, examination of the scrotal sac demonstrates the absence of a testis on that side.

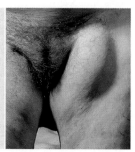

Figure 22.6.
Left femoral hernia. The lesion is larger than usual; it also demonstrates how it bulges upwards over the inguinal ligament making the differential diagnosis with inguinal hernia more difficult. However, an inguinal hernia would have passed more medially, into the region of the labia majora.

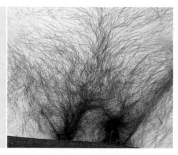

Figure 22.7.
Malignant lymph nodes secondary to a malignant melanoma. Comparison with the right femoral hernia in Figure 22.5 illustrates the potential difficulty of differential diagnosis.

A psoas abscess (p. 65; *Figure 4.6*), tracking along the psoas sheath towards the insertion of the psoas major muscle, emerges in the groin lateral to the femoral artery. Examination of the back and iliac fossa clarifies the diagnosis. A psoas bursa lies deep to the pectineus muscle and communicates with the hip joint.

A hydrocele of a femoral hernial sac is always brilliantly translucent.

Epigastric hernia

An epigastric hernia is a protrusion of extraperitoneal fat, and sometimes also a small peritoneal sac, through a defect in the midline linea alba between the xiphisternum and the umbilicus. Often, the smaller the hernia the greater the symptoms, which may mimic those of peptic ulceration with postprandial epigastric discomfort, possibly due to gastric distension pushing on the hernia. An epigastric hernia may be seen in an oblique light with the patient standing. The hernia is palpable as a firm, often tender, nodule. It rarely has a cough impulse and is only occasionally reducible.

Rectal divarication

Weakness of the linea alba may result in the rectus muscles separating by up to several centimetres. This is not a true hernia as there is no protrusion of a viscus through its wall, but rather attenuation of the wall.

Umbilical hernia

Congenital umbilical hernias (*Figure 22.8a, b*) appear at the site where the foetal umbilical vessels enter the abdomen. When the condition is associated with a failure of mid-gut development it is termed 'exomphalos' (p. 331). When it is due to a weak umbilical scar the hernia is variably sized, but on examination there is a palpable collar of fibrous tissue continuous with the linea alba. The hernia usually appears after a few weeks and is noted during crying. Complications are extremely rare and most disappear spontaneously within a few months. The condition is commonest in children of African descent and these cases are more likely to persist.

Most adult umbilical hernias are **para-umbilical**, in which about half of the fundus of the sac is covered by the umbilicus and the remainder by the adjacent abdominal skin. **Para-umbilical hernias** usually persist and may steadily enlarge. As the neck does not enlarge proportionally, these hernias do give rise to intermittent abdominal pain, although strangulation is uncommon. The omentum usually becomes adherent within the sac and these hernias are often irreducible. Women

are affected five times more often than males; the subjects are often multiparous and obese. Acquired umbilical hernias often result from chronically raised intra-abdominal pressure, the cause of which should be sought.

Incisional hernia

Incisional hernia (*Figures 22.9* and *22.10*) arises through a weakness in an acquired scar in the abdominal wall, usually

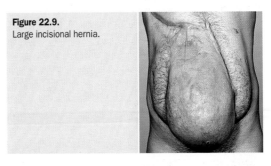

Figure 22.8.
a, A small umbilical hernia.
b. The hernia has become prominent due to filling of the associated ascites.

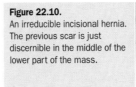

Figure 22.9.
Large incisional hernia.

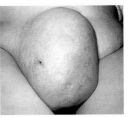

Figure 22.10.
An irreducible incisional hernia. The previous scar is just discernible in the middle of the lower part of the mass.

caused by previous surgery or trauma, especially if there was a complication such as a haematoma or wound infection. The hernia is usually large although the neck may be surprisingly small. The smaller the neck, the higher the risk of the hernia becoming irreducible and then strangulating.

Rarer forms of hernia
Obturator hernia

This can only be recognized when it strangulates, usually in elderly females. The swelling is often overlooked, as the hernia is covered by the pectineus muscle, but it may be felt as a swelling below the pubic ramus (in contrast to a femoral hernia). The patient often holds the ipsilateral leg in semi-flexion to limit the pain.

Lumbar hernia

This arises through the potential site of weakness in the triangle formed by the posterior aspect of the iliac crest, the latissimus dorsi medially and the quadratus lumborum muscles laterally.

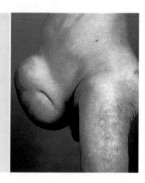

Figure 22.11.
Spigelian hernia.

Spigelian hernia

Spigelian hernia (*Figure 22.11*) occurs through the linea semilunaris, lateral to the rectus abdominus, usually a few centimetres above the inguinal ligament.

Interstitial hernia

This is a hernial sac passing between the layers of the abdominal wall and which is often associated with an inguinal hernia.

23 Non-acute abdominal conditions

Introduction

The diagnosis of abdominal disease poses many problems for the clinician. The abdominal wall is an effective diagnostic barrier and, although it can be traversed by ultrasonic probes of increasing portability, imaged by CT and MRI, and breached by the laparoscope, it can still retain many secrets which may only be revealed by an evolving disease pattern. A detailed history and examination remain the cornerstone on which to base a presumptive diagnosis and to direct appropriate investigations.

The symptoms are usually suggestive of the organ involved, such as a change in appetite or bowel habit for disease of the stomach or large bowel, and signs of organomegaly or tenderness, as in an abdominal aortic aneurysm or an inflamed appendix. Well-established patterns of investigation are available for each organ and system.

Another important consideration, however, is the **rate** at which the disease is progressing. A ruptured viscus or vessel requires urgent intervention once suspected, regardless of whether a definitive diagnosis has already been made. In surgical practice, therefore, it is common to separate non-acute and acute abdominal conditions, the latter requiring urgent management and often a laparotomy to both diagnose and treat an acute emergency.

This practice has been followed in the next two chapters. There is, naturally, overlap and 'cold' conditions may become acute. Cross-references are, therefore, freely given between the two chapters and also between them and the chapters on diseases of the alimentary tract and abdomen in children, and the chapter on tropical diseases, where common conditions encountered in the tropics have been grouped together rather than dispersed throughout the text.

Examination of the abdomen

Despite rapid advances in diagnostic investigations, clinical appraisal by careful history and examination remains the basis of good patient management. A thorough clinical approach leads to a realistic list of differential diagnoses that can then be refuted or strengthened by special investigations. The latter

are chosen to answer a specific question. Examination of any system involves firstly inspection, then palpation, percussion and auscultation.

Inspection

There is a great tendency to omit this most rewarding part of abdominal examination in one's enthusiasm to palpate, but much information can be obtained by simple observation, both about the patient's general health and any specific area of pathology. The patient must be sufficiently exposed to allow inspection of the whole abdomen, though modesty may be afforded by a sheet over the genitalia when these and the groins are not being examined specifically (but they must always be examined; *Figure 23.1*). The patient must be relaxed and comfortable; examination in the supine position with the head supported by a pillow in a warm environment yields most information. Good light is essential – daylight is best especially if coming in through a window to land obliquely on the abdomen, as this highlights any asymmetry.

Inspection begins with the hands, looking for clubbing, anaemia, jaundice, abnormal nails; spider naevi, palmar flush and Dupuytren's contracture. It proceeds to the mouth, tongue and dentition, assessment of the conjunctivae for anaemia and sclerae for jaundice, the state of hydration and examination for enlarged supraclavicular nodes.

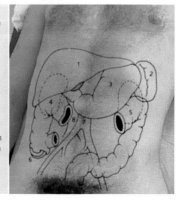

Figure 23.1.
Surface markings of the abdominal viscera.

1 Liver
2 Spleen
3 Stomach
4 Hepatic flexure of colon
5 Splenic flexure of colon
6 Appendix
7 Aortic bifurcation
8 Inferior vena cava

In the abdomen the most important signs are the presence of a visible swelling or distension. Striae caused by distension and erythema from the application of hot water bottles – erythema ab igne – may be visible; the latter is usually a sign of severe pain (p. 267; *Figure 21.2*). The presence of dilated superficial veins may indicate portal hypertension or inferior vena caval obstruction (p. 386; *Figure 29.7*).

Abdominal movement is noted during respiration and again when the patient has been asked to cough, to determine the presence of abdominal wall muscle rigidity. Voluntary guarding or involuntary rigidity are important physical signs; involuntary abdominal rigidity is associated with significant intra-abdominal pathology as it indicates parietal peritoneal irritation. Asking the patient to draw the abdomen right in and then blow it out as far as it can go demonstrates limitation of movement due to pain before any manual contact (*Figure 23.2*). Ascites (*Figure 23.3*) and large intra-abdominal masses or organomegaly (p. 284; *Figure 23.17*) may be easily apparent on inspection, especially through changes in the abdominal appearance during the various phases of respiration. The presence of any visible pulsation is also recorded, though this may be present in thin subjects from a normal aorta.

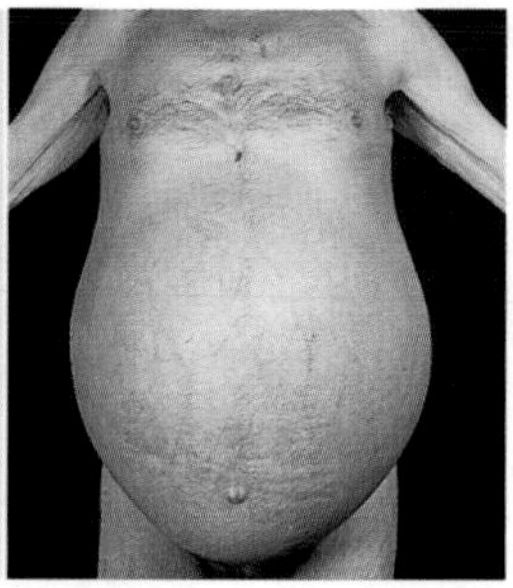

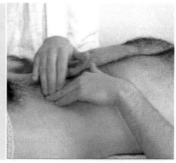

Figure 23.3.
Ascites.

Palpation

As palpation often provides the most information it is imperative that it be performed in a way which leads to the maximum amount of reproducible and accurate information. Confidence of the patient is paramount as, should this be lost, further useful examination is almost impossible.

Initial self-palpation by the patient (*Figure 23.4*) increases confidence and indicates the amount of tenderness and the depth of palpation that can be undertaken without discomfort. The flat of the hand should be used initially to palpate the abdomen superficially (*Figure 23.5*), the palmar surfaces

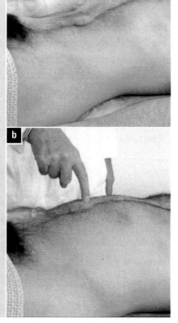

Figure 23.2.
a. Drawing in and b. blowing out of the abdomen demonstrates the limitation of movement due to tenderness and provides a good deal of information without any manual contact.

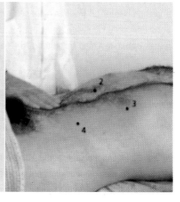

Figure 23.4.
Asking the patient to point out tender spots and examining them personally indicates the degree of local tenderness and is particularly useful in children.

Figure 23.5.
Initial palpation begins with the superficial assessment of the four quadrants of the abdomen, looking for tenderness, guarding, rigidity and obvious masses, always watching the patient's facial expression during the procedure.

of the fingers gently assessing the abdominal wall and contents. In order to avoid digging the finger tips into the substance of the abdomen, the forearm and wrist must be horizontal; this may be achieved by sitting at the same height as the patient on a chair, or preferably by kneeling at the bedside. The patient's abdominal wall must be as relaxed as possible. This can be augmented by asking the patient to breathe in and out through the open mouth, and even further by casual conversation between examiner and patient.

If pain is present the patient should be asked where the pain is arising, and the examination should begin at a site away from this area, only reaching it after the rest of the abdomen has been palpated. Start with light palpation whilst watching the patient's face – any wince or grimace is an indication of possible pathology and the area of tenderness and underlying structures that may be implicated noted. Following this, if the patient allows, deeper palpation is continued in the same fashion, the extent determined by the findings of the previous superficial examination. Deep palpation (*Figure 23.6a*) requires the hand to be placed on the abdominal wall at a slight angle, depending on the depth of the structure to be palpated. Very deep palpation may require both hands to be used, one on top of the other (*Figure 23.6b*). This is only possible if there is no

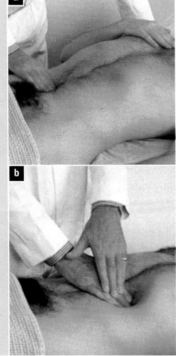

Figure 23.6.
a. Deep palpation is by firm pressure through the lax anterior abdominal wall, noting the size, shape, consistency of any organ or mass, and any associated tenderness.
b. Additional pressure can be applied, if needed, with the use of two hands.

marked tenderness and if previous parts of the examination did not result in loss of the patient's confidence.

It is convenient to have a regular format of examination such that all areas of the abdomen are examined, the epigastrium and right and left hypochondria in the upper abdomen, the umbilical and lumbar regions in the mid-abdomen and the hypogastrium and iliac fossae in the lower abdomen. Guarding and rigidity suspected on observation are confirmed by palpation. Guarding is a voluntary contraction of the muscles over a tender area, whereas rigidity is involuntary due to inflammation of the parietal peritoneum. It can be intense – 'board like' – after a perforated peptic ulcer and acute pancreatitis.

After general palpation for the presence of tenderness and masses, enlargement of specific intra-abdominal organs is determined, again watching the patient's face for signs of discomfort. The **liver** enlarges from the right costal margin towards the right iliac fossa and examination of the liver accordingly starts in the latter area, with the hand placed lateral to the rectus sheath – which can obscure the liver edge if well developed – and with fingers pointing towards the left axilla. The hand remains stationary while the patient inspires deeply through the open mouth, inspiration moving the liver down towards the right iliac fossa to touch the examining hand (*Figure 23.7a–e*). On expiration the examining hand is moved cephalad towards the right costal margin. Unless the patient has hyperinflated lungs, normally only the very edge moves below the costal margin on inspiration, except in the infant, where a two finger liver edge is normal. Riedel's lobe – an extension of the right lobe of the liver below the costal margin along the anterior axillary line – is a normal anatomical variation. An enlarged and inflamed gall bladder is also detected during this manoeuvre, the latter having a positive Murphy's sign (p. 287).

The **spleen** is not normally palpable, being hidden by the ribs, it enlarges from the left costal margin towards the right iliac fossa. Examination therefore commences in the right iliac fossa and proceeds towards the left costal margin (*Figure 23.8a–c*). The palpating hand is kept stationary during inspiration as the spleen, like the liver, moves with respiration. Only the lower edge can be palpated; it has a notched border. Although the spleen cannot be ballotted from behind, it can be displaced by pressure on the posterolateral aspect of the left costal margin which may allow the splenic tip to be felt subcostally in the posterior axillary line.

The **kidneys** are not normally palpable except in very thin patients. When palpable they are most easily felt using both hands, one pressing the organ anteriorly intermittently through

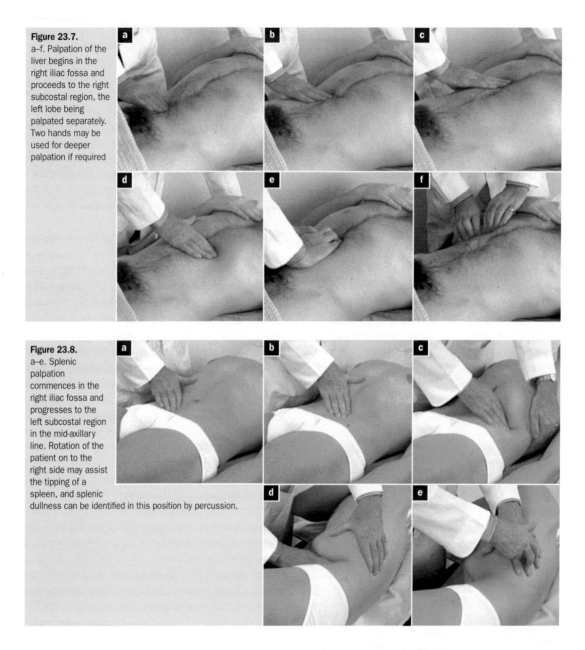

Figure 23.7.
a–f. Palpation of the liver begins in the right iliac fossa and proceeds to the right subcostal region, the left lobe being palpated separately. Two hands may be used for deeper palpation if required

Figure 23.8.
a–e. Splenic palpation commences in the right iliac fossa and progresses to the left subcostal region in the mid-axillary line. Rotation of the patient on to the right side may assist the tipping of a spleen, and splenic dullness can be identified in this position by percussion.

the loin (ballotting) to the other hand which is deeply palpating the mid-abdomen on either side of the midline (*Figure 23.9*). The kidneys also move craniocaudally on respiration.

The normal caecum may be palpable in the right iliac fossa and, on deep palpation, may even be heard to 'gurgle'. A loaded transverse colon may be palpable almost anywhere within the abdomen whereas a loaded sigmoid is felt in the left iliac fossa unless the sigmoid mesocolon is unusually long. The normal abdominal aorta may be felt in a thin subject.

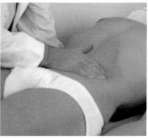

Figure 23.9.
The kidney is palpated bimanually, the left hand being placed posteriorly.

Percussion

The size of the liver may be established by percussion. Start over the resonant right anterior chest wall and descend through the dullness of the solid liver, until the resonance of the gas-containing bowel is reached below. An enlarged spleen is dull to percussion but percussion over even enlarged kidneys usually reveals resonance due to overlying bowel. Percussion should always be performed on any intra-abdominal swelling to determine its nature, whether solid, fluid filled or gas filled, or overlain by gas.

A general fullness of the abdomen may be due to **f**at, **f**luid, **f**latus, **f**aeces or **f**etus. The presence of intra-abdominal fluid may be best demonstrated by percussion. Ascites may be initially suspected on inspection as a fullness of the flanks or frank abdominal distension. The patient is asked to roll slightly on to their left side and the left side of the abdomen is percussed from the umbilicus laterally. The point at which the percussion note changes from resonant (bowel gas) to dull (fluid or retroperitoneum) is noted and marked. The patient then reverts to the supine position, and after a few seconds, percussion repeated; if fluid is present, the site of change from resonant to dull is more anteriorly placed (shifting dullness; *Figure 23.10a, b*). An alternative method for determining the presence of ascites is by eliciting a fluid thrill (*Figure 23.11*), which is based upon the vibration conductance of liquid. A third hand (the patient's or an assistant's) is placed vertically over the umbilicus and gentle pressure applied towards the spine. The examiner places one hand on a flank and taps gently and firmly on the other side – if fluid is present in sufficient volume, a vibration is felt by the stationary hand.

Figure 23.10.
a, b. Shifting dullness. The fluid level is identified by percussion in the supine position. The patient is then rotated through 45°. The abdominal fluid level changes, as does the surface marking of the level of dullness.

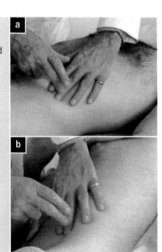

Figure 23.11.
Fluid thrill. Vibration of fluid is produced by tapping one side of the abdomen and feeling the other. The patient's or another observer's hand is placed in the midline to prevent vibrations of the abdominal wall and misinterpretation.

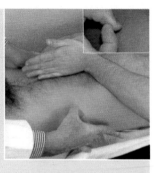

Auscultation

This consists of two parts. The first concentrates on sounds emanating from the bowel, the second on any resistance to normal vascular flow. Bowel sounds are rarely abnormal in the non-acute abdomen unless there is impending large bowel obstruction, in which case they may be increased in frequency, low-pitched in tone and cavernous in quality. Bruits due to turbulent flow may be heard in intra-abdominal vascular diseases such as mesenteric atheroma, renal artery stenosis and vascular tumours of intra-abdominal organs, as well as aortic disease.

Examination of an intra-abdominal swelling

Inspection alone of the abdomen may reveal an intra-abdominal swelling and, apart from its location and size, other information such as attachments to the abdominal wall or to deeper structures such as the aorta may be gleaned. Movement of the swelling with respiration is important to note and expansile pulsation may be visible with aortic aneurysms.

The whole abdomen is then **palpated** in the orthodox manner but with special attention paid to the swelling with regard to its size, shape, surface, consistency and whether it is of a homogeneous or heterogeneous nature. Note whether the swelling is freely mobile or attached to posterior or anterior abdominal walls, or to any intra-abdominal organ. Movements in relation to respiration are of special importance in this regard. If the swelling appears to pulsate, it is important to determine whether this is vascular in origin or is transmitted. An aortic aneurysm is expansile as well as pulsatile. If the pulsation is transmitted, this can sometimes be verified by the patient adopting the knee–elbow position which allows the swelling to fall anteriorly away from the aorta, and also allows easier palpation from either side.

Swellings arising from the small bowel mesentery are unusual in that they may move freely in one axis, i.e. in a line drawn from the right upper quadrant to the left iliac fossa, but not in the perpendicular axis, the latter being the line of attachment of the root of the mesentery. When there is the possibility of the swelling arising from the pelvis it is important to perform bimanual vaginal and rectal examinations to assess the intrapelvic component to the swelling, its mobility, and to assess the other pelvic organs. The bladder must be empty during pelvic examination.

Careful **percussion** should allow accurate assessment of the physical nature of the swelling.

Examination of a case of upper abdominal pain

In cases of upper abdominal pain the history and appropriate investigations are often more contributory than the physical examination; on occasion, however, careful examination can be most rewarding and is obligatory in all cases.

Common surgical causes of upper abdominal pain:

- Hiatus hernia.
- Oesophagitis.
- Gastritis.
- Gastric ulcer.
- Gastric carcinoma.
- Duodenal ulcer/duodenitis.
- Cholecystitis.
- Pancreatitis.
- Abdominal aortic aneurysm.
- Mesenteric vascular insufficiency.
- Oesophageal lesions – see p. 249.

Examination of the stomach

Non-acute peptic ulcer disease coincides with the acute complications of the disease on p. 300.

The history, and the findings at upper gastrointestinal endoscopy and barium meal examinations, usually yield more information than physical examination but the latter may be valuable and is essential.

Carcinoma of the stomach may arise in a polyp and in patients with pernicious anaemia; smoking is a risk factor

(*Figure 23.12a, b*). The disease is often insidious in origin and must be considered in every individual of over 40 with an alteration in appetite. Pain may be present and is constant, lacking the periodicity of benign disease; it is accentuated by gastric distension. The most obvious physical sign in patients with advanced disease is the generalized wasting, from the associated weight loss and reduced nutritional intake. Anaemia may be apparent, secondary to either overt or covert bleeding from the tumour. Bleeding is usually mild but small amounts of blood are denatured by the stomach, producing a brownish sediment (coffee ground appearance); the abnormality becomes apparent once the patient begins to vomit. The passage of upper alimentary blood per rectum is as melaena, a tarry black stool caused by the digestion of blood as it passes through the digestive tract. On occasions a mass can be felt arising from the stomach if the tumour extends below the costal margin; in most cases, though, the patient presents before a mass becomes palpable. If palpable, a gastric malignancy is characteristically hard and irregular, and the examining hand cannot get above it. The mass should move with respiration.

In advanced cases there may be signs of metastatic spread, both within and without the abdomen. Examination of the neck may demonstrate supraclavicular lymphadenopathy – Troisier's sign. Sister Joseph's nodule is an umbilical deposit associated with lymphatic spread along the falciform ligament. An irregular hard liver edge indicates hepatic involvement by the malignant process. Ascites may arise either from hepatic dysfunction or from peritoneal deposits seeded through transperitoneal spread. If deposits are situated in the rectovesical pouch or the pouch of Douglas they may be palpable on rectal examination – Blumer's shelf. The malignancy may be brought to light through an associated area of superficial thrombophlebitis – Trousseau's sign.

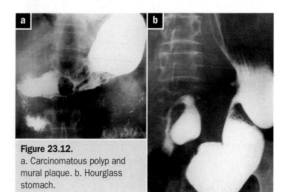

Figure 23.12.
a. Carcinomatous polyp and mural plaque. b. Hourglass stomach.

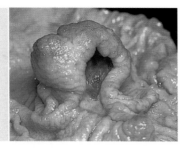

Figure 23.13.
Leiomyoma of the stomach with associated ulceration.

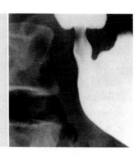

Figure 23.14.
Hypertrophic pyloric stenosis.

Benign neoplasms of the stomach include leiomyomas, neurilemmomas and neurofibromas, as well as adenomatous polyps (*Figure 23.13*). A rare glomus tumour at the distal end of the stomach may reach 5–10 cm, compared with the 5–10 mm diameter of superficial lesions. Other malignant lesions include sarcomas and lymphomas. Duodenal neoplasms are very rare and, when located, have usually arisen from the head of the pancreas. Symptoms of these neoplasms include haemorrhage, perforation and obstruction.

Gastric mucosal hypertrophy may develop in response to increased gastrin production in the **Zollinger–Ellison syndrome**. This is usually related to a tumour in the head of the pancreas; more than half of these are malignant and they may be associated with other endocrine abnormalities, particularly hyperparathyroidism. The symptoms are those of severe peptic ulcerative disease, with or without diarrhoea.

Giant mucosal hypertrophy may develop in **Ménétrier's disease**, when there is associated protein-losing enteropathy and, in the later stages, hypochlorhydria. It may produce diffuse upper alimentary symptoms and peripheral oedema from hypoprotinaemia.

Pyloric stenosis

Pyloric stenosis may be congenital (p. 333) or acquired (*Figure 23.14*). Pyloric stenosis leading to gastric outlet obstruction may arise from fibrosis secondary to chronic distal gastric or proximal duodenal ulceration (especially if there are 'kissing ulcers'), from gastric and duodenal malignancy or from extrinsic compression from a malignant growth in an adjacent organ. There is abdominal distension, fullness and discomfort. Vomiting can be profuse, usually frothy, and containing undigested old food from meals 1–2 days before. Suspicion should be aroused from the history and may be evident on careful inspection of the abdomen, which reveals peristaltic waves running from left to right. The presence of fluid in a dilated stomach may be determined by eliciting a **succussion splash**. This is done by laying the patient supine, holding either side of the rib cage and rocking the patient from side to side whilst listening with the ear close to the epigastrium (or through a stethoscope placed on the epigastrium); a splash is only significant if audible after three hours' fasting.

A wide variety of **foreign bodies** are swallowed by children and psychiatrically disturbed adults (*Figure 23.15*). The most common are coins, nuts and bolts, pins and safety pins. These may impact at the level of the cricopharyngeus or in the oesophagus but once they have reached the stomach they can usually pass through the remainder of the gut and can be managed conservatively. Complications include mucosal ulceration or perforation by sharp objects such as pins or fish bones. Occasionally ingested material can mould into a stomach mass (bezoar). An example is the trichobezoar following the chewing of hair (*Figure 23.16a, b*), usually in females; the mass may produce pyloric obstruction. Trichobezoars, like metal objects, are radiopaque and so can be diagnosed radiologically.

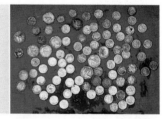

Figure 23.15.
Loose change from a collector's stomach.

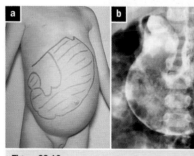

Figure 23.16.
a. Pyloric obstruction due to trichobezoar. b. Radiological appearance.

Examination of the liver (also see p. 303)
Hepatomegaly

Hepatomegaly (*Figure 23.17*, *Table 23.1*) arises in a variety of conditions and together with jaundice is one of the cardinal signs of liver disease.

The character of the enlarged liver is important in the determination of the cause. As the liver is examined by inspection, palpation and percussion, special attention should be given to the edge. It must be remembered that some causes of hepatomegaly – notably hydatid cyst and amoebic abscess – may result in enlargement into the thoracic cavity as often as into the peritoneal cavity.

Liver tumours are a common cause of liver enlargement. In the west, metastases are commonest, especially those from a colorectal primary. In parts of Africa, where there is a high prevalence of hepatitis, hepatocellular carcinoma is the commonest liver tumour; in areas of liver fluke infestation, cholangiocarcinomata are more common. Malignant neoplasms of the liver usually give rise to a stony-hard irregularity of the liver edge. When multiple they are of differing sizes. In advanced disease or when the tumour impinges on the major bile ducts, jaundice becomes an accompanying feature. A bruit may be heard over some large primary liver neoplasms and vascular tumours.

Cirrhosis of the liver

Cirrhosis is hepatic fibrosis and nodular cellular regeneration following widespread hepatocellular necrosis. The commonest causes of liver necrosis world-wide are viral hepatitis and alcohol toxicity but a wide variety of other conditions may be involved:

- Congenital abnormalities, including congenital hepatic fibrosis and cystic fibrosis.
- Drug toxicity, including carbon tetrachloride, paracetamol, cytotoxic drugs and repeated halothane anaesthetics.
- Metabolic causes, including haemochromatosis, hepatolenticular degeneration (Wilson's disease), galactosaemia and α_1-antitrypsin deficiency.
- Primary and secondary biliary cirrhosis.
- Primary sclerosing cholangitis.
- Chronic active hepatitis.
- Schistosomiasis is often the prime cause in endemic areas.

Symptoms range from mild lethargy to the extremes of ascites, portal hypertension and liver failure; malignant changes can occur.

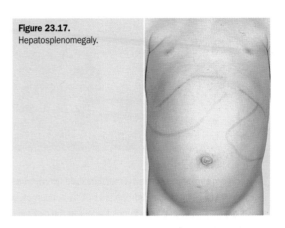

Figure 23.17.
Hepatosplenomegaly.

Table 23.1. The causes of hepatomegaly.

Infection	Viral	Hepatitis A, B, C, D, E
		Hepatitis non-A, non-B, non-C, non-D, non-E
		Infectious mononucleosis
	Protozoal	Hydatid disease
		Amoebic abscess
		Schistosomiasis
	Bacterial	Abscess
		Cholangitis
		Portal pyaemia
Cellular proliferation		Leukaemias
		Lymphoma
		Polycythaemia rubra vera
Metabolic		Haemochromatosis
		Wilson's disease
		Galactosaemia
		Drugs
Cellular infiltrative		Amyloidosis
		Sarcoidosis
		Reticuloses
Congestive		Right-sided heart failure
		Budd–Chiari syndrome
Space-occupying lesions		Abscess
		Simple cyst
		Polycystic disease
		Syphilitic gumma
		Haemangioma
Neoplastic disease	Benign	Adenoma
	Malignant	Hepatocellular carcinoma (hepatoma)
		Cholangiocarcinoma
		Metastatic, e.g. colorectal; breast; stomach; melanoma

Jaundice

This is shown in *Figure 23.18* and *Table 23.2*. Although in surgical practice obstructive jaundice is the type most commonly seen, there are many causes, and a careful history, examination and simple investigations should indicate the type. Obstructive jaundice is associated with itching of the skin which may cause intense scratching, pale stools and dark urine.

Liver enlargement associated with portal hypertension is accompanied by splenomegaly.

Portal hypertension may be due to pre-, intra- or post-hepatic obstruction of the portal vein. Prehepatic obstruction usually occurs in childhood and is due to congenital aplasia of the portal vein, or portal vein obstruction following omphalitis of the newborn. There is splenomegaly but not usually hepatomegaly; the child presents with anaemia due to gastrointestinal haemorrhage or hypersplenism. Prehepatic obstruction of the portal vein in the adult is usually due to chronic pancreatitis or pancreatic and other malignancies around the pancreas and porta hepatis.

Most portal hypertension is due to intrahepatic obstruction from cirrhosis. The signs may be of gastrointestinal haemorrhage – oesophageal varices – and liver failure, haemorrhage

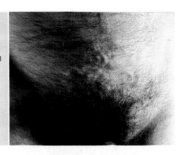

Figure 23.19. Visible veins over the lower abdominal wall in a patient with inferior vena caval obstruction.

accentuating the latter. There is extensive collateral venous development, particularly at the oesophagogastric (p. 250; *Figure 19.25*) and anorectal junctions, and over the posterior and anterior abdominal walls (*Figure 23.19*). The latter may be demonstrable as a caput medusae around the umbilicus.

Post-hepatic obstruction is rare and associated with Budd–Chiari syndrome, tricuspid valve incompetence and constrictive pericarditis. Budd–Chiari syndrome is obstruction of the hepatic veins and is usually due to neoplastic infiltration and usually a terminal event. Rare causes that need to be identified are congenital webs, clotting disorders – such as in polycythaemia – and certain hormonal therapies. It is also associated with herbal tea drinking in Jamaica.

Liver failure

This may result from any cause of liver disease and is therefore associated with other signs according to the particular cause. The degree of hepatic reserve has important consequences if surgery is contemplated, since the latter may precipitate total liver failure. Functional reserve can be assessed by investigation but the degree of liver failure can also be assessed by clinical examination. Indeed, Child's classification depends in part upon the clinical findings. Early signs include:

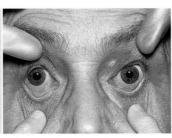

Figure 23.18. Yellow scleral discoloration of jaundice.

- Hyperdynamic circulation.
- Bounding pulse.
- Body hair loss.
- Spider naevi (*Figure 23.20a*); more than nine new crops indicates progressive disease.
- Palmar erythema (*Figure 23.20b*), particularly the thenar and hypothenar eminences.
- 'Liver palms'.
- Dupuytren's contracture (p. 457; *Figure 36.9 a,b*).
- Leukonychia.
- Clubbing (*Figure 23.20c*).

Table 23.2. The causes of jaundice.

Haemolytic disorders (pre-hepatic jaundice)	Hereditary spherocytosis	
	Hypersplenism	
Liver dysfunction (hepatic jaundice)	Hepatitis	
	Cirrhosis	
	Metabolic disorders	Gilbert's disease; Dubin–Johnson and Rotor's syndromes
Obstructed biliary tree	In the lumen	Gallstones
	In the wall	Strictures: benign; malignant
		Sclerosing cholangitis
	Outside the wall	Pancreatic, ampullary, hepatic and porta hepatis tumours

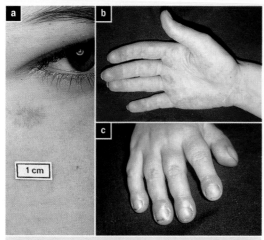

Figure 23.20.
Signs of liver failure. a. Spider naevi. b. Liver palms. c. Clubbing.

Later signs include:

- Ill-looking, wasted patient.
- Fetor hepaticus – a sweetish, musty odour.
- Jaundice.
- Gynaecomastia.
- Testicular atrophy.
- Ascites.
- Liver flap.
- Encephalopathy with cogwheel limb rigidity.
- Disorientation.
- Intellectual change.
- Convulsions.
- Coma.

Ascites

Ascites (*Figure 23.21a–d*) is the generalized accumulation of fluid in the peritoneal cavity, and may be a transudate or an exudate. The symptoms and signs are abdominal distension, dullness in the flanks and shifting dullness. Approximately 1500 mL of fluid is required before ascites is demonstrable clinically. A fluid thrill (*Figure 23.11*) may be demonstrable across the abdomen by tapping one side and palpating along the other; a third hand – usually the patient's – is placed on the abdomen in the midline to prevent false positives from vibration of the abdominal wall. With large amounts of fluid, mobile organs float on the surface and can be bounced (balloted) and felt through the abdominal wall. Among the many causes of ascites, malignancy and liver disease are the most common (*Table 23.3*).

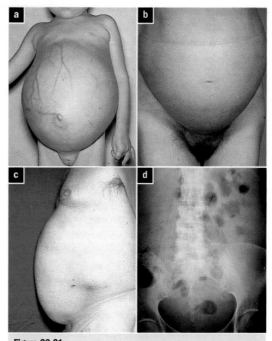

Figure 23.21.
Ascites. a. Cirrhosis. b. Due to ovarian carcinoma. c. Chylous ascites. d. Radiological appearance, the generalized opacity obscuring and separating the gut gas shadows.

Table 23.3. The causes of ascites.

Infection	Tuberculous peritonitis
Congestive	Right-sided heart failure
	Constrictive pericarditis
	Budd–Chiari syndrome
Hepatic	Cirrhosis with portal hypertension
	Hypoalbuminaemia (from any cause)
Others	Chylous ascites (lymphatic obstruction or transection)
	Meigs' syndrome
	Pseudomyxoma peritonei
	Pancreatic disease
	Intra-abdominal malignancy (especially with peritoneal seedlings)

Examination of the gallbladder

The gallbladder is a sac attached to the undersurface of the liver and it therefore moves with the liver in respiration. An enlarged gallbladder is palpable below the costal margin in the midclavicular line, impinging upon the examining hand on inspiration.

Pathology of the gallbladder usually results from the growth of stones (*Figure 23.22a, b*) within it; these may be associated with inflammation, obstruction and infection. The stones are usually mixed – cholesterol and bilirubin – but black pigment stones occur in haemolytic disorder and cirrhosis. The passage of stones out of the gallbladder down the biliary tract can cause further pain, jaundice and pancreatitis. A stone impacted in Hartmann's pouch and thereby occluding the cystic duct can lead to the development of a **mucocele** of the gallbladder from distension by mucus secreted by the gallbladder epithelium. Superadded infection may lead to an **empyema** of the gallbladder and perforation. More chronic inflammation may lead to a **fistula** with adjacent small bowel; a large gallstone may then obstruct the small bowel, usually the distal ileum. Cholecystitis (p. 302) may be acute, chronic or recurrent. A stone blocking the common bile duct can give rise to **ascending cholangitis**, typically presenting with Charcot's triad of symptoms: pain (similar to that of cholecystitis), jaundice and rigors. Impaction at Vater's ampulla may give rise to acute pancreatitis (p. 303).

Murphy's sign is a useful way of determining whether an inflamed gallbladder is the source of upper abdominal pain. This involves exerting mild pressure at the point beneath the costal margin where the gallbladder fundus would lie (in the midclavicular line). The patient is asked to take a deep breath in and, as the inflamed gallbladder descends, it impinges upon the examining hand causing the patient to stop inspiring as this causes more discomfort. Chronic cholecystitis is only rarely a cause of gallbladder enlargement because of postinflammatory fibrosis and shrinkage.

Obstruction of the biliary tree – often from pancreatic malignancy – gives rise to jaundice and an enlarged gallbladder.

Courvoisier's Law states that 'when the gallbladder is palpable and the patient is jaundiced, the obstruction of the bile duct causing the jaundice is unlikely to be a stone because previous inflammation will have made the gallbladder thick and nondistensible.' This law holds in the majority but there are exceptions, e.g. a stone occluding the cystic duct and a synchronous obstruction of the distal common bile duct; stones can form in the bile duct and the gallbladder is distensible. The converse – jaundice without a palpable gallbladder – certainly does not implicate stones in the aetiology. Carcinoma of the gallbladder – with or without associated jaundice – is rare, but locally invasive; it is felt as a hard mass.

Biliary strictures may be benign or malignant; 80% of the former are due to surgical damage during cholecystectomy. Stenosing inflammatory cholangitis is associated with infection by the Chinese liver fluke *Clonorchis sinensis*. This parasite is endemic in the Far East and is transmitted in raw fish; it is also associated with biliary stones, a dilated gallbladder, cirrhosis and, occasionally, bile duct carcinoma.

Malignant strictures may be due to cancers of the bile duct or within the head of the pancreas. **Carcinoma of the bile duct** is commoner than that of the gallbladder; it is associated with pre-existing gallstones in one-third of patients. There is an association with primary sclerosing cholangitis, clonorchiasis and ulcerative colitis. There is a slight male preponderance and patients are usually aged. Presentation is usually with jaundice.

For more on the acute gallbladder see p. 302.

Examination of the spleen

The spleen is rarely a source of symptoms *per se* except when massively enlarged (*Figure 23.23a, b*). Pain resulting from trauma or infarction is referred to the left scapula or shoulder

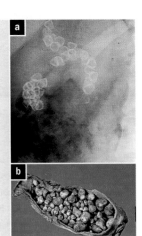

Figure 23.22
a. Plain radiograph demonstrating stones within the gall bladder and throughout the length of the common bile and hepatic ducts. b. Operative specimen following cholecystectomy for cholelithiasis.

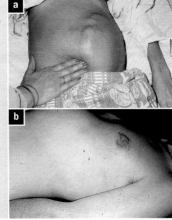

Figure 23.23.
Splenic enlargement.
a. Egyptian splenomegaly (due to schistosomiasis).
b. Splenic cyst.

as a result of diaphragmatic irritation (p. 304). A venous hum, maximal on inspiration, may be heard over the splenomegaly of schistosomiasis (Egyptian splenomegaly), heard loudest beneath the xiphoid process on inspiration – Kenawy's sign – and other types of portal hypertension. Although the majority of causes of splenomegaly (*Table 23.4*) are treated medically, hypersplenism or idiopathic thrombocytopenia may be indications for splenectomy. Splenic enlargement is almost always uniform.

Table 23.4. The common causes of hypersplenism.

Infection	Viral	Infectious mononucleosis
	Bacterial	Typhoid
		Typhus
		TB
		Septicaemia/abscess*
	Spirochaetal	Syphilis
		Leptospirosis
	Protozoal	Malaria
		Schistosomiasis*
		Trypanosomiasis
		Tropical splenomegaly*
		Hydatid cyst*
		Kala-azar
Congestive		Portal hypertension
		Hepatic vein obstruction
		Right-sided heart failure
Cellular infiltration/metabolic		Amyloidosis
		Gaucher's disease*
		Porphyria
Cellular proliferation/blood dyscrasias		Leukaemia
		Myelofibrosis*
		Polycythaemia rubra vera
		Pernicious anaemia
		Hereditary spherocytosis†
		Thalassaemia*
		Sickle cell disease*
		Idiopathic†
		Thrombocytopenic purpura†
Collagen disease		Felty's syndrome
		Still's disease
Space-occupying lesions		Solitary cyst†
		Polycystic disease†
		Angioma†
		Lymphoma*
Infarction		Embolic*
		Splenic artery/ vein thrombosis*

* Benefit from splenectomy. † Possible indication for splenectomy

Examination in pancreatic disease

The pancreas, lying posteriorly in the retroperitoneum, is impalpable and the diagnosis of pancreatic disease relies heavily on special investigations, notably ultrasound, CT and endoscopic retrograde cholangiopancreatography. The commonest complaints arising from disorders of the pancreas are pain and jaundice. The pain is constant and deeply placed, radiating through to the back, sometimes eased by sitting forwards and worsened by lying with the back extended. Jaundice results from obstruction of the common bile duct as it runs through the pancreatic head. Disease affecting the distal pancreas may remain relatively asymptomatic for a long time as it is distant from the bile duct and also from the nerves of the superior mesenteric plexus – the 'solar plexus'. The commonest chronic conditions affecting the pancreas are neoplasms – usually malignant although benign tumours are not uncommon – and chronic pancreatitis. The former usually present with jaundice and the latter with pain but this is certainly not absolute. Pancreatic neoplasms may present with superficial thrombophlebitis (Trousseau's sign). Widespread disease of the pancreas leads to diabetes mellitus and malabsorption due to pancreatic exocrine insufficiency.

Hormone-secreting tumours arising in the pancreas present with the effects of the excess secretion of hormone rather than pancreatic signs. These tumours (such as gastrin-secreting tumours causing intractable peptic ulceration in the Zollinger–Ellison syndrome (p. 300) and insulin secreting tumours causing symptoms and signs of hypoglycaemia) are not palpable and can be very difficult to locate even with special investigations. Hypoglycaemic symptoms of insulinomas often wake the patient in the early morning and are precipitated by starvation or exercise. There is hunger, malaise and vague abdominal pain, with sweating, trembling, dizziness and blurred vision. Severe symptoms include incoordination, slurred speech, diplopia, hallucinations, altered consciousness and epilepsy. Symptoms can be mistaken for those of intracranial pathology and the diagnosis rests on finding a very low blood sugar during an attack.

One of the few pancreatic conditions in which abdominal examination may be very rewarding is that of pancreatic pseudocyst, a complication of acute pancreatitis. A firm, usually vaguely tender swelling is palpable in the epigastrium which the examining hand can get below but not usually above. Although filled with heterogeneous secretions, percussion may be resonant due to the overlying stomach.

For more on acute pancreatic disease see p. 303.

The adrenals

The adrenal glands are deeply placed in the abdomen, adjacent to the upper pole of each kidney and are, therefore, rarely large enough to produce local abnormal signs (*Figure 23.24*). However, malfunction of their hormone secretion has profound systemic effects. Acute destruction of the gland usually results from haemorrhage or sepsis. Haemorrhage may occur at birth and is usually fatal. In later life it may follow meningococcal septicaemia and is followed by hyperpyrexia and profound shock – Waterhouse–Friderichsen syndrome.

Chronic destruction of the glands may follow TB infection or replacement by metastatic deposits. The clinical effect of hyposecretion is Addison's disease (p. 40). Hypersecretion is due to hyperplasia, or benign or malignant neoplasms; hyperplasia is usually secondary to a pituitary disorder and the clinical picture is usually that of Cushing's syndrome (p. 39). A tumour may also produce aldosterone – Conn's syndrome. In this syndrome there is sodium retention and increased potassium loss, the clinical presentation being with muscle weakness, polydipsia, polyuria and hypertension.

Tumours of the adrenal medulla may be neurogenic, or neoplasms of chromaffin cells. Neurogenic tumours may be benign ganglioneuromas or malignant neuroblastomas. The latter occur in children, grow rapidly to a large size and metastasize early. They may secrete vasoactive intestinal polypeptide (VIP) but the clinical picture is usually that of weight loss, abdominal pain, distension, ascites, fever and anaemia.

Figure 23.24.
Large left phaeochromocytoma.
a. Displacement of the stomach. b. Tumour blood supply.

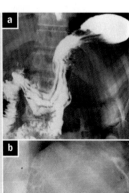

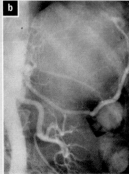

Chromaffin tumours are phaeochromocytomatas, which make up 10% of adrenal tumours, 10% being bilateral and are 10% malignant; 10% are also found outside the adrenal medulla and 10% have a familial history. The tumours secrete adrenergic substances, particularly noradrenalin, producing sustained, marked hypertension that can give rise to fatal cerebral haemorrhage and cardiac dysrhythmias. The patient complains bitterly of feeling unwell with headache, palpitations, dyspnoea, vomiting and generalized weakness. There may be associated hyperparathyroidism and medullary carcinoma of the thyroid, in the multiple endocrine neoplasia syndrome (MEN II). Many of these symptoms are non-specific and the diagnosis must always be kept in mind, especially when hypertension is not a prominent feature.

Multiple endocrine adenomas may occur in the same patient in the **multiple endocrine neoplasia syndrome** (**MEN**). These tumours have a common cell type, characterized by amine precursor uptake and decarboxylation cells; MEN syndromes have two main varieties, MEN I and II, and are inherited as an autosomal dominant – members of the same family have the same variety of the syndrome.

The commonest variant is MEN type I which is made up as follows:

- Parathyroid tumours (80%).
- Islet tumours of the pancreas, producing gastrin (Zollinger–Ellison syndrome), insulin, glucagon, somatostatin and VIP.
- Pituitary chromaffin adenomas (65%), producing prolactin or giving rise to acromegaly.
- Thyroid and adrenocortical tumours.

In MEN type IIa there is a 50% incidence of parathyroid tumours, together with medullary carcinoma of the thyroid, producing calcitonin and phaeochromocytomas. Type IIb, in addition, has neurological components with the presence of neuromas of the eyelids and lips, and ganglioneuromatosis, together with marfanoid facial appearances and megacolon.

The small bowel

The small bowel (see also p. 307) is the site of absorption of most nutrients, hence extensive small bowel disease leads to a malabsorptive state. Small bowel obstruction – usually from adhesions after previous abdominal surgery or due to hernias – gives rise to midgut colic, felt periumbilically. Inflammation of the small bowel may be evident as a tender palpable mass in the right iliac fossa. Malignancies of the small bowel are rare and usually present as obstruction, perforation or bleeding.

Peutz–Jeghers syndrome

This manifests as pigmentation of the lips and intestinal poly-posis. The syndrome is characterized by spots, varying from brown to black, on and about the vermilion surfaces of the lips (*Figure 23.25*). The condition is strongly familial and is the outward sign of adenomatous polyposis of the small intes-tine. The polyps may bleed, intussuscept and, on rare occa-sions, become malignant. Occult blood is present in the stool and attacks of melaena are common.

Crohn's disease

Although most commonly a disease affecting the small bowel, this disease of unknown aetiology may affect any part of the gastrointestinal tract from the mouth to the anus. Crohn's is grouped with ulcerative colitis as **inflammatory bowel dis-ease** because of the clinical similarities but they differ histo-logically in their depth of lesion – ulcerative colitis only involves the mucosa and submucosa. The full thickness of inflammation of the bowel wall in Crohn's disease classically occurs as skip lesions with macroscopically normal bowel between the areas of chronic inflammation (*Figure 23.26*). Ulceration, fissures, perforation with abscess formation or peritonitis, fistulae (p. 295; *Figure 23.36*) with adjacent structures (gut; urinary tract; vagina; skin) and obstruction, either due to active inflammation or fibrosis of a previously inflamed segment of bowel, are all classic features.

Diarrhoea is less constant in Crohn's disease than with ulcerative colitis but colicky abdominal pain is more prominent and there is often a 'food fear' of precipitating symptoms with consequent weight loss. Fulminating toxic colitis (p. 312) may occur. The disease usually commences in the age range 15–40 and there is a slight female predominance. Physical signs depend upon the disease activity and site. In the abdomen, a mass is a common finding, and perianal disease (*Figure 23.27*) is usually observable, either as acute abscess and fis-tula formation or as residual perianal tags and fissuring.

Tuberculous enteritis

Although rare in the western world, tuberculous enteritis (*Figure 23.28a, b*) is similar to Crohn's disease of the ileum. Involved tuberculous nodes may present with a periumbilical mass, most commonly seen in children, and accompanied by central mild but constant pain. Extra-intestinal manifestations of TB may be present in the lungs or renal tract.

In the assessment of patients with suspected inflamma-tory bowel disease, it is important to examine the stools to exclude abnormal bacteria – e.g. *Salmonella*, *Shigella*, *Yersinia* and *Giardia* spp. – and parasites (amoebiasis). *Clostridium difficile* should be identified to exclude the pos-sibility of **pseudomembranous colitis**, the growth of this organism becoming prolific and causing the disease follow-ing the administration of certain antibiotics.

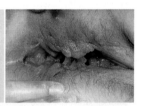

Figure 23.27.
Perianal Crohn's disease.

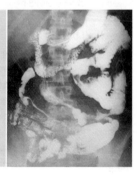

Figure 23.25.
Perioral pigmentation in a patient with Peutz–Jeghers syndrome.

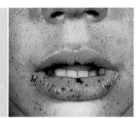

Figure 23.26.
Crohn's disease of terminal ileum demonstrating the sting sign of Cantor.

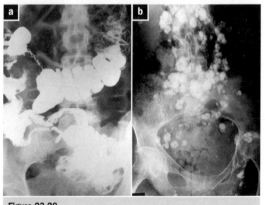

Figure 23.28.
Abdominal TB. a. Stricture of the hepatic flexure of the colon.
b. Calcification in tuberculous lymphadenitis.

Colonic and rectal disease

Alteration in bowel habit

Individuals vary considerably in the number of times they evacuate their bowels, a quoted range being from three times a day to every third day. Thus, in assessing diarrhoea and constipation, it is essential to establish what is the normal frequency for each individual. Also determine what a patient means by the terms diarrhoea and constipation since this not only implies changes in frequency but also the quantity and consistency of the stool and ease or difficulty in evacuation. A key feature, however, is always **change** from an individual's normal pattern. Everyone has experienced this change since modification of diet, alcohol intake and overseas trips affect dietary flora and bowel habit, as do changes in daily routine, such as reduced mobility and dietary change, due to confinement to bed at home or in hospital.

Diarrhoea is most commonly due to infection, either endemic or epidemic. Organisms in temperate climates are commonly *Salmonella* sp. and *Escherichia coli* whereas in tropical areas a wide variety of bacterial, viral and parasitic agents may be involved (p. 150). Ingestion of purgatives and antibiotics may precipitate diarrhoea while pancreatic disorders, such as chronic pancreatitis and cystic fibrosis, can give rise to steatorrhea (*Figure 23.29*) as can small gut abnormalities such as gluten-induced or protein-losing enteropathy. Diarrhoea is a common symptom of inflammatory bowel disease, particularly ulcerative colitis. Surgical interventions producing the symptom include gastrectomy, vagotomy, blind loop syndromes and small bowel resection, while fistulae and stomas both decrease bowel transit time. Systemic diseases producing diarrhoea include thyrotoxicosis, uraemia, and carcinoid and Zollinger–Ellison syndromes.

Spurious diarrhoea is the leakage of faecal fluid around impacted faeces. Subacute obstruction due to stenotic bowel lesions, such as large bowel malignancy, may produce alternating diarrhoea and constipation (p. 327). It is for this reason that any change in bowel habit in an individual over 45 years old must be considered as due to malignant large bowel disease until proved otherwise (in the same way that change in appetite should be ascribed to a gastric neoplasm).

Constipation is a cardinal sign of acute intestinal obstruction, together with vomiting, abdominal distension and colicky abdominal pain; vomiting predominates in high, and constipation in distal, bowel obstruction (p. 307). In obstruction, the patient may open their bowels after the onset of symptoms and an enema may produce a good result. However, there is no further passage of flatus and no response to a second enema, whereas obstruction from faecal impaction responds to repeated enemas. Lack of food and fluid, as in starvation and cachexia, reduces stool content and frequency of bowel action. Non-obstructive and subacutely obstructing large bowel stenotic lesions, such as malignancy and diverticulitis, produce alteration in bowel habit and possibly alternating diarrhoea and constipation (see above).

Peritoneal inflammatory disorders, such as appendicitis, pelvic inflammatory disease, peritonitis, perforation, and biliary and renal colic are usually accompanied by constipation. Transit time is delayed by drugs (analgesics and ganglion blockers) and adynamic disorders – such as Hirschsprung's (p. 312; *Figure 24.11b*) and Chagas' megacolon – produce aganglionosis of the large bowel (Chagas' – American trypanosomiasis – also produces megaoesophagus). Other causes of constipation include disorders of the spinal cord and myxoedema. Pelvic masses such as pregnancy, fibroids and uterine ovarian tumours inhibit defecation, as do painful anal lesions such as fissures, abscesses and complicated haemorrhoids.

Bleeding may be overt or covert and the latter may present with the associated symptoms of anaemia. Other symptoms are abdominal pain, weight loss and the passage of mucus per rectum. The nature of these symptoms are to a large extent determined by the site of the pathology. Thus fresh bleeding is more often seen with left-sided colon disease, and covert bleeding and anaemia with right-sided tumours. As the right colon is more capacious than the left, lesions on the right produce non-specific symptoms of postprandial fullness or heaviness, whereas left-sided lesions result in obstructive type symptoms of colicky abdominal pain and a more definite change in bowel habit.

Common disorders affecting the large bowel include colorectal cancer, the second most common malignancy in both males and females in the UK. Ulcerative colitis is a mucosal disease limited to the large bowel. Ulcerative colitis and Crohn's disease are collectively grouped as **inflammatory**

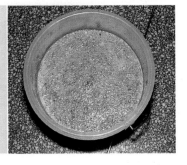

Figure 23.29.
Stool from a patient with steatorrhoea.

bowel disease since their symptoms are similar and they are both of unknown aetiology. Diverticular disease is a condition seen more commonly in the western world; it is associated with increased intraluminal pressures consequent upon eating highly refined foodstuffs with little indigestible fibre. Although investigations – usually by double contrast barium enema, instant water soluble contrast enema or colonoscopy – are necessary to confirm clinical suspicion, a detailed history and clinical examination often yield useful information. Clinical examination is incomplete without digital rectal examination and proctosigmoidoscopy.

Carcinoma of the colon and rectum

Large bowel cancer is the second commonest malignancy in males and the fourth in females. It usually occurs after the age of 50 but can occur in the young adult, when it has a poor prognosis. The lesion usually starts in a benign polyp and these frequently coexist; a second carcinoma is present in 5% of patients. The lesion is usually an adenocarcinoma, there being a raised, everted edge to the ulcer and an indurated base. On presentation the ulcer is usually confined to the wall (Dukes' A), spread through the wall (Dukes' B) and nodal involvement (Dukes' C) taking 1–2 years to develop depending on whether the tumour is well, moderately or undifferentiated. Poor differentiation is associated with an increased number of mucin-producing cells.

In **familial adenomatous polyposis** the large bowel is carpeted with polyps, and long-term malignancy is inevitable unless the lesions are excised, usually by proctocolectomy. The condition is due to a genetic abnormality involving the short arm of chromosome 5; it is transmitted as an autosomal dominant. Sporadic cases do occasionally occur and the condition may be associated with multiple lipomas, fibromas and exostoses in Gardner's syndrome.

The symptoms of colorectal cancer are related to the site of the disease. Right-sided lesions and those in the transverse colon present with anaemia and malaise; a palpable mass may be present. Caecal lesions can act as the apex of an intussusception. Left-sided (*Figure 23.30a, b*) lesions present primarily with alteration in bowel habit, faeces impacting in a malignant stricture but then being propelled by the build-up of proximal bacteria-produced gas, there thus being a cycle of constipation and diarrhoea. Approximately 20% of lesions are treated as an emergency for obstruction and perforation.

Rectal lesions present with fresh bleeding that may mimic that of haemorrhoids; there is also tenesmus (a feeling of incomplete evacuation). Weight loss is a bad prognostic sign in large bowel carcinoma as it usually indicates liver metas-

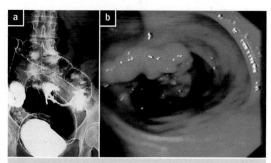

Figure 23.30
a. Typical 'apple core' appearance of barium indenting by colonic carcinoma with a thin stream of contrast medium passing through the stenosed lumen. b. Colonic neoplasm as viewed through a colonoscope showing the elevated, rolled edge and adjacent normal mucosa.

tases. Pain may be due to intestinal obstruction or invasion of adjacent pelvic structures.

The majority of colonic tumours are impalpable but may have an associated mass while 90% of rectal tumours can be felt on digital examination or seen at sigmoidoscopy. If the lesion is obstructive and the ileocaecal valve competent, a fullness may be felt in the region of the caecum; this is more evident if the right and left iliac fossae are compared. An advanced tumour may be palpable as a mass. Tumours of the caecum, and ascending and descending colons are relatively immobile whereas those occurring in the transverse or sigmoid colon may be palpable in most areas of the abdomen due to their longer mesenteries. In thin patients, stool within the left colon may be palpated in the left iliac fossa and mistaken for a mass; re-examination after the patient has evacuated should allow a distinction between the two. Colonic malignancies most commonly spread to the liver so this organ should be carefully examined in all cases.

Benign large bowel tumours

Large bowel polyps are common (*Figure 23.31*) and, as already indicated, adenomas have malignant potential. They can be divided into tubular, villous or tubulovillous. Tubular adenomas usually grow to 2 cm in diameter and are firm, sessile or pedunculated. The softer villous, frondiform adenomas are larger and usually carpet one wall of the bowel. They are common in the distal rectum, often have malignant potential and usually present with a mucous diarrhoea which, if profuse, can lead to a reduced serum potassium.

Rarer tumours include lipomas, fibromas, leiomyomas and haemangiomas. In addition, metaplastic and hamartomatous

Figure 23.31.
Colonic polyps outlined by barium enema with air insufflation.

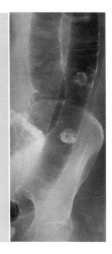

polyps occur and, in inflammatory bowel disease, ulceration can leave islands of mucosa with a pseudopolypoid appearance. **Juvenile polyps** occur in infants and children, are pedunculated and grow to 1–2 cm in diameter. They bleed and cause pain on prolapse; one-third are multiple.

Diverticular disease

Diverticulosis (*Figure 23.32*) is a common condition in the western world thought to arise through a diet low in roughage and high in refined foods. The small volume of gut contents passing through the colon requires increased pressures for the stool's passage; this results in a thickening of the gut wall and outpouchings of mucosa through the wall at sites of relative wall weakness. Such diverticula may be innocent and remain asymptomatic or they may be associated with the complications of inflammation and infection, perforation with pericolic abscess formation, localized or generalized purulent or faecal peritonitis, the formation of fistulae between bowel and adjacent structures (urinary tract; vagina) and bleeding.

Patients with uncomplicated diverticular disease may complain bitterly of left iliac fossa pain, variable bowel habit and food intolerance, probably relating to chronic muscle spasm. Scarring from previous episodes of inflammation may result in stricture formation and obstructive symptoms. Patients with vesicocolic fistula commonly complain of passing wind with the urine (**pneumaturia**). Examination of cases of diverticular disease often mimic those of colonic malignancy, and even with special investigations the pathology may remain in doubt until the segment of bowel has been resected and examined histologically.

Pneumatosis intestinalis is a condition of multiple submucosal epithelial-lined gas cysts of 1–2 cm diameter. They may be mistaken for multiple polyposis on a barium enema if the lucencies are not recognized (*Figure 23.33*). On rare occasions the lesions may occur in the small bowel or be sited submucosally. The aetiology of the lesions is ill determined although the high hydrogen content of the gas suggests a bacterial involvement. The condition is often associated with obstructive airways disease although a pathway by which the air can track through the diaphragm and retroperitoneum has not been established. Other associated lesions are enteritis, diverticulitis or following colonoscopy.

The condition is usually asymptomatic and a chance finding on plain abdominal radiographs. The lesions, however, may produce diarrhoea, malabsorption and flatulence, and may bleed, or bunches may produce intestinal obstruction.

Ulcerative colitis

This inflammatory disease may afflict patients at any age but classically it has its onset in early adult life. There is a fifteenfold increased incidence of the disease in first degree relatives but no genetic pattern has been established; altered mucosal metabolism, deficiency of the mucosal barriers and immunological abnormalities have been considered as aetiological factors. The pathological changes are

Figure 23.32.
Operative specimen demonstrating multiple diverticula of the colon.

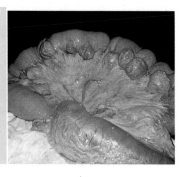

Figure 23.33.
Pneumatosis coli. Note the multiple lucent gas shadows indenting the barium column.

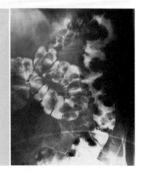

limited to the gut mucosa and submucosa and start in the rectum, spreading proximally to involve part or all of the colon (*Figure 23.34*) although changes may be seen in the terminal ileum (backwash ileitis) and extra-intestinal manifestations may be evident.

The main symptoms of the colonic disease are lethargy, malaise and the frequent passage of loose, watery stools with blood and slime; this may occur up to twenty times a day with anaemia as a persistent problem. The symptoms are variable in intensity and may be classified as mild, moderate or severe; pain is initially absent but may accompany complications. In the extreme state, toxic megacolon may develop in which the patient is severely ill, with septicaemia – the colon is dilated and the abdomen is distended. Abdominal pain and diarrhoea are present.

Patients are usually thin though they may have the stigmata of chronic steroid use. Examination should be thorough to look for the extra-intestinal manifestations listed in *Table 23.5*. The abdomen in mild disease is not usually tender but there is often deep left iliac fossa and pelvic tenderness. Rectal examination is uncomfortable and sigmoidoscopy reveals an empty rectum with mucosal changes reflecting disease activity. Complications include toxic megacolon (p. 312) and malignant change after many years of active inflammation.

Extra-intestinal manifestations of inflammatory bowel disease

These are shown *Figure 23.35a–f*. Both Crohn's disease (p. 290) and ulcerative colitis can give rise to a number of complications outside the gastrointestinal tract which are common to both diseases but the incidence varies. These effects are probably due to activation of inflammatory mechanisms against other tissues and they may continue despite adequate treatment of the intestinal pathology.

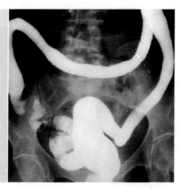

Figure 23.34. Barium enema of a patient with ulcerative colitis showing the featureless, 'pipestem' bowel wall with loss of the normal colonic haustral pattern.

Fistulae

A fistula is an abnormal tract between two epithelial surfaces. It may be an epithelial-lined congenital remnant such as a tracheo-oesophageal, umbilical or branchial fistula, and cloacal abnormalities or spinal dysraphism. Most fistulae, however, are the result of disease, particularly inflammation and malignancy, preventing normal healing of ducts and tracts, and allowing misrouting of their contents.

In the vascular system the term fistula is applied to abnormal communications between arteries and veins – e.g. congenital or acquired arteriovenous fistulae and caroticocavernous

Table 23.5. Extra-intestinal manifestations of inflammatory bowel disease.

Liver disease (These conditions may only be apparent on liver function tests or may present with jaundice or with the signs and symptoms of liver failure)	Sclerosing cholangitis
	Pericholangitis
	Bile duct carcinoma
	Fatty infiltration
	Chronic active hepatitis
	Postnecrotic cirrhosis
	Cholelithiasis
Haematological disorders	Iron deficiency anaemia
	Haemolytic anaemia
	Leukocytosis
	Thrombocytosis
Thromboembolic disease	Deep vein thrombosis
Arthropathy	Ankylosing spondylitis
	Sacroiliitis
	Migratory monoarthropathy
	Peripheral arthritis (in children)
Ocular lesions	Iritis/uveitis
	Episcleritis
	Superficial keratitis with blepharitis
	Retinitis
	Retrobulbar neuritis
Dermatological disease	Erythema nodosum (raised, tender erythematous swellings, 2–5 cm diameter, usually on the extensor surfaces of the limbs)
	Pyoderma gangrenosum (this may become gangrenous and can lead to fatal septicaemia)
	Drug reactions, e.g. erythema multiforme
	Finger clubbing
Renal disease	Pyelonephritis (immune mediated; dehydration)
	Nephrolithiasis (deranged calcium metabolism, dehydration and recumbancy)
	Glomerulonephritis
	Hypokalaemic nephritis (prolonged diarrhoea)

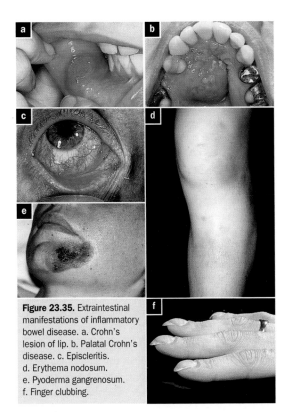

Figure 23.35. Extraintestinal manifestations of inflammatory bowel disease. a. Crohn's lesion of lip. b. Palatal Crohn's disease. c. Episcleritis. d. Erythema nodosum. e. Pyoderma gangrenosum. f. Finger clubbing.

Factors that influence the production and persistence of fistulae include:

- Inadequate drainage of an intervening abscess.
- Persistent large gut organisms, e.g. colorectal and colovaginal fistulae, secondary to diverticulitis.
- Chronic and granulomatous infection, e.g. Crohn's disease, TB, persistent foreign bodies, actinomycosis and amoebiasis.
- Radiation necrosis, e.g. rectovaginal fistulae post-radiotherapy for cervical carcinoma.
- Duct obstruction, e.g. residual gallstones blocking common bile and pancreatic ducts after surgical procedures.
- Poor healing of surgical closures, e.g. the breakdown of colonic anastamoses or duodenal and appendix stumps; such defects may be related to poor technique, ischaemic bowel, strangulated bowel or trauma.
- Malignant invasion, e.g. colocutaneous fistulae.

fistulae – or between a vessel and the gut – aortoenteric fistulae – or between lymphatics and other organs, e.g. chyluria, chylothorax and chyloperitoneum.

Fistulae are most commonly associated with the gut, joining two loops, a loop and another organ (bladder or vagina) or a loop and the exterior. Secondary tracts and sinuses (blind ending tracts) may also be present (*Figure 23.36*).

Systemic symptoms of bowel fistulae include those related to coexisting disease such as sepsis, nutritional abnormalities and malignancy. Local symptoms depend on the fistula site. Enterocutaneous fistulae are considered as high output when loss is greater than 1 L per day, resulting in fluid volume depletion, electrolyte imbalance and shock. Persistent infection of the tract – Crohn's disease and perianal fistulae – is accompanied by loss of pus and blood and recurrent abscess formation. Colovesical fistulae are accompanied by recurrent urinary tract infection. High enterocutaneous fistulae are rich in the digestive juices of the bile, pancreas and small gut, and lead to extensive skin excoriation.

Stomas

Stomas may be temporary or permanent. Temporary stomas may be required to protect a distal anastomosis, often a transverse **loop colostomy** being raised in the right hypochondrium. For more effective defunctioning the loop is divided – a **double-barrelled colostomy** – and the ends may be separated by a skin bridge. Such total defunctioning is desirable when treating difficult colonic anastamoses and complicated high perianal fistulae. The term **ileotransverse colostomy** is applied to an anastamosis between the terminal ileum and the transverse colon bypassing an obstructing lesion of the ascending colon. In this situation the term does not denote a stoma as elsewhere.

Figure 23.36. Abdominal wall sinuses following surgery in Crohn's disease.

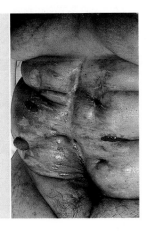

Permanent colostomies (*Figure 23.37a, b*) are of a single end of bowel, circumferentially sutured to the skin, as required after excision of the rectum. They are usually placed along a line joining the umbilicus to the left anterior superior iliac spine, at the lateral border of the rectus sheath. Complications of colostomies include oedematous stomas, haemorrhage and ulceration from the divided end, ischaemic stenoses, detachment of the cutaneous suture line, prolapse and paracolic hernias.

Ileostomies (*Figure 23.38a, b*) are usually end stomas placed to the right of the umbilicus and fashioned after proctocolectomy for inflammatory bowel disease. Because of the fluid content of the efflux, a 4 cm spout is fashioned to prevent skin excoriation. Complications of ileostomy are similar to those of colostomy but, in addition, diarrhoea and high output may lead to dehydration and electrolyte disturbance. The gut usually adapts to these changes but certain foodstuffs, such as onions, have to be avoided and appropriate dietary requirements considered long term.

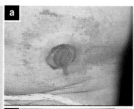

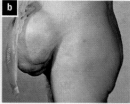

Figure 23.37
a. End colostomy.
b. Parastomal hernia in a patient with an end colostomy.

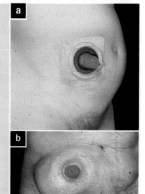

Figure 23.38
a. Typical ileostomy showing the ileal spout. This is fashioned to divert the small bowel contents into a bag and away from the adjacent skin.
b. Parastomal hernia in an ileostomy.

Peritoneal cavity

The peritoneum is the largest cavity in the body and its surface area almost equals that of the skin. It has an abundant blood and lymphatic supply and has the potential for copious fluid production, both by exudation and transudation. Usually, however, there is only enough peritoneal fluid to allow smooth gut contact during peristalsis. The peritoneum can act as a semipermeable membrane, as demonstrated by its use in peritoneal dialysis. Changes in hydrostatic and colloid osmotic pressure – as seen in cardiac failure and hypoproteinaemia – result in ascites (p. 278). Fluid collections are dull to percussion and their position influenced by gravity, so they can be diagnosed by shifting flank dullness (p. 281). Peritoneal fluid and fluid leaked through perforations gravitates to the pelvis and the paracolic gutters, but the small gut mesentery, the transverse mesocolon and the greater omentum tend to localize fluid collections, for example in subphrenic spaces (p. 304) or the lesser sac. Air in the peritoneal cavity – e.g. postoperatively and after a gut perforation – rises and can be demonstrated under the diaphragm on an erect abdominal radiograph.

Abdominal visceral carcinomas can spread and seed in the peritoneal cavity. This is particularly seen in carcinomas of the stomach, ovary and colon; secondary deposits from the bronchus and breast are also common. Extensive peritoneal carcinoma can present as seedlings over the peritoneal cavity or as infiltrating, dense plaques, producing gut adhesion and intestinal obstruction. A particular problem is infiltration across the pelvic floor, causing a **frozen pelvis**. This can be palpated rectally across the pouch of Douglas, and is termed a Blumer's shelf. Peritoneal carcinomatosis is accompanied by a variable amount of ascites. It is usually a terminal event but in a few slow-growing malignancies, particularly carcinoid tumour, nutrition is maintained, symptoms are mild and survival may be for a number of years. The differential diagnosis of infiltrating peritoneal carcinoma includes peritonitis, (particularly TB), fat necrosis and widespread hydatid daughter cysts.

Mucoceles of the gallbladder and appendix, and pseudomucinous cysts of the ovary can give rise to **pseudomyxoma peritonei**, the cavity being filled by extensive yellowish, jelly-like material. The primary pathologies are often malignant. Other peritoneal neoplasms include a **mesothelioma** which is a highly malignant neoplasm associated with exposure to asbestos. **Desmoid tumours** are usually part of Gardner's syndrome, which is familial adenomatous polyposis associated with lipomas, fibromas and exostoses; it is transmitted as an autosomal dominant.

The **retroperitoneum** is subject to haematoma formation in trauma, over-anticoagulation and rupture of abdominal aortic and visceral artery aneurysms, the latter being particularly seen during pregnancy. Malignant masses may be extensions of neoplasms of the kidney and adrenal glands, or primary sarcomas and neurogenic tumours. Secondary nodal involvement occurs, for example, in testicular tumours.

Retroperitoneal fibrosis is an uncommon idiopathic disease, which causes particular problems when it involves the ureters; it is considered on p. 345.

Mesenteric cysts are usually congenital anomalies such as urological remnants and enterogenous cysts. The latter are partial duplication of the gut and may undergo torsion or become infected. They are also subject to the complications of peptic ulceration as they often contain ectopic gastric mucosa, giving rise to haemorrhage and perforation. Chylolymphatic cysts are some of the commonest mesenteric abnormalities. They are filled with milky chyle and are usually solitary but may be loculated. Chylolymphatic cysts have an independent blood supply and, therefore, can be enucleated. This differs from enterogenous cysts which have a common blood supply with the gut, and removal usually involves adjacent gut resection. **Mesenteric tumours** include desmoids, teratomas and fibromas. The latter are usually benign although extensive encroachment on mesenteric vessels can impair the gut blood supply, as can extension of carcinoid masses.

Disorders of the female genitalia

Gynaecological disorders are not the prime concern of this book but fibroids, and ovarian and uterine malignancies are common, as are acute gynaecological emergencies (p. 317). They thus form an important differential diagnosis in both the acute and non-acute abdomen, and the surgeon has to be aware of their presentation.

Uterine disorders

Uterine disease – which includes malignancy of the body and cervix, fibroids and infection (*Figure 23.39*) – most commonly presents with intermenstrual bleeding. Uterine pain is experienced as a constant ache in the lower abdomen and pelvis, and as low backache.

Cancer of the cervix occurs primarily in the fourth decade and there may be menorrhagia as well as intermenstrual bleeding. Cytological surveys aim to diagnose the early *in situ* lesion before invasion occurs. The latter can be into the broad ligament and involve the vaginal vault and adjacent ureters,

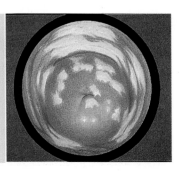

Figure 23.39. Candidal infection of the cervix.

possible complications being urinary and faecal fistulae as well as painful involvement of the sacral plexus.

Cancer of the body of the uterus usually occurs postmenopausally in the fifth and sixth decades, heralded by bleeding and pain. The bloody discharge is not usually foul smelling, and if this is present alternative diagnoses of sarcoma, sloughing of a fibroid or tuberculous endometriosis should be considered. Bimanual examination reveals a bulky uterus, usually a smooth enlargement, compared to the irregular enlargement of multiple fibroids. Rapid enlargement is unusual so when this is present, sarcomas, choriocarcinomas or cystic degeneration in a fibroid are more likely diagnoses. Choriocarcinoma always occurs post-pregnancy although this may be a number of years before.

Uterine fibroids are tumours of the uterine smooth muscle. They are usually benign, about 6 cm in diameter and can give rise to pain and mimic other causes of an acute abdomen. A pedunculated fibroid can twist, giving rise to torsion, presenting in a similar fashion to torsion of the ovary or, if right sided, it can mimic appendicitis. Fibroids tend to enlarge and give rise to symptoms in pregnancy. In the older, post-menopausal woman fibroids may degenerate, and this in itself may give rise to pain. However, fibroids are common and are usually asymptomatic, and the mere presence of a large fibroid uterus must not preclude the diagnosis of an acute abdomen from other causes.

Endometriosis is the deposition of endometrial tissue outside the uterine cavity. This is usually in the region of the uterus, commonly in the fallopian tubes, broad ligaments or beneath the serosa. Other sites include the ovary, peritoneal cavity, omentum, bladder and umbilicus. About 4% of cases of endometriosis occur in the gut and, in rare instances, the breast and pleural cavity. Acquired endometriosis is due to the deposition of endometrial tissue during uterine surgery, such as Caesarean section, deposits usually being in abdominal scars.

The condition is thus relatively common, occurring in 8–10% of women, usually between 30 and 40, and regressing post-menopausally. Symptoms are unusual but there may be low backache, particularly the week before menstruation, and in severe symptomatic patients this may progress and become continuous. Menorrhagia may be present, particularly with ovarian deposits. Bleeding from the lesions of endometriosis is uncommon; however, it is reported, such as in umbilical deposits and pleural collections. Occasionally endometriosis of the gut can cause intestinal obstruction through tumour masses and adhesions.

Ovarian tumours

Ovarian tumours (p. 317) have a great variety of cell origins, including germ cells, sex cord, epithelial and connective tissue. As many as 10% of these lesions are secondary deposits, usually being carried in the blood stream but they may be transperitoneal implantation, particularly from the stomach – Krukenberg tumours. The diagnosis of cell type is often only made after histological examination.

Tumours present at any age but are mainly post-menopausal. Epithelial tumours are more evenly distributed throughout adulthood, and dermoid tumours are commoner in the young. Approximately 80% of lesions are cystic; of these 15% are malignant whereas 60% of solid tumours are malignant. Any lesion larger than 8–10 cm across is likely to be malignant or have malignant potential and should be excised; 20% of lesions are bilateral. Other functional ovarian lesions include cysts of the corpus luteum (p. 318) and deposits of endometriosis.

Ovarian tumours are usually asymptomatic, the mass being found at routine examination or post-mortem. Malignancies, therefore, usually present late, possibly with cachexia and emaciation. They may also present as acute abdominal problems such as with torsion, bleeding, rupture, infection or infarction (p. 317). The swelling associated with these tumours may be massive (*Figure 23.40*), both from the size of the tumour and associated ascites. Specific forms of ascites include pseudomyxoma peritonei – from a ruptured pseudomucinous cyst (p. 296) – and Meigs' syndrome, in which a solid fibroma, usually small and benign, gives rise to a pleural effusion and ascites, these complications disappearing after removal of the tumour.

Pain may be due to the weight of the tumour, abdominal distension and pressure, and invasion of abdominal organs. Other symptoms include urinary retention, invasion of the sacral plexus, intestinal obstruction from omental and peritoneal seedlings, and adhesions, faecal fistulae, urinary incontinence and a swollen leg. Intermenstrual bleeding and menstrual abnormalities are not usually a feature of ovarian disease. However, menorrhagia does occur in ovarian endometriosis and with granuloma cell tumours. Amenorrhoea during the childbearing years is not a feature of ovarian tumours. Tumours can be palpated bimanually and move independently of the uterus unless fixation has occurred; this is in contrast to primary uterine tumours.

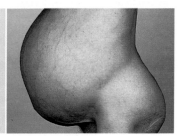

Figure 23.40. Abdominal distension from an ovarian malignancy.

24 The acute abdomen

Introduction

Acute abdominal conditions are common and of multiple and diverse aetiologies. The prevalence of specific diseases depends upon sex, age and country of origin. The clinician has to determine whether the patient should undergo a laparotomy before the onset of generalized peritonitis becomes established, with its attendant significant mortality and morbidity, or whether it is safe to wait, observe, and undertake further investigation. A detailed history is essential and the examination is central to the decision making process.

The pain is usually from an inflamed intra-abdominal viscus. Initially the visceral peritoneum is involved and the pain is referred to the body wall, dependent on its origin from the fore-, mid- or hindgut. As the condition develops the parietal peritoneum may become involved and the pain then localizes accurately to the site of the disease. Two important questions to ask are 'When did the pain start?' and 'Where is it?', i.e. at the time of examination. Patience in the examination of the patient (usually a child), together with experience and perhaps repeated examination, are required to make a diagnosis. If in doubt it is wise to have the patient admitted to hospital where a rising pulse rate noted over several hours indicates the necessity for laparotomy.

Two cardinal signs of intraperitoneal inflammation are rigidity of the abdominal wall and guarding. In both cases there is reflex contraction of the abdominal wall muscles in the first instance at rest and in the secondly to provocation from the pressure of the examining hand.

A number of signs may be of use in distinguishing serious from not so serious conditions:

- The pointing sign – Ask the patient to point to the site of maximum pain. If this is also the site of maximum tenderness, the underling viscus is very likely to be the site of the problem.
- The cough test – The patient is asked to cough. If this causes the patient to experience pain in the abdomen, there is inflammation affecting the parietal peritoneum; if the pain is experienced in the chest, the inflammation is affecting the parietal pleura.
- The bed shaking test (Bapat's sign) – The bed is shaken which, in the presence of peritoneal inflammation, causes pain at the site of the inflammation.
- Percussion rebound – Gentle percussion over the abdomen is sufficient to identify and localize severe inflammation without the need for potentially painful palpation. This is particularly valuable in children.
- Rebound tenderness (release sign; Blumberg's sign) – If the pain and tenderness are vague, and there is doubt about the possibility of early peritonitis, sudden complete withdrawal of the hand after gentle deep palpation produces pain. This is useful in suspected cases but should not be used when there is obvious tenderness as it then produces severe pain and an unhappy relationship.

When diffuse peritonitis is present, the patient lies still and looks obviously unwell, with a rigid abdomen and generalized tenderness. Respiration is shallow and rapid. Bowel sounds are absent and the patient may draw their knees up and refuse abdominal palpation. To ensure that the abdomen is the site of the tenderness, the anterior aspect of the thighs should be palpated to show that no tenderness is present until the hand is gently advanced over the inguinal ligament, when the tenderness is elicited. Ask the patient firstly to palpate tender areas themselves as this provides an indication of the degree of tenderness and how vigorous subsequent examination can be. This is particularly important in children, as is using the child's own hand for palpation.

Acute abdominal pain is due to many causes; the more common are listed in *Table 24.1*. The table order gives some indication of relative frequency in the UK but this is very variable in different localities world-wide. The subsequent order of disease entities therefore follows an anatomical rather than a relative incidence pattern.

Table 24.1. Causes of acute abdominal pain.

Adults	Appendicitis
	Acute colonic diverticulitis
	Perforated peptic ulcer
	Acute cholecystitis
	Intestinal obstruction
	Ureteric colic
	Dyspepsia
	Acute pancreatitis
	Inflammatory bowel disease
	Regional ileitis
	Meckel's diverticulum
	Rectus sheath haematoma
The elderly	Colorectal cancer (obstruction; perforation)
	Vascular disease (mesenteric infarct; ruptured aortic aneurysm)
	Medical causes
Children (p. 333)	Appendicitis
	Non-specific abdominal pain
	Mesenteric adenitis
	Intussusception
	Urinary tract infection
	Hernia
	Upper respiratory tract infection
Women	Pelvic inflammatory disease
	Ovarian cyst
	Ectopic pregnancy

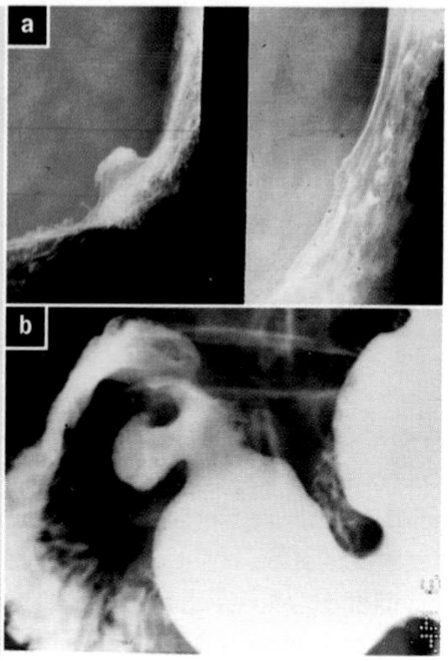

Figure 24.1. Peptic ulceration demonstrated on barium studies. a. Gastric ulcer. b. Large duodenal ulcer.

Peptic ulcer disease

Acute multiple gastric erosions

Acute multiple gastric erosions are particularly related to non-steroidal, anti-inflammatory drugs, while in stress ulceration follows hypovolaemic, endotoxic or cardiogenic shock, the reduced tissue perfusion gives rise to mucosal ischaemia. Stress ulcers can also follow neurosurgical procedures, cerebral trauma and extensive burns. In these patients, however, the mechanism of ulceration is linked to a raised serum gastrin level.

Peptic ulceration

Peptic ulceration (*Figure 24.1a, b*) of the stomach and duodenum is due to either an excess of acid and digestive enzymes or a lack of the mucosal defence systems protecting the stomach and proximal duodenum from their actions. The underlying causes vary from endocrine dysfunction to

drugs and the presence of the ulcer-associated bacteria *Helicobacter pylori*. The disease is often familial and increased in patients with blood group O. Other risk factors are smoking, alcohol and vitamin deficiency, and there is often a marked geographical variation in the incidence. Specific underlying causes are tumours of the non-β-islet cells of the pancreas – as seen in Zollinger–Ellison syndrome – and in hyperparathyroidism and some multiple endocrine abnormalities.

The site of the ulcer influences symptoms. Chronic gastric ulcers have periodic bouts of pain every few months, lasting for a few weeks. The pain comes on soon after meals so there is a fear of eating and a consequent weight loss. Pain is relieved by lying down and vomiting. Fried food is avoided, and the common diet is of fish and dairy products. In duodenal ulcers there is less periodicity in the exacerbations of pain. Pain comes on 2 hours after a meal and is relieved by eating, hence the patient's weight is usually maintained. Depending on the location of the ulcer the acute conditions that they can cause are haemorrhage (if the ulceration erodes into a blood vessel) and perforation (if the ulceration proceeds through the viscus and into the peritoneal cavity).

Perforated peptic ulceration

Perforation results in the passage of gastric or duodenal contents into the peritoneum where it causes peritonitis. Although the perforation may be self limiting – and on occasion may be best managed without recourse to operation – there is a risk of untreated peritonitis leading to death. There is often, but not always, a history of previous peptic ulcer disease. This varies from simple indigestion to previous serious episodes of haemorrhage – haematemesis or melaena – or perforation. There may be other risk factors involved such as a history of taking non-steroidal, anti-inflammatory drugs, steroids or anticoagulants. Smoking, alcohol and stress are also recognized risk factors.

There is usually a sudden dramatic history of epigastric pain, which may spread down the paracolic gutters and later involve the whole abdomen, and occasionally vomiting. The patient may already be shocked if peritonitis has been swift in onset. However, if the omentum is able to seal the perforation early on and limit the volume of fluid released into the peritoneal cavity, the symptoms may be relatively mild and the patient may appear fairly well. The general condition, and in particular the pulse and blood pressure, are important in judging the seriousness of the problem. For the first 6 hours the pulse rate is often practically unaltered. Tachycardia on presentation with a pulse greater than 100 is associated with a graver prognosis. There is rarely a pyrexia and more commonly the patient feels cold, especially if shocked.

The abdomen is usually held rigidly still, with painful respiratory movements resulting in the patient breathing with a characteristic shallow grunting sound. On palpation the abdomen usually has a generalized 'board-like rigidity' which is a cardinal sign of generalized, chemically induced peritonitis. As the peritonitis becomes more established the abdomen becomes more distended and, with this, rigidity and the severe pain may diminish. There may be slightly more tenderness and guarding in the epigastrium but usually all the abdomen is affected. In late cases the presence of bowel gas in the peritoneum gives rise to increased resonance to percussion, most especially in the midaxillary line on the right where there is normally dullness from the liver; in a very late case this may actually become tympanic. Auscultation reveals absent bowel sounds. Rectal examination can occasionally give rise to tenderness in the rectovesical pouch.

The presence of the perforation is usually confirmed on an erect chest radiograph showing the presence of gas under the diaphragm (*Figure 24.2a, b*) and, after resuscitation, the source of the perforation is sought at laparotomy and treated appropriately.

Perforated gastric ulcers are seldom difficult to diagnose but may be confused with myocardial infarction and other thoracic problems, giving rise to diaphragmatic inflammation, pancreatitis and leaking or dissecting aortic aneurysms. Gastric carcinomas may present as a perforated ulcer.

Perforated duodenal ulcers – the commoner type of peptic ulcer – are usually indistinguishable from perforated gastric ulcers on examination. One diagnostic pitfall is known as the

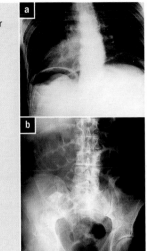

Figure 24.2.
Perforated peptic ulcer. a. Air under the right dome of the diaphragm. b. Air tracking between loops of gut.

right paracolic gutter phenomenon. This occurs after a duodenal perforation; the leaking duodenal fluid is directed downwards, alongside the ascending colon into the right iliac fossa where it gives rise to a more localized peritonitis. This can be confused with appendicitis. The tenderness elicited in such a condition tends to be more generalized and slightly higher than in 'classic' appendicitis. A perforation into the lesser sac may limit the abdominal signs.

Bleeding from peptic ulceration

If the ulceration erodes into a blood vessel, the signs and symptoms are from haemorrhage and, if enough blood is lost, from shock. The likely presenting complaints following epigastric pain are haematemesis or melaena (depending on the location and rate of bleeding), shock or anaemia. Gastric ulcers have a higher incidence of haematemesis and a lower incidence of melaena than their duodenal counterpart.

For more on peptic ulcer disease see p. 283.

Bleeding from other locations in the alimentary canal, such as oesophageal or gastric varices, Mallory–Weiss tears of the lower oesophagus, multiple gastric erosions, ectopic gastric mucosa in Meckel's diverticulum or a duplicated gut, or rarely conditions such as aortoduodenal fistulae present in a similar way. Management is determined largely by the anatomical location of the bleeding and early endoscopy is mandatory.

If the rate of bleeding is sufficient, the patient is shocked, as evidenced by their mental state, pallor, peripheral vasoconstriction, sweating and dry mucous membranes. The pulse and blood pressure should be noted and recorded at regular intervals depending on the urgency of the case. The signs of

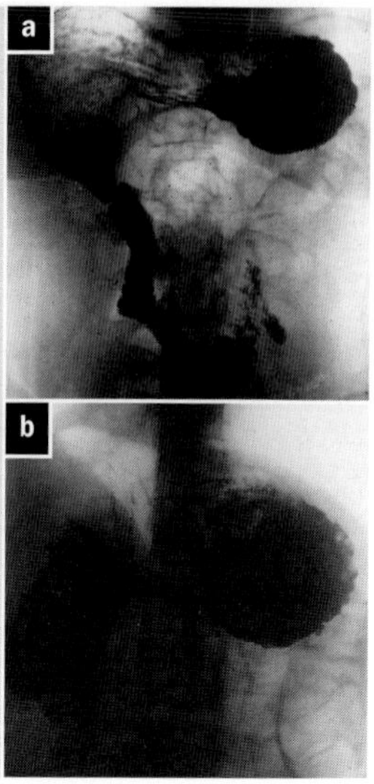

Figure 24.3.
Volvulus of the stomach.
a. Organoaxial.
b. Mesenterioaxial.

upper gastrointestinal malignancy, liver disease and portal hypertension should be sought. The rectum is examined to look for melaena stool caused by the digestion of blood, which has a characteristic jet black, tarry appearance and an equally characteristic smell. The rest of the abdominal examination is usually normal.

Volvulus

The stomach is fixed at one end by the oesophagus passing through the diaphragm, and at the other by the first part of the duodenum passing retroperitoneally. Occasionally the organ can rotate between these points – either along its axis (organoaxial; *Figure 24.3a*) or at right angles to this plane (mesenterioaxial; *Figure 24.3b*) – producing a volvulus. The condition is usually associated with eventration (p. 248) of the diaphragm but may also occur if the stomach has entered the chest in a rolling hiatus hernia (p. 250). The colon is usually taken up with the greater curve under the diaphragm but it is uncertain whether this is primary or secondary to the volvulus.

The patient complains of fullness after small amounts of food and of abdominal distension. Vomiting, particularly retching, are prominent, with abdominal pain; a stomach tube cannot be passed. The gas shadows on a plain abdominal radiograph or a barium meal demonstrate the twisted stomach and the high colon.

Acute dilatation of the stomach

This rare complication can follow any operation or trauma, such as long bone or spinal fracture. The patient vomits copious amounts of brownish-black fluid and displays the signs of hypovolaemic shock. There is discomfort from the increasing size of the abdomen, the pulse rate rises insidiously, the urine output falls and the patient may complain of nausea or hiccough before the onset of vomiting. The dilated stomach may reach the pelvis and may be evident on examination, a succussion splash is present. Once the condition has been suspected, a nasogastric tube should be passed to decompress the stomach of large amounts of gastric fluid, since vomiting may be accompanied by a lethal inhalation.

Acute cholecystitis

Gallstones (p. 287) can cause pain through chemical inflammation of the gallbladder wall, usually by obstruction of the cystic duct by a stone impacted in Hartmann's pouch. This may proceed to infection giving rise to acute cholecystitis. Pain from the biliary tree is usually felt in the right upper quadrant, radiating to the right subscapular or interscapular regions. Frequently there is a history of biliary colic, with self-limiting right upper quadrant pain that starts suddenly – often precipitated by certain foods – and may be severe. As acute cholecystitis develops the pain becomes duller and more localized. This is followed by the onset of nausea, retching and then vomiting. The temperature rises and the pulse rate increases with the onset of infection.

Examination of the abdomen usually elicits tenderness and rigidity in the right upper quadrant, and Murphy's sign (p. 287) is very easy to elicit. Obstruction of the common bile duct produces jaundice, either directly by a stone within it or indirectly by inflammation caused by impaction of a stone in the cystic duct (Morizzi's syndrome type 1). Infected bile within an obstructed system leads to Charcot's triad of pain, jaundice and rigors, and can lead to septicaemia and septic shock, which may develop at an alarming speed. Occasionally a palpable swelling is found in the right upper quadrant, usually caused by the greater omentum sealing the inflamed area. Other causes of right upper quadrant pain that may be mistaken for acute cholecystitis are acute appendicitis, right-sided pyelonephritis, perforation of a peptic ulcer (especially if this perforation has been walled off by the omentum) and rectus sheath haematoma. Thoracic causes include myocardial infarction, right lower lobe pneumonia and right-sided heart failure. The last condition can cause a sudden enlargement of the liver, the patient is short of breath and the JVP markedly increased, though the temperature is normal.

Acute pancreatitis

The majority of cases of acute pancreatitis are due to alcohol consumption or gallstones. Other causes include viral infection, trauma (especially blunt upper abdominal trauma), upper gastrointestinal or splenic surgery, or following endoscopic retrograde cholangiopancreatography. Rare causes include congenital abnormalities of pancreatic development, autoimmune disease (polyarteritis nodosa), hyperparathyroidism, hypolipidaemia, diabetes mellitus, porphyria, and secondary to steroids and diuretics. Nevertheless, in a proportion of cases no underlying cause is found. In acute pancreatitis there is oedema, haemorrhage and necrosis of the organ, at least in part due to autodigestion. At the end of an attack the pancreas returns to normal but the condition may recur. Although the condition can arise at any age it is commoner after the third decade.

Pancreatitis presents with severe abdominal pain usually sited in the upper abdomen and often radiating to the back or the left loin. The pain is usually constant, deep and agonizing, and slowly increases. The patient can find relief occasionally by either sitting up and leaning forward or lying on the side in the knee–chest position. The onset of pain is frequently followed by retching or even vomiting. Diaphragmatic irritation causes hiccoughs.

On examination there may be evidence of shock with tachycardia, hypotension and cyanosis with cold clammy extremities; jaundice is not uncommon. The abdomen is not as rigid as with gastroduodenal perforation, which can give rise to a similar degree of pain and shock. The area of maximum tenderness is usually the central abdomen and epigastrium, with guarding and rebound. In mild pancreatitis tenderness to deep epigastric palpation may be evident and inflammation from the tail of the pancreas gives rise to tenderness at the left costovertebral angle. Ileus commonly develops after a few hours giving rise to abdominal distension. Retroperitoneal haemorrhage may lead to discoloration in the flanks (Grey Turner's sign, p. 267, *Figure 21.3*) or around the umbilicus (Cullen's sign, p. 268, *Figure 21.4*). From the seventh day onwards a pancreatic pseudocyst may develop in the epigastrium. The examining hand cannot get above the mass, it is usually tender and resonant to percussion, due to overlying gastric gas.

Initial management of pancreatitis is conservative whereas the management of the main intra-abdominal conditions that mimic pancreatitis – such as gut perforation or a leaking abdominal aortic aneurysm – require urgent laparotomy. For this reason it is important to confirm the clinical suspicion of pancreatitis by estimation of the blood amylase level, which is raised in acute pancreatitis to a far greater degree than in other acute abdominal conditions.

Chronic pancreatitis

Chronic pancreatitis, like the acute version, is an inflammatory disease but differs in that irreversible morphological changes are present. There is usually, but not invariably, abdominal pain sited in the epigastrium, radiating to the back and to each hypochondrium. The pain is usually exacerbated by alcohol. The appetite is poor and this, together with malabsorption from pancreatic dysfunction, gives rise to weight loss. Jaundice is occasionally present and diabetes mellitus is a late feature.

Acute pyogenic liver abscess

This condition can be confused with right-sided subphrenic abscesses. In the UK the commonest cause is infection from the biliary tract, as portal pyaemia following appendicitis is now rare. Other sources of liver abscesses include the gut, the umbilicus and a general septicaemia. Local spread may be from penetrating injuries, subphrenic abscesses or an empyema. These lesions are often multiple. The gut sources may be due to infection (typhoid; actinomycosis; TB; hydatid), inflammatory bowel (ulcerative colitis; Crohn's disease) or neoplasia (colonic carcinoma). Biliary infection often follows the impaction of a stone in the common bile duct, and umbilical infection can occur in the newborn (p. 332).

The patient complains of a fever with rigors and of fullness in the right upper quadrant, due to an enlarged liver; jaundice is not uncommon. There may be weight loss and anaemia if the condition is long standing. As with a subphrenic abscess, there may be inflammatory changes in the right lower pleural cavity and lung. The signs of liver abscesses may be minimal but they can rapidly change and develop into a fulminating septicaemia as well as rupture into the biliary tree or peritoneum.

Amoebic liver abscess

This is a complication of amoebic dysentery, usually, but not always, a disease of the tropics. The amoebae, having invaded the bowel wall, are carried to the liver where they give rise to an abscess, producing pain over the area of the liver. The pain is characteristically worse after the ingestion of alcohol and on jarring movements. There is usually a history of fevers and rigors, most often at night. The liver may be slightly enlarged and is tender. The abscess may displace the liver downwards, and upward pressure may collapse the right lung; a reactive right pleural effusion may also result. If untreated, the abscess may burst into the peritoneum (giving acute peritonitis), into the pleural cavity (giving rise to empyema), into the lung (causing the patient to cough up chocolate-coloured pus) or into the intestines.

Amoebic dysentery can also give rise to a granulomatous reaction, producing a mass known as an amoeboma. If in the caecum, the right iliac fossa mass may be mistaken for an appendix mass or a caecal neoplasm; if in the rectum, it is most often mistaken for rectal cancer. Treatment with antibiotics gives a speedy resolution of the signs and symptoms.

Subphrenic abscess

A subphrenic abscess (*Figure 24.4*) follows an intraperitoneal disease, usually after leakage of infected or infective fluid from a viscus. The cause is often known but may have resolved, and the subphrenic abscess may be the presenting complaint. The commonest causes are a perforated peptic ulcer, abdominal trauma, perforation of the biliary tree, perforation of the stomach, perforation of the colon and acute appendicitis. Perforation may be due to an inflammatory or malignant lesion or may be iatrogenic, such as during instrumentation or an operation.

Patients with subphrenic abscesses look and feel ill, with nausea and anorexia. They usually have upper abdominal or back pain, which may radiate to the shoulder. There is a swinging pyrexia that may wax and wane over the course of a few days. Rigors are uncommon, unless there is a coexisting liver abscess. There is a tachycardia which may be out of proportion to the recorded temperature. Unless there is coexisting liver or biliary tract disease, such patients are rarely jaundiced. Occasionally hiccoughs are present, due to diaphragmatic irritation.

Figure 24.4.
Large subphrenic abscess with air fluid level and a highly displaced right dome of the diaphragm.

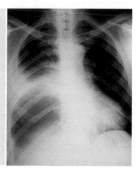

On examination, any postoperative wound is usually infected. There may be tenderness around the right or left upper quadrant but usually the tender point is only found over the posterior intercostal spaces, the commonest site being the 11th intercostal space; this may only be detected with the patient lying prone. On examination of the chest, signs of pneumonia or atelectasis may be found from the accompanying pleurisy or pleuropneumonia. On percussion, characteristic findings are the mixture of liver dullness, resonance from gas in the abscess, dullness in a collapsed lung or pleural effusion, and resonance in the normal lung.

Acute appendicitis

Acute appendicitis (*Figure 24.5*) was first described as a clinical entity approximately 100 years ago, as was its surgical management by appendectomy. The incidence increased after its description but is now diminishing. It can occur at any time during life but is commoner in young to middle-aged adults. The aetiology is still not entirely understood but usually involves obstruction of the appendix by a faecolith, a worm or one or more of its abundant lymphoid follicles, causing acute inflammation with oedema, venous engorgement and later arterial insufficiency. Inflammation of the appendix may be self limiting but may progress until the appendix perforates, which occurs in 25–30% of patients. The subsequent course of the disease depends on the action of the omentum and adjacent intraperitoneal tissues. If the perforation is successfully walled off, an **appendix mass** is clinically evident, usually after the third day, and may become an **appendix abscess**. If the perforation is not successfully isolated, generalized peritonitis occurs, leading to shock and even death. As the omentum is less well developed in the infant, the morbidity and mortality is higher in this group.

The classic history is of the gradual onset of central colicky abdominal pain over 24 hours associated with anorexia, nausea, occasionally vomiting and usually constipation. The pain may change when the parietal peritoneum becomes

Figure 24.5.
Operative photograph of an acute appendicitis.

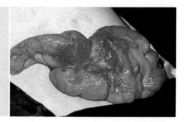

involved in the inflammation, localizing to the right iliac fossa. Pain is aggravated by moving or coughing. Unfortunately only half the patients give this typical history. In a third of cases the pain presents over 1–2 days and it may present in the right iliac fossa. Vomiting may be absent and diarrhoea occurs in 20% of patients. An atypical presentation is commoner in the very young and elderly. Confirmation of the diagnosis is attempted by examination. There is often difficulty in palpating the inflamed appendix because it can vary in its length and only the terminal part may be inflamed, hence producing signs and symptoms in the pelvis. The diagnosis is also complicated in the very young, the elderly and during pregnancy.

On examination the patient looks unwell, may have a facial flush and usually has a mild pyrexia (also mild leukocytosis). There is often halitosis – fetor oris – and a slight tachycardia. On examination of the abdomen, signs of generalized peritonitis are sought as already described. The patient is asked to indicate the point of maximum pain – in appendicitis this should correspond with McBurney's point which lies at the junction of the lateral third and medial two-thirds of an imaginary line drawn from the umbilicus to the anterior superior iliac spine. Classically there is right iliac fossa tenderness with guarding, again maximal at McBurney's point, and mild but persistent rigidity. If these symptoms are absent or equivocal, rebound tenderness can be elicited, together with other signs for peritonitis. The appendix is retrocaecally sited in approximately 75% of cases. A partially or wholly retrocaecal appendicitis may present with symptoms and signs referable to the right flank and posterior aspect of the abdominal wall, lateral to the sacrospinalis muscle. The patient is asked to roll over on to the left side when tenderness may be elicited just medial to the right anterior superior iliac spine. The tenderness may be even higher with a high caecum, due to malrotation. A pelvic appendicitis – in 20% of cases – is best diagnosed on rectal examination.

Other signs of peritonitis include Rovsing's sign. This is elicited by pressing in the left iliac fossa and the patient complaining of pain in the right iliac fossa. It is probably due to moving loops of small bowel against the inflamed appendix in the right iliac fossa. The bowel sounds are listened for as their absence confirms the suspicion of generalized peritonitis. Other signs that may be useful include the psoas test – where inflammation adjacent to the psoas muscle is diagnosed by active flexion of the right hip, giving rise to discomfort – or, in cases of psoas spasm, pain is produced by hyperextending the hip with the patient on their left side. Where inflammation is adjacent to the obturator internus, stretching this muscle by flexing and internally rotating the hip causes tenderness.

Acute appendicitis in pregnancy

Appendicitis complicates approximately 1 in 2000 pregnancies; it also carries the additional risk of inducing abortion. Appendicitis in early pregnancy presents in the typical fashion although the differential diagnosis is complicated by a number of complications of pregnancy, notably a urinary tract infection. In later pregnancy the enlargement of the uterus displaces the caecum and hence the appendix. The pain and tenderness produced by an inflamed appendix is therefore more superior and lateral, and is also difficult to palpate as it is overlaid by the uterus. The gravid uterus may become inflamed and hence tender in cases of concealed haemorrhage or necrosis, or torsion of a uterine fibroid. To distinguish between a uterine cause and appendicitis, having located the area of maximal tenderness. mark it on the skin and then ask the patient to roll on to the left side and wait for a minute. If the cause of the pain is uterine the point of maximal tenderness shifts with the uterus to the left.

Appendicitis in the elderly

Although appendicitis is not uncommon in the elderly population its diagnosis can be difficult. This is in part due to the relative increase in incidence of other causes of abdominal pain, such as intestinal obstruction. It is also due to differences in the way in which elderly patients respond to appendicitis. Abdominal rigidity may be absent either due to lax abdominal muscles or due to the rapid onset of overwhelming infection.

For **appendicitis in infancy and childhood** see p. 335.

The differential diagnosis of acute appendicitis

The number of conditions in the differential diagnosis are legion (*Table 24.1*). Any pain arising from the organs on the right side of the abdomen and thorax can mimic the pain arising from the appendix. Intrathoracic inflammation, arising for instance from pneumonia, may, by irritating the diaphragmatic peritoneum, mimic peritonitis arising from appendicitis; an anaesthetic in these circumstances is undesirable. In such cases abdominal or rectal tenderness is minimal or absent, chest examination and a chest radiograph reveals pneumonia. When doubt still exists, especially in children, compression of the lower thorax – the thoracic compression test described by Dott – produces pain when the problem is intrathoracic.

A common cause of diagnostic confusion is inflammation arising from the right kidney and ureter. Not only can similar pain arise from a right urinary stone, but the signs may also be very similar, while an inflamed appendix next to a ureter can produce pyuria and haematuria. Although removing a normal appendix in a case of urinary colic is embarrassing, failure to remove an inflamed appendix because of doubt in diagnosis can have more serious consequences. For these reasons, if doubt exists, radiological diagnosis by plain or contrast radiology must be used to confirm the presence of the urinary stone.

Women, especially in the childbearing years, by virtue of their generative organs, pose even more problems in the diagnosis of right iliac fossa pain. The main gynaecological pathologies in the differential diagnosis are acute salpingitis, ruptured or twisted ovarian cysts and ectopic pregnancy. In order to prove these diagnoses it is necessary to perform a pelvic examination and it is mandatory to perform a pregnancy test. Ultrasound examination of the pelvic organs can be very useful in determining the cause. Despite this it is not unusual to diagnose these conditions at laparotomy through a right iliac fossa incision.

Appendix mass

Where the diagnosis is delayed by a few days it is not unusual to find a mass in the right iliac fossa. This is due to the omentum and small bowel mesentery walling off the inflamed appendix. The appendix may have perforated but the perforation can be contained by the action of the omentum and surrounding bowel. The outline of the resulting mass should be drawn on the abdominal wall with a marker pen so that its progress can be monitored, since a conservative course of action is usual until the inflammation has settled. An appendix mass may also extend to the pelvis and be palpable per rectum. The differential diagnosis of a mass in the right iliac fossa includes the following:

- Infection of a solitary caecal diverticulum.
- Infection of the caecum (TB; actinomycosis; amoebiasis).
- Caecal lymphadenitis.
- Caecal carcinoma.
- Crohn's disease.
- Tubovarian abscess.
- Cysts, torsion or neoplasms of the ovary.

Tumours of the appendix

Tumours of the appendix are rare and are usually of the carcinoid variety, derived from neuroendocrine cells. These tumours may secrete vasoactive peptides (particularly 5-hydroxytryptamine), producing the **carcinoid syndrome** – reddish-blue

cyanosis, flushing, diarrhoea, asthma attacks and, in the later stage, tricuspid and pulmonary valve stenosis. The tumours are slow growing but some have an invasive and metastatic potential. Carcinoma of the appendix does occur, especially of a mucinoid variety which, if it perforates, may seed over the peritoneum, giving rise to pseudomyxoma peritonei – large quantities of yellow jelly-like material loculated throughout the peritoneal cavity, which also occurs after rupture of a pseudomucinous cyst of the ovary.

Meckel's diverticulum

If the appendix is normal in a patient with suspected appendicitis, the terminal ileum must be examined for a Meckel's diverticulum (*Figure 24.6*), classically occurring in 2% of patients, 60 cm from the ileocaecal valve and being 5 cm long. This remnant of the vitellointestinal duct is subject not only to inflammation but can be the apex of an intussusception or the site of an umbilical band, giving rise to intestinal obstruction or a volvulus. It may also contain gastric mucosa, which is subject to haemorrhage and perforation. The diverticulum has been reported in inguinal and femoral hernial sacs – Littré's hernia.

Other rare **small gut** diverticuli occur around the mesenteric border of the duodenum in its second and third parts, and the antimesenteric border of the jejunum, where they are often multiple and may give rise to inflammation and malabsorption syndromes. Tumours of the small bowel are exceedingly rare, a unique syndrome being familial intestinal hamartomatous polyposis, affecting the jejunum and accompanied by melanosis of the mucous membrane of the lips – Peutz–Jeghers syndrome. Malignant tumours, when they do occur, are usually lymphoma or myeloma.

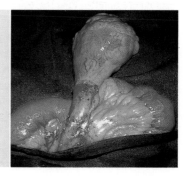

Figure 24.6. Operative photograph of a Meckel's diverticulum.

Regional ileitis

Due to the proximity of the terminal ileum to the appendix, inflammation of the terminal ileum may easily be mistaken for appendicitis. This can be due to a number of conditions. *Yersinia* sp. infection gives rise to an acute regional ileitis but may also affect the caecum when it is known as typhlitis. Because the signs and symptoms mimic those of appendicitis the diagnosis is usually made at laparotomy.

Crohn's disease

Crohn's disease (p. 290) frequently affects the terminal ileum and may mimic appendicitis. The patient can present without a previous diagnosis of the disease but usually there is a history of repeated abdominal pain and diarrhoea. Other manifestations of Crohn's disease, such as perianal disease and malabsorption, may be evident. Often the appendix is removed before the diagnosis is proved. If a mass from the affected inflamed ileum is present, and treated conservatively as for an appendix mass, it may not decrease in size with time and further investigations are necessary to make the diagnosis. Occasionally the ileal inflammation is great enough to cause intestinal obstruction and failure of this to resolve leads to laparotomy. If there is perforation and peritonitis, the clinical symptoms and signs indicate the need for urgent laparotomy.

Terminal ileitis can also be caused by tuberculous infection of the ileum which is now rare in the UK due to the pasteurization of milk.

Typhoid

The diagnosis of typhoid is usually made before perforation of the small bowel occurs. However, due to the general poor state of the patient, the signs and symptoms of this complication are similar to a postoperative peritonitis or peritonitis in the elderly, rather than the more obvious and florid presentation of a perforated peptic ulcer. There tends to be only mild, generalized tenderness, with few bowel sounds.

Intestinal obstruction

Intestinal obstruction may be dynamic or adynamic in origin. **Dynamic** obstruction is a mechanical problem, due to obstruction of the lumen (e.g. faecal impaction), an abnormality of the wall (e.g. an inflammatory stricture or neoplasm) or external compression (such as adhesions, obstruction within a hernial sac, an intussusception or a volvulus). **Adynamic** obstruction is due to a paralysed bowel, as in postoperative paralytic ileus or in acute mesenteric ischaemia.

The cardinal symptoms of simple intestinal obstruction are vomiting, colicky abdominal pain, abdominal distension and absolute constipation. These are present to a greater or lesser degree according to the level of obstruction. If the obstruction becomes compromised, with bowel ischaemia, and then perforates, the symptoms and signs change to those of peritonitis. Intestinal obstruction in children is considered on p. 333.

With **high intestinal obstruction**, vomiting is of rapid onset and profuse, leading to early and profound dehydration. With more distal obstruction, vomiting is delayed and may take a day or two to appear. Pain is usually of sudden onset; its various features are described below.

Abdominal distension may be minimal with high obstruction but progressive with more distal lesions (*Figure 24.7*). Distension is due to gas, which is swallowed (70%) or produced by digestion and bacterial decomposition. Large quantities of fluid may be sequestrated in the small bowel since more than 8 L are produced each day through oral intake and from digestive juices; this is normally absorbed in the large bowel. Fluid loss through vomiting and sequestration in intestinal obstruction accounts for the rapid dehydration and the onset of hypovolaemic shock.

The gas and fluid are demonstrated radiologically as fluid levels within the small gut loops on an erect plain abdominal film. In small bowel obstruction the radiological picture is of transverse gas patterns, stacked like coins, the indentations being due to contraction of the valvulae conniventes. In large bowel dilatation the caecum is distended and there is asymmetry of the colon due to the haustral folds. Gas shadows may also demonstrate the cause of the obstruction, such as loops of bowel entering the neck of a hernial sac, or the 'apple core' appearance of a circumferential large bowel cancer.

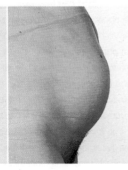

Figure 24.7.
Abdominal distension in a patient with intestinal obstruction.

Acute obstruction of the small intestine

The commonest causes of small bowel obstruction are adhesions from previous surgery and incarceration of the intestine in hernias. The principal symptoms are abdominal pain and vomiting. The pain is usually felt over the whole abdomen, worse in the epigastrium and around the umbilicus. It usually occurs as bouts of increasing colicky pain, varying from 3 to 10 minutes in length depending in part on the level of the obstruction, the more proximal the obstruction the shorter the duration of the bouts of colic and the shorter the interval between bouts. Obstruction causes retrograde peristalsis up to and including the stomach; the contents of the stomach, duodenum, jejunum and/or ileum down to the level of the obstruction are then vomited. The vomit includes undigested food and fluid, digestive juices and later increased mucosal secretion. With distal small bowel and large bowel obstruction the vomit looks and smells like fluid faeces due to the action of bacteria. It is termed faeculent vomiting as the presence of true faeces in vomiting requires a short circuit in the bowel such as in a gastrocolic fistula. As there is decreased absorption, and fluid intake is inhibited, water and electrolyte loss is considerable; if left untreated it ultimately leads to the patient's demise. The more distal the obstruction the longer it takes for severe dehydration to occur. In jejunal obstruction it is possible to suffer fatal water and electrolyte loss in one or two days, whereas terminal ileal obstruction may take a few days to become evident.

Constipation is not a constant feature in small bowel obstruction and takes at least 24 hours to develop. In cases of mesenteric vascular occlusion, Richter's hernia and pelvic abscess causing adhesions or pelvic colonic irritation, diarrhoea may be a prominent feature.

On examination the patient appears ill. The pulse and blood pressure should be monitored to identify and treat shock before it becomes irreversible. The patient, if dehydrated, has papery skin and dry mucous membranes. After prolonged dehydration the tongue becomes brown, furred and dry. The abdomen is carefully examined for evidence of abdominal scars and hernias, as these are the commonest causes of small bowel obstruction. The patient usually provides a history of previous surgery or of inguinal or umbilical hernias. Note particularly the femoral hernial orifices as femoral hernias are the commonest missed sign of importance by both patient and clinician. This part of the examination requires complete exposure of the patient for its duration.

In early obstruction little else can be seen on inspection. As the condition progresses the abdomen becomes slightly distended. Later signs include visible peristalsis. This requires patience on the part of the examiner as it may take a considerable amount of time to detect one visible contraction – occasionally it can be provoked by gently flicking the abdominal wall. Other signs include the 'ladder pattern' where the distended intestine is visible through the anterior abdominal wall.

Palpation occasionally reveals the causative factor, such as an intussusception, small bowel tumour or even a coil of distended intestine entrapped by an internal hernia. If peristalsis has not been easily visible it may be palpable. If the examining hand is rested flat upon the abdominal wall the underlying bowel alternately hardens and softens with the action of peristalsis like a pregnant uterus. Localized tenderness denotes the possibility of strangulation and ensuing perforation and is therefore an important sign to elicit. Laparotomy should be undertaken before perforation leads to generalized peritonitis. Gaseous distension arising from the obstructed loops of intestine can be confirmed by a resonant percussion note.

The sounds emitted from the obstructed loops of bowel provide the cornerstone of the diagnosis of intestinal obstruction. At first these are heard with a stethoscope placed over the abdominal wall slightly to the right of the umbilicus. The sounds start as a low-pitched gurgling but this rapidly changes to the characteristic high-pitched tinkling. These sounds are produced by the enteric fluid splashing against the resonant, taught intestinal walls of the gas-filled distended intestinal loops. Eventually the sounds become obvious without the aid of a stethoscope. The sounds of the fluid filled intestinal loops can also be heard, with or without a stethoscope, by eliciting a succussion splash.

Rectal examination rarely contributes to the diagnosis unless the distended loops of intestine, or a palpable cause of the obstruction, are present in the pelvis. The rectum is empty if the gut distal to the obstruction has been evacuated.

Gallstone ileus

Gallstone ileus is an uncommon cause of small bowel obstruction usually found in elderly subjects; it is easily cured by simple surgical removal and decompression. The gallstone enters the bowel from an inflamed gallbladder wall which had become adherent to a loop of intestine, perforating through the walls and passing into the lumen of the bowel to cause obstruction. There is a history of right upper quadrant pain becoming more generalized with intermittent symptoms of small bowel obstruction. The plain abdominal radiograph nearly always shows an air cholangiogram as bowel gas passes through the cholecyst–enteric fistula into the bile ducts; it occasionally shows the gallstone as well.

Acute obstruction of the large intestine

Causes of large bowel obstruction:

- In developed countries – Carcinoma of the colon or rectum; chronic diverticulitis.
- In developing countries – Faecal impaction; colonic volvulus; idiopathic intussusception.
- Uncommon causes – Inflammatory bowel disease (p. 290); ischaemic colitis; endometriosis (p. 297); carcinoma peritonei (p. 296); megacolon; pseudo-obstruction; anastomotic stricture.

The signs and symptoms depend upon the cause of the obstruction. A history of change in bowel habit (due to chronic incomplete colonic obstruction) together with weight loss, anorexia, and possibly a history of rectal bleeding (or occult blood loss leading to the signs and symptoms of anaemia) point to a carcinoma of the colon. The place of origin of the patient may point towards the diagnosis of a volvulus, in which case the history is particularly acute in onset.

The other determining factor in the pattern of signs and symptoms in acute colonic obstruction is the competence of the ileocaecal valve. Normally this valve prevents reflux of the caecal contents into the terminal ileum but it may not act effectively in otherwise healthy subjects. If the valve retains its normal function in colorectal obstruction, the pressure in the colon and particularly the caecum rises as the normal peristaltic activity of the ileum adds enteric fluid and gas to the caecum through the valve. The rise in intracolonic pressure may lead to rapid distension of the caecum, interruption of the blood supply of the caecal wall, mural necrosis and finally perforation. If the valve is or becomes incompetent, the obstructed colon is able to decompress by first the caecal fluid and then the colonic fluid flowing back into the ileum. In this case the signs and symptoms of obstruction become apparent much later that when the valve is competent and the signs are also more like those of ileal obstruction.

The course of the condition, although variable, is somewhat slower in onset and progression than that found in small bowel obstruction, with slower, more prolonged, less regular bouts of colic and hyperperistalsis. The time taken for vomiting to follow the pain is also longer.

If presentation is early, the patient appears less unwell than an equivalent case of small bowel obstruction. On inspection of the abdomen, unless the ileocaecal valve is incompetent, there is abdominal distension which is most marked in the right iliac fossa and this may seem to rise with each wave of peristalsis. Palpation of the abdomen for a mass

is generally not fruitful as an obstructing carcinoma is usually impalpable. Hepatomegaly is a sinister sign of possible metastatic spread.

Percussion of the abdomen yields hyperresonance, most noticeably in the right iliac fossa. Examination of the rectum is of paramount importance as a rectal tumour may give rise to large bowel obstruction. Faecal impaction may also be evident on rectal examination; it may be the cause of or a compounding factor in an obstruction, the latter occurring relatively early in a non-obstructing carcinoma. Polypoid colonic tumours may be palpable on rectal examination if they intussuscept to this level. In colonic obstruction the rectum is usually empty.

Volvulus of the sigmoid colon

Volvulus of the sigmoid colon is a condition affecting the middle-aged and elderly male particularly in Africa, Eastern Europe, parts of South America, Scandinavia and India. There is a history of attacks of abdominal pain with constipation followed by the relief of the pain with the passage of watery stools and copious volumes of flatus. These episodes are due to a volvulus of the sigmoid colon which spontaneously untwists. The vessels may be twisted in the root of the mesentery at the base of the volvulus, and also rotated into the compressed knuckles of bowel, with resultant strangulation and perforation of the involved bowel segment.

The onset of the pain is sudden and severe, and frequently occurs when the patient is straining at stool. The abdomen rapidly distends and the patient may retch and hiccup; vomiting occurs at a relatively late stage. The rectum is empty and its wall oedematous.

Caecal volvulus

Caecal volvulus (*Figure 24.8*) only occurs in those whose whole right colon has a mesentery continuous with that of the small bowel and so the caecum does not occupy its normal

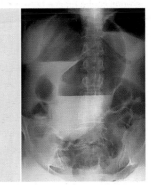

Figure 24.8.
Caecal volvulus.

position in the right iliac fossa. Usually there is a distended, tense, palpable, resonant mass in the centre of the abdomen with an empty, concave right iliac fossa. Both sigmoid and caecal volvulus have characteristic plain radiological appearances. Volvulus of the midgut due to developmental malrotation can occur in neonates (p. 333).

Intussusception

An intussusception is the invagination of a segment of bowel into an adjacent loop. The resulting compression usually gives rise to intestinal obstruction. The mesentery is drawn in between the two loops, and the blood supply may thus be compromised, leading to strangulation and perforation. The cause of an intussusception is usually a lesion at the apex of the inverted loop (the intussusceptum). It is massaged distally by the peristalsis of the outer loop (the intussuscipiens; *Figure 24.9a, b*). The lesion may be a malignant or benign polyp (e.g. Peutz–Jeghers syndrome), a colonic cancer or a gut abnormality, such as a Meckel's diverticulum (in adolescence).

Most commonly the condition is due to an enlarged Peyer's patch. This may be in response to a viral or bacterial infection of the gut. It is also seen in infants changing from human to cow's milk, probably related to an associated change in the gut's dietary flora. Occasionally the intussusception can progress over a substantial length of bowel and can protrude through the anus: it has to be differentiated from a rectal prolapse. This is more likely to occur if the intussusception commences in the left side of the colon.

Symptoms usually commence as a sudden onset of colicky abdominal pain. In infants – usually a male of 6–24 months – the pain causes drawing-up of the legs and screaming attacks, occurring every 15–30 minutes and lasting for 1–2 minutes. The pain, however, becomes more severe and prolonged as the disease progresses. Vomiting can take 24 hours to appear but may be copious, as can progressive distension. A diagnostic feature in children is the appearance of a classical 'red currant jelly' stool, which is a fluid stool containing much mucus and blood.

On abdominal examination of the infant there is typically a sausage-shaped lump to the left of the umbilicus, with emptiness in the right iliac fossa (*signé de dance*). In adults a mass may be palpable over the intussusception If the intussusception involves the lower colon, it can be palpated on rectal examination; digital palpation resembles the cervix. Perforation is due to gangrene at the neck of the intussusception, where the intussusceptum enters the intussuscipiens. A natural cure can occur by sloughing of the intussusceptum, and sealing and healing of the surrounding gut, but this is a rarity.

Obstruction due to **adhesions** usually follows a surgical procedure. It may occur within the first few months postoperatively but can be delayed for many years. Adhesions may be generalized or confined to a single loop of gut, or attenuated down to a fibrous band. The latter, like congenital bands, such as a persistent vitellointestinal duct, can become the site of compression or the apex of a volvulus. Obstruction due to generalized adhesions is likely to recur following any further surgery. It is, therefore, often managed conservatively with intravenous fluids and gastric suction to overcome acute exacerbations.

Internal hernias

Internal hernias may pass through congenital or acquired defects. Congenital pockets exist under the duodenum (under the superior mesenteric artery and inferior mesenteric vein), beneath the terminal ileum or the caecum and through the diaphragm. Obstructive disease of the small bowel wall is usually due to Crohn's disease, while obstruction of the small bowel lumen in children is not uncommonly due to large collections of the roundworm *Ascaris lumbricoides* or, in adults, a gallstone (see above).

Intestinal pseudo-obstruction

This is a condition where there is stasis of the bowel due to a disorder of colonic motility of either indeterminate or specific but variable aetiology – metabolic; hormonal; severe trauma; burns; septicaemia. The condition presents with

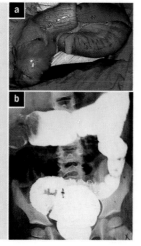

Figure 24.9.
Intussusception. a. Operative photograph of small bowel intussusception. b. Barium radiological study in a colocolonic intussusception.

considerable abdominal distension and a history of complete constipation, and it is frequently recurrent. There may be difficulty with respiration as the distension affects the diaphragm, an unusual feature of organic obstruction. The patient appears otherwise fairly well, and abdominal examination reveals little other than a very distended and resonant abdomen. On rectal examination there is usually a very dilated rectum, with or without faeces.

Occasionally caecal distension leads to perforation, and right iliac fossa pain and tenderness are ominous symptoms and signs, especially if associated with tachycardia and hypotension. Other than in this circumstance, laparotomy is not helpful and is best avoided. Plain abdominal films show a distended colon but no small bowel dilatation. A limited contrast enema is useful to exclude an obstructing lesion and allow a conservative approach to be adopted until the pseudo-obstruction resolves.

Adynamic obstruction

Paralytic ileus

A short period of ileus is common after abdominal operations and is characterized by abdominal distension, and silent or sparse bowel sounds, with nausea or vomiting. Paralytic ileus is an extreme of this condition and can both cause and be aggravated by imbalances in the serum electrolytes. It usually commences after the third postoperative day and may last for a week or more. Abdominal discomfort is present, due to distension, but the patient is usually happy with the postoperative course. They may complain of thirst only to find that any fluids taken orally are vomited back soon afterwards. The condition is marked in retroperitoneal and intraperitoneal haemorrhage – e.g. ruptured abdominal aortic aneurysms, spinal and abdominal trauma – and may accompany peritonitis, particularly in the terminal phases.

On examination the patient is dry. There is an increase in the pulse rate, in keeping with the degree of dehydration and abdominal distension. The abdomen is resonant to percussion. Auscultation is the key to the diagnosis as the characteristic absence of bowel sounds can only be diagnosed if no bowel sounds are heard during three minutes of listening just to the right and below the umbilicus (the most sensitive spot), in relatively quiet surroundings.

Ileus in renal failure

Ileus in renal failure may cause the symptoms of vomiting, hiccup and abdominal distension which may lead to confusion with intestinal obstruction. It is also possible in cases of intestinal obstruction at a late stage to develop renal failure, complicating the issue further. The absence of increased bowel sounds from peristaltic activity and the lack of evidence of obstruction on plain abdominal radiographs, together with high blood urea and creatinine levels, point to a metabolic rather than mechanical cause.

Mesenteric arterial occlusion

Mesenteric arterial occlusion is usually due to embolic disease but is occasionally due to local atherosclerosis (p.367; Figure 28.9). There is a history of sudden onset of central abdominal colic, which fairly rapidly becomes an agonizing generalized abdominal pain with copious repeated vomiting. The vomit is initially bile but becomes faeculent. There may be a history of recent myocardial infarction or atrial fibrillation, or a history of previous intermittent pain following meals (see mesenteric angina, p. 374). On examination the patient looks unwell and there is pronounced shock at an early stage. Nevertheless, the severe pain is out of all proportion to the paucity of physical signs. There may be abdominal distension but tenderness and the signs of generalized peritonitis are delayed until later, when perforation occurs; ileus is present. There may be an area of tender rigid abdominal wall adjacent to the infarcted bowel and an indeterminate lump which shifts with the position of the patient. Haematemesis and/or melaena occur in a third of cases.

Mesenteric venous occlusion results from intra-abdominal infections or portal hypertension and it is occasionally seen in sickle cell disease and in women taking the contraceptive pill. It has a slower onset and progression than arterial occlusion, when infarction becomes massive, the signs becoming very similar to those of arterial infarction. An enema often produces a stool containing much dark blood.

Ischaemic colitis

Ischaemic colitis occurs in cases where the vascular occlusion is incomplete or where the collateral supply, principally through the marginal artery of Drummond, is able to provide enough blood to allow the ischaemic bowel to recover. The signs and symptoms are similar to those of other causes of colitis, namely the passage of bloodstained diarrhoea and left-sided abdominal pain with tenderness along the course of the descending colon. The commonest site for this condition is at the watershed between the superior and inferior mesenteric arteries in the region of the distal transverse colon and the splenic flexure. The condition is sometimes associated with stricture formation and intestinal obstruction.

Acute colonic diverticulitis

Colonic diverticulosis is common, especially in populations eating highly refined western-type diets. Although diverticula (p. 293) are usually asymptomatic, they may give rise to complications that cause acute abdominal pain. A diverticulum may become inflamed producing signs and symptoms resembling acute appendicitis, but on the left rather than right side of the lower abdomen.

The location of the tenderness and the subsequent possible course of the condition depends in part on the location of the affected diverticulum; most diverticula are in the sigmoid and descending colon but they may rarely occur, although usually singularly, in the ascending colon or caecum. Right-sided diverticulosis, usually solitary, is seen in populations who do not eat highly refined foods; it presents with symptoms at an earlier age and probably has a different aetiology. Whether the affected colon is retroperitoneal or intraperitoneal determines the subsequent course of the condition. In non-retroperitoneal diverticulitis there is a much higher likelihood of free peritoneal perforation and peritonitis. Where perforation occurs, it can also perforate into another viscus such as the bladder, the colon or occasionally through the abdominal wall.

The symptoms of acute diverticulitis mirror those of acute appendicitis. The pain usually starts around the umbilicus and then localizes around the area of the individual diverticulum, normally this is the left iliac fossa and the maximum tenderness is elicited around the area of the inflammation. Where the tenderness is maximal on pelvic examination it may be difficult to distinguish between acute diverticulitis and acute appendicitis. Left-sided lesions can obstruct the passage of flatus and subsequent caecal distension can give rise to local tenderness mimicking appendicitis.

Where **acute free perforation of a colonic diverticulum** occurs the signs are of rapid diffusing peritonitis and these commonly occur without much in the way of premonitory symptoms.

Where perforation occurs retroperitoneally or into the mesocolon the perforation is contained and a **localized peridiverticular abscess** results. The surrounding oedema may give rise to large bowel obstruction and, where this abscess encroaches on to the peritoneal cavity, the omentum and the small bowel mesentery separate off the inflammation, producing a peridiverticular mass. A tender mass may be palpable on deep palpation in the left iliac fossa but it may also be masked by overlying rigidity.

Toxic megacolon

Toxic megacolon (*Figures 24.10a, b* and *24.11a, b*) is life threatening and merits early surgical intervention if optimum medical treatment fails to settle the inflammation, or if the patient has signs of peritonism indicating impending colonic perforation; the latter carries a 50% mortality. The severity of symptoms in inflammatory bowel disease usually mirrors the extent of the disease. Bad prognostic signs are a severe initial attack, late onset disease and involvement of the whole colon. Persistent inflammatory changes over many years can *predispose* to malignant change, the patient presenting with symptoms and signs of large bowel cancer (p. 292).

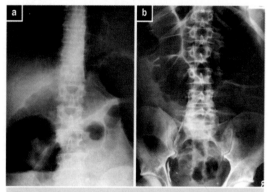

Figure 24.10
a, b. Toxic megacolon.

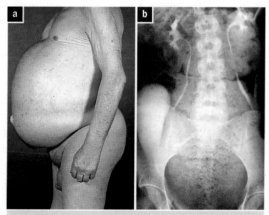

Figure 24.11
Megacolon. a. Gross abdominal distension. b. Gross dilatation of the distal large bowel in a previously undiagnosed youth with Hirschsprung's disease. The bladder has been displaced to the right and the whole of the central abdomen is filled with the dilated, faeces-filled rectum.

Abdominal aortic catastrophes

Severe abdominal or thoracic pain and hypotension may be due to:

- Perforated peptic ulcer.
- Myocardial infarction.
- Pancreatitis.
- Ruptured aortic aneurysm.
- Dissecting aortic aneurysm.
- Spontaneous oesophageal rupture (rare).

All of these most commonly occur in middle-aged and elderly men. Ruptured aortic aneurysms (*Figure 24.12*) most commonly occur in the abdominal aorta and are usually secondary to atherosclerosis. The condition is commonly fatal and is a common cause of sudden death in this group of patients. There may already be a diagnosis of aortic aneurysm but this is likely to have been asymptomatic and found on routine examination, or the patient may have noticed a pulsation in the epigastrium. When large (greater than 6 cm diameter) these aneurysms are repaired electively.

A leaking aneurysm causes severe epigastric, central abdominal or back pain as blood leaks into the retroperitoneum. The patient who is usually hypertensive becomes hypotensive. On abdominal examination the aneurysm is usually palpable but if bleeding has been extensive widespread abdominal rigidity and a mass, due to haematoma formation in the retroperitoneum or peritoneal cavity, may be palpable. The distal pulses may be reduced from hypovolaemia, but are usually patent and possibly dilated. Although bleeding may be temporarily halted by retroperitoneal tamponade, interventional measures are urgently required to prevent a fatal outcome.

Dissecting aortic aneurysms usually originate in the proximal thoracic aorta or aortic arch. As the dissection begins it causes excruciating chest pain, and if the ostia of the coronary arteries are occluded the patient may suffer a myocardial infarction. The pain radiates to the shoulders, occasionally down the arms and down the back. Upper abdominal pain commences as the dissection reaches the abdominal aorta.

On examination the patient is usually, but not always, shocked. Blood pressure in the arms may be different due to different involvement of the brachiocephalic and left subclavian arteries. Abdominal signs are usually absent but the dissection may affect the mesenteric vessels producing infarction or rupture, which is usually fatal. Involvement of the renal arteries may lead to anuria. The dissection stops at the aortic bifurcation, often occluding one or both common iliac arteries, producing acute limb ischaemia and requiring urgent intervention.

Medical causes of acute abdominal pain

There are several non-surgical causes of abdominal pain that can mimic the 'surgical abdomen'. Usually the features of the disease simplify the diagnosis. It must not be forgotten, however, that surgical pathology may occur in patients with known medical conditions that cause abdominal pain, and the clinician must always consider these possibilities. Cardinal signs are the presence of percussion or deep rebound tenderness during these assessments.

Ischaemic heart disease

Ischaemic heart disease gives rise to intermittent chest pain from coronary ischaemia and this may be referred or perceived as abdominal pain. As the pain is usually associated with exercise or stress, the diagnosis may be fairly easy to distinguish from abdominal pain. When the ischaemia is severe and sudden enough to cause acute coronary thrombosis, the resulting myocardial infarct is associated with severe central chest pain, usually radiating to the jaw or arms. Occasionally the pain is felt in the upper abdomen and may be confused with pain from peptic ulceration or pancreatitis. The diagnosis is made from an electrocardiogram and by the estimation of the enzymes characteristically released by ischaemic cardiac muscle. Treatment may involve the administration of thrombolytic enzymes: as these are contraindicated after surgery, accurate diagnosis is essential.

The pleura

The pleura is innervated in a similar way to the peritoneum and intrathoracic conditions causing pleural irritation cause pain that characteristically is worse on inspiration and can be provoked by asking the patient to cough. Causes of pleurisy include viral infection of the pleura and underlying

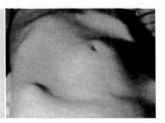

Figure 24.12.
Ruptured abdominal aortic aneurysm. The central mass is produced by both the aneurysm and the surrounding haematoma.

bronchopneumonia. Where the diaphragmatic or lower thoracic pleura are involved, the pain can be referred to the abdomen and confuse the diagnosis.

The somatic nerves and nerve roots

These can mimic pain originating from the abdomen. A condition that can cause such pain and confusion is herpes zoster infection (*Figure 24.13*). This affects nerve root ganglia; pain may occur many years after the initial infection. The condition is to be suspected if there is hyperaesthesia in the distribution of a somatic nerve. There is no rebound or guarding over the affected area and the characteristic vesicular eruption occurs, in the affected dermatome, a few days after the pain starts. Other causes of spinal nerve root irritation, such as degenerative disease of the thoracic spine, and tumours and abscesses in the thoracic spinal canal, can cause abdominal pain.

Disease of the distal oesophagus

Disease of the distal oesophagus (p. 249) can give rise to abdominal pain, usually epigastric, as well as chest pain; the latter may be mistaken for angina or the pain of myocardial infarction. Conditions which can give rise to confusion include reflux oesophagitis, infective oesophagitis from organisms such as *Candida* and, most alarmingly, oesophageal perforation.

Diabetic crises

Patients in a ketotic hyperglycaemic state of metabolic disorder may complain of abdominal pain. The diagnosis rests on estimation of the blood sugar and the abdominal symptoms should disappear on its return to normal. If they do not, a surgical cause is likely – the metabolic derangement must still be corrected as part of the resuscitation.

Porphyria

Porphyria is a congenital abnormality of haemoglobin metabolism. It can present with photosensitivity and anaemia, hypersplenism and constipation. It may also provide a difficult differential diagnosis of acute intestinal colic. Abdominal crises are characterized by violent intestinal colic and constipation and

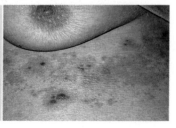

Figure 24.13. Resolving vesicles of abdominal herpes zoster. Pain precedes the eruption and can be mistaken for that of an acute abdominal event.

may be precipitated by alcohol, steroids, oestrogens or sulphonamides. Previously barbiturates were a common precipitant. The abdomen is distended but not rigid, and the spleen may be palpable. Motor weakness leading to flaccid paralysis may occur. The diagnosis rests on biochemical tests of the urine. An unusual physical finding is the colour change of urine to a port wine shade after a few hours on exposure to light.

Sickle cell anaemia

Sickle cell anaemia is a recessive hereditary disorder of haemoglobin, causing it to crystallize abnormally in the presence of low oxygen partial pressures. The heterozygote condition confers a protection against malarial infection and the disorder arose in endemic areas, notably central Africa. Descendants of people originally from these areas may carry the gene, and the homozygote gives rise to sickle cell anaemia. The crystallization of the haemoglobin leads to the formation of aggregates of affected red blood cells, which may occlude small vessels.

The mesenteric vessels are commonly affected and a crisis may present with severe generalized abdominal pain from the ischaemia. The abnormal red blood cells are removed in the spleen and may give rise to splenomegaly and hypersplenism. Enlarged spleens may undergo spontaneous infarction, giving rise to abdominal pain, predominantly in the left upper quadrant where the tender, enlarged spleen may be easily palpable. Patients may also suffer attacks of abdominal pain from excess haemolysis of red cells within the (enlarged) spleen, and right upper quadrant tenderness from biliary tract pain, with or without gallstones.

Haemophilia

Patients with haemophilia who complain of abdominal pain are likely, though not invariably, to have suffered a retroperitoneal haematoma; a palpable loin mass and a femoral nerve palsy may be present. The diagnosis should be confirmed by ultrasound or CT assessment. The condition may also be seen in patients taking anticoagulants.

Malaria

Although rare in the UK, malaria may be seen in residents and visitors to malarial zones. Haemolysis in the spleen may cause left upper quadrant pain though generalized abdominal pain with diarrhoea and vomiting may also occur. Diagnosis is confirmed by examination of a thick blood film.

Hyperlipidaemia

Hyperlipidaemia may cause attacks of abdominal pain, usually left sided, associated with a raised serum amylase concentration. There is usually a positive family history of the disorder, and signs of hyperlipidaemia such as arcus senilis, xanthelasmata and xanthomata, are often present.

Lead colic

Ingestion of lead in small amounts can give rise to mental impairment, especially in children and, in larger amounts, death. Of surgical relevance is the occasional symptom of colicky abdominal pain. There may be a history of exposure to lead, although medicines and paints now rarely contain it. The diagnosis can also be suspected by the appearance of a characteristic blue line on the gums, which consists of many small grey/blue/black dots 1 mm from the free margin of the gums.

Tabes dorsalis

Syphilis has become less common through the ages but its reputation as the great mimic of other diseases should not be forgotten (p. 69). Of relevance to the abdomen is the occasional symptom of acute abdominal pain in tabes dorsalis – tabetic crisis. The pain is of neurogenic origin in the absence of abdominal pathology. Look for other signs of tertiary syphilis such as the Argyll Robinson pupil – small, irregular and non-responsive to light – and the absence of tendon reflexes.

Munchausen's syndrome

This is the syndrome of patients who mimic illness, often very skillfully, in order to undergo some medical treatment. The diagnosis must always be considered when dealing with a patient whose complaints seem to be out of proportion to the findings on examination or investigation. However, never ignore the risks of missing real disease in unusual patients.

There are three types of Munchausen's patients: those with abdominal pain, the bleeders, and those with fits, faints and palsies. Abdominal pain and bleeding types present to surgeons. The experienced hoaxer may have an impressive array of scars and often has a long, convoluted history involving a large number of different hospitals. The patients are often, but not always, rather aggressive and threaten litigation.

Although well versed in giving an excellent history for a significant and dangerous disease, and skilled in the production of clinical signs such as tenderness, guarding and rebound, their control over involuntary bodily functions, such as their pulse and

bowel sounds, may let them down. Investigations may help but skill in contaminating urine with blood from elsewhere, or claiming allergy to contrast media can fool the unwary. Similarly, the practice of taping objects to the back to appear in plain radiographs has caused unnecessary alarm. Mental state examination and detailed psychiatric review usually reveal nothing. A syndrome of **Munchausen's syndrome by proxy** is where parents use or abuse their children to obtain medical treatment for the child. This in turn can result in direct or iatrogenic injury.

An assortment of **foreign bodies** are encountered, and may require removal, from any body orifice. These include swallowed items (p. 283) and those such as are illustrated in *Figure 24.14*.

Peritonitis

Infection of abdominal organs, such as appendicitis, cholecystitis, pelvic inflammatory disease and strangulated hernias, also involves the overlying peritoneum. The peritoneum, in addition, may be infected by organisms carried by the bloodstream or by direct spread from perforations, trauma and surgical procedures.

The severity of any infection is dependent both on local and systemic factors. The greater omentum plays an important role in the localization of abdominal infection. It is brought to an inflamed area by gut peristalsis and chemotaxis, and fibrin adhesions develop between it and gut loops, sealing off the area. The greater omentum has been aptly termed 'the

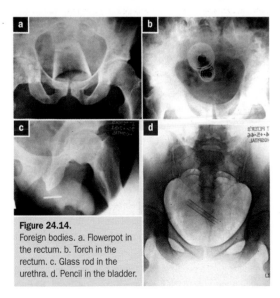

Figure 24.14.
Foreign bodies. a. Flowerpot in the rectum. b. Torch in the rectum. c. Glass rod in the urethra. d. Pencil in the bladder.

abdominal policeman' for its ability to arrive at trouble spots, localizing an infection and plugging perforations or potentially dangerous hernial orifices. Omentum is poorly developed in children and, therefore, less efficient in these functions.

Other factors influencing localization of an infection are the number and virulence of the organisms involved, the duration of the infection, and the contents and quantity of fluid leaking from any perforation. Some collections of perforated fluids are initially sterile – gastric and pancreatic juices; bile; urine; blood – but become secondarily infected within 6–12 hours due to transmigration of organisms from the adjacent gut. Foreign material, such as undigested food, takes longer for the body's defence mechanisms to remove.

Systemic resistance is influenced by the age and nutrition of the patient, coexisting diseases (such as malignancy and generalized infection) and altered immune responses. Steroids can diminish the inflammatory reaction and also mask local signs of disease.

The clinical features of peritonitis are related to the degree of localization of the disease. Pain is usually a prominent feature and may be severe; it is usually constant but, in chronic adhesive peritonitis, it may be colicky in nature. If only the visceral peritoneum is involved, pain from the fore-, mid- and hindgut is referred respectively to the epigastrium, umbilicus and suprapubic areas, whereas subdiaphragmatic pain may be referred to the shoulder tip; once the parietal peritoneum is involved, pain and tenderness are accurately localized. There may be diarrhoea or constipation in the early phases but constipation, associated with paralytic ileus, is usual in advanced disease. Weight loss is common; 20% of peritoneal abscesses may be silent, particular examples being subphrenic (p. 304) and pelvic collections.

Peritonism is usually present – i.e. palpation of the abdomen demonstrates involuntary muscle rigidity and voluntary guarding (muscle contraction) – the patient complaining of local tenderness. Board-like rigidity is a feature of a perforated peptic ulcer and, to a lesser extent, acute pancreatitis. In this situation local tenderness may be minimal as the sensitive peritoneum cannot be displaced by palpation.

The importance of anticipating the site and degree of tenderness before palpation cannot be overemphasized. This is obtained from the patient's history, their ability to draw the abdomen in and blow it out, their response to a cough, and the amount of self-abdominal palpation that they are willing to demonstrate. The use of a child's hand for palpation is valuable in gaining their confidence.

Initial gentle percussion of the whole abdomen identifies tender areas prior to palpation (percussion rebound); rebound tenderness, i.e. deep palpation and sudden release, should only be used if peritoneal signs are doubtful. Other signs are dependent on the underlying cause of the peritonitis. A palpable mass may be present, due to rolled-up omentum, an abscess or distended loops of inflamed gut; these features may also be visible. Abscesses may be palpable in the right or left iliac fossae, the paracolic gutters or on pelvic examination, and may be suspected from subphrenic referred pain or pain on compression of the lower thoracic cage.

The patient is likely to be pyrexial and tachycardic. Respiratory movements are reduced to limit pain from diaphragmatic descent, the patient looks unwell and toxic, and vomiting may be present. In the intermediate stages of peritonitis the local and systemic symptoms and signs may improve but if the infection progresses the patient develops terminal signs of swinging pyrexia, tachycardia, tachypnoea, hypotension and oliguria. The patient's face is drawn and anxious (Hippocratic facies), paralytic ileus is present, and the toxaemia is accompanied by electrolyte imbalance, renal dysfunction, bone marrow suppression and multiorgan failure.

Primary, blood-borne peritoneal infections include pneumococcal and TB. The latter may be acute, generalized or loculated, or may present as a low-grade infection producing extensive fibrous adhesions; palpable masses and rolled omentum are common. Talc or starch peritonitis, with foreign body granulomas, have been largely eradicated once it was recognized that they were due to contaminants from surgeons' gloves. Meconium peritonitis, following perforation in meconium ileus, carries a high mortality (p. 334). Other diseases to consider in generalized peritoneal masses include fat necrosis and hydatid disease, where daughter cysts have been disseminated through the peritoneal cavity. Mesenteric lymphadenitis may accompany a peritoneal infection or be present as a non-specific lymphadenopathy (p. 335) or as specific infection, such as TB.

The acute abdomen in women

In addition to the disorders common to both sexes, women are prone to a number of other conditions that may give rise to abdominal pain and should be considered in its management. These conditions arise for the most part from the organs of reproduction and usually affect women in the childbearing years. Important differential diagnoses in the acute abdomen are an ectopic pregnancy, complications of fibroids (p. 297), pelvic inflammatory disease and torsion of, or bleeding from, an ovary.

Ectopic pregnancy

This is a relatively common disorder occurring about 15–20 times per 1000 normal deliveries. A fertilized egg implants in a site outside the body of the uterus, usually in a fallopian tube although other sites include the outside of the fallopian tube, uterus or ovary, or elsewhere in the peritoneal cavity. The fertilized ovum grows as normal initially until it presents in one of two ways:

- Tubal abortion – After some intermittent lower abdominal pain, which may localize to the side of the affected fallopian tube, and vaginal bleeding, the embryo is aborted through the uterine os.
- Tubal rupture – As the embryo grows the tube ruptures; this is accompanied by haemorrhage. There is intermittent abdominal pain that increases in severity. The patient feels faint although usually there is no actual syncope. The abdominal signs and symptoms change with time as the bleeding continues to fill the peritoneal cavity. Initially the signs and symptoms are confined to the pelvis and lower abdomen, as the blood irritates the peritoneum. Blood in the pelvic peritoneal cavity, characteristically gives lower abdominal pain that gets worse on coughing, going to the toilet, or during sexual intercourse. The pain may also be referred to the rectum (the toilet sign) as the peritoneum around the upper rectum becomes irritated by blood. As blood fills the abdomen, the pain becomes widespread until the diaphragmatic peritoneum is irritated, usually when the patient is supine, giving rise to shoulder tip pain.

The patient may know or suspect that she is pregnant, but she may not. There may be breast tenderness, morning sickness or urinary frequency. The menstrual history of a woman complaining of abdominal pain is vital, amenorrhoea being a cardinal sign of pregnancy. However, the patient may have had a period following ectopic implantation although in retrospect, this may have been different from normal, or bleeding from a tubal abortion may have been mistaken for a normal period. Very sensitive pregnancy tests may detect pregnancy before a period is missed, but are not infallible, and if the fetus has died they are negative.

Previous or ongoing fertility problems, with a history of investigations and treatments such as tubal or pelvic surgery, the presence of an intrauterine contraceptive device and a previous history of ectopic pregnancy are all associated with an increased rate of ectopic pregnancy.

On examination, the pulse may be raised. As the patients are young, the blood pressure may be maintained for a long period of time following the initiation of bleeding and hypotension is a serious sign, as it is the herald of decompensation. The abdomen may be slightly distended and initially signs are confined to the lower abdomen; usually there is unilateral iliac fossa or suprapubic tenderness that later spreads across the abdomen.

On rectal examination there is generalized pelvic tenderness, the uterus being very tender. Vaginal examination is important and on inspection there is usually bleeding from the os; the blood is characteristically dark ('prune juice' blood). The cervix is redder and more heterogeneous than usual and is extremely sensitive to palpation, especially if the uterus is tipped forwards (cervical excitation). The fornices are tender and a mass may be palpable around the affected fallopian tube. The pelvic signs are usually critical in the diagnosis and, as pelvic examination can aggravate haemorrhage, it is essential that an experienced clinician is involved. If the diagnosis is still in question further investigation may be required, including diagnostic laparoscopy, prior to surgical intervention.

Acute salpingitis

Acute salpingitis usually occurs in sexually active women or following sexually transmitted disease, childbirth or abortion; very occasionally haematogenous spread can occur in young girls. It is commonly recurrent. Common organisms include *Neisseria gonorrhoeae*, coliforms and *Chlamydia trachomatis*. The lower abdominal and pelvic pain is commonly bilateral and intermittent, becoming constant later. It is exacerbated by coughing and sexual intercourse. Characteristically pain starts at the end of a period and menorrhagia may be present. There is usually a history of vaginal discharge, and commonly associated nausea and vomiting. On examination there is pyrexia and often tachycardia. The lower abdomen is usually tender with associated rebound tenderness and there may be an associated peritonitis. On vaginal examination there is a vaginal discharge and an adnexal mass may be present: this may be due to a pyo- or hydrosalpinx, or a tubovarian abscess. Cervical movement in every direction produces severe discomfort. Unilateral pelvic inflammation, such as with a pelvic appendicitis, gives rise to unilateral pain on cervical excitation.

Ovarian cysts

Ovarian lesions are common, and their complications may give rise to acute abdominal pain. These include torsion, bleeding, rupture, infection and infarction. Ovarian cysts (also see p. 298) undergoing torsion are pedunculated and usually

8–10 cm in diameter. The pain is of acute onset and there may be associated low grade fever, with vomiting. Tenderness is in the right or left iliac fossa and the lesion is usually palpable, either within the abdominal cavity or bimanually.

Ruptured luteal cyst

During the course of a normal menstrual cycle the mature luteal cyst ruptures, releasing the ovum into the fimbriae of the fallopian tube or into the peritoneal cavity in their vicinity. This may be accompanied by a small haemorrhage or the release of fluid from the cyst. The process may irritate the peritoneum and give rise to sufficient pain for the young woman to seek medical advice. The patient is usually otherwise well and there is little to find on examination. The key to the diagnosis is the timing of the onset of the pain in relation to the menstrual cycle. Midcycle pain or *Mittelschmerz* are alternative names given to this condition. If there is marked bleeding from the right ovary the condition can be identical to acute appendicitis and, if the bleeding is excessive, it can mimic an ectopic pregnancy.

Abdominal trauma

The abdomen is subject to penetrating and blunt trauma. The former is primarily from surgical exploration but it may also be due to bullets, shrapnel and other injuries. Blunt trauma is most commonly encountered after road traffic accidents and falls. The presence of abdominal wall bruising indicates that there was a reflex contraction to the injury, and this helps to dissipate the force, reducing the injury to deeper structures. A body imprint of the injuring force, such as bruising in the shape of a tyre tread, is an indication of a severe injury and probable underlying visceral damage.

Although they are enclosed within the lower rib cage, the **liver** and **spleen** are particularly susceptible to all forms of trauma. An enlarged spleen is more fragile in patients with infective mononucleosis and malaria, the latter being known to ancient assassins who developed a specific implement, called a larange, to inflict lethal rupture in malarial regions. Bleeding from both liver and spleen may be fatal, there being a 20% mortality with a damaged liver, rising to 50% if four organs are involved. Liver tears bleed and release bile into the peritoneal cavity, while intrahepatic haematomas undergo secondary rupture into the peritoneum or biliary tree. Deep lacerations may devitalize liver segments. Pain from both organs may be referred to their respective shoulders and there may be local tenderness over fractured ribs or a bruised abdominal wall.

Intraperitoneal bleeding may produce signs of hypovolaemic shock, accompanied by guarding, rigidity, paralytic ileus and distensions (meteorism). Blood collections of more than 1500 mL may be detected by shifting dullness, and blood tracking down to the pelvis produces tenderness in the pouch of Douglas on digital examination. The spleen, in particular, is subject to delayed rupture, in which a haematoma and capsular tear are temporarily sealed off, only to leak when the sealing blood clot haemolyses 10 to 16 days later, producing signs of haemorrhage and local pain from peritoneal irritation. Suspicion that such a lesion is a potential complication is essential, since these patients are likely to have been discharged before the secondary event.

The **pancreas** is deeply seated across the upper posterior abdominal wall but it is still susceptible to penetrating injuries, and a direct blow to the relaxed abdomen can split the pancreas over the vertebral column at the level of its neck, in line with the aorta. Blows from the right side can damage the duodenum and the head of the pancreas, while iatrogenic injuries to the tail occur in gastric and splenic surgery, to the duct during sphincterotomy and to the body during enucleation or resection of tumours. Pancreatic damage causes pain from haemorrhage and leakage of digestive enzymes. It may be complicated by early acute pancreatitis or later development of fistulae into the peritoneal cavity, adjacent viscera or on to the abdominal wall. Another late complication is a pancreatic pseudocyst. Renal, ureteric and bladder injuries are considered on p. 361.

The **intestines** may be perforated by gun shot, shrapnel and knife wounds, and iatrogenic injuries during surgical procedures. Blunt trauma from blows, or crushing injuries to the abdomen, may tear the gut against the vertebral column, while deceleration injuries may produce a perforation at the duodeno–jejunal flexure. The presenting signs of gut perforation are similar to those described in other pathology (pp. 301 and 315). The diagnosis, however, may be masked by the pain of abdominal wall bruising or other injuries, and unconsciousness. The clinician must, therefore, remain awake to the possibility of gut perforation from the history of the trauma and the distribution and severity of other injuries.

The **small gut** and, to a lesser extent, the **transverse** and **sigmoid colonic mesenteries**, can be torn in deceleration injuries, particularly if a seat-belt is being worn. Initially the signs are those of intraperitoneal haemorrhage but devitalized gut may perforate at a later time and the patient's abdomen must be monitored for changing peritoneal signs.

25 Anorectal and vaginal examination

Introduction

Rectal and vaginal examination are part of the routine examination of the abdomen. Omission has often proved to be the cause of diagnostic delay, embarrassment to the physician who failed to perform them, and regret to all concerned.

Anorectal examination can be made with the patient in one of four positions:

- **The left lateral (Sims') position** – The patient is positioned comfortably with the trunk across the bed rather than parallel to it and the buttocks projecting well over the edge of the bed. The legs should be flexed at the hips and knees.
- **The knee–elbow position** – This is adopted more commonly in the USA and is especially useful for examining anteriorly located perianal pathology, the prostate and seminal vesicles.
- **The dorsal position** – This is used when either the patient cannot be moved laterally, because of possible spinal injury, or because the patient is too ill to turn into the left lateral position. The patient lies semirecumbent with the knees flexed and the examiner passes his or her arm under the patient's right thigh to gain access to the anorectum. Digital examination is used in conjunction with the other hand upon the lower abdomen, such that pelvic swellings can be assessed bimanually and that access to the rectovesical or rectouterine pouches can be made with minimal disturbance of the patient.
- **The lithotomy position** – This allows the most thorough examination of the pelvis and allows lesions high in the rectum to be felt which might not be so in the other positions. Normally this position is adopted for examination under anaesthesia (EUA). The buttocks project beyond the end of the operating table and the hips are flexed beyond the right angle with legs in stirrups outside the poles.

Anorectal examination includes inspection, careful palpation – both within and without the anal canal – with an adequately lubricated digit, rigid sigmoidoscopy and proctoscopy. If pain or other factors preclude a full examination in the awake patient, and there is doubt about the diagnosis, arrangements must be made for the patient to undergo an EUA.

Surgical anatomy

The anatomy of the anal sphincter is shown in *Figure 25.1*. The pelvic floor is formed by the levator ani group of muscles, the components named according to their attachments, with the most important in terms of anorectal anatomy being the puborectalis. Through this muscular diaphragm pass the rectum and anal canal posteriorly and the urethra and vagina anteriorly. It is important, especially in the assessment of anorectal sepsis, to realize that the pelvic floor is not a flat sheet but a funnel. The puborectalis envelopes the lower rectum on all sides, except anteriorly, and is continued inferiorly as the external sphincter of the anal canal. The puborectalis muscle is responsible for the forward angulation of the anorectal junction and is easily felt in the conscious patient as a posterior ridge, but less easily under anaesthesia. Because of the arrangement of the

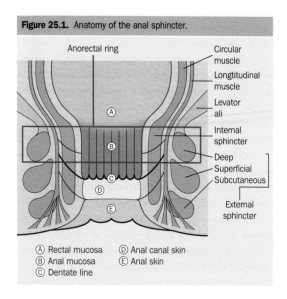

Figure 25.1. Anatomy of the anal sphincter.

Anorectal ring

Circular muscle

Longtitudinal muscle

Levator ani

Internal sphincter

Deep
Superficial
Subcutaneous
External sphincter

Ⓐ Rectal mucosa   Ⓓ Anal canal skin
Ⓑ Anal mucosa   Ⓔ Anal skin
Ⓒ Dentate line

puborectalis sling, the length of the anal canal surrounded by striated muscle is less anteriorly than posteriorly.

The classic description of the external sphincter as three distinct bundles – subcutaneous; superficial; deep – is somewhat arbitrary, but the subcutaneous portion may be regarded as anatomically separate from the remainder by virtue of the terminal ramifications of the conjoined longitudinal muscle that encloses it, as the latter inserts into the perianal skin.

The internal anal sphincter is a direct continuation of the circular smooth muscle coat of the rectum, which has developed specialized properties. The lower edge of the internal sphincter may be easily felt under anaesthesia, with an anal retractor opened in the anal canal, as a tight band rather like a thick guitar string, which forms the upper border of the anal intermuscular groove. The internal sphincter is crossed by fibroconnective tissue fibres derived from the medial aspect of the conjoined longitudinal muscle as this runs down the intersphincteric space; these fibres intermingle with those of the subepithelial space and support the overlying anoderm and mucosa. There is a condensation of these supporting fibres at the level of the dentate line which Parks named the mucosal suspensory ligament. This description is important since it separates the vessels of the superior haemorrhoidal plexus (related to internal haemorrhoids) from those of the inferior haemorrhoidal plexus (related to thrombosed external piles) as well as separating the marginal space from the submucous space.

Between the internal and external sphincters lies the intersphincteric space, which is clinically important as it contains the anal glands and is thought to be responsible for the majority of 'idiopathic' anal fistulae. Infection of the anal glands is probably responsible for the majority of cases of acute anorectal sepsis. Bacteria pass retrogradely up the anal ducts from the crypts at the dentate line to create an abscess in the gland in the intersphincteric space; this cannot spontaneously discharge back into the anal lumen because of the tone of the internal sphincter. Anal glands may also be found superficial to the internal sphincter but these are not important clinically since infection in such glands is able to drain and resolve spontaneously.

The skin of the perineum is stratified, squamous, hairy, keratinized epithelium. This contains apocrine glands which may become the site of chronic infection (**hidradenitis suppurativa**). The distal end of the anal canal is lined by stratified, squamous, non-keratinized epithelium to the level of the dentate line, which line may be regarded as the site of fusion of the embryological proctodeal ectoderm and the hindgut. In practical terms it is the site of the anal crypts at which point the anal gland ducts open into the anal lumen, and is the site of the majority of internal openings of cryptoglandular or idiopathic anal fistulae.

The **dentate line** is so called because of its likeness to a row of teeth (or pectinate: akin to a comb), the sides of the teeth passing cephalad as the rectal columns of Morgagni. The dentate line is also a watershed for lymphatic drainage; this drainage – which accompanies the arteries – passes upwards to the inferior mesenteric nodes above the dentate line but downwards to the inguinal nodes below the dentate line. It is in the region of the line that there is the highest concentration of sensory nerve endings; the sensory component of the anal canal is important, not only in the conscious discrimination of gut contents passing over it but also in the unconscious reflex in which the internal sphincter relaxes to allow 'sampling' of the rectal contents.

Above the dentate line is the so-called transitional zone of the anal canal (not to be confused with the transitional epithelium of the urinary tract). This area represents a gradual change from flattened squamous type cells to the true columnar epithelium of the rectum. Above the dentate line the epithelium is relatively insensitive although an appreciation of stretch can be elicited.

The arrangement of muscular and supporting tissues of the anal sphincter complex means that there are several well-defined anatomical spaces in relation to them. As these spaces are important in the spread of sepsis, accurate identification of the site of sepsis is fundamental to correct management.

Inspection of the perineum is extremely important. Soiling may be a result of incontinence or poor local hygiene. Minor anal seepage from haemorrhoids, fissure, fistula, proctitis, rectal polyp, prolapse or malignancy, from minor incontinence secondary to anal surgery, and from liquid stool from whatever cause may lead to itching, scratching and excoriation of the perianal skin. Excoriation may also result from primary skin disorders which may affect the perineum, fungal, viral and parasitic infections, and, not uncommonly, hypersensitivity reactions to washing agents, toilet paper and even those topical agents applied in the hope of relieving the itching.

Inspection of the skin of the perineum may reveal one or more external openings of anal fistulae, of multiple sinuses due to underlying hidradenitis, scars from previous infection or surgery, or warts which may also be present on the external genitalia and inside the anal canal. Look closely at the anal margin itself – look for the olive-shaped subcutaneous perianal haematoma, resulting from thrombosis of one of the veins of the external (superficial) haemorrhoidal venous plexus, the external skin components of true haemorrhoids, the sentinel tag of a fissure and simple anal skin tags.

Look closely at the anus, i.e. its position in relation to the ischial tuberosities at rest and on straining – perineal descent. If there is a history suggestive of prolapse – of piles, a polyp, malignancy or of the rectum itself – and this is not demonstrable by inspection in the left lateral position, observe the anus whilst the patient is sitting on a lavatory. This is easiest if the patient is crouched forward and the examiner leaning over to look from behind. This simple manoeuvre can be most informative.

Palpation includes feeling the skin of the perineum as well as actual digital examination of the anorectum itself; tracks leading from external openings of fistulae may course superficially and may then easily be traced by using a well-lubricated, gloved digit. Rectal examination, although often embarrassing to the patient, should be a painless process. The left lateral position is adopted. Always warn the patient about what you are going to do and what sensation this action may result in before proceeding. Lay the pulp of the index finger flat upon the anal verge and slowly introduce the tip of the digit into the anal canal with the pulp facing posteriorly.

If an acute fissure is present, entry of the digit is not tolerated by the patient and the examination should be abandoned with arrangements made for an EUA. On initial insertion, the anal intermuscular groove can be felt; an assessment of internal sphincter tone can be made digitally with the patient at rest, and of the external sphincter when the patient is asked to squeeze the examining finger. Rotating the pulp of the finger around the circumference of the anal canal and asking the patient to squeeze allows a clinical assessment of external sphincter integrity. This takes much experience, especially the anterior sphincter aspect in females. Feel for induration around the anal canal; above the levators, induration feels bony hard like the sacrum lying posteriorly and can be best appreciated by comparing one side with the other.

Anteriorly, in the male the prostate should be felt and assessed for size, consistency and the presence of the median sulcus. A long digit may reach the seminal vesicles, especially if the patient is in the knee–elbow position.

In the female, the cervix uteri can be felt projecting through the anterior rectal wall. Assessment of the cervix transanally is difficult for the inexperienced, and occasionally the experienced, examiner because of its variety in size and shape, and it is not unusual for a normal cervix to be thought a rectal neoplasm. Only practice and experience gives an appreciation of what is clinically normal and what is pathologically valid. Above the prostate or cervix uteri, the rectovesical pouch (in males) and the pouch of Douglas (in females) should be assessed digitally.

Haemorrhoids

Patients with rectal bleeding may complain of true 'piles', i.e. lumps that appear at the anal orifice during defecation and which return spontaneously up into the anal canal (second degree piles), or have to be replaced manually (third degree piles; *Figure 25.2*) or which lie permanently outside the anus. The term 'first degree piles' is applied to painless rectal bleeding from the potentially prolapsing mucosa. Many so-called fourth degree piles cannot be reduced because it is the external skin component of the haemorrhoids that represents the irreducible components. These tags arise through intermittent congestion and oedema when the internal components prolapse. True strangulated haemorrhoids (*Figure 25.3*) usually present via the A & E department and are associated with severe, constant, unremitting pain with large pile masses protruding from the anal orifice with gross oedema and later ulceration.

A **perianal haematoma** (*Figure 25.4*) is a 5–10 mm thrombosed vein in the subcutaneous perianal venous plexus. The lesion is usually of sudden onset and exquisitely painful. The lump is blue and tender, and visible on the anal verge. The pain takes 4–5 days to resolve and the lesion slowly fibroses, often leaving a palpable, persistent nodule.

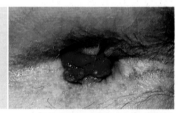

Figure 25.2. Third degree haemorrhoids.

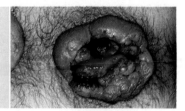

Figure 25.3. Strangulated haemorrhoids.

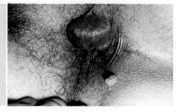

Figure 25.4. Perianal haematoma.

Acute perineal sepsis

Acute anorectal sepsis is common. An understanding of aetiology and anatomy is fundamental to correct management. Patients with acute anal sepsis present with a story of increasing pain in the region, usually a lump, and occasionally a purulent or bloody discharge and fever. The condition of high intermuscular abscess is uncommon but must be considered in the differential in a patient with fever, vague deep anorectal pain, perhaps difficulty in passing urine, but in whom although no abscess is visible digital examination of the anorectum is extremely painful.

For the most part anorectal sepsis may be divided into that which has nothing to do with the anorectum – e.g. simple boils; pilonidal abscess; hidradenitis suppurativa – and that which is intimately related to the anorectum (*Figure 25.5*). Pilonidal disease and hidradenitis are usually simple to recognize. Cutaneous boils can present as both perianal and ischiorectal abscesses. The key to their distinction, from those associated with anal problems, can often be found in the microbiology and the smell of the pus. The incidence of anorectal sepsis due to skin organisms – and nothing to do with fistulae – is equally divided between the sexes, whereas sepsis due to gut organisms is more common in men, reflecting the similar [unexplained] male predominance of the chronic condition, the anal fistula. A history of previous sepsis at the same site is also indicative, but not diagnostic, of a communication with the anorectal lumen.

Most cases arise spontaneously and are not associated with underlying diseases but are occasionally a presentation of established inflammatory bowel disease and can be associated with underlying diabetes and other immunosuppressed states, which should be revealed on history and examination.

Anal fistula

The vast majority of anal fistulae seen in surgical practice are due to persisting infection of the anal glands in the intersphincteric space – the cryptoglandular hypothesis. However, anal fistulae are also seen in association with other specific conditions such as inflammatory bowel disease, TB, malignancy, actinomycosis, lymphogranuloma venereum, trauma and foreign bodies. Anal fistulae (*Figure 25.6*) are those that communicate between the anal canal and the perianal skin and may be considered the chronic sequel of the parent condition, acute anorectal sepsis, although many years may elapse between the two clinical conditions.

Patients with anal fistulae complain of intermittent anal pain and discharge, either purulent or mixed with blood; the two symptoms are often inversely related, with the pain increasing until it eases off when the pus drains out through the external opening. There is often a history of acute anal sepsis, either treated surgically, or which has settled after spontaneous discharge of pus or which settled insidiously leaving an opening on the perianal skin.

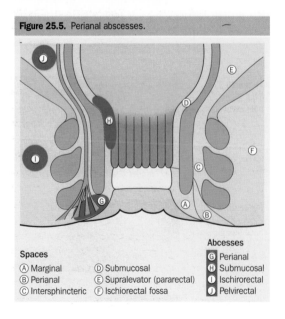

Figure 25.5. Perianal abscesses.

Spaces

Ⓐ Marginal   Ⓓ Submucosal
Ⓑ Perianal   Ⓔ Supralevator (pararectal)
Ⓒ Intersphincteric   Ⓕ Ischiorectal fossa

Abcesses

Ⓖ Perianal
Ⓗ Submucosal
Ⓘ Ischirorectal
Ⓙ Pelvirectal

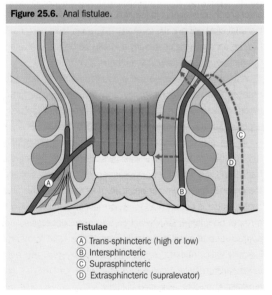

Figure 25.6. Anal fistulae.

Fistulae

Ⓐ Trans-sphincteric (high or low)
Ⓑ Intersphincteric
Ⓒ Suprasphincteric
Ⓓ Extrasphincteric (supralevator)

Surgical management of anal fistulae depends upon an accurate knowledge of both anorectal sphincter anatomy and the course of the fistula through it. According to Parks' classification, there are four main fistula types: trans-sphincteric, intersphincteric, suprasphincteric and extrasphincteric, each of which may be further subdivided according to the presence and course of any secondary tracks (*Figure 25.7*):

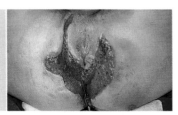

Figure 25.7.
Surgical laying open of anal fistulae indicating the extent of its various channels.

- **Trans-sphincteric fistula** – The primary track of this fistula passes through the external sphincter at varying levels into the ischiorectal fossa. Such fistulae may be uncomplicated, consisting only of the primary track opening on to the skin of the buttock, or can have a high blind secondary track that ends either below or above the levator ani muscles.
- **Intersphincteric fistula** – This passes from the anal canal across the internal sphincter, downwards between the internal and external sphincters and opens on to the perineal skin. Such fistulae are most commonly simple but others end with a high blind track, or have an internal opening into the rectum, or no perineal opening, or even have a pelvic extension or arise through pelvic disease.
- **Suprasphincteric fistula** – Suprasphincteric fistulae run up in the intersphincteric plane to loop over the top of the puborectalis muscle thence to pass down through the levator ani and ischiorectal fossa to reach the skin of the perineum.
- **Extrasphincteric fistula** – This is a fistula that runs without relation to the sphincters and is classified according to aetiology. Some are iatrogenic in origin, arising from overzealous probing of the ischiorectal fossa in a patient who presents with an ischiorectal abscess. The underlying fistula in this circumstance is usually trans-sphincteric.

It is important to understand the basic primary tracks of the four recognized types of anal fistula. Superimposed on these primary tracks are extensions or secondary tracks which may be blind or which may open on to the perineal skin or back into the anorectal lumen (usually because of injudicious probing). Besides vertical and horizontal spread, sepsis may also spread circumferentially in any of the three tissue planes: intersphincteric (or intermuscular, which implies no restriction to below the anorectal ring), ischiorectal and pararectal.

Parks' classification does not include those low intersphincteric fistulae which result from an anal fissure, and sub-cutaneous tracks arising from superficial infection, two types which although relatively minor are seen much more commonly in local hospitals than tertiary referral centres.

The differentiation of fistulae into 'high' and 'low' is often a point of confusion. A sensible and useful way of implementing such terminology is to describe all those fistulae which, if laid open at a single stage fistulotomy would cause significant functional morbidity, as high; and the remainder, in which laying open would not cause major incontinence, as low. This does not mean that laying open of 'low' fistulae is not associated with functional morbidity but rather that the incidence and degree of symptoms are less.

Clinical assessment of anal fistulae involves five essential points: the location of the external and internal openings; the course of the primary track and any secondary tracks ('lateral burrowings'); and the presence of other diseases complicating the fistula. The relative positions of the internal and external openings indicate the likely course of the primary track and the presence of any palpable induration, especially supralevator, alerts the surgeon to a high secondary track.

The distance between the external opening and the anal verge may assist the differentiation between an intersphincteric and a trans-sphincteric fistula; and the greater the distance, the more the likelihood of a complicated upward extension.

The position of the external opening also gives a clue as to the likely site of the internal opening. **Goodsall's rule** states that for openings anterior to a transverse mid-anal line, the fistula usually runs radially into the anal canal; for openings posterior to this imaginary line, the track is usually curvilinear to open into the anal lumen in the posterior midline. The exceptions to this rule include anterior openings more than 3 cm from the anal margin, which may be anterior extensions of posterior horseshoe fistulae, fistulae associated with Crohn's disease and those arising from carcinoma of the anal glands.

The internal opening may be felt digitally as an indurated nodule or pit, or seen at proctoscopy, aided if necessary by gentle downward retraction of the dentate line which may expose openings concealed by prominent anal valves. Outpatient assessment must include sigmoidoscopy, but beyond this more information can only safely and comfortably be obtained from EUA or special investigations. Probing fistulae in the clinic is both painful and dangerous. Special investigations are generally reserved for 'difficult' – i.e. recurrent or complex – fistulae.

Anal fissure

An anal fissure (*Figure 25.8*) is a cutaneous tear in the ectodermal portion of the anal canal and is usually found in either the 12 o'clock or 6 o'clock positions around the anal circumference (orientation of the anus is conventionally described in the lithotomy position: 12 o'clock is then sited anteriorly – towards the scrotum or vagina). It commonly occurs after a bout of constipation and is very painful. Patients find themselves in a vicious circle where they appreciate that the next bout of defecation will be painful, hence they avoid passing a stool and become progressively more constipated. When the bowel is eventually opened the tear is made worse. Fresh bleeding is common and this is the commonest cause of rectal bleeding in a child.

A diagnostic feature of an anal fissure is anal pain after defecation and, in chronic cases, the skin at the lower part of the fissure becomes swollen and can be used as a marker of an anal fissure – the 'sentinel pile'. This may be the only sign of a chronic anal fissure as it is often too painful to examine the patient proctoscopically.

Pruritus ani (*Figure 25.9*) is an insatiable itch around the perianal region; it may extend to the introitus in the female.

Common causes are listed in *Table 25.1*. The skin is usually moist from anal or vaginal discharge of infected material, mucus or faeces. There is erythema, maceration, excoriation and lichenification, and one of the lesions listed in *Table 25.1* may be visible. In the female, pruritus vulvae may be associated with pruritus ani. Thrush is common and urinary leakage may be due to a cystocele or an ectopic ureter (p. 349).

Every baby develops a nappy rash (*Figure 25.10*) at some point and this is usually due to prolonged contact with urine or faeces but may be due to a fungal infection or a reaction to an emollient.

Table 25.1. Causes of pruritus ani.

Generalized causes of itching	Obstructive jaundice
	Diabetes mellitus
	Hyperparathyroidism
	Myeloproliferative disorders
	Lymphoma
Local disorders	Excess sweating; poor hygiene; woollen underwear
Skin conditions	Eczema
	Allergy
	Contact dermatitis (to detergent and other local applications)
	Lichen planus
	Psoriasis
Infections/infestations	STDs
	Fungal
	Scabies
	Lice
	Threadworms
Diarrhoea/incontinence	Leakage of liquid paraffin
	Sphincter malfunction
	Rectal prolapse
Anal pathology	Piles
	Fissures
	Fistula in ano
	Warts
	Crohn's disease/TB
	Polyps/cancer
Pathology of the lower rectum and anal canal giving diarrhoea and mucous discharge	Villous adenoma/carcinoma
	Solitary ulcer
In women	Candida infection (thrush)
	Trichomonas vaginalis
	Urinary leakage
Psychological causes	
Nappy rash	Infrequent nappy changes
	Reaction to local applications

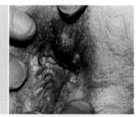

Figure 25.8.
Anal fissure.

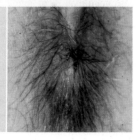

Figure 25.9.
Skin changes in pruritus ani.

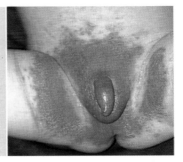

Figure 25.10.
Nappy rash.

Prolapse of the rectum

This encompasses both prolapse of the rectal mucosa through the anus and full-thickness prolapse of the rectum (*Figure 25.11*). The two can be distinguished by feeling one wall of the prolapse between index finger and thumb – a full-thickness prolapse feels like a double-layered tube. Prolapse may be caused by straining excessively at stool, especially if the pelvic floor muscles are weak. Although the young and the elderly are most frequently seen with the condition, any age group can be affected. In children it may be associated with malnutrition and chronic diarrhoea. If present for a long time the prolapse may ulcerate and the patient then present with bleeding and discharge of mucus. Occasionally a prolapse can become ischaemic and present as a surgical emergency.

Perianal Crohn's disease

Perianal Crohn's disease – PACD (*Figure 25.12*) – may be found in up to 75% of patients with Crohn's disease, the incidence relating to the site of gastrointestinal pathology with higher rates the more distal the disease. It is important to remember however that PACD may precede Crohn's

disease elsewhere in the gastrointestinal tract by many years. The spectrum of PACD may be clinically divided into those primary conditions – fissures; ulcerated piles; cavitating ulcers – whose activity reflects that of the intestinal disease, and secondary lesions – either mechanical (skin tags; strictures; epithelialized fistulae) or infective (abscesses; fistulae) – for which local treatment should be determined by local severity.

Perianal warts

The incidence of perianal warts – condylomata accuminata (*Figure 25.13*) – caused by the human papilloma virus, is increasing in the population. The highest rates are seen in homosexual males although heterosexuals are certainly not immune, the condition being almost invariably sexually transmitted. For this reason there is often a history of other sexually transmitted diseases (STDs). Patients with perianal warts usually complain of itching, bleeding and perianal lumps; there may also be symptoms from warts elsewhere on the genitalia. The appearance of the warts is variable, ranging from one or two discrete excrescences, which may be both within and without the anal canal itself, to massive cauliflower-like lesions totally obscuring the anal orifice. Warts may occasionally have the appearance of frank malignancy.

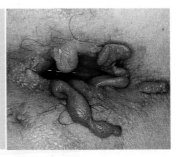

Figure 25.12.
Perianal Crohn's disease.

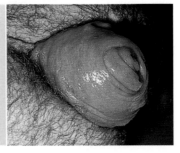

Figure 25.11.
Prolapse of the rectum.

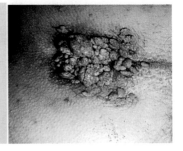

Figure 25.13.
Perianal warts.

Pilonidal disease

A pilonidal sinus (*Figure 25.14a, b*) is a chronic inflammatory disorder comprising a midline epithelialized pit between the buttocks which extends as a granulation tissue-lined track, usually in a cranial direction, for a variable distance and which ends either as a cul-de-sac or at another orifice, and which almost invariably contains a nest of hair. The condition is not seen before puberty and rarely over the age of 45 years.

The aetiology of the condition is unclear. It is possibly congenital but a traumatic aetiology is suggested by the fact that the opening is in the natal cleft between the ischial tuberosities at a site of maximum shearing stresses when seated. An attractive hypothesis is that shed hairs 'drill' into congenital midline pits. Such pits are commonly seen as incidental findings on examination and may never be associated with pilonidal disease, which is characteristically seen in hairy truck drivers. Abscess formation within the sinus leads to the development of secondary lateral tracks since discharge through the midline is prevented by the fibrous septa connecting the skin to the fascia over the sacrum. Such lateral tracks may pass caudally and create an appearance which may resemble hidradenitis suppurativa or fistula in ano, both of which may coexist with pilonidal disease.

Patients usually present with an acute abscess or with a chronic discharging sinus. The acute abscess usually lies to one side of the midline although a midline pit is always present.

Rarer versions of the condition are seen in the hands, the umbilicus and axillae. Pilonidal sinuses of the hand are seen in barbers where hair clippings enter the web of the right hand between the index and ring fingers. A small black spot is present and a palpable lump – barber's nodule – both of which may become infected. The condition is also reported from wool clippings in sheep shearers.

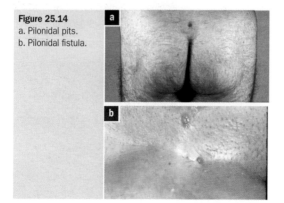

Figure 25.14
a. Pilonidal pits.
b. Pilonidal fistula.

Hidradenitis suppurativa

This (*Figure 25.15*) is a chronic recurring suppurative disease of apocrine gland-bearing skin – apocrinitis. It usually affects the axillae but may involve the back of the neck, the areola of the breast, the groins and perineum. Although more common in women, those cases involving the perineum – the apocrine circumanal Gay's glands – are more often seen in men. Like pilonidal disease, hidradenitis is not seen before puberty and most patients present in the age range 16–40 years. Its aetiology is unknown although obesity, acne, poor hygiene and excessive sweating have been suggested as predisposing factors. It may be seen in a variety of endocrine disorders, suggesting that a relative androgen excess or increased target organ androgen sensitivity may be implicated.

Occlusion of the apocrine gland ducts leads to bacterial proliferation within the glands, and rupture and spread of infection to adjacent glands. Secondary infection causes further local extension, skin damage and fibrosis, eventually leading to multiple communicating subcutaneous fistulae. In the primary stages it presents with multiple, tender, raised, red lesions around the perianal region but in its chronic form multiple sinuses are seen, with secondary infection leading to gross fibrosis and scarring. Rarely it may extend into the anal canal but never above the dentate line.

Sexually transmitted diseases of the rectum and anus

Anal receptive intercourse is not uncommonly practised by both sexes and may lead to disease that is evident on examination of the anus and rectum. Although it is not uncommon for drugs to be used as an adjunct to the practice of anal intercourse to relax the anal sphincters, anal intercourse can still give rise to tears of the anal and rectal mucosa and the underlying musculature. This leads to bleeding, problems with continence, and also allows easier entry of potential pathogens.

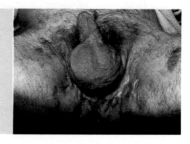

Figure 25.15.
Hydradenitis suppurativa.

Anorectal gonorrhoea

Anorectal gonorrhoea is caused by the gonococcus, a Gram-negative coccus, transmitted sexually. The infection can be asymptomatic or may give rise to constipation, tenesmus and the passage of mucus or pus. Little is likely to be seen on inspection although the anal and rectal mucosa may look inflamed, congested and covered with discharge.

Anorectal syphilis

Anorectal syphilis gives rise to a chancre (*Figure 25.16*) that may be confused with a fissure in ano but is usually not in the characteristic midline position. It has the appearance of a well-defined indurated ulcer.

Herpes simplex

Herpes simplex is a viral infection caused by the herpes simplex virus. It gives rise to painful vesicles that may ulcerate. The patient usually presents with pain, especially on defecation and also constipation and discharge.

Perianal disease in the HIV-positive patient

The rise in prevalence of AIDS sufferers and the anorectal lesions associated with the syndrome mean that more such patients are attending the general surgical or colorectal outpatients' clinics. In addition to the STDs seen in the general population – especially those associated with anoreceptive intercourse, e.g. gonorrhoea; syphilis; chlamydia – various viral infections and tumours, both benign and malignant – e.g. squamous cell and cloacogenic carcinomata; lymphoma; Kaposi's sarcoma – are more or less restricted to this group.

Anorectal pathology in the HIV positive or AIDS patient includes conditions common to all patients, i.e. haemorrhoids, fissures and fistulae, as well as those more prevalent in the HIV positive group, namely herpes simplex virus (HSV), cytomegalovirus (CMV), *Mycobacterium avium-intracellulare* (MAI), *Candida*, condylomata accuminata and non-specific, primary, HIV positive-induced anal ulcer.

Most patients seen in the surgical clinic are already under the care of an immunologist. A thorough history should include an evaluation of the anorectal symptoms, age, HIV status, CDC classification, previous and current STDs, previous anorectal conditions and treatments, and current medication. Examination should be carried out with all precautions taken, and specific pathology such as warts, vesicles, ulcers, fissures, fistulae and abscesses looked for. Proctoscopy and sigmoidoscopy should be performed and intra-anal/rectal ulcers biopsied. Biopsies should be sent for routine microscopy, viral cultures (including HIV, HSV and CMV), acid-fast stain for MAI, and indian ink stain for cryptococcus. Anal condylomata of various viral types are probably the most frequent pathology seen, and there may be a higher incidence of dysplasia and *in situ* neoplasia than in non-HIV positive homosexuals with warts.

For more on perianal disease in the HIV-positive patient see p. 95.

Tumours of the rectum and anus

Adenocarcinoma of the colon and rectum (p. 292) is one of the commonest causes of cancer death in the western world. Most tumours are found in the distal colon and rectum where they are often detectable by digital and sigmoidoscopic examination (*Figure 25.17*). The presenting complaint is usually one of a change in bowel habit, as the obstructing lesion causes constipation or overflow diarrhoea, although rectal bleeding and tenesmus – the sensation of the desire to empty the rectum caused by a tumour in the rectum mimicking the presence of faeces – are other common symptoms. Adenomatous tumours are also common and are clinically important as they may give rise to malignant tumours if they

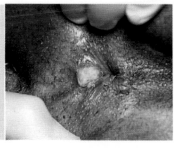

Figure 25.16.
Syphilitic anal ulcer.

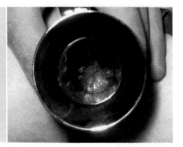

Figure 25.17.
Melanoma of the anal canal.

grow over a certain size. Anal tumours are not as common as rectal and colonic tumours and present as either painful or painless lumps in the anus, usually with bleeding. Arising from skin, they are of different cellular origin and are usually squamous cell carcinomas or melanomas.

On inspection, only the most distal of anal tumours are evident. Anal squamous cell carcinomas (*Figure 25.18*) can appear warty, as an indurated plaque or as an ulcer. Anal basal cell carcinomas have an appearance similar to that of other basal cell carcinomas, that is a pearly ulcer with a rolled edge. Melanomas are usually wart-like, pigmented tumours. Spread from anal malignant tumours is commonly to the inguinal lymph nodes, which therefore should be palpated if an anal tumour is suspected.

Digital examination may bring to light the presence of a tumour in the anus or proximal rectum. Colorectal tumours are either sessile, that is arising without a stalk – in which case they can extend part or all the way round the lumen of the bowel – or polypoid. Whether the tumour is benign or malignant can only be determined with certainty by microscopic examination of the whole tumour.

Benign tumours tend to be more homogeneous with an intact, velvety mucosal surface that can make the tumour quite difficult to feel, compared to the heterogeneous consistency and ulcerated surface of the frankly malignant tumour. Invasion through the rectal wall may be determined by the degree of fixity of the tumour to the pelvic wall. Although usually only the distal 10 cm of the rectum can be examined digitally it may be possible to examine tumours in the sigmoid colon through the rectal wall, as it is also possible to examine tumours of other pelvic organs through the rectal wall.

Other tumours of the rectum include lipomas, leiomyomas, leiomyosarcomas and melanomas. Tumours of the colon and rectum usually spread to the liver and the presence of hepatomegaly should be sought if a malignant tumour of the colon or rectum is suspected.

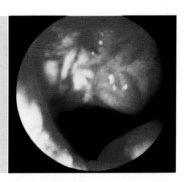

Figure 25.19.
Solitary ulcer of the rectum.

The **solitary ulcer syndrome** (*Figure 25.19*) is characterized by an ulcer of the anterior rectum just above the anal canal. The ulcer is usually 2–3 cm across but there may be just a reddened, oedematous area or even more than one ulcer. The area may be elevated or polypoid, increasing the difficulty of differential diagnosis from Crohn's disease or carcinoma of the rectum.

The syndrome occurs in patients who have difficulty in defecation, with straining and incomplete evacuation, producing an internal intussusception of the rectum or, occasionally, a prolapse. There is a weakness of the pelvic floor muscles but it is uncertain whether this is primary or secondary to the development of the ulcer. An earlier theory that the ulcer was due to the trauma of the digital evacuation used to overcome the defecation problem may also be a factor in some instances. The ulcer may bleed and a good deal of mucus is produced. This, and associated incontinence, may produce soiling and often pruritus ani.

Vaginal examination

Although the vagina is mainly the province of the gynaecologist, diseases of the female reproductive organs can mimic conditions that present to general surgeons and vaginal examination is invaluable in the evaluation of these diseases. A clinician can gain further access to the pelvis and the organs within it, enabling more information to be gathered about their involvement in these diseases. For these reasons vaginal examination is a skill that should be acquired by those managing surgical conditions.

The hands should be washed and a glove worn. In the general surgical setting the vaginal examination is carried out before or after rectal examination. For this reason the glove should be changed to avoid cross-contamination and it is

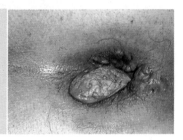

Figure 25.18.
Anal squamous cell carcinoma.

Figure 25.20.
Lipoma of the vulva.

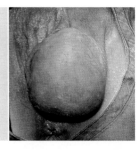

Figure 25.21
a. Bartholin's cyst.
b. Bartholin's abscess due to gonococcal infection.

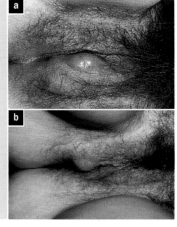

Figure 25.22
a. Vaginal procidentia. b. Vaginal procidentia and rectal prolapse.

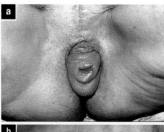

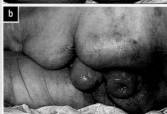

usual for the surgeon to use the left lateral position rather than the usual lithotomy position used by gynaecologists.

The **vulva** and **introitus** are firstly inspected. They are subject to all lesions found on the penis – primary chancre, the primary lesion of lymphogranuloma inguinale, chancroid, herpes simplex, leukoplakia, cancer and other subcutaneous lesions (*Figure 25.20*) . Papillomatous warts can be prolific, and sebaceous and Bartholin's cysts (*Figure 25.21a, b*) are also common. A **vaginal discharge** from the above conditions or uterine abnormalities may give rise to pruritus vulvae and there may be visible erythema, eczematous changes, excoriation and scratch marks.

A small amount of whitish mucous vaginal discharge is normal, as well as bloodstained discharge due to menstruation, but bleeding is also present from an impending or recent abortion, ectopic pregnancy or uterine carcinoma. A profuse whitish or purulent discharge denotes salpingitis, endometritis, cervicitis or, most commonly, vaginitis. *Trichomonas vaginalis* infection causes profuse, watery, pale yellow, sometimes frothy discharge with intense pruritus. Thrush – *Candida albicans* infection – leads to thick, yellowish discharge which is particularly excoriating. In gonorrhoea, the discharge is purulent.

At this stage ask the patient to strain down, when a **cystocele** – descent of the bladder through the anterior vaginal wall – or a **rectocele** – descent of the rectum through the posterior vaginal musculature – becomes apparent. When the pelvic diaphragm and the ligaments supporting the uterus are defective, the cervix appears at the introitus on straining, and becomes extruded to a varying degree – **procidentia** (*Figure 25.22a, b*). Ask the patient to cough several times, when the competence of the sphincter urethrae is noted, as urine is spilled in cases of **stress incontinence.**

On palpation, the forefinger and, if the vagina comfortably allows, the middle finger are introduced into the vagina until the cervix is encountered. The shape, size and surface of the os are assessed and irregularities noted for subsequent visualization. The size, position and attitude of the corpus of the uterus are noted and the fornices are examined in turn, through which the pelvic contents are palpable. Abnormalities are then palpated bimanually, both through the vagina and the lower abdominal wall. This establishes the relations of any abnormality, especially fixity to the pelvic wall or other pelvic organs. The ovaries may be palpable and the mobility of any ovarian mass is assessed. The fallopian tubes cannot usually be palpated but tenderness in the lateral fornices is marked in acute salpingitis, as is lateral movement of the cervix. A hydro- or pyosalpinx may be palpated. Other abnormalities of the uterus are considered on p. 297.

In gynaecological practice at this stage a speculum is introduced and samples of secretions and any discharges taken for culture and cytology, and a cervical smear taken for cytological examination.

26 The alimentary tract and abdomen in children

Introduction

The alimentary tract is formed in the early embryo as a tube of endoderm. The gut undergoes a number of changes during development, including the formation of the pancreas and liver. The midgut develops outside the abdominal cavity in the umbilical cord and returns into the abdomen in the 14th week, undergoing rotation as it does so, to assume the normal adult configuration. The gut begins to function in the 12th week and after the 20th week of intrauterine life around 500 mL of amniotic fluid is swallowed and excreted each day. Digestive enzymes are present at birth and allow the newborn baby to adequately digest milk. Following birth the gut soon becomes colonized with bacteria and although the indigenous immunological defences of the neonate are poor, IgA from the mother's milk assists in the maintenance of an effective barrier to infection. By the time the baby is 48 hours old it is able to survive on the nutritional benefits of its mother's milk.

One of the commonest and most dangerous consequences of disease of the alimentary tract is dehydration from the excess loss of water and electrolytes in vomiting or diarrhoea (*Figure 26.1*, *Table 26.1*). It is vital that the degree of dehydration is adequately assessed as the management of any of the conditions causing dehydration should be tempered by the need to adequately rehydrate and resuscitate the child. Assessment is hardest in the neonate and young infant.

Exomphalos

Exomphalos (*Figure 26.2*) is the partial or total persistence of the midgut within the umbilical cord where it usually undergoes development between the 6th and 14th weeks of intrauterine life; it occurs once in every 6000 births. Exomphalos minor is the herniation of one or two loops of bowel into the base of the cord whereas exomphalos major is the complete failure of the return of the midgut. In the latter there is a huge swelling in the centre of the abdomen produced by the whole midgut covered by a membrane.

Another related condition is gastroschisis, where loops of bowel herniate through an opening in the abdominal wall to the right of the umbilical cord; it has no coverings. Surgical repair is the treatment of choice, although this can be difficult, especially in exomphalos major in which there may be insufficient development of the anterior abdominal wall to close the abdomen without respiratory embarrassment.

Congenital umbilical fistula

Congenital umbilical fistula (*Figure 26.3*) is usually associated with local infective dermatitis. It may arise through failure of closure of the urachus – urachal fistula – in which case urine leaks from the umbilicus, or through failure of closure

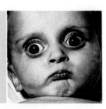

Figure 26.1.
Facies of a baby with acute dehydration.

Table 26.1. Signs of dehydration.

Physical sign	5% dehydration	10% dehydration
Mental state	Lethargy; lassitude	Prostration; coma
Skin	Loss of turgor	Poor capillary return; mottled
Fontanelle	Depressed	Deeply depressed
Eyes	Sunken	Deeply sunken; sticky
Peripheral pulses	Normal	Tachycardia; thready

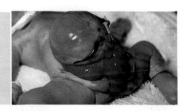

Figure 26.2.
Exomphalos.

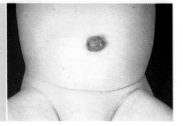

Figure 26.3.
Umbilical polyp associated with urachal fistula.

of the vitellointestinal duct, in which case ileal contents leak. Partial persistence of the embryonic ducts may lead to intermittent discharge of mucus and pus.

An umbilical adenoma or polyp – enteroteratoma – is a remnant of omphalomesenteric duct epithelium which presents as a pedunculated, raspberry-coloured mass. A similar, somewhat paler protuberance can arise from granulation tissue after separation of the cord (umbilical granuloma), this may be effectively treated by the application of silver nitrate sticks.

Omphalitis is an infection of the umbilical cord at the cutaneous line of separation, usually due to lack of aseptic precautions. This may spread along the umbilical arteries to the pelvis, with possible peritonitis, or through the umbilical vein to the liver, causing jaundice and septicaemia. Long-term sequelae are stenosing intrahepatic cholangitis and portal vein thrombosis.

Jaundice in infancy

It is extremely common for the newborn baby to develop jaundice in the first week of life, especially if the delivery is premature. The rest of the examination is normal – the liver is not enlarged, the stools are normal in colour and the urine is not dark. This so-called physiological jaundice – icterus neonatorum – usually fades in a few days. Any infection either in utero at the end of pregnancy or in the immediate neonatal period may give rise to jaundice. If there has been significant bruising from a difficult birth this may give rise to a haemolytic jaundice. Haemolytic disease of the newborn (p. 31) is accompanied by varying degrees of jaundice.

In congenital biliary atresia – agenesis of the bile ducts (*Figure 26.4*) – jaundice may be present at birth but usually develops on the second or third day. The jaundice becomes progressively worse until the saliva and tears become yellow.

The stools are pale at birth but over a few weeks may darken. This is due to bile pigments passing through the intestinal wall, not through the biliary tree. The liver may be enlarged at birth and becomes progressively enlarged and hard. Pruritus, osteomalacia, clubbing and skin xanthelasma are common. Untreated the condition is fatal but, surprisingly, the child may survive for a number of years.

Congenital atresia of the oesophagus

The trachea develops from the primitive oesophagus and, in abnormal development, different configurations of oesophagus and trachea can result (*Figures 26.5* and *26.6*). The commonest is a proximal blind-ending pouch of oesophagus with the distal oesophagus connected to the trachea. This stops the child swallowing effectively and every time it tries it regurgitates the whole feed immediately. Feeding is always associated with coughing and if the feed enters the lungs, pneumonia may develop. The baby has frothy saliva drooling most of the time, which is the key sign of oesophageal

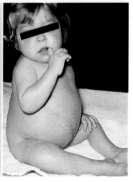

Figure 26.4.
Jaundiced infant with congenital biliary obstruction.

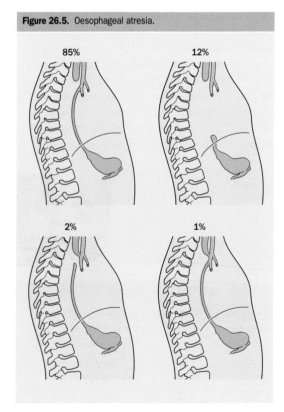

Figure 26.5. Oesophageal atresia.

85%   12%

2%   1%

Figure 26.6.
Barium swallow demonstrating oesophageal atresia with tracheal fistulae.

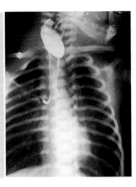

Figure 26.7.
Visible peristalsis in a neonate with intestinal obstruction.

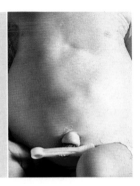

atresia; in no other condition does it occur. If a patent distal fistula is present, the abdomen swells as the stomach distends with swallowed air, and the presence of the oesophageal atresia is confirmed by the failure of attempted passage of a fine nasogastric tube down the oesophagus into the abdomen. Feeding is stopped, intravenous fluid replacement commenced and preparations made for surgical correction.

Infantile pyloric stenosis

This condition, commoner in boys, the firstborn and those with a family history, geographical and seasonal variations exist. The condition is caused by the hypertrophy of the pyloric sphincter. It characteristically takes 3 to 6 weeks to develop. The baby vomits milk soon after each feed and the vomiting becomes progressively more common, more prolonged, more complete and more violent, until the characteristic projectile vomiting and the onset of dehydration are encountered. The physical signs that can be elicited are those of the vomiting of milk with no bile after each feed. The hypertrophied pylorus may be palpated in the right of the epigastrium at rest, and is 1.5–2 cm in diameter. After the feed, peristalsis of the stomach can be seen and felt prior to the projectile vomiting. Following vomiting the baby is often very hungry. Surgical treatment is by pyloromyotomy after fluid and electrolyte imbalances have been corrected.

Intestinal obstruction of the newborn

Babies frequently vomit. After birth it is common for a baby to vomit amniotic fluid, vaginal secretions, blood and its first feeds. Frequent and continuous vomiting in the neonatal period is usually due to one of three things: intracranial

haemorrhage, severe infection and intestinal obstruction (*Figure 26.7*). The presence of bile in the vomit, imparting a yellow or green colour, increases the likelihood of the cause being intestinal obstruction. The vomiting of green fluid in the neonate should be taken very seriously. The consequences of untreated neonatal intestinal obstruction include perforation of the bowel and infarction of the whole midgut in cases of malrotation.

The causes of intestinal obstruction in the new born are:

- Duodenal atresia.
- Duodenal bands.
- Annular pancreas.
- Ladd's band.
- Midgut volvulus.
- Meconium ileus, secondary to cystic fibrosis (*Figure 26.8*).
- Strangulated hernia (*Figure 26.9*).

Figure 26.8.
Meconium ileus.

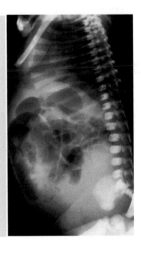

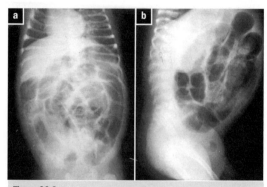

Figure 26.9.
a. Strangulated inguinal hernia in a neonate. Note the gas shown in the right groin. b. Lateral view.

To the above list can be added oesophageal atresia, pyloric stenosis, Hirschsprung's disease and anorectal agenesis (all considered elsewhere in this chapter). The physical signs include abdominal distension. This may not be obvious initially because the neonate's abdomen is usually protuberant.

Pronounced fullness of the abdomen at birth may be due to:

- Intestinal obstruction.
- Distended bladder secondary to urethral obstruction.
- Congenital cystic kidneys.
- Fetal ascites (*Figure 26.10*).
- Meconium peritonitis (*Figure 26.11*).

Figure 26.10.
Neonatal ascites.

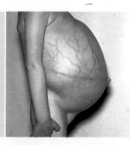

Figure 26.11.
Meconium peritonitis.

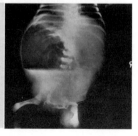

In all these cases, except the last, the abdomen is dull to percussion. If there is tympanic distension at birth with dilated abdominal wall veins, the cause is almost certainly meconium ileus. This is caused by cystic fibrosis which affects the pancreatic secretions and causes the meconium to become inspissated leading to blockage of the ileum. Distension from other causes increases gradually following birth from the swallowing of air.

Another sign associated with intestinal obstruction in the neonate is the failure to pass meconium rectally; however in at least 40% of cases meconium is still passed. Rectal examination in proximal intestinal obstruction reveals a narrow rectum and anus and, after the finger is withdrawn, only rarely does the normal passage of meconium result.

The neonate with obstruction appears otherwise well for 24 to 48 hours unless the cause is midgut volvulus which, if untreated, leads to rapid dehydration and death. This initial good health in most cases is misleading and may lead to a delay in definitive treatment. This is followed by a rapid deterioration as the intestine becomes gangrenous, leading to either perforation, or inhalation of vomit and pneumonia.

Intussusception

This condition affects male more often than female infants and usually occurs between the ages of 6 months and 2 years. Its peak incidence is in the spring and autumn and is thought to arise due the increase in size of lymphatic tissue in the small intestine. This forms a polyp-like intrusion into the bowel lumen, the bowel tries to propel the polyp down the lumen by peristalsis and in so doing inverts the bowel into itself (p. 310). There is obstruction of the bowel proximal to the intussusceptus and, in extreme cases, the bowel may be passed through the anal canal.

The characteristic history is of an infant who has been crying intermittently from attacks of colic and is getting progressively more distressed. The infant may have had previous episodes which have resolved spontaneously. There is often a history of vomiting. On abdominal examination, a sausage-shaped mass is often present, usually in the upper right quadrant; conversely, the right lower quadrant may appear to be hollow on inspection and palpation. This sign – *signe de Dance* – may only be apparent when the child is sedated or anaesthetized. Visible peristalsis may be present.

After a while the child develops a fever and signs of dehydration. Abdominal distension and the passage of a red jelly-like stool – the classic redcurrant jelly stool – are late signs.

If the intussusception involves the lower colon it can be palpated on rectal examination; digital palpation resembles the cervix of the adult uterus.

Necrotizing enterocolitis

This condition – where an infection of the colon spreads throughout the bowel wall causing necrosis and sometimes perforation – is increasing in incidence. The aetiology may be due to invasive bacterial infection or infection following mucosal damage from hypoxia and/or poor tissue perfusion.

The baby presents with vomiting, usually of bile-stained vomit, diarrhoea that characteristically contains blood, and abdominal distension. The baby appears lethargic and in severe cases there is a bradycardia and episodes of apnoea. An ominous sign is of erythema of the abdominal wall, associated with full thickness enterocolitis. If the condition continues unabated a picture of disseminated intravascular coagulation occurs with collapse and a haemorrhagic rash.

Appendicitis in infancy and childhood

The diagnosis of appendicitis in infancy and childhood is complicated by the fact that infants and children are often not specific as to the nature of their symptoms, and are also susceptible to other causes of abdominal pain, such as intussusception. Perforation occurs early, and directly into the peritoneal cavity, because of a relative lack of omentum.

In the infant the signs of appendicitis include pyrexia, abdominal pain, vomiting and diarrhoea, of which all or none may predominate. Pyrexia in the young may reach a higher level than the usual low-grade pyrexia associated with the adult disease, and is more effectively dealt with by the administration of antibiotics or antipyrexials, thus masking the onset of peritonitis. Appendicitis may complicate respiratory infection or gastroenteritis and it is essential to perform repeated abdominal examinations in doubtful cases in order not to miss the diagnosis.

In later childhood, although the history and initial physical examination may be more like the adult condition (p. 304), the physical examination of the abdomen may prove difficult due to the child's fear of the pain that is to be elicited. If necessary it is useful therefore to use the child's own hand to palpate the abdomen. Percussion rebound is a valuable means of identifying peritonism and is the least painful.

Non-specific mesenteric lymphadenitis

Mesenteric adenitis is termed non-specific to differentiate it from tubercular – or specific – adenitis. It is inflammatory enlargement of the ileocaecal lymph nodes, which are slightly erythematous and oedematous, but not adherent to adjacent structures. The condition may follow an upper respiratory tract infection but no organism has been implicated. Mesenteric adenitis occurs under the age of 15 and, like acute appendicitis, is common in the first decade, producing a difficult differential diagnosis. Both conditions present with central abdominal pain, and mild pyrexia and leukocytosis. In mesenteric adenitis the pain is colicky and between attacks, unlike acute appendicitis, the pain may resolve. Also, vomiting occurs at the beginning of the illness rather than later on. Patients have a perioral pallor and a malar flush, which are not common features of appendicitis. The tenderness of mesenteric adenitis is higher than in appendicitis and does not later move to the right iliac fossa. Rigidity is present, but, with gentle perseverance, it is possible to undertake deep palpation over the right iliac fossa, again not a feature of appendicitis. Rectal examination is always normal. By re-positioning the patient from side to side, the root of the mesentery and associated tender nodes may be shifted in position and, if shifting tenderness can be demonstrated, it is diagnostic of the condition.

Hirschsprung's disease

This condition is due to a failure of the myenteric plexus of the bowel to migrate, leading to aganglionosis of the bowel. The condition always starts in the distal rectum but may spread into the small intestine. Inability of the bowel to adequately contract leads to a failure in peristalsis and then constipation. Hirschsprung's disease is the commonest cause of intestinal obstruction in the newborn, with a 4:1 male predominance and in 90% of cases presents in the first three days of life. Although usually apparent in the neonatal period, occasionally, if the defect is short enough, the condition may not be diagnosed until adult life; there will however be a history of lifelong constipation. The history in the neonate is of a failure to pass meconium in the first two to three days of life. Meconium is usually passed after the passage of a finger into the rectum. The rectum is empty and contracted, and the anus normal.

If the obstruction is low, the finger may enter the dilated normal rectum. After removing the finger there is a large gush of flatus and meconium and there may be intermittent passage of stool for a short while before constipation returns. The abdomen becomes increasingly distended, and borborygmi and visible peristalsis become ever more obvious. In many cases the proximal colon becomes increasingly enlarged, i.e. a megacolon (*Figure 26.12*), and may in time perforate. The initial treatment is to raise a stoma of normal colon to allow decompression and passage of stool from the colon; restorative surgery is performed later.

Anorectal agenesis

This (*Figure 26.13*) encompasses a large number of different anatomical malformations, which can be divided into the high variety, where the bowel ends above or at the level of the pelvic floor muscles (these may fistulate into the vagina

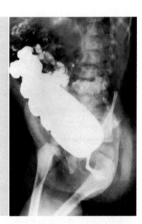

Figure 26.12.
Hirschsprung's disease. Note the narrow aganglion segment

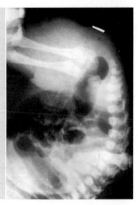

Figure 26.13.
Imperforate anus demonstrating the gap between the lowest gas shadow and the coin placed over the anus. Radiograph taken in head down position to fill the rectum with air.

in girls, and in boys invariably fistulate into the bladder), and the low variety, ending below the pelvic floor. About a third of these infants also have genitourinary abnormalities. Definitive surgical correction is delayed; a defunctioning colostomy is raised soon after birth. The tell-tale sign at examination after birth is the absence of the anus, or that meconium is being discharged from an abnormal exit. Isolated agenesis of the rectum with an anus present is extremely rare.

Recurrent abdominal pain

This is a very common condition in childhood and in the vast majority of instances there is no cause found after history, examination and simple investigation. Causes that can be identified include:

- Peptic ulceration – This usually manifests itself as the interruption of sleep by nocturnal pain; the cause is more likely to be duodenal than gastric ulceration.
- Urinary tract infection – This usually results in loin or suprapubic pain, together with frequency and dysuria. The diagnosis can be excluded by microscopy and culture of the urine and, if persistent, by imaging the renal tract to exclude hydronephrosis.
- Childhood abdominal migraine – This is a precursor to classic migraine where children, usually with a family history of classic migraine, develop episodes of prolonged midline abdominal pain with nausea and vomiting.
- Haemolytic disease of the newborn – This is caused by blood group incompatibility, usually from the rhesus group, although this is now uncommon in the UK due to a programme of immunization with anti-D immunoglobulin. The baby is born jaundiced and high levels of circulating bile acids can lead to kernicterus. In this condition, the basal ganglia are fixed with bile acids, causing first abnormal behaviour, then fits leading to opisthotonus (arched spastic contraction of the spine), mental retardation and, in extreme cases, death. Treatment is by phototherapy unless the levels of circulating bilirubin are too high, in which case exchange transfusion is required.

27 The genitourinary system and genitalia

Introduction

The urinary tract in non-pathological states is relatively inaccessible to physical examination, owing to the anatomical position of its various components. In pathological states however, diseased organs can be identified, thus examination is an essential part of diagnosis. In particular, urinary tract disease may have widespread systemic manifestations and these signs and their significance need to be recognized. For example, renal failure, peripheral vascular disease and disseminated malignancy can all be associated with primary urinary tract pathology, and a high index of suspicion must be maintained during the diagnostic process if a full appreciation of the entire disease process is to be made.

Specific to the urinary tract, the urological examination is looking for hypertension, enlargement of a kidney or the bladder, abnormalities in the inguinal region and genitalia, abnormalities of the prostate and evidence of pelvic disease. A full history is mandatory and this, combined with the physical signs, directs the appropriate special investigations to be requested and an accurate diagnosis made.

Examination of the urine

Examination of the urine is an essential physical sign in any patient and is of particular importance in patients suspected of having urinary tract pathology. Ideally a fresh specimen should be passed so that the colour, presence of blood or blood clots and/or sediment can be evaluated immediately.

A red colour, which may be interpreted as blood by the patient or clinician, appears if the urine of a patient with porphyria is left standing for a few hours. Rifampicin, an antituberculous drug, similarly produces a port wine colour of the urine, and red/purple urine may occur after eating rhubarb or beetroot. Bile pigments darken urine, giving it a greenish hue, and chyle (*Figure 27.1*) produces a milky-white colour with fat globules. The latter may be due to malignant infiltration of the thoracic duct or cisterna chyli, but may also be spontaneous in origin.

Dipstix

Often the results of a urine dipstix is available to the clinician at the time of examination. The results are not always to be relied upon but, used in conjunction with other symptoms and physical signs, can help to formulate a diagnosis and direct the choice of special investigations. Urine dipstix can indicate:

- Glycosuria – An important finding, especially in the presence of symptoms of urinary frequency and nocturia, and any physical signs suggesting the onset of diabetes mellitus.
- Haematuria – Can be an indicator of intrinsic renal disease or any lower urinary tract pathology (*Table 27.1*).
- Pyuria – An inflammatory process within the urinary tract; it is nearly always present if there is significant urinary infection as opposed to a contaminated specimen.

Midstream urine

The taking of a catch of urine midway through the stream reduces the risk of bacterial contamination from the perineum. A significant bacterial count, suggesting genuine urinary tract infection, is usually taken to be 105 colonies per millilitre. This is associated with the presence of white cells in the urine.

Haematuria
Microscopic

The routine use of dipstix testing of the urine has led to a number of people being diagnosed as having microscopic haematuria. Although not necessarily indicating any serious pathological process, persistent microscopic haematuria can

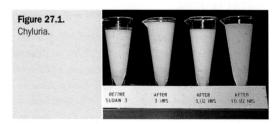

Figure 27.1. Chyluria.

BEFORE SUDAN 3   AFTER 3 HRS   AFTER 5.1/2 HRS   AFTER 10.1/2 HRS

Table 27.1. Causes of haematuria.

Renal	Carcinoma of the kidney
	Carcinoma of the renal pelvis (urothelium)
	Stone
	Trauma
	Intrinsic renal disease, e.g. glomerulonephritis
	Polycystic kidney
	TB
	AV malformations
Ureteric	Carcinoma of the urothelium
	Stone
Bladder	Carcinoma of the bladder
	Stone
	Trauma
	Cystitis (infective and other inflammations)
	Schistosomiasis
Prostate	Carcinoma of the prostate
	Benign prostatic hyperplasia
	Prostatitis
Urethra	Carcinoma of the urothelium
	Stone
	Trauma
	Urethritis
	Stricture
Others	Blood dyscrasias and coagulopathies

signify intrinsic renal disease urinary tract infection, stone disease or malignant disease anywhere along the urinary tract. It always warrants investigation.

Macroscopic

Frank haematuria indicates a urological malignancy until proven otherwise. Careful examination and imaging of the upper tracts followed by cystoscopic visualization of the lower urinary tract is essential in all patients with this symptom.

Renal failure

Renal failure may occur as the result of underlying urinary tract disease or, alternatively, a diagnosis of urinary tract disease may bring to light unsuspected renal impairment, together with its associated clinical features. Intrinsic renal disease as a cause of renal failure is not further considered here but obstructive renal failure is either due to urinary tract pathology or extrinsic compression of the urinary tract from some other

pathological process. It may be acute or chronic in onset and may result from pathology anywhere along the length of the urinary tract, from kidney to external urethral meatus. For these reasons the clinical features of renal failure are considered before those associated with individual urinary tract organs.

Acute or chronic renal failure can be due to pre-renal (renal hypoperfusion), renal (renal parenchymal damage) and post-renal (acute obstruction to renal flow) causes. The predominant cause related to urinary tract disease is the gradual onset of post-renal failure resulting from obstruction to the excretion of urine.

Acute renal failure

Acute renal failure is often clinically dramatic in onset and, because of the high frequency of associated problems, has a high mortality. It has a tendency to appear in patients with pre-existing renal disease, especially chronic vascular ischaemia. It is a potentially reversible syndrome, characterized by an abrupt loss of renal function, causing retention of nitrogenous waste products. There are many causes but perhaps those most commonly seen are sepsis, drug toxicity and obstruction to urine flow.

Causes of acute renal failure

Pre-renal:

- Sepsis.
- Haemorrhage, e.g. surgical.
- Burns.
- Gastriintestinal fluid loss.

Renal:

- Drugs, e.g. aminoglycosides; non-steroidal anti-inflammatory.
- Hypertension.
- Eclampsia.
- Bacterial interstitial nephritis.
- Other toxins – myoglobinuria.

Post-renal:

- Benign prostatic hyperplasia.
- Pelvic tumours.
- Stones.
- Retroperitoneal fibrosis.
- Papillary necrosis.

The clinical state of patients presenting with acute renal failure ranges from those in whom only a biochemical abnormality has been detected, to the gravely ill with multiple organ failure. Initial assessment depends on the clinical situation encountered. However, all patients should have an assessment of their fluid status made by examining their blood pressure, skin turgor, central venous pressure and by looking for signs of pulmonary, ankle and sacral oedema. It is also useful to review the records of urine output and fluid balance for the preceding hours or days, and the recent drug history. Investigations to document the degree of uraemia, hyperkalaemia and acidosis should be urgently undertaken as early treatment may be imperative.

Chronic renal failure

Chronic failure of renal function results in a number of clinical manifestations which relate to functions of the kidney, namely the failure of body salt and water homoeostasis, a reduction in urea excretion and a failure of normal red blood cell production. The onset is gradual, over many months or years, and the patient typically passes through three clinical stages:

1. Renal insufficiency – Usually asymptomatic but with mildly abnormal serum and plasma biochemical investigations, and at risk of acute renal decompensation.
2. Renal failure – Persistent malaise, nocturia invariably present and osteomalacia.
3. Uraemic – Unwell, anaemic, acidotic, hypocalcaemic, hypophosphataemic and hyperkalaemic.

There are a number of clinical features that develop during the gradual onset of chronic renal failure. These are all related to the loss of renal function and should each be considered when examining these patients. An obvious cause for the renal failure should also be considered during this examination. Features to assess include:

- Signs of chronic uraemia – Skin excoriation, brown arcs of nails, pigmentation, anaemia, neuropathy and pericardial rub, restless leg syndrome.
- Acidosis – As demonstrated by rapid shallow breathing: Kussmaul breathing.
- Fluid status – Skin turgor, venous pressure, and peripheral and pulmonary oedema.
- Signs of urinary tract obstruction.

If the chronic renal failure persists, the patient ultimately reaches end stage renal failure and requires some form of renal replacement therapy. The aetiologies of end stage renal failure in the UK are:

- Glomerulonephritis (30%).
- Pyelonephritis (reflux) (20%).
- Polycystic kidneys (10%).
- Hypertension (10%).
- Renal vascular disease (10%).
- Drugs (10%).
- Unknown (10%).

Renal transplantation

Of the forms of renal replacement therapy available – haemodialysis, continuous ambulatory peritoneal dialysis and renal transplantation – transplantation offers the most cost effective treatment and the greatest improvement in quality of life for patients. Successful transplantation has become a reality for an increasing number of patients with end stage renal disease, as a result of the expanding knowledge of the immunological mechanisms and the ability to manipulate the immune response using immunosuppressive drugs. One year graft survival rates are 80% for cadaveric transplants and over 90% for living related transplants if there is a good antigen cross-match. There is a continuous attrition rate after the first year with the mean graft half-life being 7.5 years for cadaveric transplants. The technique for transplant has changed little since it was first performed over 40 years ago. The donor kidneys are harvested with efforts made to keep the warm ischaemic time to a minimum and, once harvested, are preserved in solutions, such as hyperosmolar citrate, that minimize tubular cell damage.

The potential recipient is selected by blood group and human leukocyte antigen typing. These histocompatibility antigens occur in two classes and evidence suggests that the Class II antigen, designated by DR loci-matching, has a greater influence on graft survival than class I antigens. Class I (DR) antigen matching has a greater influence on graft survival than the Class II antigens. Traditional barriers to transplantation such as age, coronary heart disease, hypertension and diabetes are no longer considered contraindications. The transplant kidney is placed extraperitoneally in the left or the right iliac fossa, where there is access to the iliac vessels, for direct vascular anastomosis, and to the bladder for implantation of the ureter. Immunosuppression begins immediately with cyclosporin, azothiaprin or prednisolone or any combination of these. Cyclosporin is the main ingredient in most immuno-suppressive protocols and is the single most important cause for the improved transplant survival figures seen over the last decade. The transplanted kidney can easily be palpated in the iliac fossa below the scar and it should not be mistaken for a pathological mass.

The kidney

The kidneys lie high up in the retroperitoneum with psoas and quadratus lumborum muscles posterior to them and the peritoneal contents anterior. They are surrounded by perinephric fat and Gerota's fascia and are thus relatively mobile, fixed only by their vascular attachments at the hilum. They move normally in a cranio/caudal direction on respiration.

Renal pain

Renal pain is a persistent fixed ache in the angle between the lowest rib and the lumbar spine. The patient typically describes this by putting their hand on the waist with the thumb forwards and the fingers spreading backwards. If there is significant renal enlargement, stretching of the peritoneum may localize the pain more anteriorly to the upper outer quadrant of the abdomen. Renal colic pain – usually caused by a stone – is more spasmodic and severe and is due to obstruction of either a calyceal infundibulum within the kidney or the pelviureteric junction of the renal pelvis, producing collecting system distension and increased peristaltic muscular activity.

Renal examination

Unless a patient is very thin the normal kidney is not easily felt (p. 280; *Figure 23.9*), thus examination usually involves the search for an enlarged organ. Classically, the enlarged kidney is a mobile, smooth mass, palpable bimanually, that can be moved into the loin, moves on respiration and which one can get above. Percussion is usually resonant due to the overlying colon. In order to identify a renal mass the patient should lie on their back and they must be relaxed and comfortable to minimize abdominal wall muscle tone. One hand, usually the left, is placed beneath the patient in the lumbar region and the other on the upper outer quadrant of the abdomen. As the patient breathes out the kidney can be palpated between the two examining hands and felt to move on inspiration. The kidney is thus ballottable between the hands; this feature helps to distinguish it from other structures such as the spleen.

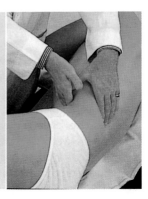

Figure 27.2. Alternative method for the examination of the kidney. (Also see *Figure 23.9*, p. 280). Palpation of the left kidney with the patient lying on their right side.

An alternative method of palpating a kidney is to turn the patient on their side with the affected side uppermost and repeat the bimanual examination (*Figure 27.2*). Another physical sign – Murphy's 'kidney punch test' – is performed by jabbing the kidney area under the ribs to examine for renal tenderness. This can be painful to the patient and is an unnecessary physical sign to elicit.

It is essential when examining any patient with suspected renal pathology that the blood pressure reading be taken and recorded. Hypertension can be a cause or consequence of renal disease and serial values should be recorded. Renal artery stenosis, which itself can represent either a cause or consequence of hypertension, can be detected clinically by auscultation for a bruit over the lumbar areas adjacent to the lumbar spine at the level of L2.

Polycystic kidneys

Infantile polycystic kidney disease is a hereditary autosomal recessive condition and is often fatal in the neonate/infant child.

Adult polycystic disease (*Figure 27.3*) is an autosomal dominant condition and typically presents in middle adult life (30–40 years old). The condition accounts for up to 10% of

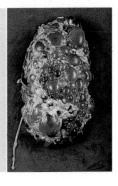

Figure 27.3. Operative specimen of an excised polycystic kidney.

patients on long-term renal replacement therapy. The clinical features are:

- Pain (due to enlargement of the kidney).
- Haematuria (present in 25% of patients).
- Infection (presents with pyelonephritis).
- Hypertension.
- Chronic renal failure.
- Abdominal mass (a knobbly, enlarged kidney).

Solitary cysts of the kidney are usually asymptomatic but, when large, they may cause renal pain and a palpable mass. They are common and usually do not require any treatment so long as they can be reliably distinguished from other renal masses. Adenocarcinomas can appear in the walls of cysts and, if suspected on ultrasound or CT scanning, should be managed as renal cell carcinomas.

Other congenital abnormalities include a horseshoe kidney, a duplex pelviureteric collecting system and aberrant renal vessels compressing the renal pelvis.

If the normal ascent of the kidneys is incomplete the two sides may fuse, producing a mid-line **horseshoe** kidney below the umbilicus. This kidney is palpable and can be mistaken for malignancies of other systems. The kidney is also prone to infection, the ureters descending anteriorly over the body of the organ. The ureters are subject to pelviureteric obstruction.

A kidney may be **absent**. This factor is of extreme importance if surgery is being considered on the other side. In this condition, in males, the testis on the affected side may also be absent or poorly developed.

Duplication of the pelvis and/or ureter occurs in 3% of the population and is usually a chance radiological finding. The upper ureter, however, is always inserted distally below the lower ureter (*Figure 27.4*) and, in females, this ectopic origin may be below the urethral sphincter. This situation produces a history of urinary leakage; this is not always admitted by the patient and the condition takes many years to diagnose and treat.

Pelviureteric junction obstruction

Chronic obstruction of the kidney at the pelviureteric (*Figure 27.5*) junction is usually congenital in origin and leads to hydronephrosis of the kidney. This can cause the kidney to enlarge to many times its normal size and results in diminished function. The patient typically complains of intermittent pain, especially after drinking large amounts of fluid, but may also have haematuria or hypertension. If the kidney is hydronephrotic it can often be palpated. The cause of the obstruction at the junction of the ureter and renal pelvis remains unknown although a number of suggestions have been proposed, including the presence of crossing aberrant lower polar renal vessels, a failure of propagation of the peristaltic wave across the junction and an excess of collagen at the pelviureteric junction.

The condition is diagnosed in patients from birth to any age. The diagnosis is often made *in utero* since, with the routine use of antenatal ultrasound, dilatation of the fetal renal collecting system can be easily observed. The management of these babies post-partum is to avoid surgery if possible as the condition may correct itself with time.

Neoplasms
Wilms' tumour/nephroblastoma

This is the commonest abdominal tumour in children, accounting for about 10% of all childhood malignancies. The peak incidence is between 2 and 4 years but cases can occur into adolescence. Presentation is most commonly the finding of an abdominal mass (*Figure 27.6*) by a parent, though haematuria occurs as the first symptom in about

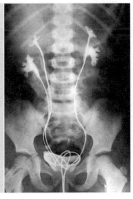

Figure 27.4.
Duplex collecting system. Note that the upper ureter enters the bladder at a lower level.

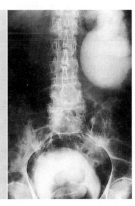

Figure 27.5.
Intravenous urogram showing a typical pelviureteric junction obstruction.

Figure 27.6.
Nephroblastoma (Wilms') tumour.

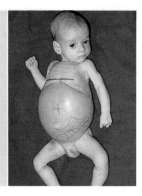

25% of cases. Metastases to the liver and lung are not uncommon at the time of diagnosis and bilateral tumours occur in 5% of cases.

Renal cell carcinoma

Renal cell adenocarcinoma (*Figure 27.7a, b, c*) – also known as a Grawitz tumour, hypernephroma and clear cell carcinoma – is by far the commonest solid neoplasm of the kidney. This tumour typically presents with one or more of a triad of clinical features: haematuria (40%), abdominal pain (30%) and abdominal mass (20%), though only 10% of patients have all these symptoms. An increasing number of renal tumours are found incidentally due to the increased use of imaging modalities such as ultrasound and CT scanning, up to 20% of all renal tumours being found in this way. The mass associated with a renal cell carcinoma tends to grow anteriorly and, if large, can readily be palpated per abdomen. About a third of patients present with non-urological features or para-neoplastic syndromes.

Figure 27.7.
Renal cell carcinoma.
a. Tumour of the upper pole of the left kidney showing distortion of calyceal system. b. Operative specimen of the tumour demonstrated in a. c. CT scan showing a right-sided carcinoma.

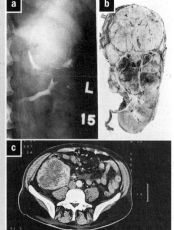

These can be either non-specific manifestations of malignant disease, such as loss of weight, or more specific endocrine or metastatic abnormalities.

The most commonly used clinical staging system is that devised by Robin:

- Stage I. Tumour within the capsule.
- Stage II. Tumour invasion of perinephric fat but within Gerota's fascia.
- Stage III. Tumour involvement of regional lymph nodes and/or renal vein.
- Stage IV. Tumour involvement of adjacent organs or distant metastases.

The commonest site for metastases to appear is the lungs; the tumour spreads via both the lymphatic and venous systems, and tumour cells reach the pulmonary vascular capillaries via the heart. The patient typically develops a number of isolated lesions within the lung fields, known as cannonball metastases. Renal cell carcinoma is one of the tumours that commonly metastasizes to bone and renal imaging remains one of the investigations necessary in people who present with a pathological fracture. The acute development of a left-sided varicocele in a middle-aged or elderly man can indicate obstruction of the renal vein and the presence of tumour from a renal cell carcinoma within it (*Figure 27.8*).

Renal cell carcinomas may produce renin and thus cause hypertension; 60% of patients with these tumours have a raised level of erythropoietin although only 10% have evidence of polycythaemia. Other ectopic hormones produced include parathyroid hormone, a parathyroid hormone-like substance which also gives rise to hypercalcaemia, adrenocorticotropic hormone and human chorionotropic hormone. Production of other kinin substances by the tumour can give rise to a pyrexia, and renal cell carcinoma is one of the differential diagnoses of a pyrexia of unknown origin. Renal tumours can spread by growth along the renal vein and subsequently into the inferior

Figure 27.8.
CT scan showing a left renal cell carcinoma spreading along the renal vein and expanding in the inferior vena cava.

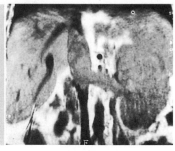

vena cava. Patients may thus present with the signs and symptoms of obstruction to the vena cava such as gross distension of the subcutaneous veins on the abdomen and a swollen leg.

Renal calculi

Infection in the renal pelvis produces an environment that encourages the deposition of debris and minerals, and these can form the nidus on which stones can develop (*Figure 27.9*). Other risk factors are dehydration and starvation; vitamin A deficiency in the latter produces desquamation of urinary tract epithelium. Prolonged immobility, such as in paraplegia, increases skeletal decalcification, with the deposition of urinary calcium phosphate. Other suggested aetiological factors are calcification of areas of papillary erosion, and endocrine and metabolic abnormalities, giving rise to the deposition of oxalates, phosphates, urates, calcium, cystine and xanthine.

Clinically, small calculi and even large calculi that fill the pelvis – staghorn calculi – may be asymptomatic. The commonest symptom is loin pain but there may be pain from secondary infection (p. 347) and microscopic haematuria. The pressure and obstructive effects of large calculi cause destruction of renal substance and eventually renal failure.

Perinephric abscess

With the current minimally invasive techniques for the treatment of renal stones, perinephric abscesses (*Figure 27.10*) are less common in the UK than previously. Nevertheless, they still occur and, if severe morbidity is to be prevented, an early diagnosis is essential. The patient is typically septic, toxic, dehydrated, shocked and anaemic, with flank tenderness; a mass is palpable in 50–60% of cases. The abscess

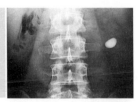

Figure 27.9.
Plain abdominal radiograph showing a calcium oxalate stone in the left renal pelvis.

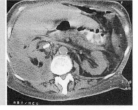

Figure 27.10.
CT scan demonstrating a large right perinephric abscess. The renal outline is destroyed although the stone that caused the problem can be seen in the renal pelvis.

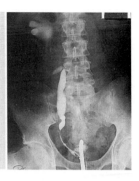

Figure 27.11.
Right renal genitourinary TB showing dilated calyces and a dilated ureter from a ureteric stricture.

may track down the psoas muscle and present as a swelling in one or other iliac fossa. Scoliosis of the spine with the concavity to the affected side is almost invariably present and is a well-recognized feature on a plain abdominal radiograph.

Genitourinary tuberculosis

Tuberculosis – TB; *Figure 27.11* – can affect the whole of the urinary tract and include the testis, but is most commonly seen in the upper urinary tracts. Males are affected more than females and 80% of sufferers are between 20 and 40 years old. The commonest presenting symptom is persistent urinary frequency. Renal pain is usually mild but general symptoms include weight loss and night sweats. On examination the kidney may be palpable and there may be, in male patients, associated tubercular thickening in the prostate, seminal vesicles and the scrotal contents.

The urine is sterile but exhibits pyuria of 20+ cells per high power field and haematuria may be present. The diagnosis depends on the isolation of *Mycobacterium tuberculosis* in three consecutive early morning urine samples. An intravenous urogram is an important investigation to perform to identify the affected parts of the pelvicalyceal system and ureter, and to assess the renal damage.

The ureter

The ureter runs from the renal pelvis along the psoas muscle, entering the pelvis at the common iliac bifurcation, anterior to the sacroiliac joint. It descends to the level of the ischial spine before turning forwards and medially to enter the bladder. In the female it is closely related to the lateral fornix of the vagina.

Ureteric pain

This is typically caused by a ureteric stone, or possibly a tumour. The pain of ureteric colic is severe, gripping and spasmodic. The patient often describes rolling around on the floor during an attack. The pain may be referred to cutaneous areas innervated from the same segments of the spinal cord, namely T11–L2. It thus typically commences in the loin and radiates down into the scrotum or labia majora and even into the upper thigh via the genitofemoral nerve.

Ureteric examination

The anatomical depth of the ureter and its high degree of mobility make it impalpable even when significantly dilated. A stone however, lodged at or just above the vesicoureteric junction can be palpated in the anterolateral fornix of the vagina. Indeed it can be surgically removed through this route. If ureteric obstruction is suspected the physical signs of a hydronephrosis or pyonephrosis must be sought as these findings may alter the initial management. In particular, a tender kidney in the presence of a pyrexia are indications of an obstructed and infected system. The common causes of ureteric obstructions are listed in *Table 27.2*.

Ureteric stone

Stones formed in the collecting system of the kidney may drop down into the ureter (*Figure 27.12a, b*) and give rise to the typical symptoms of ureteric colic; 90% of these stones contain calcium and can be seen on plain radiography to lie along the expected path of the ureter (the transverse processes of the lumbar vertebrae, the line of the sacroiliac joint and the pelvis). If 5 mm or less, 90% of these stones pass down the ureter spontaneously but if larger usually get stuck and cause complete or partial ureteric obstruction. There are three points along the length of the ureter where stones tend to become lodged: the pelviureteric junction, the sacral promontory and

the vesicoureteric junction. Intravenous urography remains the most useful investigation to determine the size and position of the stone and to assess the degree of renal obstruction.

Ureteric tumour

Transitional cell tumours can affect any part of the transitional cell epithelium, which lines the whole of the urinary tract. The chances of a tumour developing are approximately related to the length of time that the urine – which contains the carcinogen – has been in contact with the epithelial surface. They are thus more likely to appear in the bladder (p. 346) than the ureter (*Figure 27.13a, b*), and also more likely in the renal pelvis (*Figure 27.13a, b*) than the ureter. In fact about 5% of urothelial tumours present in the renal pelvis and 1% in the

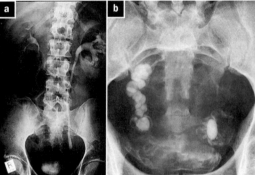

Figure 27.12
a. Ureteric stone near the lower end of the left ureter, causing obstruction, dilating the whole length of the ureter above it and producing dilatation of the calyces. b. Extensive ureteric calculi in a patient with *Bilharzia*.

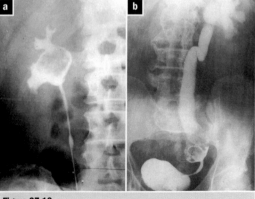

Figure 27.13.
Transitional cell tumours of the urothelium. a. In the renal pelvis. b. Tumour in the lower end of the left ureter.

Table 27.2. Common causes of unilateral/bilateral ureteric obstruction.

Extramural	Abdominal and pelvic neoplasms (caecum; colon; rectum; bladder; prostate; uterus; cervix)
	Retroperitoneal fibrosis
Intramural	Pelviureteric obstruction
	Ureterocele
	Tuberculous stricture
	Stricture secondary to schistosomal infection
	Surgical damage (colectomy; excision of the rectum; procedures on the bladder and prostate; hysterectomy)
Intraluminal	Renal and ureteric stones
	Sloughed renal papilla
	Blood clot

ureter alone. Ureteric tumours present with haematuria or even symptoms of ureteric obstruction and the diagnosis is confirmed by a combination of urine cytology and radiological imaging.

Idiopathic retroperitoneal fibrosis

Retroperitoneal fibrosis involves both ureters, drawing them medially and producing a progressive obstructive hydro-nephrosis, leading to renal failure. In some instances the fibrosis is related to an inflammatory abdominal aortic aneurysm, malignant infiltration or occurs in a patient taking the drug methysergide.

In the majority of instances, however, the cause is unknown. Various theories linking it to an autoimmune disease, urinary leakage, sepsis, haemorrhage and trauma, have proved unsatisfactory.

There may initially be no symptoms, the diagnosis being a chance finding. However, as obstruction progresses, there is severe backache and systemic disturbances of malaise, weight loss and anorexia, progressing to anuria and renal failure.

The bladder

The bladder lies deep in the pelvis, posterior to the pubis and when empty is impalpable. The majority of the bladder is extraperitoneal though the dome which expands on filling has a peritoneal covering.

Bladder pain

Pain in the bladder is typically a dull, midline suprapubic pain which may be exacerbated on micturition. This is also the pain of acute urinary retention and is accompanied by an intense desire to micturate. Strangury is the painful desire to micturate combined with the inability to completely void the bladder.

Bladder examination

On filling, the bladder rises up out of the pelvis and above the symphysis pubis (*Figure 27.14*). When enlarged, or in the thin patient, it can be palpated in the lower abdomen as a smooth

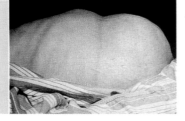

Figure 27.14. Chronic prostatic obstruction producing a distended bladder that has risen beyond the umbilicus.

mass arising from the pelvis. It is usually symmetrical but occasionally is more easily palpable on one side of the mid-line. When less distended, or in the obese patient, palpation can be more difficult and it may then be identified by percussion. Percussion of the bladder should be from above downwards, the bladder appearing as a dull area usually between the umbilicus and symphysis pubis. Other useful clinical signs include its hemiovoid shape, smoothness and immobility. It may extend up to and past the umbilicus. Other pelvic masses that need to be differentiated from the bladder include an ovarian cyst, the pregnant uterus and a fibroid uterus. If doubt remains examination should be repeated after passage of a urethral catheter. When very large, the bladder may rest on the abdominal aorta and transmitted pulsations may be felt. This should not be mistaken for an aneurysm.

Retention of urine

In infants and children the bladder is more of an abdominal organ and can be palpated without the child being in retention of urine. If associated with difficulty or the inability to pass urine the cause is most likely to be neurological in origin, or due to obstruction from the presence of posterior urethral valves.

In the adult male the finding of a distended bladder associated with the inability to micturate should provoke a search for the possible cause. The foreskin and urethral meatus are examined for a phimosis and meatal stenosis, and the length of the urethra as far as the bulb can be palpated for a stricture, peri-urethral abscess, or the presence of a stone or foreign body, and the presence of a urethral discharge noted. The prostate must be examined as prostatic disease is the commonest cause for retention of urine in the male. A full assessment should include examination of the CNS to exclude a neurogenic cause for the retention. The bladder sensation/micturition reflex arc can be inhibited or obliterated by a disease of the CNS which is localized at the level of the midsacral neural outflow.

The physical signs associated with nerve damage at this site are an absent ankle jerk and diminished or absent cutaneous sensation in the perineum and perianal regions. This examination is essential in all younger patients who present with retention of urine and those with any other physical signs of neurological disease. When retention of urine is due to prostatic enlargement it is preceded by the typical symptoms of bladder outflow obstruction.

If these symptoms are untreated a proportion of these men develop acute retention, which is the painful inability to micturate. However, in another though smaller proportion of men, the bladder continues to enlarge as the obstruction increases and the condition of chronic retention follows.

The chronic retention of urine produces similar physical signs but is quite painless to the patient. He may also complain of dribbling 'overflow' incontinence; firm palpation of the enlarged bladder may induce leakage at the urethral meatus. Chronic retention is more likely to produce upper tract hydronephrosis and thus renal impairment – the appropriate physical signs may be present. Why some men with bladder outflow obstruction from prostatic hyperplasia suffer acute retention, while others develop chronic enlargement of the bladder and upper tract dilatation, remains unclear.

In the female, retention of urine can also occur. In the younger woman this is usually neurological in origin and may represent the onset of a more widespread neurological disease such as MS. In the older woman difficulty with micturition due to obstructed voiding can result from a urethral stenosis. This may develop in the postmenopausal woman as part of atrophic vaginitis due to poor oestrogenization of the vulval tissues.

Bladder cancer

Unless a bladder tumour is large (Figure 27.15) it is not usually palpable above the symphysis on abdominal examination. Depending on its position in the bladder, it may be palpable per rectum or per vagina. The majority (80%) of bladder tumours are superficial – i.e. not involving the muscle of the bladder wall – at the time of first diagnosis and cannot be detected on clinical examination, except for the observation of haematuria. The remaining 20% are invasive at presentation with the tumour invading the bladder wall and sometimes the surrounding structures, such as the ureter, leading to obstruction and hydronephrosis. These advanced tumours are palpable on bimanual examination under an anaesthetic, when the size, position and mobility of the tumour need to be assessed. The clinical staging of the disease at the time of initial assessment is crucial in determining subsequent treatment and predicting the prognosis. Staging is achieved by a combination of cystoscopic excision biopsy of the tumour and examination under anaesthetic.

Superficial:

- Ta – Papillary.
- T1 – Subepithelial connective tissue.

Invasive:

- T2 – Superficial muscle.
- T3a – Deep muscle.
- T3b – Perivesical fat.
- T4 – Invading prostate, uterus, vagina or pelvic wall.

Bladder stones

Historically a common ailment in the UK, bladder stones (*Figure 27.16a, b*) now rarely reach the size at which they become symptomatic. If they do so, they usually occur as a consequence of recurrent urinary tract infection. As the patient stands, the stone falls to the trigone of the bladder producing urinary frequency. As the patient micturates, the bladder contracts around the stone, producing pain. Haematuria, macroscopic or microscopic, is also a commonly associated symptom. Large stones can be palpated on bimanual examination.

Urinary tract infection

The urinary tract of both sexes is usually sterile, the commensal flora of the distal urethra protecting against invading organisms. The presence of micro-organisms in the tract is termed urinary tract infection (UTI) and is a common problem

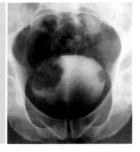

Figure 27.15.
Filling defect on the right side of the bladder.

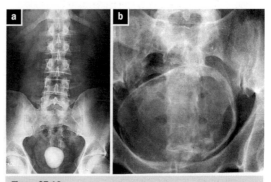

Figure 27.16
a. Plain radiograph of the abdomen, showing a midline bladder calculus. b. Large bladder calculus in a patient with *Bilharzia*.

at all ages and in both sexes. However, after the first month of life the incidence is much higher in the female, particularly young women, and often related to intercourse.

The condition may be asymptomatic but distressing symptoms are common, and UTIs cause considerable morbidity and also mortality from septicaemia and renal failure. The organisms involved are usually gut flora, particularly *Escherichia coli* (60%), *Pseudomonas aeruginosa*, *Proteus mirabilis*, staphylococci and streptococci. Chronic infection can be from TB and, of particular note in endemic areas, *Schistosoma* sp. A variety of other organisms may be implicated and mixed flora may be present, particularly with gut/urinary fistulae; hospital-acquired infection (nosocomial) may introduce resistant strains.

Once infection is present in the urinary tract it may ascend to the kidney or descend into the prostate, epididymis, testis and urethra. Urinary stasis is an important risk factor for UTI and is produced by outflow obstruction (prostatic and urethral strictures), incomplete emptying of the upper urinary tract (vesicoureteric reflux) and neurogenic abnormalities of the bladder. The presence of renal calculi or bladder stones serves as a nidus for persistent infection. Mucosal abnormalities due to trauma, such as instrumentation and surgery, and tumours, serve as entry points for infection from the urine or from bloodstream spread.

Nosocomial infection – following catheterization or instrumentation – may be due to poor technique, the infection and reflux of infected urine from an open drainage system, or organisms passing along the outside of a catheter. Specific patterns of infection occur in different patient populations. Urinary tract infections in childhood are particularly associated with the presence of vesicoureteric reflux, but congenital posterior urethral valves, ureteroceles and neuropathic abnormalities also occur.

Vesicoureteric reflux is prevented in the normal ureter by the narrow angle at which it enters the bladder and by a long, submucosal tunnel. Congenital ureteric anomalies include a laterally placed ureter, with a wider angle of entry, and short submucosal tunnels. Surgical procedures, such as tumour resection, can also damage a ureteric orifice and render it incompetent. Infection ascending to the kidney produces a pyelonephrosis and this, in turn, may be followed by interstitial and glomerulonephritis, hypertension and renal failure, the abnormality being termed reflux nephropathy (*Figure 27.17*).

Urinary tract infections and stress and urge incontinence are common in pregnancy. Infection has an association with maternal anaemia and carries a high risk of pyelonephritis. Bacteriuria thus needs to be investigated to prevent harmful effects on mother and fetus.

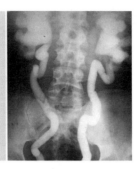

Figure 27.17.
Late effects of bilateral vesicoureteric reflux, showing hydronephrosis and hydroureters.

Interstitial cystitis is a chronic idiopathic pancystitis, occurring predominantly in women in their third and fourth decades. There is mucosal ulceration, with contact bleeding and marked muscular fibrosis, which leads to a contracted bladder with reduced functional capacity.

The **urethral syndrome** is acute urethral pain in young, sexually active women, that mimics UTI but in the absence of bacteriuria.

The clinical picture of a patient with a UTI is very variable in its severity. Lower urinary tract symptoms include frequency and urgency of micturition, this occurring often every few minutes and accompanied by nocturia. Suprapubic pain may be severe and this is accompanied by local tenderness over the bladder. Dysuria is present and the pain radiates into the labia or the tip of the penis. The urine is cloudy and offensive, and haematuria may be present. Systemically, the patient is unwell, with fever, rigors and vomiting.

In upper UTI, these lower tract symptoms are usually present and, in addition, there is loin pain and tenderness; there may also be a swinging pyrexia and general septicaemia.

Tuberculosis (TB)

Genitourinary TB can affect the whole of the urinary tract from the kidney to the testis. When TB affects the bladder there is invariably evidence of infection in the upper tracts. If the bladder is involved, attention should be drawn to the prostate and epididymis as these structures may also be involved. The patient suffers from urinary frequency, bladder pain and haematuria, and the chronic infection and inflammation lead to loss of bladder compliance and capacity; this may be only 50 mL. Symptoms of systemic infection may also be present, such as fever and weight loss. Even when treated, the subsequent scarring often leaves a small volume, non-compliant bladder which is neither able to store or void urine and is thus of little value. The lower ureters may also become involved by the process of healing and fibrosis, leading to obstruction.

Schistosomiasis

There are an estimated 200–300 million people in the world infected with schistosomiasis. Only malaria exceeds the prevalence of this disease world-wide even though most cases of schistosomiasis are centred around North and West Africa, and the Middle East. Urinary tract schistosomiasis is caused by infestation with a trematode fluke, genus *Schistosoma*, with the commonest species being *S. haematobium*, *S. mansoni* and *S. japonicum*. Infection is the result of direct penetration of the skin by free-swimming cercariae released from freshwater snails. The cercariae enter the venous system, traverse the pulmonary circulation and migrate to the perivesical veins. There, each adult female (about 2 cm long) produce 50–300 eggs per day. These migrate into the lumen of the bladder before being shed into the urine. On their way they induce a granulomatous response leading to ulceration of the mucosa on release of the eggs into the lumen.

The clinical manifestations depend on the egg load, the immune status of the patient and the degree of secondary infection. However, most infected patients exhibit haematuria and on cystoscopic examination have typical perioval granuloma visible on the mucosal surface. They later develop ulceration, fibrosis and calcification. Lower ureteric involvement is a feature of heavy or prolonged infection, and leads to obstruction and hydronephrosis. Chronic infection has also been shown to be a risk factor for the development of bladder cancer, especially squamous cell carcinoma of the bladder, which is an uncommon variant in non-endemic areas.

Urinary incontinence

Urinary continence is not established until after the age of two, daytime continence usually being present by four, but some degree of enuresis – the failure to suppress detrusor muscle activity during sleep – may continue into adolescence. Normal micturition requires normal bladder sensation to assess need, involves choosing a socially acceptable time and place, requires normal detrusor activity to provide bladder capacity (filling under low pressure and complete bladder emptying on contraction) and a normal urethral sphincter that can both maintain continence and relax when micturition is initiated. A large number of disorders can interfere with these mechanisms and are outlined in *Table 27.3*.

Psychological disorders interfere with a normal, socially acceptable choice of the time and place for micturition. They include parenchymatous and multi-infarct dementia.

Abnormalities of the urethral sphincter may be due to congenital anomalies such as hypospadias and ectopia vesicae.

Genuine stress incontinence is due to lax pelvic floor muscles with weakness of the urethral sphincter. It occurs in women after multiple pregnancies or prolonged labour, with possibly the need for forceps extraction. There is a varying degree of anterior vaginal wall prolapse, with a cystocele or a urethrocele, but detrusor muscle tone is normal. Incontinence is brought on by any increase in abdominal pressure such as coughing, laughing, sneezing or straining. Stress incontinence may also occur when the intra-abdominal pressure is raised from other causes such as ascites, ovarian tumours and pregnancy.

Damage to the urethral sphincter can occur with infiltrating tumours, trauma and surgical procedures. Notable in the latter are rectal excision and prostatectomy. The innervation of the sphincter may be damaged by malignancy, trauma or surgery, or by neurological abnormalities, particularly MS and spinal cord damage.

Abnormalities of the detrusor muscle include idiopathic detrusor instability. This is a common disorder, giving rise to frequency, urgency and urge incontinence. The condition also accompanies an irritating lesion of the bladder, such as cystitis, and when there is a small bladder capacity. The latter may be due to interstitial cystitis, TB, radiotherapy or surgical procedures, but may also be secondary to increased detrusor tone or hyperreflexia, such as occurs in Parkinson's and cerebrovascular diseases.

Outflow obstruction, such as in prostatic disease, a urethral stricture or bladder neck hypertrophy, produces a large bladder, stretching the detrusor muscle and resulting in only a small functional bladder capacity. Obstructive symptoms

Table 27.3. Urinary incontinence.

Psychological	
Abnormalities of the urethral sphincter	Congenital abnormalities
	Genuine stress incontinence
	Trauma
	Surgery
	Malignancy
	Damage to nerve supply
Abnormalities of the detrusor muscle	Idiopathic detrusor instability
	Small capacity bladder
	Outflow obstruction
Drugs	
Fistulae	

are hesitancy, poor stream and terminal dribbling, while over-activity of the stretched detrusor muscle produces incontinence overflow. Neurological damage may interfere with detrusor activity as well as sphincter innervation and give rise to a large, incontinent bladder. A number of drugs, such as some antihypertensives, anticholinergics and tricyclics, can give rise to urinary retention and overflow incontinence, while drugs with extrapyramidal side effects, such as phenothiazine, may produce urinary frequency and incontinence.

Urinary incontinence occurs in duplex systems (p. 341) when the ectopic orifice is below the level of the urethral sphincter.

In the history, enquire whether incontinence is limited to episodes of raised intra-abdominal pressure (stress induced), whether there is urgency (urge incontinence) and whether the leakage is continuous (due to a fistula). Obtain some idea of the amount of soiling and how the patient manages the problem. The obstetric history should identify difficulties of labour and, in the past history, note previous prostatic or pelvic surgery.

On examination look for general signs of sepsis or malignancy, any abdominal scars and distension from a large bladder, ascites or masses. Perineal and pelvic examination determine abnormalities of the penis, scrotum and vulva. Rectal and vaginal digital examination may identify pelvic inflammatory or malignant disease, while vaginal speculum examination can demonstrate anterior wall prolapse of the bladder or urethra. Urine should be examined and cultured, and a full blood count, and measurement of blood urea and electrolytes. Further studies include cystoscopy, urodynamics and radiological assessment of the urinary tract.

Urinary fistulae

These lesions occur between the urinary tract and the exterior, or communicate with another hollow viscus, such as the colon. Congenital anomalies of the urinary tract include a patent urachus (p. 331), an ectopic ureter and cloacal abnormalities, giving rise to an abnormal bladder and urethra, such as hypospadias and ectopia vesicae.

Vesicovaginal or **ureterovaginal fistulae** occur in untreated obstructed labour and are common in developing countries. They can occur in gynaecological surgery, where the damage can be of the bladder or the ureters, which are closely applied to the lateral vaginal fornices. Radiotherapy to pelvic neoplasia or the infiltration of the primary disease are common causes of these lesions.

Vesicocolic fistulae (*Figure 27.18a, b, c*) occur in diverticulitis, carcinoma of the colon, Crohn's disease, and after trauma or radiotherapy.

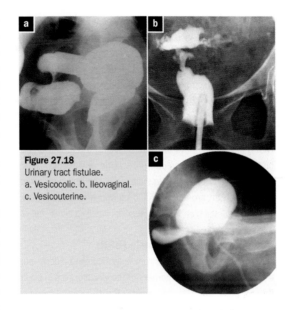

Figure 27.18
Urinary tract fistulae.
a. Vesicocolic. b. Ileovaginal.
c. Vesicouterine.

The prostate

The prostate is a gland whose function is related to the promotion of fertility and sits at the base of the bladder. It encompasses the first part of the urethra, into which drain the prostatic glands, and through which pass the ejaculatory ducts to open adjacent to the verumontanum.

Prostatic pain

Prostatic pain from inflammation – prostatitis – is a persistent pain felt in the perineum, usually associated with difficulty in passing urine.

Prostatic examination

The prostate can be palpated through the rectum. The examination should be performed with the patient in the left lateral position, though some prefer the patient to be in the knee–elbow position. The bladder should be emptied prior to examination. The index finger is used and should be turned to face the anterior surface of the rectum where the lobes of the prostate can be felt through the rectal mucosa. Superior to the prostate, on either side of the midline, are the seminal vesicles which are impalpable in the normal individual. Inferior to the prostate lobes, the membranous urethra can be felt. The normal prostate is firm, rubbery, bilobed and 2–3 cm across. Its surface should be smooth and there is an obvious central median sulcus between the lateral prostatic lobes. The rectal mucosa moves freely over the surface of the gland. Features of the prostate that should be assessed include the size, consistency, texture, degree of tenderness and the presence of any asymmetry or nodules.

Digital rectal examination is an important screening examination in men over 50 years old. Although its sensitivity and specificity as a test for prostatic malignancy are less than ideal, it is cheap and easy to perform – it should be a part of all health checks in men of this age. Used in combination with a measurement of the serum level of the prostate-specific antigen and transrectal ultrasound and biopsy, these tests have led to a dramatic increase in the number of men diagnosed with prostatic carcinoma and a reduction in the average age at which it is diagnosed.

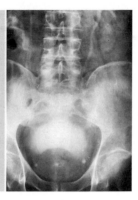

Figure 27.19.
Enlarged prostate producing a central median lobe impression in the opacified bladder.

Benign prostatic hyperplasia (BPH)

Histological BPH is an almost universal finding in elderly men and some palpable enlargement of the gland occurs in about 60% of men over 70 years of age. The two lateral lobes of the gland can be felt to bulge into the rectum though the central sulcus is retained. There may be some asymmetry of the enlargement though both lobes retain their smooth texture. The size of the gland may be falsely exaggerated if the patient has a full or enlarged bladder at the time of palpation, and this should be avoided. An assessment of the total prostatic volume is made by passing the examining finger from base to apex and also from side to side, however, the size of the gland does not always correlate with the degree of obstruction that the gland causes. Benign prostatic hyperplasia predominantly affects the central zone of the prostate and thus the prostatic lobes of the gland protrude into the urethral lumen, obstructing urine flow during voiding (*Figure 27.19*). Symptoms arise from either this obstruction to urine flow or from the consequent effects that this obstruction has on the muscle function of the bladder (detrusor). These prostatic symptoms are thus categorized as being either 'obstructive' or 'irritative' in nature:

- Obstructive – Slow stream; hesitancy; terminal dribbling.
- Irritative – Frequency; nocturia; urgency.

Clinically, the prostate is divided into three lobes, two lateral and one median. Although the histological process of BPH usually affects all lobes equally, sometimes the median lobe grows more than the lateral lobes. This lobe cannot be felt per rectum but can be seen cystoscopically as it grows up into the bladder lumen. This tends to give rise to predominantly irritative symptoms.

Carcinoma of the prostate

In Europe, 13% of all cancers diagnosed in men are prostate cancer and nearly 3% of all men over 50 alive today will die of carcinoma of the prostate. About 50% of all cases of cancer of the prostate diagnosed in Europe have metastases at presentation and, of those clinically localized to the prostate, over half have spread beyond the prostatic capsule. Clinical and pathological staging of the disease influences treatment and the overall prognosis of the patient. The commonest system used is based on the TNM system.

Incidental

- T1 – Clinically inapparent; not visible on imaging.
  1a –Incidental histological finding in <5% of resected tissue.
  1b –Incidental histological finding in >5% of resected tissue.
  1c –Needle biopsy; histologically positive.

Palpable or visible on ultrasound; confined to prostate

- T2 – Extends to capsule.
  2a – Involves <50% of one lobe.
  2b – Involves >50% of one lobe.
  2c – Involves both lobes.

Locally extensive

- T3 – Tumour penetrates through capsule.

Tumour fixation or invasion of neighbouring organs

- T4 – Tumour invasion of adjacent organs, e.g. seminal vesicles, rectum or pelvic walls.

Examination of the prostate may not only suggest the diagnosis of prostate cancer but also allows an assessment of the clinical stage of the disease. The hallmark physical sign of a malignant prostate is the asymmetry of the gland. Around 70% of malignant prostatic tumours arise in the periphery of the gland and thus in their early stages do not obstruct the prostatic urethra or urine flow. The finding of a patient with a relatively early prostate cancer is suggested by a firm nodule within one of the prostatic lobes. As it enlarges it may occupy the whole of one lobe and/or extend posteriorly to invade one or both of the seminal vesicles, giving extensions shaped like the horns of a bull. The central sulcus may be distorted or lost altogether and the rectal mucosa may become fixed to the gland. As the disease becomes more extensive it may also involve both prostatic lobes and be felt as a hard, irregular, nodular structure with extensions of tumour laterally to the pelvic walls; these fix the position of the gland within the pelvis. Rarely, the tumour may invade the rectum, and even encircle the rectum and anal canal, to cause an anal stenosis and obstruction.

Other physical signs that may be associated with a diagnosis of advanced prostate cancer include a hydronephrotic kidney, due to unilateral or bilateral ureteric obstruction, and thus the signs of renal impairment. About half of all men presenting with prostatic cancer have metastases at the time of diagnosis, the commonest site for these being in the bones. The lumbar spine is often affected and deposits of metastatic tissue may invade or compress the spinal cord and give rise to lower limb neurological signs. Prostatic examination is therefore an imperative examination in all men with unexplained lower limb neurological signs as treatment must be initiated before permanent damage occurs. Other manifestations of malignant disease, such as blood dyscrasias, are not uncommon, especially if there is widespread disease.

Prostatitis

Acute or chronic prostatic inflammation is characterized by perineal pain and strangury, but is associated with a number of other symptoms such as ejaculatory disturbance and low back pain. In the acute situation, the prostate may be slightly enlarged, smooth and acutely tender on palpation. If the patient allows it, massage of the gland can result in the passage of prostatic secretions into the urethra which appear as a urethral discharge and can be used for diagnostic analysis. Specimens of urine should be taken both before and after the expressed prostatic secretion so that localization of the source of any infection within the lower urinary tract can be made – the Stamey localization test. The finding of an acutely tender, boggy swelling within the substance of the prostate suggests the presence of an abscess.

In chronic prostatitis, the prostate may be firm with a granular texture and can be confused with carcinoma. Once again a sample of expressed prostatic secretions should be obtained.

Prostatic calculi

These stones vary in size and usually appear on the periphery of the gland. They can often be felt as hard nodules in a firm fibrotic gland and this also can be confused with a malignancy. They are usually of little clinical significance.

The female urethra

The female urethra is about 2 cm long and contains the urethral sphincter mechanism.

Examination

This should begin with the patient in the lithotomy position when the urethral orifice can be observed on parting of the labia majora (*Figure 27.20*). The whole length of the urethra can be palpated through the anterior wall of the vagina. Vaginal examination determines the capacity of the vagina and the presence of any degree of vaginal vault descent, as well as the presence of any gynaecological pathology. For a full interpretation of the integrity of the anterior and posterior vaginal walls the patient should be turned into the left lateral

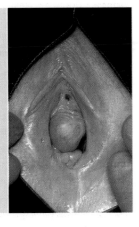

Figure 27.20.
Suburethral cyst bulging into the vagina.

position and a Sims speculum used to look for anterior and posterior wall vaginal prolapse.

Caruncle

This lesion presents with pain and urethral bleeding. Examination reveals it to be a red, tender mass about the size of a pea on a broad pedunculated base that arises from the posterior wall of the urethra.

Carcinoma of the urethra

This is a rare tumour but one that is twice as common in females as males. It is usually larger, harder and more irregular than a caruncle, the only certain way of differentiating it being by excision biopsy. Examination may reveal a localized area of induration or a mass extending into the vagina or bladder neck. These tumours metastasize to the inguinal lymph nodes and they must be included in the examination.

Urethral descent

This usually presents as genuine stress incontinence, when the patient complains of urine leakage after any manoeuvre that raises the intra-abdominal pressure, such as laughing, coughing and sneezing. Examination involves observation of the urethral meatus when the patient has a full bladder and is asked to cough. The urethral orifice is seen to descend from its resting position and urine usually leaks out. At cystoscopy this can be demonstrated by filling the bladder and then gently pressing the suprapubic area. The urethra is seen to descend and angulate upwards, which can be shown by placing a cotton bud in the urethral orifice. The descent can be prevented by placing two fingers inside the vagina alongside the bladder neck and holding them in a fixed position – the Bonney or Marshall test. This position mimics the action of a bladder neck suspension operation and is a guide to the potential efficacy of that operation. The presence of anterior or posterior vaginal wall and vault prolapse should also be sought in these women, who often have generalized pelvic floor laxity.

Urethral diverticulum

Although quite uncommon the incidence of urethral diverticula in females is increasing, probably as a reflection of the increased prevalence of sexually transmitted diseases, though they may be congenital in origin. They cause symptoms of recurrent urinary tract infection, dysuria, frequency and dyspareunia. They can be felt as a palpable tender lump behind the urethral meatus and occasionally pus can be seen to exude from the meatus on palpation.

The penis and male urethra

Examination of the penis

Examination of the penis and genitalia usually causes a certain degree of embarrassment for the patient and he should be kept at ease, and have confidence in the examiner. It is, however, an essential part of every examination of the urinary tract and should not be neglected. Examination should focus on conditions of the foreskin (prepuce) if present, the glans penis, the shaft of the penis and the urethra.

The foreskin should be retracted in all adults and the glans inspected; if it is at all difficult to retract, the prepuce and frenulum should be examined looking for a specific cause. The glans can be the site of a number of inflammatory conditions, and benign, premalignant and malignant neoplasms. In children the foreskin is adherent to the glans at birth and remains so until 1 year old, though there may still be preputial adhesions up to the age of 5. The shaft of the penis should be palpated and the two corpora cavernosa identified. Fibrous plaques within one or both of these represents Peyronie's disease which can cause pain on erection and/or angulation.

The male urethra is anatomically divided into four parts: the prostatic and membranous (the posterior urethra), and the bulbar and penile (the anterior urethra). Only the penile urethra can be examined externally. The urethral meatus should be examined and opened, looking for abnormalities of position, neoplasms and meatal stenosis. The remainder of the penile urethra can be palpated down the ventral aspect of the penis, between the testes and into the perineum. Along this line urethral diverticula, tumours or periurethral abscesses may be identified and sometimes the indurated tissue around a urethral stricture.

Hypospadias

Hypospadias (*Figure 27.21*) is the premature opening of the urethra anywhere along its length on the ventral surface of

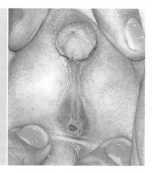

Figure 27.21.
Perineal hypospadias.

the penis or in the perineum. It is a relatively common congenital abnormality, occurring in 1 in 300 male births. The abnormality is a combination of various degrees of urethral and corpus spongiosal deficiency. The skin over the ventral surface of the urethra is thin and the prepuce is deficient ventrally giving the characteristic hooded appearance. The abnormality is associated with chordee – ventral angulation of the penis – due to replacement of the normal Buck's fascia with fibrous tissue; 70% of hypospadiac urethras open in the glandular, coronal or subcoronal areas, 15% along the shaft of the penis and 15% in the penoscrotal or perineal areas. Patients with hypospadias should be examined for other associated anomalies such as undescended testes and inguinal hernias which occur with an incidence of about 15%.

Epispadias

Opening of the urethral meatus on to the dorsal surface of the penis, in males, represents an epispadiac deformity (*Figure 27.22*). Occurring in 1 in 40 000 live births, it is twice as common in males as females. The condition is classified according to the position of the urethral opening, being glandular, penile or total, when it may also be associated with extrophy of the bladder. In females it is recognized by the presence of a bifid clitoris.

Phimosis

Fibrous constriction of the prepuce preventing retraction is a phimosis (*Figure 27.23*) and should not be confused with the normal adherence of the foreskin to the glans in the infant. At 6 months old only 20% of boys have fully retractile foreskins, increasing to 90% at 3 years. A true phimosis can occur in the child as the result of balanoposthitis – balanitis is inflammation of the glans and posthitis is inflammation of the prepuce – but also commonly affects the elderly as a consequence of long-standing balanitis.

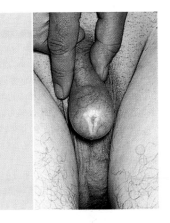
Figure 27.23. Phimosis.

Paraphimosis

This is the entrapment of the prepuce proximal to the coronal margin. If the foreskin is tight, prolonged retraction over the glans can lead to constriction and oedema of the glans and the development of a paraphimosis. The cause is usually iatrogenic and frequently occurs after failing to replace the foreskin after urethral catheterization. The vast majority can be reduced by simple compression of the glans to reduce the oedema followed by advancement of the foreskin.

Balanitis xerotica obliterans

Also known as lichen sclerosus et atrophicus, balanitis xerotica obliterans (*Figure 27.24*) often presents with the urinary symptoms of meatal stenosis or with a phimosis. It typically presents in men aged 20–40 years old. The aetiology is unknown although men with this condition have a higher than average incidence of associated autoimmune disorders. The lesions appear as white plaques on the surface of the glans and prepuce and the foreskin is often thickened, fibrous and difficult to retract. Involvement of the meatus leads to the stenosis.

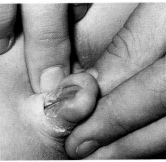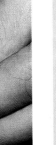
Figure 27.22. Epispadias.

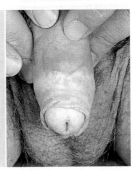
Figure 27.24. Balanitis xerotica obliterans producing phimosis and white plaques over the glans.

Urethral strictures

Patients with a urethral stricture (*Figure 27.25*) present with similar symptoms to those with prostatic enlargement. They are, however, usually younger and often overcome their poor urinary flow by abdominal straining. They suffer from repeated urinary tract infections. There are many causes of urethral strictures but the main ones are iatrogenic (instrumentation), infection (sexually transmitted diseases) and trauma.

Causes of urethral strictures:

- Congenital – Meatal stricture; bulbar stricture; posterior urethral valves.
- Traumatic – Instrumentation, e.g. catheterization; direct injury; foreign body.
- Inflammatory – Gonococcus; non-gonococcal urethritis; balanitis xerotica obliterans.
- Neoplastic – Transitional cell carcinoma; squamous cell carcinoma of the penis.

Iatrogenic and traumatic strictures tend to be short and situated in the bulb of the urethra, while infective strictures often involve longer lengths of the anterior urethra. Examination and subsequent investigations – radiological imaging – aim at determining the exact site and length of the stricture as subsequent management is dictated by these two factors.

Carcinoma of the penis

An uncommon urological malignancy, carcinoma of the penis (*Figure 27.26*) appears on the glans of the penis and occurs almost exclusively in uncircumcised patients. The incidence is thus considerably higher in populations who do not partake in this practice, such as Hindus and Chinese, and is almost unknown in Jews who circumcise at birth. The lesions are often covered by a phimotic prepuce and may present as a penile discharge. They appear on the glans as either an ulcer with raised edges or as a sessile papilliferous tumour. Premalignant changes of the skin of the glans may be identified before the disease forms these characteristic tumours. They include leukoplakia and erythroplasia of Queyrat, the latter appearing as a red, shiny, flat area on the glans of the penis and the former as white, flat hyperkeratotic plaques; both should be considered as carcinoma *in situ*. Another premalignant condition is the cutaneous horn which is an overgrowth and cornification of the epithelium. The base should be biopsied as it may demonstrate squamous cell carcinoma.

If a carcinoma is suspected, the shaft of the penis should be examined looking for extension of the tumour down the corpora cavernosa and regional lymph nodes palpated (the inguinal nodes drain the glans). About 50% of patients with invasive carcinoma have palpable nodes though only 50% of these are due to metastases, and 50% are due to reactive inflammation.

Carcinoma *in situ* of the penis is termed **erythroplasia of Queyrat** (*Figure 27.27*). This is an intraepidermal lesion that equates to Bowen's disease at other cutaneous sites. The ulcer is clearly defined, with a velvety floor. The penis is also subject to cutaneous and subcutaneous lesions encountered elsewhere in the body (*Figure 27.28a, b*).

Priapism is painful, persistent erection due to thrombosis of blood in the corpora cavernosa, the glans and corpora spongiosum always being spared. The condition may be a complication of leukaemia, sickle cell disease and haemodialysis. On rare occasions the thrombosis may be precipitated by malignant infiltration of extensive pelvic tumours or metastatic disease around the base of the penis. The condition can also occur as a complication of intracavernous injection of agents used in the treatment of impotence and after a spinal cord injury.

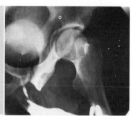

Figure 27.25.
Urethral stricture at the junction of the bulbous and membranous urethra.

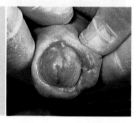

Figure 27.26.
Squamous cell invasive carcinoma of the penis.

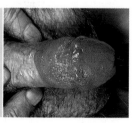

Figure 27.27.
Erythroplasia of Queyrat.

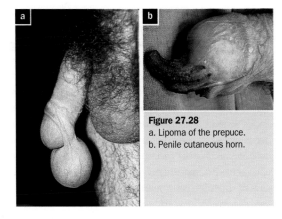

Figure 27.28
a. Lipoma of the prepuce.
b. Penile cutaneous horn.

Peyronie's disease is a condition of unknown aetiology in which dense fibrous plaques develop along one side of the penis in the tunica albuginea or the adjacent corpora cavernosa. A relation has been noted between the condition and Dupuytren's contracture. The condition is painless in the flaccid penis but produces pain and deformity on erection and may make intercourse impossible.

Sexually transmitted diseases
Gonorrhoea
The incubation period is 4–7 days and the predominant symptom is a urethral discharge. This may be thick and creamy, and yellowish in colour. The external meatus is red and the patient complains of dysuria, frequency and urgency of micturition.

Non-specific or non-gonococcal urethritis (NSU)
This is now the commonest form of sexually transmitted disease in the UK; it has an incubation period of 2–3 weeks. The patient usually complains of urinary frequency and dysuria, and a discharge. The discharge is more watery than gonorrhoea and may contain mucus. Inguinal lymphadenopathy is a less common finding, occurring in about 10% of sufferers.

Genital herpes (Figure 27.29)
The virus herpes simplex type 2 is responsible for genital infection. The attacks are like other herpes infections, being intermittent and involving groups of small papules that become irritating and then painful. These develop into small, clear or yellow vesicles which erode and remain until healing occurs. The diagnosis can be confirmed by a complement fixation test which determines the presence of the herpes simplex antibody.

Figure 27.29.
Genital herpes.

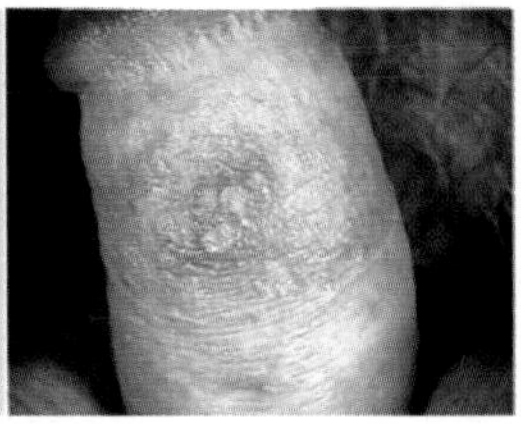

Genital warts (condylomata acuminata)
Caused by the human papillomavirus, infection gives rise to exophytic genital warts (Figure 27.30). These appear on the frenulum, glans and coronal sulcus and also inside the urethral meatus. They occur in areas subject to trauma during sexual intercourse. Infection has been associated with changes in the cervical epithelium which may progress to cervical intraepithelial neoplasia and later to invasive carcinoma.

Other lesions
The primary lesions of syphilis, chancroid, lymphogranuloma inguinale and granuloma inguinale (*Figure 27.31a–d*), together with genital herpes and warts, occur on both the penis and the labia.

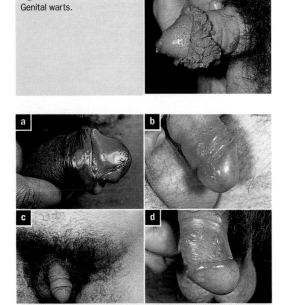

Figure 27.30.
Genital warts.

Figure 27.31
a. Primary syphilitic lesion. b. Chancroid. c. Lymphogranuloma venerium bubo. d. Granuloma inguinale.

Behçet's syndrome

Behçet's syndrome (*Figure 27.32a, b*) is a disease of unknown origin but having an immunological basis, presenting with oral and genital ulceration, occasionally uveitis, arthritis, transient neurological symptoms and thrombosis.

The scrotum and its contents

The scrotum contains the testes and spermatic cords. The testis and cord together form the testicle. The subcutaneous tissue of the scrotum has no fat but contains the dartos muscle which gives rise to the characteristic rugosity. The scrotal skin should at all times be freely mobile over the testes. Because of this laxity the contents of the scrotum can be examined with relative ease.

General examination of the scrotum

In examination of the genitalia the patient needs to be warm, comfortable and relaxed, and should be examined both lying and standing. Scrotal skin abnormalities are not uncommon and include sebaceous cysts (*Figure 27.33*), intertrigo, ulcers, cellulitis and tumours. Carcinoma of the scrotum (*Figure 27.34*) is notable in that Sir Percivall Pott's 18th century description of the lesion – due to soot in children chimney sweeps – was the first description of a carcinogenic agent. Although tar, pitch and mineral oil used in cotton mule spinners have been likewise implicated, the reduced contact with these agents makes the condition now a rarity.

Scrotal skin abnormalities can also be a manifestation of systemic conditions such as primary lymphoedema (p. 396) and generalized oedema; scrotal oedema from heart failure and immobility is a very common sign. Other causes of generalized scrotal swelling include surgical emphysema (from a pneumothorax), spreading cellulitis (or even gangrene in the case of Fournier's gangrene, *Figure 27.35a, b*), extravasation of urine and, in young boys, there is the condition of idiopathic scrotal oedema.

One of the first important features to determine about scrotal masses is whether the pathology is from within the scrotum (testicular) or whether it has descended through the inguinal canal to lie within the scrotum (i.e. a hernia). This can usually be achieved easily by attempting to get above the scrotal mass. If there is a palpable upper limit to a scrotal mass, it must arise from the scrotum. If, however, there is no upper border, the mass may be descending down the inguinal canal. Masses descending down the inguinal canal also usually exhibit a positive cough impulse.

Figure 27.32.
Behçet's syndrome.
a. Penile ulceration. b. Mouth ulceration.

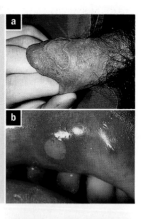

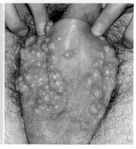

Figure 27.33.
Sebaceous cysts of the scrotum.

Figure 27.34.
Carcinoma of the scrotum.

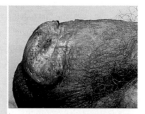

Figure 27.35.
Fournier's gangrene.
a. Acute. b. Following debridement.

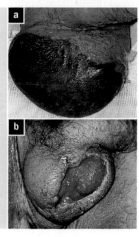

Another important part of any examination of a scrotal swelling is to look for transillumination. This should distinguish solid scrotal masses from cysts of the epididymis and cord structures, and a hydrocele. To examine for translucency the swelling should be made tense by the application of pressure at the neck of the scrotum, a torch is then placed to the distal side of the swelling.

The entire contents of the scrotum – i.e. the testes, epididymis and cord structures – need to be considered individually and each structure should be checked firstly for its presence and secondly its normality. Any individual component may be absent congenitally and this needs to be established at the outset. If it has been proven that a particular testis or even the vas of a testis is absent, the presence of a kidney on that side should be determined by ultrasound as there is an association with renal agenesis.

The testes

The testes can be palpated as smooth ovoid structures within the scrotum. They vary in size both between individuals and within individuals and can be 'sized' according to Prader's orchidometer (*Figure 27.36*). This may be useful when considering possible causes of male factor infertility. Generally the left testis hangs lower than the right.

When examining testes, the 'normal' side should be looked at first so that an idea of the size, shape and smoothness of the unaffected side can be assessed before moving to the affected side. The texture, firmness, shape, tenderness and general lie of the affected side need to be considered. This can only be achieved by examining the patient in both the lying and standing positions.

In the male child the presence of two testes must be confirmed by careful palpation. Both testes should be present in the scrotum at 1 year old and, if not, palpation along the normal line of descent should be made. Distinction should be made between retractile testes, which are able to be manipulated into the scrotum, and undescended testes which are fixed in an elevated or abnormal position. To achieve this the child should be as relaxed as possible and the fingers of the examining hand sweep from the area of the deep ring down and medially in an attempt to coax the testis down into the scrotum. If so, the testis can then be held between thumb and forefinger and its position in the scrotum clearly demonstrated. If the testis does not appear in the scrotum at all, it is undescended or possibly absent. If it can not be palpated at all its presence should be sought in various ectopic places such as the perineum and suprapubic areas (p. 359).

Testicular tumours

Testicular tumours (*Figure 27.37*) make up 1–2% of male cancers. They may be related to cryptorchidism (which accounts for 7% of these tumours), environmental factors, gonadal dysgenesis and ethnic factors. Enlargement of the testis occurs in 90% of testicular tumours, the vast majority of which are painless. The remaining 10% present with various manifestations of metastatic disease (*Figure 27.38*); 95% occur between the ages of 18 and 45 years. The testicular mass is firm and nodular and can be felt to arise from the body of the testis itself. If any clinical doubt as to the diagnosis exists, an ultrasound examination or even a surgical exploration is indicated. If the diagnosis is ever considered, blood should be taken for α-fetoprotein and β-subunit human chorionic gonadotrophin as these tumour markers are able

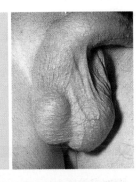

Figure 27.37.
Left testicular teratoma.

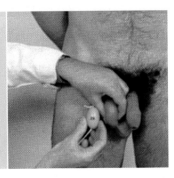

Figure 27.36.
Testicular sizing by comparison with a standard set of oval beads.

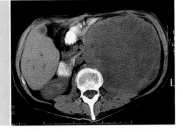

Figure 27.38.
CT scan of para-aortic lymphadenopathy from a testicular teratoma.

to help with diagnosis, prognosis and later monitoring of disease progress.

Metastatic para-aortic lymph nodes may present behind or above the umbilicus. There may be hepatic enlargement and supraclavicular lymphadenopathy or pulmonary metastases.

The diagnosis of testicular tumour must always be considered with some degree of urgency as the cell doubling time of the tumour can be very short (10–30 days). Although the majority of men can now be cured, long-term prognosis is dependent on the disease stage at diagnosis and any delay at this time may result in significant disease progression; 95% of testicular tumours have a germ cell origin. There are two principal types of germ cell tumours: seminomas and non-seminomatous tumours. The non-seminomatous tumours can further be divided according to their histological characteristics, although there are a number of different classification systems for these tumours in use around the world. Essentially there are two systems most often used, the British and American (*Table 27.4*).

There are likewise a number of different clinical staging systems used but these are all variations of the original system devised by Boden and Gibb:

- I. Tumour confined to the testis.
- II. Spread to regional lymph nodes – retroperitoneal, para-aortic nodes – below the level of the diaphragm.
- III. Spread beyond the retroperitoneal nodes, to the mediastinum or extralymphatic metastases.

Hydrocele

Fluid within the tunica vaginalis – a **vaginal hydrocele** – lies in front of, and surrounds the body of, the testis (*Figure 27.39*). The testis itself can not usually be palpated. The hydrocele is either primary, or secondary to some other condition of

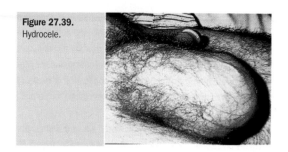

Figure 27.39. Hydrocele.

the testis, such as infection or malignant transformation, when it is an effusion into the tunica.

A **congenital hydrocele** presents in the neonate and is due to failure of the processus vaginalis to obliterate. Peritoneal fluid collects within the sac although movement in and out of the sac makes the hydrocele intermittent.

An **infantile hydrocele** occurs when the processus vaginalis closes at the level of the deep inguinal ring but remains unobliterated lower down. Fluid collects and remains in this sac until treated.

A **hydrocele of the cord** is a smooth, oval swelling attached to the spermatic cord, which can be mistaken for an inguinal hernia. A similar condition can occur in females, being attached to the round ligament, where it is palpated in the inguinal canal; it is called a **hydrocele of the canal of Nuck**.

Torsion

Torsion (*Figure 27.40*) is a notoriously difficult diagnosis to make with confidence, but one which needs to be considered in all patients who present with acute scrotal symptoms. Typically, the story is of a sudden onset, short duration pain which is severe, occurring between the ages of 10 and 30 years, most commonly 12–18, though these observations are not always universal. Nausea and vomiting are common associated features. The patient should be questioned about the presence of urinary symptoms and the urine should be

Table 27.4. The two main classification systems for testicular tumours.

British (Pugh)	American (Mostofi and Price)
Seminoma	Seminoma
Teratoma	Teratoma, differentiated (TD)
Embryonal carcinoma with teratoma	Malignant teratoma, intermediate (MTI)
Embryonal carcinoma (adult type)	Malignant teratoma, undifferentiated (MTU)
Choriocarcinoma	Malignant teratoma, trophoblastic (MTT)
Embryonal carcinoma (juvenile type)	Yolk sac tumour

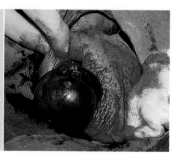

Figure 27.40. Operative picture of a testicular torsion.

tested for the possibility of infection. On examination the normal testis may be shown to have a horizontal lie, the 'bell-clapper testis', which are known to be more susceptible to torsion. The scrotal skin overlying the affected testis may be reddened and swollen. The spermatic cord is thickened and the testis elevated in the scrotum, due to either twisting of the cord but more likely cremasteric spasm. The testis is acutely tender and difficult to examine. Torsion can also occur in a maldescended testis and if such a testis is found to be tender on palpation, surgical exploration should follow.

A number of differential diagnoses need to be considered in men with suspected testicular torsion but the one that provides the greatest diagnostic difficulty is epididymo-orchitis. In this condition the onset is less acute and may be associated with other urinary tract symptoms such as frequency and dysuria. On examination the epididymis is initially the site of maximal swelling and tenderness, and the testis remains in the normal position. In the presence of torsion the testis occupies an elevated position and is itself tender on palpation.

Another condition that mimics torsion of the testis is torsion of the testicular appendage or Morgagni's hydatid which is a müllerian duct remnant. It usually gives rise to very similar but much less severe symptoms; this diagnosis can often be made by visualizing the torted appendage which is blue-black in colour and 3–5 mm in size when transilluminated through the scrotal skin, at the upper pole of the testis.

Undescended testis

Cryptorchidism (*Figure 27.41*) means hidden testis and is one of the commonest of all congenital disorders of childhood, occurring in 3.5% of all full term infants and 30% of premature infants. By 1 year old the overall incidence has fallen to about 1%, showing that many spontaneously descend. A **maldescended testis** – one that fails to descend normally – may be intra-abdominal, canalicular (within the inguinal canal), ectopic (outside the normal pathway of descent, such as suprapubic, femoral or perineal) or retractile. The commonest

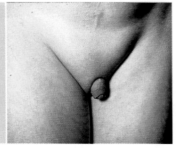

Figure 27.41.
Cryptorchidism.

place to find an undescended testis is in an ectopic position, just anterior to the inguinal canal in the superficial inguinal pouch. The testis descends through the canal normally and then, instead of descending into the scrotum, flips forward and forms a small fascial pouch in which it sits. The reasons for attempting to place testes in the scrotum instead of leaving them in an undescended position are:

- Cosmetic.
- Function – The higher and longer the testis resides away from the bottom of the scrotum the greater the likelihood of damage to the seminiferous tubules.
- Risk of malignancy – The undescended testis is 40 times more likely to undergo malignant transformation than a normal testis, though this risk remains even after repositioning.

The epididymis and cord structures

These should be carefully examined for their presence. Congenital absence of parts of the epididymis or vas are not uncommon – about 2% of all subfertile males – and have obvious consequences on fertility. The epididymis can be palpated behind the body of the testis. Parts or all of the epididymis can be congenitally absent or nodular and scarred from previous infection. Engorgement can indicate some form of ductal obstruction although the commonest cause of this is previous vasectomy. The vas is felt as a cord like structure and can be followed up into the neck of the scrotum.

Epididymal cyst

These are common, usually quite small, often multiple or bilateral and usually quite easy to distinguish from other testicular swellings. They may give rise to some discomfort as they get bigger but generally are asymptomatic. Epididymal cysts appear as cystic swellings usually above, behind and separate from the upper pole of the testis. They are tense, often lobulated and transilluminate. Because they often contain septa, and their brilliant translucency, they give rise to the appearance of a Chinese lantern. When they get bigger they may encroach downwards, further into the scrotum and mimic a hydrocele, although the cyst actually lies behind the testis rather than in front, as in the case of a hydrocele.

An epididymal cyst in the adult contains sperm and is termed a **spermatocele** (*Figure 27.42*). This is sited above and behind the testis. However the position is not constant and spermatoceles can occasionally be enclosed within a hydrocele sac.

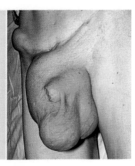

Figure 27.42.
Right-sided spermatocele. There is also a small hydrocele present around the testis.

Epididymitis

Epididymitis is a common form of scrotal swelling, occurring in a wide age range but typically increasing in frequency with age. This mirrors the incidence of urinary tract infection which is often a consequence of bladder outflow obstruction as the infection passes retrogradely along the vas to the epididymis. The condition is usually unilateral but may be bilateral and is also seen in a younger group of men who are infected with a sexually transmitted disease, usually NSU.

The clinical history is usually of a gradual onset of increasing discomfort, often associated with other urinary symptoms suggestive of infection such as frequency, dysuria and fevers. The scrotal skin is red, hot and swollen and the epididymis is enlarged and acutely tender. The body of the testis remains relatively normal, at least in the early stages of the condition. The most relevant investigation to perform is dipstix of the urine, followed, if necessary, by culture. The differential diagnosis is often torsion of the testis but the history and age of presentation are often good indicators of the likelihood of an infective origin.

Chronic epididymo-orchitis can occur as a consequence of tuberculous infection (*Figure 27.43*). The patient may have systemic infection including pulmonary disease or involvement of other parts of the urinary tract. The epididymis is not tender but hard and irregular, and the vas may feel like a 'string of beads'.

Varicocele

A varicocele (*Figure 27.44*) is an engorgement of the pampiniform plexus and occurs in up to 15% of the male population. The patients typically present with a chronic dull ache in the scrotum, worse on standing for prolonged periods. A varicocele has also been associated with oligospermia though it remains unclear whether this is cause or effect. The condition is nearly always left sided and is due to incompetence of the valve mechanism of the testicular vein as it enters the left renal vein. The diagnosis can only be made on standing the patient erect, when the engorged veins become visible as the characteristic 'bag of worms'. This sign disappears on laying the patient down. The onset of a varicocele in a middle-aged or elderly man may occasionally represent the presence of a left-sided renal tumour. This is due to obstruction of the renal vein by tumour growth from the kidney along the vein, to the point where the testicular vein enters on its left side.

Injuries of the genitourinary tract

Renal injuries are usually blunt and due to road traffic accidents, falls or crush accidents. Penetrating injuries can occur with knife and gunshot wounds but of prime importance are iatrogenic problems from percutaneous biopsy and surgical procedures, when haemorrhage and possibly AV fistulae may result. Injuries of the renal substance may be minor, tearing neither the capsule nor the renal pelvis. Major injuries lacerate the capsule and/or the renal pelvis, while critical injuries are those involving the renal vessels or shattering the kidney.

Clinical examination may reveal superficial bruising, with pain and tenderness, but these signs may be absent and are not a good indication of the underlying damage. Of more value is flattening of the normal subcostal concavity on the affected side, and rigidity of the anterior abdominal wall, the latter being a consistent sign in severe retroperitoneal haemorrhage. A loin mass may be palpable in spite of the rigidity.

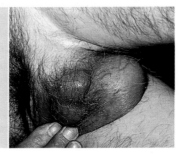

Figure 27.43.
Tuberculous epididymo-orchitis showing inflamed epididymis above a hydrocele surrounding the inflamed testis.

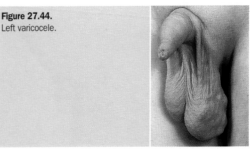

Figure 27.44.
Left varicocele.

Abdominal distension or meteorism is common within 36 hours of retroperitoneal haemorrhage and is probably an autonomic reflex, as ballooning is also present on rectal examination. When shock is profound and fails to respond quickly to resuscitative measures, one should suspect the possibility of concomitant splenic or liver injury. Although most lesions can be managed conservatively, progressive blood loss and an expanding loin haematoma require radiological assessment and, possibly, surgical intervention.

Haematuria is an important sign of major injuries but may not appear for a few hours, and the urine must be examined serially. Absence of haemorrhage may indicate avulsion of the renal pelvis, and severe haemorrhage may be delayed for 3 to 5 days due to clot sealing the haematoma, with subsequent rupture. Clot in the ureter or bladder may produce colic. The pain in the former radiates from the loin to the groin and occurs usually within 48 hours of the injury; the pain is less severe than with a calculus. Bladder colic can be severe and radiates to the external urethral meatus. It usually occurs between 3 to 5 days after the injury.

Ureteric injuries are usually iatrogenic in origin, related to surgical procedures, particularly hysterectomy, damage being where the ureters lie adjacent to the lateral vaginal fornices. The lesion may also occur in large bowel resection and in the surgery of abdominal aortic aneurysms. In these procedures the ureter may be crushed, devascularized, ligated, divided or excised.

The injury may be recognized and treated at the time but an unrecognized ligation may lead to asymptomatic atrophy of the kidney. The obstructed system, however, may give loin pain or become secondarily infected, and renal function depends on the competence of the second kidney. Urinary leak from division of a ureter or delayed necrosis may be into the peritoneal cavity, producing peritonitis, or a fistula may develop into the vagina or through the wound.

Bladder injury

The bladder may be ruptured intraperitoneally (20%) or extraperitoneally. An **intraperitoneal rupture** occurs when a blow is applied to a full bladder. The classic history is of an inebriated individual involved in a fight. The distended bladder is ruptured through the vault by a blow or a kick, there being minimal abdominal wall guarding against the injury. The vault of the bladder may be inadvertently opened in a lower abdominal incision, or penetrated during a cystoscopic resection.

The bladder may enter a femoral or hernial sac and be damaged during hernial repair, and intra- or extraperitoneal damage may occur in hysterectomy or in rectal excision.

In the conscious individual there is initially agonizing suprapubic pain, accompanied by hypotension and tachycardia but there is rapid recovery. The patient has no desire to micturate and may return to his or her previous activity. The abdomen gradually distends, partly from accumulation of urine and partly from the distended bowel of paralytic ileus; there is a variable amount of abdominal rigidity. Suprapubic dullness is absent although the patient has not micturated, but shifting dullness may be present. Rectal examination may reveal bulging and a boggy sensation in the rectovesical pouch. If left untreated, the signs of progressive peritonitis and uraemia supervene over the next 24 to 48 hours. If the patient is not seen until 24 hours after the accident, the diffuse signs of peritonitis may be misinterpreted as rupture of another hollow viscus and the anuria explained as a feature of general septicaemia.

Extraperitoneal rupture of the bladder and intrapelvic rupture of the **posterior urethra** (prostatic – in the male – and membranous) are considered together as they can be produced by similar injuries and have similar signs. The usual cause is a comminuted fracture of the pelvis (p. 461) in which a fragment of bone may pierce the bladder, or the puboprostatic ligaments are torn, resulting in prostatourethral dislocation, the prostate being widely separated from the perineal membrane. The commonest injury at this level is due to transurethral resection of the bladder or prostatic capsule. Full thickness resection of bladder tumours into the adjacent fat may be deliberately undertaken and treated by catheter drainage. In the other injuries described, however, there is urinary leakage into the retroperitoneal space that rises up beneath the anterior abdominal wall.

The patient complains of severe pain from both visceral and bony injuries. There is a desire to micturate but this increases extraperitoneal urinary leakage and pain. On examination there may be visible bruising and dullness over the lower abdomen up to the umbilicus. Rectal examination may reveal displacement of the prostate but this can be difficult to interpret as there is invariably a boggy haematoma which may also be present with bladder and other pelvic injuries. An important sign is the presence of blood at the external urethral meatus. Urethral injuries at this site present difficult management problems, and likely late sequelae include stricture, incontinence and, in the male, impotence.

The **extrapelvic (anterior) urethra** includes the bulbous and penile urethra. It may be damaged by forceful catheterization or instrumentation, tears being partial or complete, and false passages (*Figure 27.45*) may be produced. The bulbous urethra may be crushed against the pubic arch, typical causes

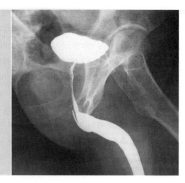

Figure 27.45. Iatrogenic false passage in the bulbous urethra.

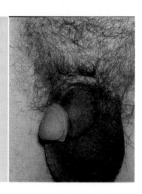

Figure 27.46. Scrotal bruising, with a haematocele following local trauma.

being a kick, or a fall astride the crossbar of a bicycle, a length of scaffolding or a gymnasium beam. The symptoms are of pain from the injury, perineal haematoma, urinary extravasation and inability to urinate. There are a few drops of blood passed from the external urethral orifice. The penile urethra is only damaged in the erect state, the signs being those of haemorrhage, extravasation and urethral bleeding. Bleeding into the superficial perineal pouch is contained by Colles' fascia and produces a characteristic 'butterfly wings' pattern of bruising across the perineum.

Perineal extravasation of urine is beneath Colles' fascia. This is attached posteriorly to the perineal membrane and laterally to the pubic rami. Urine thus extravasates over the scrotum and penis and up onto the abdominal wall. In the latter site, Colles' and Scarpa's fasciae are continuous and, as Scarpa's fascia is attached to the fascia lata in the region of the groins, extravasation is thus extended over the lower abdomen producing a boggy oedema which later produces cellulitic changes.

Scrotal trauma is usually due to a kick, a sports injury or sustained in a road traffic accident. The injury may be an avulsion of the scrotum or trauma to the testis and other scrotal contents. There is usually marked bruising and a secondary hydrocele or haematocele (*Figure 27.46*). Secondary infection can occur; this may be severe, such as in Fournier's gangrene (p. 356). As self-examination after minor trauma may, for the first time, identify other scrotal lesions, it is important to consider other diagnoses such as a testicular tumour, a torsion of the testis or epididymitis.

28 Arterial disease

Introduction

Diseases of the circulatory system affect the heart, arteries, capillaries, veins and lymphatics. Cardiac problems are considered on p. 255. Congenital diseases of the arteries, veins and lymphatics may involve all these elements but other pathological conditions of the components differ widely and are considered separately (veins, p. 381; lymphatics, p. 395).

Pathogenesis of arterial disease

Arteries may bleed or block. Bleeding is usually due to trauma but may also be due to rupture of an abnormally thin wall, such as an aneurysm, or arterial erosion by inflammation or malignancy.

The majority of arterial problems in the western world are due to **atherosclerosis**. This is a subintimal deposition of fatty material, giving rise to narrowing and damage to the intimal surface. The latter may ulcerate, discharging atheromatous embolic material into the blood stream, and stimulate thrombus formation.

Atherosclerotic disease, and other diseases, can also give rise to arterial dilatation. There may be generalized arteriomegaly of major vessels, as well as focal aneurysmal dilatation (p. 349). The common sites of aneurysm formation are the abdominal aorta and the common iliac and popliteal arteries.

Buerger's disease (thromboangiitic obliterans) has a similar pathology to atherosclerosis but affects medium-sized arteries, especially in the lower leg and forearm. It is accompanied by superficial venous thrombosis and is rarely seen in non-smokers.

Atherosclerosis becomes less common as one travels from Europe to Asia but the number of forms of **arteritis** increases. Most notable is **Takayasu's disease**, a pan-arteritis producing marked thickening and causing occlusion of the branches of the aorta. An arteritis of the proximal cerebral vessels is also seen in Japan and has been termed **moya moya disease** on account of the diffuse collateral formation around the base of the brain that shows the typical 'puff of smoke' on cerebral angiography.

Fibromuscular dysplasia is a degenerative disease of the arteries that is particularly seen in renal and carotid vessels where there is disruption of the arterial wall with sacculation and narrowing, as well as associated intraluminal thrombus formation.

General history and examination of the arteriopath

Atherosclerosis makes up well over 90% of arterial diseases in the west. It mostly affects the coronary, carotid and lower limb vessels. The history is, therefore, directed mainly at these regions but being sensitive to other areas, since no large- or medium-sized artery is exempt. Risk factors including hypertension, smoking and diabetes. Hypercholesterolaemia, obesity and a strong family history are also noted.

Incapacity from accompanying cardiac, cerebral and lower limb disease may have profound socio-economic effects, both on wage-earning and the nursing requirements after a stroke or an amputation. The number, closeness and physical fitness of relatives, and the accessibility and layout of the patient's home, need to be fully evaluated.

Examination of the arteriopath, like the history, pays particular attention to the heart, central nervous system (CNS) and lower limbs. In the general impression, note rest pain from the feet, the presence of anaemia or dyspnoea and signs of congestive cardiac failure (raised jugulovenous pressure, oedema, basal creps, pleural effusion and ascites). The heart is considered on p. 255. Blood pressure is taken in both arms. In the examination of each pulse, the sides of the body are compared, and the rate, rhythm, volume, character and the vessel wall are assessed. There may be a palpable thrill and/or an audible bruit or, on occasions, the machinery murmur of an arteriovenous (AV) fistula. The vessel may be graded into prominent, normal, weak and absent pulsation, the hardness of the wall and any enlargement being noted. A hand-held doppler probe provides a simple means of identifying blood flow in a vessel and, with a blood pressure cuff, provides a means of measuring systolic blood pressure in the upper and lower limb arteries.

In assessment of the cerebrovascular system, examine the common carotid arteries and their bifurcation, and the facial and superficial temporal vessels over the skull. Note the patient's mental status and speech abnormalities, visual defects, and use fundoscopy to identify cholesterol emboli in retinal vessels and changes of hypertension or diabetes. Examine for evidence of motor or sensory disorders.

In the upper limbs the subclavian, axillary, brachial, radial and ulnar pulses can be localized, together with any nutritional changes of the fingertips or hands. In the abdomen, the aorta is usually palpable in thin subjects, when compressed against the vertebral column. The size of any enlargement can be roughly gauged by dipping the fingers of the hands on either side and measuring the horizontal distance between the fingertips. Listen for aortic, renal, coeliac and iliac bruits. Although these are commonly found in normal individuals, coarse bruits are usually indicative of stenotic disease.

In the lower limbs, pulses should include the femoral, popliteal, dorsalis pedis, posterior tibial and perforating peroneal arteries, together with the nutritional status of the feet, particularly pressure points between the toes and their tips. Subsequent sections consider specific atheromatous problems of the CNS and the limbs, followed by the assessment of aneurysm and small vessel arterial diseases.

Coronary arteries are considered on p. 255.

Carotid arteries

Stroke accounts for more than 10% of deaths in western society, and a great deal of disability. The major aetiological factors are hypertension – producing intracranial haemorrhage (*Figure 28.1*) – and atheromatous carotid artery disease. A common site for the latter is at the carotid bifurcation and as this is surgically accessible it is also potentially correctable. The main problem is, therefore, to identify patients at risk prior to the onset of irreversible stroke symptoms. This has been found partly possible as 50% of atheromatous strokes are preceded by a **transient ischaemic attack (TIA)**, in which emboli from a tight stenotic area in the internal carotid artery (*Figure 28.2*) pass to the brain and then break up, producing only temporary symptoms. Even asymptomatic disease of greater than 70% stenosis carries a high risk of subsequent stroke symptoms.

A TIA takes the form of a hemiparesis contralateral to the affected carotid artery (*Figure 28.3*) or a visual loss in the ipsilateral eye, usually lasting less than a few minutes or up to 1–2 hours. (By definition a TIA lasts for less than 24

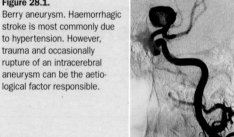

Figure 28.1.
Berry aneurysm. Haemorrhagic stroke is most commonly due to hypertension. However, trauma and occasionally rupture of an intracerebral aneurysm can be the aetiological factor responsible.

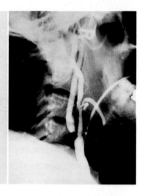

Figure 28.2.
Very tight stenosis of the origin of the internal carotid artery. This is a typical site for carotid atheromatous disease.

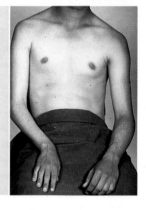

Figure 28.3.
Hemiparesis affecting mainly the upper limb.

hours.) Questions should cover the four areas of **motor, sensory, speech** and **vision**. Motor symptoms range from a dense hemiplegia affecting the contralateral leg, arm and face, to a transient, almost unnoticed, mild weakness of the hand or face. Ask patients if they drop things or catch their toes when they walk, and whether they have had recent trouble with their writing. There is a similar range of severity and distribution of sensory symptoms. There may be mild sensory disturbance of a few fingers, which can be difficult to differentiate from symptoms related to cervical osteoarthritis.

Speech problems are usually expressive in nature. There is often aphasia, which lasts from a few minutes to a few hours. An expressive dysphasia, in which patients know what they want to say but cannot say it, is an exasperating symptom and is likely to be remembered. A degree of nominal aphasia may continue. Sensory dysphasia, in which the patient speaks incoherently (jargon aphasia), or a combination of expressive and sensory dysphasia (global dysphasia) are less common.

An ipsilateral temporary visual loss (**amaurosis fugax**) is usually in the form of a shutter dropping across the visual field. This may be a total loss or dimming of vision, as if looking through a haze. It may involve the whole field or be a quadrantic loss and is usually noted when reading or watching television. A permanent scotoma may persist although this is not necessarily noted by the patient. 'Floaters' are black spots crossing the visual field and disappearing; they are due to atheromatous fragments of cholesterol passing through the retinal vessels without sticking or permanently blocking them.

Less specific symptoms, such as memory loss, dizziness and headache, may be related to reduced blood flow due to bilateral extracranial disease or multi-infarct dementia due to recurrent emboli. These non-specific symptoms, however, are also associated with other neurological disorders and are less valuable in the specific diagnosis of cerebrovascular disease.

Occlusive distal thrombosis or embolism may permanently block cerebral vessels, producing an **acute stroke** with a possibly fatal outcome or a permanent hemiplegia. Other terms applied are a **stroke in evolution** (where the stroke may progress over a number of hours or days), a **completed stroke** (which is the end result of an acute stroke) and a **prolonged, reversible, ischaemic, neurological defect** (i.e. **PRIND**, in which the stroke patient recovers but takes longer than 24 hours); the latter is possibly the result of revascularization around a small vessel occlusion.

An uncommon form of TIA or stroke is produced by a **subclavian steal**. In this condition a narrow or occluded proximal subclavian artery may be inadequate to meet the arterial needs of the arm. An alternative blood supply is obtained, particularly during exercise, through the vertebral artery thus 'stealing' blood from the circle of Willis and the cerebral circulation, with possible neurological sequelae (*Figure 28.4a, b*). The arm may also give rise to the symptoms of claudication (see below). The blood pressure should be taken in *both* arms in all patients with peripheral vascular diseases, and particularly in stroke patients.

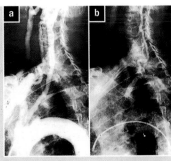

Figure 28.4.
Subclavian steal. a. Contrast medium passes up the innominate and left common carotid arteries but there is occlusion of the left subclavian. b. Delayed films show the contrast medium passing down the left vertebral artery and filling the left subclavian artery back to the occlusion, as well as passing distally.

Upper limb arteries

Upper limb ischaemia is surprisingly uncommon; this is probably related to the excellent anastamoses around the scapula, the elbow and the palm of the hand. Occlusion of the origin of the subclavian artery can give rise to the subclavian steal syndrome (as above). With subclavian artery occlusion there may be symptoms of upper limb claudication on severe exercise, this being accentuated when working above the head, such as painting ceilings.

All the supra-aortic arteries may be stenosed or occluded in the **aortic arch syndrome**. This occurs in Takayasu's arteritis, common in Japan, but also occasionally in atheromatous disease (*Figure 28.5*). There may be surprisingly few cerebral symptoms, the brain being adept at drawing on collateral blood flow; hypoxic visual symptoms may predominate. The arm is commonly the site of access for coronary artery radiological procedures and also for the formation of AV fistulae for dialysis. Upper limb vessels are also a common site for the intravascular injection of recreational drugs (*Figure 28.6*) or the inadvertent arterial injection of anaesthetic agents, particularly the toxic sodium thiopentone.

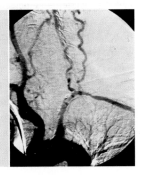

Figure 28.5.
Severe atheromatous disease of the aortic arch with occlusion of the left common carotid artery and stenosis of the left subclavian artery.

Figure 28.6.
Acute ischaemia of the left arm following intra-arterial heroin injection.

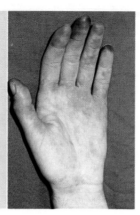

Figure 28.7.
Radiograph of bilateral cervical ribs. Note that the cervical transverse processes are directed downwards and the thoracic upwards, therefore any rib attached to a downward angled process is abnormal.

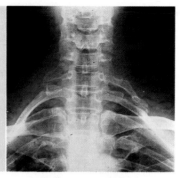

Figure 28.8.
Marked wasting of the right thenar eminence. This is due to a cervical rib pressing on the T1 root of the brachial plexus.

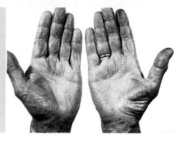

Two other groups of upper limb arterial symptoms are due to small vessel abnormalities (p. 376) and the thoracic outlet syndrome.

Thoracic outlet syndrome

The thoracic outlet syndrome is a collective term given to various anatomical anomalies that can compress the nerves and vessels of the upper limb in the root of the neck. The term embraces other conditions, such as the anterior scalene, the costaclavicular and the hyperabduction syndromes. The bony abnormalities encountered are:

- A partial or complete cervical rib (*Figure 28.7*).
- A prominent seventh cervical transverse process.
- Callus from a healed fracture of the first rib or clavicle.
- A high or congenitally abnormal first rib.

The possible sites of compression are between the first rib and the clavicle, the coracoid process, the pectoralis minor tendon, the scalenus anterior, the seventh cervical transverse process and an incomplete cervical rib; or between the scalenus anterior and the scalenus medius muscles. Also described are fibrous bands, prominent bellies of the above muscles and an aberrant scalenus minimus muscle.

The presence of these anomalies is not invariably accompanied by any symptoms, and symptoms are very rare in childhood. Often they are precipitated by abnormal posture, particularly in positions of prolonged abduction (painters and truck drivers) or downward traction (carrying heavy loads). Symptoms may be vascular or neurological or, occasionally, both. Arterial symptoms range from Raynaud's phenomenon to frank digital ischaemia. The most severe syndromes are usually secondary to recurrent emboli arising from a post-stenotic dilatation of the subclavian artery in association with a complete bony cervical rib.

Neurological symptoms predominate. These include nocturnal pain and minor sensory changes, particularly along the medial border of the hand and forearm, but weakness sometimes occurs and is most marked in the hand (*Figure 28.8*). These various symptoms are related to pressure on the lower part of the brachial plexus by a cervical rib or abnormal band. Occasionally the upper part of the brachial plexus may be involved, in which case there are symptoms along the lateral aspect of the arm, and pain is also experienced in the side of the neck and face. Venous compression is manifested by pain, swelling and cyanosis of the limb.

The diagnosis of thoracic outlet syndrome is aided by a diminished or absent radial pulse, the presence of a subclavian bruit and delayed hand flushing. Various manoeuvres have been described to make the radial pulse disappear in patients with the syndrome, but they may also do so in a normal individual. Examples are hyperabduction and hyperextension, these movements being increased passively by the examiner. The carrying of heavy weights may also alter a palpable radial pulse. These extreme manoeuvres sometimes reproduce the patient's pain, supporting the need for decompression procedures on the thoracic outlet, often by removal of the first rib.

Lower limb arteries

Lower limb ischaemic symptoms, as previously noted, are largely dependent upon the rate of onset of an arterial occlusion. **Acute occlusion** leads to gangrene unless revascularization is undertaken, whereas **chronic occlusive disease** allows time for collateral arterial formation. In the latter group, mild ischaemia gives rise to intermittent claudication but when the residual vessels are unable to provide enough blood to support the resting metabolic needs of the limb, a state of **critical ischaemia** is reached, accompanied by the symptoms of rest pain and gangrene.

Acute lower limb ischaemia

Acute ischaemia is often the result of thrombosis but may be due to embolism and can accompany trauma. Another, less common, cause is an arterial dissection.

Thrombosis of an artery can occur at sites of previous disease and may present with acute ischaemia superimposed on chronic atheromatous states. Thrombosis may also occur in an aneurysm (p. 375). Arterial **emboli** usually arise from the heart, examples being auricular thrombus proximal to a diseased mitral valve and thrombus developing on myocardial disease of the left ventricle, such as after a recent myocardial infarct. Emboli entering the aorta or another artery pass along it to its bifurcation. They can then be broken into two, passing down each branch, or, if small enough, can enter one of the branches. Eventually the embolus is too large to pass on and wedges across a bifurcation (*Figure 28.9*).

Large cardiac emboli wedge across the bifurcation of the abdominal aorta, producing the so-called **saddle embolus**. If left untreated, this lesion produces severe ischaemia, with gangrene of both legs. If the individual survives the haemodynamic and metabolic insult, the lower limb outcome is likely to be bilateral above-knee amputation; this is in marked contrast to chronic occlusion of the abdominal aorta where patients may complain of only mild claudication. It is also in marked contrast to the rapid recovery of the limbs if the embolus is lysed or surgically removed.

When tumours grow into an artery, fragments may break off. These may be of a large size; for example, a length of bronchial carcinoma entering the pulmonary vein, breaking off and blocking a femoral artery.

Smaller emboli arise from diseased mitral and aortic valves, such as in rheumatic heart disease, and from atherosclerotic disease of the arteries, from which atheromatous debris and platelet aggregations may be dislodged. Smaller emboli can give rise to focal areas of infarction, presenting as blue cutaneous patches over the lower leg and particularly the foot – the so-called **trash foot** (*Figure 28.10a, b*). Fat emboli occur after fractures of long bones; they can have marked pulmonary (dyspnoea) and cerebral (confusion, disorientation and coma) effects. Amniotic fluid emboli can produce similar symptoms.

Intra-arterial emboli may also be deliberately introduced radiologically to block bleeding arteries, tumour blood supply, AV fistulae or to reduce flow in an AV malformation. A wide variety of materials have been used, including blood clot, macerated muscle or tendon, or foreign material, such as plastic balls and metal springs (*Figure 28.11a, b*). Venous emboli are considered on p. 244.

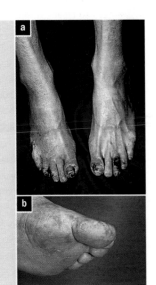

Figure 28.10.
Trash feet. a. Small emboli arising from an aortic valve prosthesis. b. Microemboli arising from an ulcerated atheromatous plaque.

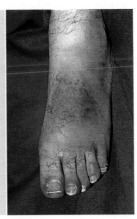

Figure 28.9.
Acute ischaemia of the left leg. This is due to an embolus blocking the division of the common femoral artery into superficial and deep branches.

Figure 28.11.
a. Arteriovenous malformation of the left shoulder. Note the enormous dilatation of the left subscapular artery feeding into an AV malformation around the shoulder joint.
b. Abnormal vessel occluded by a metal coil introduced through a percutaneous catheter.

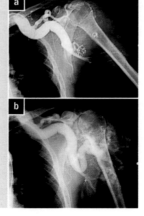

Figure 28.12. Arterial injuries.

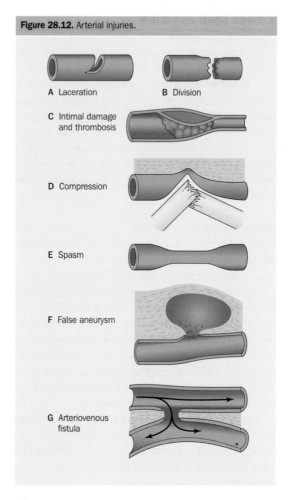

A Laceration

B Division

C Intimal damage and thrombosis

D Compression

E Spasm

F False aneurysm

G Arteriovenous fistula

Acute ischaemia in **trauma** may be due to major arterial damage with laceration or transection, or arterial ligation in the control of haemorrhage (*Figure 28.12*). Arterial occlusion may also occur due to thrombosis following intimal damage and a vessel may be compressed by surrounding oedema or by a displaced fracture or a dislocated joint. Other complications of arterial trauma are **spasm** (particularly in children), a **false aneurysm** (p. 375) or an **AV fistula** (p. 391).

Presentation of acute lower limb ischaemia

The presentation of acute ischaemia is classically with the six Ps: pulseless, pallor, perishingly cold, and the three neurological symptoms of pain, paraesthesia and paralysis. These features provide a useful reminder but the picture is not always so clear-cut, particularly in trauma where the patient may be shocked, pale, peripherally shut down and cold, from blood loss, and the limb may have local bruising and nerve injuries complicating the neurological signs. Pulses also persist in 20% of vascular injuries. Important factors to remember are, therefore, always to compare an affected limb with that on the other side, and always be suspicious of possible vascular complication of injuries near major vessels.

The presentation of non-traumatic acute ischaemia is characterized by the sudden onset of severe, constant pain. This gradually fades as tissue changes become irreversible. Paralysis is an important sign as it is easier to elicit than the associated patchy sensory loss. The limb is cold and usually pale but in a warm environment it may be a dusky blue, progressing to a blotchy white/blue appearance. At this stage it is still possible to blanch much of the limb by digital pressure but there may be deep tenderness over ischaemic muscle.

Revascularization within 6 hours of total ischaemia is usually accompanied by full recovery but there may be temporary renal failure. After 6–12 hours, mottling progresses, with cutaneous blistering. The skin becomes firmer, due to oedema, and a 'marble-like' mottling is present.

By 12 hours, totally ischaemic muscle has undergone irreversible changes. The subsequent signs of fixed [non-blanchable on elevation or digital pressure] tissue staining and muscle rigidity come on over the next 12–24 hours, indicating irreversible damage of all the tissues of the limb. These signs progress proximally to the level of propagated thrombosis.

A late sequelae (*Figure 28.13*) of muscle ischaemia is fibrosis and Volkmann's contracture (see also p. 421). This is particularly seen after trauma and may also be precipitated by tight splintage or bandaging of severely traumatized and fractured limbs.

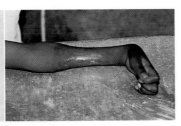

Figure 28.13. Volkmann's contracture. The ischaemia followed rigid splinting of a forearm fracture.

Chronic lower limb ischaemia

Mild ischaemia of the lower limbs gives rise to intermittent claudication whereas severe symptoms are those of rest pain, skin changes and gangrene.

Intermittent claudication is a cramp-like pain occurring on exercise. Although it occurs in any active ischaemic muscle, it is classically seen in the calf, as indicated by its Latin derivation (*claudicatio* – to limp). The pain is severe and forces the subject to stop their activity. This relieves the pain, the activity is recommended and the cycle repeated.

The cause of the pain can be explained as a response to an accumulation of acidic anaerobic metabolites due to inadequate blood and oxygen supplies to meet the requirements of the increased activity. On stopping the activity, the blood supply is replenished, anoxia abolished and painful metabolites washed away. The anoxia is not harmful and, if the pain is only mild, the patient may be able to maintain the activity through the pain without ill effect.

Although pain is usually in the calf, it may radiate to the back of the thigh and into the buttocks, indicating interference with pelvic as well as lower limb blood supply (*Figure 28.14a, b*). There may be **numbness** or **pins and needles**

of the forefoot associated with exercise; this is probably due to the shunting of an already defective forefoot blood flow into the calf.

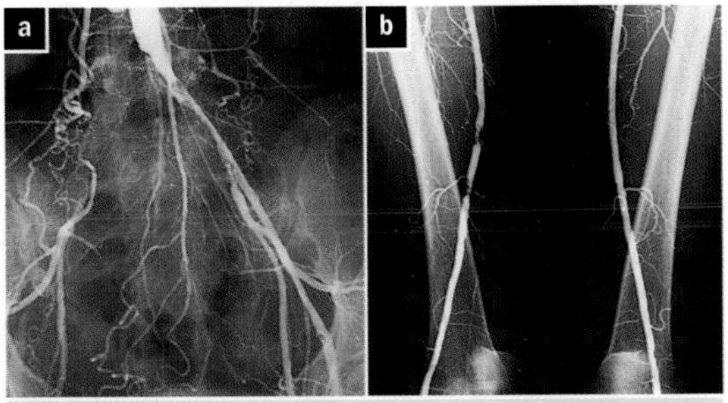

Claudication is usually of insidious and gradual onset in one leg but commonly becomes bilateral. Only 10% of claudicants progress to severe symptoms, the severity of which is largely related to the needs and expectations of each patient. In some, claudication at 50 m may not interfere with normal activity while in others this distance may prevent work or participating in sport or other social activities. These factors should be questioned, together with the time and form of onset of the symptom, its progress and the current claudicating distance.

The severe symptoms of **rest pain** and **gangrene** of the foot may occur suddenly, as well as being the end point of 10% of claudicants. To produce these symptoms in chronic disease there has to be severe stenosis or occlusion in at least two sites of the lower limb arterial tree. Severe symptoms of this nature usually require some form of intervention. Rest pain is a severe throbbing pain, affecting the toes and forefoot. It is increased by leg elevation, such as in bed at night. This is related to the reduced flow in the absence of gravity. Patients may have to get out of bed and walk about or sit with their legs hanging down, producing bilateral oedema. The patient may also hang on to the foot with the knee bent, and this can result in a fixed flexion deformity. The systemic effect of the pain may produce loss of appetite, with weight loss, and the patient usually looks unwell.

Other symptoms related to lower limb vascular disease include impotence, this usually being associated with occlusion of the abdominal aorta (**Leriche's syndrome**, *Figure 28.15*). Neurogenic pain can mimic rest pain, and the two pains can occur simultaneously. This is particularly so if the blood supply to the lower spinal cord is impaired or produc-

Figure 28.14. Typical radiological appearances of atheromatous disease. a. Occlusion of right common iliac with marked stenosis of the left common iliac. b. Stenotic disease of the superficial femoral artery (the continuation of the femoral after it has given off its deep branch). Such atheroma commonly commences at the level of the adductor hiatus.

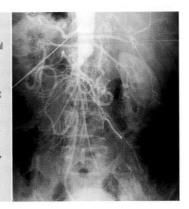

Figure 28.15. Occlusion of the infrarenal abdominal aorta. Chronic occlusion of this nature allows time for the development of extensive collaterals across the pelvis and through the mesenteric vessels, preventing acute ischaemic changes in the legs.

ing **cauda equina (neurogenic) claudication.** Non-vascular symptoms of the cauda equina can occur with standing and various other movements, as well as with walking, and tend to persist longer after stopping the activity than claudication. Straight leg raising may be reduced and there may be low back pain and neurological signs.

Examination of the lower limb vasculature starts with the abdominal aorta to exclude tenderness and enlargement, and auscultation for bruits over the aorta and iliac vessels. It is possible to palpate an external iliac pulse in thin subjects, even in the absence of a palpable femoral artery. Renal bruits are best heard posteriorly below the twelfth ribs, and coeliac axis bruits in the epigastrium.

The femoral artery may be difficult to feel in the obese subject, so palpate halfway between the anterior superior iliac spine and the symphysis pubis. Even an occluded artery may be palpable because of the pipestem, hard, atheromatous disease. Some dilatation is common in older subjects, particularly in patients with existing aneurysmal disease. Compare the two sides – the femoral artery is also a useful reference point for comparing with the radial artery to assess radiofemoral delay.

Listen over the adductor hiatus, a hand's breadth above the knee; there may be an audible bruit as this is a common site for early atheromatous disease. The popliteal arteries may be difficult to feel and, conversely, the normal arteries can appear expanded in some subjects. This is an important finding since it is a classic site for aneurysm formation. The artery is palpated against the lower femur or, more easily, against the upper tibia.

The dominant foot pulses palpable in the normal limb are the dorsalis pedis and posterior tibial arteries. The anterior tibial artery is malpositioned, usually more laterally placed over the dorsum of the foot, in 14% of individuals. The posterior tibial artery can be palpated against the medial aspect of the talus or, more proximally, against the back of the tibia. The perforating peroneal artery is palpated on the anterior aspect of the lateral malleolus.

All three arteries may be palpable in the normal limb but the peroneal artery is usually absent, unless it is dominant over the anterior tibial (5%) or is enlarged because of disease of the posterior tibial artery. Foot pulses may be preserved in patients with mild claudication but disappear if the patient exercises.

Ischaemic changes of the foot

A patient's feet provide a useful monitor for the assessment of severe ischaemia. They are placed at the end of the arterial tree and, therefore, show the first clinical signs of reduced

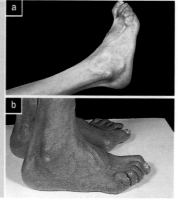

Figure 28.16.
Postural changes.
a. Elevation of the limb has produced blanching and venous emptying.
b. The patient subsequently stood up for 3 minutes, the veins filling after 1 minute, and hyperaemia developing.

perfusion. Pallor and coldness may be present, and capillary refilling after digital pressure of a nail bed is slow, compared to a normal limb.

Pallor is accentuated by elevating the limb above the heart. In severe ischaemia, gravity also empties the veins, producing a bloodless gutter along the line of the subcutaneous venous channel (*Figure 28.16a, b*). On subsequent dependency, capillary and venous refilling are delayed, taking 20–50 seconds for the foot veins to refill. A reactive hyperaemia follows, the feet taking on a pink/purplish colour over the next 2–3 minutes due to the vessels being dilated as a result of ischaemic metabolites. These postural changes are named after Buerger, as is the leg elevation angle at which the limb and nail bed capillaries blanch.

The chronically ischaemic foot undergoes nutritional or **trophic changes**. The skin is thin, of fine texture and atrophic, and there is pulp loss with withering and wrinkling; nails are brittle and deformed. The skin is easily damaged by minor trauma and painful cracks appear across the heel (*Figure 28.17*). Prolonged pressure over a bony prominence, such as when lying in bed, on the heel (*Figure 28.18a–d*) or

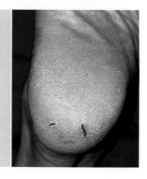

Figure 28.17.
Skin cracks over the heel.

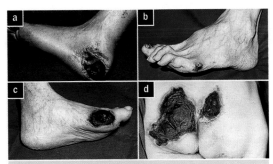

Figure 28.18.
Cutaneous pressure necrosis in severe ischaemia. a. Extensive ulcer over the heel. b. Ischaemic changes over the lateral border of the foot following 24 hours' bed rest. c. Ischaemic changes over the head of the first metatarsal. d. Large sacral ischaemic changes.

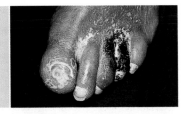

Figure 28.21.
Gangrenous fourth toe.

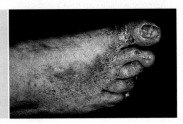

Figure 28.22.
Ischaemic changes of Buerger's disease. Note the abnormal nails, scarred skin and surrounding pigmentation.

malleoli, or a tight bandage over the tendon of the tibialis anterior or the tendo Achilles (*Figure 28.19*) can produce ulceration; ulcers may also appear over the tips and between the toes (*Figure 28.20*). The initial eschar gives way to a thin, fixed, green slough.

Once ulcers are established there is inadequate blood supply to heal them and they become full thickness, punched-out or undercut, penetrating through to the tendons, ligaments, bones and joints. Ulcers are of very variable size and are very painful. There is inadequate blood to produce bleeding or a purulent response but there may be a clear discharge.

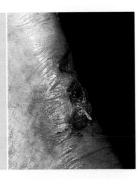

Figure 28.19.
Pressure necrosis over the tendo Achilles following the application of a tight bandage.

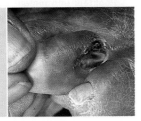

Figure 28.20.
Ischaemic ulcer between the left fourth and fifth toes. Note the punched-out edges and the exposed ligaments and tendons.

The above features indicate minimal capillary flow but there may also be occlusion of the distal small arteries. This gives rise to infarction and areas of gangrene of one or more toes (*Figure 28.21*). The line of demarcation between the gangrene and normal skin might not be very distinct, and the term **pre-gangrene** is applied to such areas. Revascularization of such a limb will produce a very clear line of demarcation between viable and dead tissue, and also produce a purulent response; this in turn eventually leads to auto-amputation. This may be more conveniently undertaken by the surgical removal of dead tissue. Buerger's disease may produce a similar ischaemic picture (*Figure 28.22*).

The diabetic foot

Diabetic patients are subject to atherosclerosis and tend to get it a decade earlier than their non-diabetic counterparts. They are, therefore, subject to the arterial changes already described. Pressure readings in the diabetic foot may be falsely raised, since the typical calcified leg and thigh arteries of the diabetic patient are not easily compressed with a blood pressure cuff. Diabetic patients are also subject to increased infection due to altered cellular and humoral responses, and to neuropathic changes.

The latter affects autonomic as well as somatic nerves. The foot is dry and deceptively pink and warm, due to the lack of autonomic vasoconstriction (*Figure 28.23*). There is often enough blood present in the foot to produce an inflammatory response (*Figure 28.24*), and purulent disease with oedema may accompany dead toes. Infection may penetrate bones and joints (*Figure 28.25*), with associated osteomyelitis and deep abscesses tracking along tendon sheaths (*Figure 28.26*).

Figure 28.23.
Gangrenous second right toe in a diabetic patient. Note the patchy hyperaemia in spite of gangrenous changes of the second and third toes.

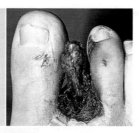

Figure 28.27.
Perforating ulcer over the heads of the third and fourth metatarsals in a neuropathic diabetic foot.

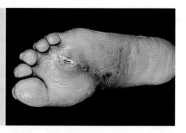

Figure 28.24.
Diabetic foot showing the combined effects of neuropathic deformity and ischaemic gangrene.

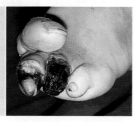

and second. There is commonly excessive callus formation around ulcers and cracks, and this inhibits epithelial in-growth and healing. In assessment of the diabetic foot, all infective, neuropathic and arterial components must be considered; the deformed, infected forefoot, with patchy gangrene, is a typical presentation.

Figure 28.25.
Ulceration in a diabetic foot extending into the metatarsophalangeal joint.

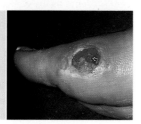

Critical ischaemia

Critical ischaemia is arterial disease that endangers the whole or part of a leg. In order to compare the management of vascular disease in different centres, it has been proposed that **critical ischaemia** should be defined by objective criteria, as follows: persistent, recurrent rest pain (requiring regular analgesia for more than 2 weeks) and/or ulceration or gangrene of the foot or toes, with an ankle systolic pressure of less than 50 mmHg.

As calcification of the arteries in diabetes and some other diseases makes measurement of the ankle pressure unreliable, absent palpable pulses are sufficient for definition of critical ischaemia in diabetics and patients with calcified arteries.

Figure 28.26.
Mid-foot sole abscess in a diabetic patient.

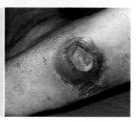

Popliteal artery disease

The popliteal artery is susceptible to atherosclerotic occlusion in the elderly male, particularly starting at its origin beneath the hiatal opening of the adductor magnus. It is also a focal point of popliteal aneurysms, which are frequently bilateral (see below), and two rare conditions, popliteal artery entrapment and cystic degenerative disease.

Popliteal entrapment must be considered when calf claudication occurs in a man in his late teens or early adulthood. The condition is due to a congenital anomaly of one of the heads of gastrocnemius or popliteus muscles, or abnormal bands, the artery being misplaced and compressed between the muscle and the femoral condyle. Although claudication is the classical presentation, there may also be acute thrombosis, producing the signs and symptoms of acute

Sensory loss means that minor, or even major, trauma to the foot can go unnoticed, and repeated trauma – e.g. walking around on bare feet or the rubbing of new shoes – should be avoided, as must radiators, hot baths, hot water bottles, hot sand and sun. The diabetic patient may also have reduced vision and altered finger sensation, reducing the ability to see changes directly or with a mirror, or to feel abnormalities.

Motor neuropathy particularly affects the small muscles of the foot. The unopposed action of the long tendons produces a high arch and hammer toes, subjecting the knuckles and the metatarsal heads to increased pressure from shoes and loading when walking. Increased loading in an insensitive foot can give rise to perforating ulcers over the heads of the metatarsals (*Figure 28.27*), particularly the first

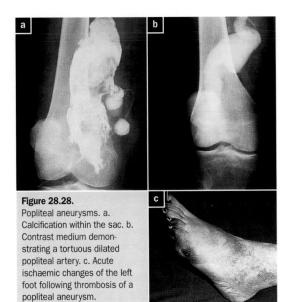

Figure 28.28.
Popliteal aneurysms. a.
Calcification within the sac. b.
Contrast medium demon-
strating a tortuous dilated
popliteal artery. c. Acute
ischaemic changes of the left
foot following thrombosis of a
popliteal aneurysm.

ischaemia. Associated embolism is rare and the condition may be bilateral. It is usually diagnosed angiographically but may be suspected in a symptomatic patient if foot pulses can be abolished by active plantar flexion or passive dorsiflexion of the foot. When chronic occlusion occurs, pulses may be palpable in collateral vessels, particularly on the medial aspect of the knee.

Cystic degeneration is a mucinous degeneration within the arterial wall, usually subadventitial but with one or more cysts growing to impinge into the arterial lumen. Histological and radiological appearances are characteristic, although the latter is obscured once thrombosis has occurred. The presentation is usually acute ischaemia. The condition is rarely bilateral.

Popliteal aneurysms are commonly bilateral and may present with a prominent, pulsating bulge behind the knee or with the symptoms of acute lower leg ischaemia due to thrombosis or embolism (*Figure 28.28a–c*). Rupture is very rare (see also aneurysms p. 374).

Intestinal ischaemia

Intestinal ischaemia is a rare but serious complication of vascular disease, and it is difficult to both diagnose and treat. Problems of diagnosis are due to the wide spectrum of clinical presentations, ranging from mild, intermittent abdominal pain

to a lethal catastrophe. The various presentations also mean that referral is to a variety of clinics, and so no-one gains a great deal of experience in the condition. The diagnosis is often by exclusion of other pathology and facilitated by a continued awareness of the possibility of this vascular complication.

Anomalies of the blood supply of the fore-, mid- and hindgut respectively (from the coeliac axis and the superior and inferior mesenteric arteries) are common. There is, however, a good collateral blood supply between the various bowel segments through the bowel wall and the marginal artery. As in arterial disease elsewhere, it is the *rate* of occlusion that is important in the type of clinical sequelae.

Acute intestinal ischaemia may be due to embolism or thrombosis, or can occur without occlusion, probably as a result of acute spasm related to gut toxins or external poisons such as ergot. Acute intestinal ischaemia is not infrequently seen in the aged and, as such, is not an uncommon way of death (*Figure 28.29*). Presentation is of the acute onset of abdominal pain, accompanied by some diarrhoea and vomiting. The patient looks acutely ill, tachycardic and hypotensive but there is not usually a fever. Although there is an ileus present, the abdominal signs are minor with no marked tenderness or palpable mass, this being in sharp contrast to the profound systemic symptoms. Abdominal tenderness and peritonism appear and progress over subsequent hours. Mortality is very high, even when the dead gut is resected or when revascularization is possible.

Acute focal ischaemia may involve the small or large bowel. **Small bowel ischaemia** may be due to bands, hernia, vasculitis, drugs, trauma, haemodynamic abnormalities or focal radiotherapy. The abdominal pain is constant and of gradual or sudden onset. It may become generalized if peritonitis supervenes, and colicky if there is associated intestinal obstruction. In the early phase there is mild diarrhoea and/or vomiting. The patient initially looks well but toxaemia and fever develop, with peritonitis and perforation. Abdominal signs are focal tenderness; hernial orifices must be carefully examined and the strangulated loop diagnosed before irreversible damage, perforation and generalized peritonitis occur.

Figure 28.29.
Acute mesenteric
ischaemia.

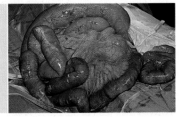

Intra-abdominal lesions may give rise to general peritonitis and perforation before a definitive diagnosis has been made. Obstructive lesions produce distension, progressive vomiting and the symptoms and signs of dehydration.

Focal **large bowel ischaemia** usually presents as an ischaemic colitis, the condition occurring in elderly males but not producing marked shock, the differential diagnosis being late onset ulcerative colitis or Crohn's disease. There is pain and tenderness on the left side and in the left iliac fossa, diarrhoea is present and contains dark, altered blood. The condition is usually self-limiting within a few weeks but may progress to perforation, particularly of the sigmoid colon, or late stricture formation. The differential diagnosis of malignancy is important.

Chronic mesenteric ischaemia

This condition is uncommon, as two of the three gut arteries can be gradually occluded without any ill effect. It is only when the third vessel becomes compromised that symptoms appear. The classic triad of symptoms is that of **food fear**, **weight loss** and **diarrhoea** but milder, vague pains are usually present. The pain is a mesenteric angina related to the increased blood flow required for digestion after meals. Patients do not eat for fear of the severe upper abdominal pain and have dramatic weight loss, accentuated by diarrhoea of pancreatic origin. Surgery can transform the lives and appearance of these cachectic individuals to normality.

Renal artery disease

Atherosclerosis accounts for two-thirds of renal artery problems in western civilization. Other diseases to which it is subject include congenital anomalies, AV fistulae and fibromuscular dysplasia. Aortic aneurysms and dissections may involve the origin of the renal arteries and, occasionally, renal artery aneurysms may be present. The latter are usually asymptomatic but, like other visceral artery aneurysms, are prone to rupture in pregnancy.

Occlusive disease of the renal arteries may present as renal failure; this usually requires bilateral renal artery disease. However, unilateral renal artery stenosis may influence angiotensin release, producing hypertension that can, in turn, damage a contralateral normal kidney.

In assessing renal artery disease it is, therefore, essential to monitor the blood pressure and examine for clinical signs of renal failure (p. 338). As renal artery stenosis is usually one manifestation of systemic arterial disease, the clinical assessment should also consider cardiac, cerebrovascular and lower limb arterial problems, diabetes and the risk factors of atherosclerosis.

Aneurysms

Aged arteries tend to become hardened, slightly wider and longer, and this gives rise to some tortuosity. If this enlargement becomes greater than 50%, the term arteriomegaly or ectasia is applied. Dilatation to double an artery's diameter is termed an aneurysm, and this may be focal (saccular) or extend along a length of the artery (fusiform). Both forms may arise in pre-existing ectatic vessels.

Any artery or arterialized vein may become aneurysmal but it is more common at certain sites, and this is also linked with the aetiology. The term aneurysm is also applied to a blowout of the wall of a cardiac atrium or ventricle.

Pathogenesis

Well over 90% of aneurysms are labelled atherosclerotic but a better term for this proportion is **non-specific** since only 25% are associated with the co-existent occlusive disease typical of atherosclerosis.

Non-specific aneurysms have similar risk factors to atherosclerosis, namely hypertension, smoking, diabetes and associated cerebrovascular and coronary heart disease; there is a familial tendency. The commonest site of non-specific aneurysms is the abdominal aorta which accounts for over 90%, one-third being associated with iliac dilatation. Suprarenal and thoracic aortic aneurysms are occasionally encountered. Other typical sites are the popliteal and, occasionally, the femoral and carotid arteries (*Figure 28.30*).

Aneurysms are found in individuals with tissue abnormalities such as **Marfan's** and **Ehlers–Danlos syndromes** and **cystic medial necrosis. Dissecting aneurysms** are due to fractures of the intima, with blood passing between the intima and the media, producing a false lumen. The commonest site of dissecting aneurysms is in the aorta distal

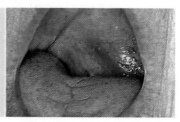

Figure 28.30.
Aneurysm of the left common carotid artery deforming the posterior aspect of the oropharynx.

to the left subclavian artery, the false passage usually missing the renal arteries and coeliac axis but occluding one or both iliac arteries. The vessel in dissecting aneurysms is not necessarily dilated but the outer wall may rupture.

Focal **congenital** (*Figure 28.31*) abnormalities of an arterial wall often produce saccular aneurysms and do not present until middle age. Examples are around the circle of Willis (Berry aneurysms; *Figure 28.1*) and of the splenic, renal and carotid arteries. **Infection** can damage the wall of an artery. It may arise from an adjacent abscess, such as in the tonsil or cervical nodes, or be disseminated through the blood stream, such as in the kidney associated with acute bacterial endocarditis. Infective aneurysms are termed **mycotic**. A previously common mycotic aneurysm was of the ascending aorta, due to syphilis (*Figure 28.32*).

Injury to a vessel usually produces haemorrhage or thrombosis but rupture may produce a haematoma that is both contained by surrounding tissues and remains in communication with the damaged vessel through the laceration. This is known as a **false aneurysm** or pulsating haematoma (*Figure 28.33a, b*); it usually continues to enlarge. The puncture sites in radiological procedures are a potential cause of false aneurysms, particularly when anticoagulation is used, such as in coronary artery stenting. Trauma may also damage a vessel wall and present as true aneurysmal dilatation, such as a post-stenotic dilatation, when the turbulent jets beyond a tight stenosis give rise to aneurysm formation.

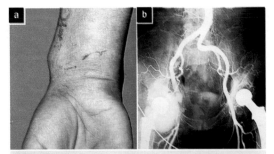

Figure 28.33.
False aneurysm. a. False aneurysm of the right radial artery.
b. False aneurysm of the right femoral artery, following arthroplasty. The contrast medium has leaked into the aneurysm sac anterior to the hip joint.

Clinical features

Many features of an aneurysm are common, regardless of their site, particularly expansion, pain and rupture. The following description, however, concentrates on abdominal aortic aneurysms as these are the commonest and give rise to the greatest morbidity and mortality. Three-quarters of abdominal aortic aneurysms are asymptomatic. They come to light as the chance findings of a lump, with or without pulsation, noted on self-examination, a routine physical check-up or on radiographs for some other reason, such as a plain abdominal film, intravenous urogram (IVU), barium, computed tomography (CT) or magnetic resonance imaging (MRI) studies. The lesion may also be found at laparotomy or post-mortem.

Pain is the commonest symptom and may be acute or chronic. Sudden onset is often associated with a complication of the aneurysm. The pain is due to stretching of the vessel wall and, in the case of the aorta, is referred through to the back. Erosion of the adjacent vertebral bodies may also produce back pain. The pain of rupture, infection and fistulae is considered below.

A quarter of non-specific aneurysms are associated with atherosclerotic distal occlusive disease and the patient may present with claudication or rest pain and gangrene. The effects of embolism of thrombotic or atheromatous material vary from small, scattered areas of infarction to acute limb ischaemia. The small infarcts may be blue, scattered spots in the foot and may go unnoticed (**trash foot**). Thrombosis of an abdominal aortic aneurysm is rare but may present with acute lower limb ischaemia. This complication is more common with aneurysms of the popliteal artery (*Figure 28.28*).

Figure 28.31.
Congenital aneurysm of the right axillary artery. Similar changes were present on the left side.

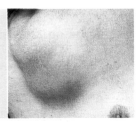

Figure 28.32.
Syphilitic aneurysm of the ascending aorta eroding the sternum.

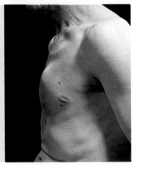

Examination

Clinical examination of a patient with an abdominal aortic aneurysm produces an accurate diagnosis in 85% of cases. The lesion may be difficult to feel in obese patients, and the differential diagnosis of a pulsating abdominal mass can be difficult with pancreatic and gastric neoplasms; the pulsation is transmitted and not expansile in these cases. Tortuous and ectatic aortas may be easily felt and are made more prominent with a lumbar lordosis or a very thin subject. Some idea of the diameter of the vessel can be obtained by pressing the fingers of each hand down either side of the aorta, this diameter should not be more than 3 cm. If the abdominal swelling extends across to the right, the pulsation is likely to be from an aneurysm.

It is usually possible to get a hand above the aneurysm underneath the costal margin and it can then be diagnosed as infrarenal in site. It is still likely to be infrarenal even when it does extend to the costal margin; 95% of abdominal aortic aneurysms are of this form. Common iliac enlargement in one-third of these patients is suspected if the dilatation extends below the umbilicus. Aneurysms of the internal iliac arteries can be palpated digitally per rectum.

In the clinical examination of the rest of the patient, note the characteristics of the pulse, particularly noting auricular fibrillation and abnormal rhythms. In the lower limb pulses, note the presence of any femoropopliteal aneurysms or absent pulses, suggesting peripheral vascular disease. Note any symptoms and signs of cerebrovascular and cardiovascular disorders, look for signs of congestive cardiac failure and measure the blood pressure in both arms. Note symptoms and signs of the diabetic patient and respiratory problems in patients where surgery is being considered.

Progressive enlargement of an aneurysm places extra tension in its wall which increases by a factor of 12 with the expansion of an aorta from 2 to 6 cm in diameter. Rupture occurs when the tangential tension at any point is greater than the strength of the wall. In rupture of the abdominal aorta there is severe central anterior abdominal pain extending through to the back and then radiating cranially and caudally or around each side. The differential diagnoses include biliary and renal colic, perforated peptic ulcers and an acute lumbar disc lesion. If the rupture is into the peritoneal cavity there is usually rapid exsanguination. Surprisingly, a number of patients initially survive a ruptured abdominal aortic aneurysm, since the tear is usually retroperitoneal, particularly on the left side, the peritoneum providing a degree of tamponade; thrombus within the wall also shifts to block the defect temporarily. The period of stability may last for a

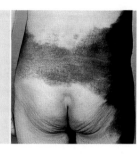

Figure 28.34.
Extensive haemorrhage in a patient following graft replacement of a ruptured abdominal aneurysm.

number of hours or even days before a second, fatal haemorrhage occurs. This period of delay, or a period of severe pain when an aneurysm is pending rupture, provides an opportunity for diagnosis and to consider surgical intervention (*Figure 28.34*).

Infection in non-specific aneurysms is usually due to the erosion of a viscus, or in a false aneurysm occurring after synthetic graft replacement. There may be pain, pyrexia and intermittent bleeding, the latter presenting as haematemesis, melaena or anaemia. Anaemia or pyrexia of unknown origin in a patient with a previous aortic graft must be considered as a graft complication until proved otherwise. An aneurysm or a replacement graft may also erode into an adjacent large vein, particularly the inferior vena cava, or renal and iliac veins. There may be no pain but acute oedema is common, due to venous hypertension, with a wide pulse pressure and possible heart failure. On auscultation, the continuous bruit of the AV fistula is heard.

Small vessel disease

A normal individual handling snow or ice for any length of time develops white hands and, on rewarming, may have pain and reactive hyperaemia (*Figure 28.35a, b*). This is because normal arterioles and capillaries close down in response to cold, blood being diverted from the capillary bed by proximal AV shunts. Shunts are particularly prominent in the fingers, where two-hundredfold blood flow changes have been recorded. This normal response is accentuated in individuals with over-reactive (**vasospastic**) vessels, small vessel disease (**vasculitis**) or who have reduced arterial in-flow due to large vessel disease.

Cold sensitivity produces a characteristic set of colour changes in the hands and sometimes the feet, known as **Raynaud's phenomenon**. The condition is in response to temperature change rather than extreme cold, and is influenced by

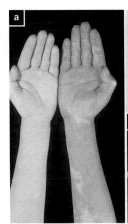

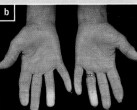

Figure 28.35
Colour changes following cooling of the hands. a. Two sides, in which the right side had been cooled before the left. b. Delayed revascularization of the index fingers following cold immersion.

to endothelial damage and thrombosis. Haemorrheological changes may also produce spasm and promote endothelial damage and thrombosis.

Raynaud's disease is the name given to the condition in individuals suffering from painful Raynaud's phenomenon, but in whom no pathological vascular changes are demonstrated. In 60–80% of cases, these are women in their late teens and early adult life. The condition primarily affects the hands rather than the feet. Pain linked with temperature change can be very disabling and the large number of remedies reflect the difficulty of its management.

Chilblains (perniosis; erythema pernio; *Figure 28.36a–c*) are painful, often multiple localized swellings due to cold injury. On exposure they become cold and white due to vasospasm, but on warming itch insatiably and are sometimes accompanied by marked pain. They are common from childhood, more frequent in women and may be familial. The swellings are usually 4–6 mm in size, sited over the toes and may be a few centimetres across when on the legs. The oedematous nodules may weep fluid and ulcerate. Histological examination demonstrates interstitial round cell infiltration.

Bazin's disease (ecchymosis crurum puellarium frigida) is a cold sensitivity, particularly over exposed areas. It is commoner in women and found in the late teens and twenties. There is dusky purplish, blotchy swelling that may progress to induration, fatty necrosis and superficial ulceration. There may be associated chilblains.

Paralysis of a limb from polio or hemiparesis is accompanied by oedema and cyanosis of the limb, and there may be an enhanced response to vasomotor changes. Altered responses are also present after peripheral nerve injuries, syringomyelia, post frostbite (p. 126) and after limb crush

autonomic activity and emotional changes. The sequence starts with paroxysmal blanching. The cold **white** changes to the **blue** cyanosis on rewarming and finally the **red** of reactive hyperaemia. Rewarming is usually accompanied by pain and this can be severe – it is usually the patient's presenting complaint.

Everyone suffering from Raynaud's phenomenon is said to have **Raynaud's syndrome** regardless of its aetiology. The term **Raynaud's disease**, named after Maurice Raynaud, who first described the characteristic colour changes in 1865, is reserved for a group of individuals who have Raynaud's phenomenon with no associated vessel pathology.

Small vessel diseases comprise a wide variety of diverse abnormalities that differ markedly from the predominant atheroma of large arteries. They are considered under vasospastic and vasculitic disorders.

Vasospastic disorders

It has already been intimated that cold sensitivity is an extension of a normal response. What is not known is whether the abnormality is in the autonomic supply, the receptor, oversensitivity of smooth muscle or elastic tissue, or whether cold agglutinins, cryoglobulins or other mediators are involved in the response. Emotional and hormonal changes do play a role.

Damage of a small vessel, such as vibration white finger disease, or the nerve supply, such as in polio, can give rise to Raynaud's phenomenon and in some of these conditions pathological changes do occur thus blurring the division between vasospastic and vasculitic disorders. Drugs administered both systemically and intra-arterially can also have marked vasospastic effects and vasculitic consequences due

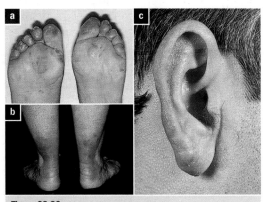

Figure 28.36.
Chilblains. a. Toes. b. Legs. c. Right ear.

injuries. If a limb is not used and left to hang dependent, there is progressive oedema, cyanosis, muscle wasting and the development of a progressively useless appendage. This occurs in *oedem bleu*, a psychiatric problem that is very difficult to treat. The problem is complicated by the application of a proximal tourniquet. The line of application may be visible or palpable, although not admitted.

Vibration white finger disease (**VWF**) is an occupational disorder following the use of chainsaws, grinders, pneumatic chipping tools and the swaging of copper pipes. Only tools of specific frequency produce these effects and each has a characteristic pattern of digital distribution. There is cold sensitivity with blanching and there may be accompanying pain and loss of dexterity. Tissue damage, if present, is usually mild. However, the condition can interfere with work and recreational activity. Its severity is linked to the individuals susceptibility and the length of time of exposure. In the UK, VWF is recognized for industrial compensation purposes.

Drugs and poisons may affect small vessels, both by systemic administration and by inadvertent intra-arterial injection. **Ergot** (*Figure 28.37*) is a potent example of the former, and it can produce intense spasm followed by thrombosis and gangrene. It can occur in the overdosage of ergotamine tablets prescribed for migraine and is produced by the fungus *Claviceps purpurea* contaminating grain. Nicotine and heavy metals also have vasospastic effects. Inadvertent intra-arterial injection of thiopentone into the brachial artery during anaesthesia produces intense spasm, and crystallization in small vessels, producing severe hand ischaemia. Similar effects can follow the introduction of a varicose vein sclerosant, inadvertently injected into an artery, and the intra-arterial injection of recreational drugs. Hypertonic solutions used for flushing intra-arterial lines may also produce focal spasm and ischaemia.

Haemorrheological changes give rise to hyperviscosity, capillary sludging and thrombosis. Hyperfibrinaemia and platelet abnormalities, and the by-products of sickling episodes, are examples producing these effects. The latter can produce diverse symptoms such as strokes and abdominal perforation, linked with cerebral and gut small vessel occlusion.

Acrocyanosis is a persistent, cold cyanosis of the hands and, occasionally, the feet due to arteriolar spasm, although the capillary bed remains perfused and dilated (*Figure 28.38*). It is usually but not invariably initiated by cold, and the palms are often moist. There is not usually any associated pain and the diagnosis is based purely on the colour changes. It occurs mainly in young women and, once attacks wear off, the hands become red, warm and swollen. At this stage there may be discomfort.

Livido reticularis (*Figure 28.39*) is a cyanotic blotching and mottling of the skin similar to a normal cold response but is associated with autoimmune disease and, in particular, antiphospholipid syndrome.

Erythromelalgia (**erythralgia**; *Figure 28.40*) is a painful rubor affecting the feet and, more rarely, the hands. The skin is flushed with venous congestion, and distended veins are accentuated by dependency. There is hyperasthaesia which may be extreme, patients being unable to bear the touch of bed clothes and having to get out of bed to walk on a cold floor or immerse their feet in cold water. The condition occurs in older individuals, usually with no precipitating cause but it

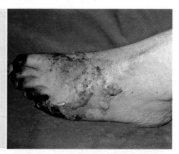

Figure 28.37.
Ergot poisoning demonstrating severe ischaemic changes of the left foot.

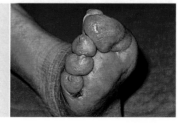

Figure 28.38.
Acrocyanosis of the toes.

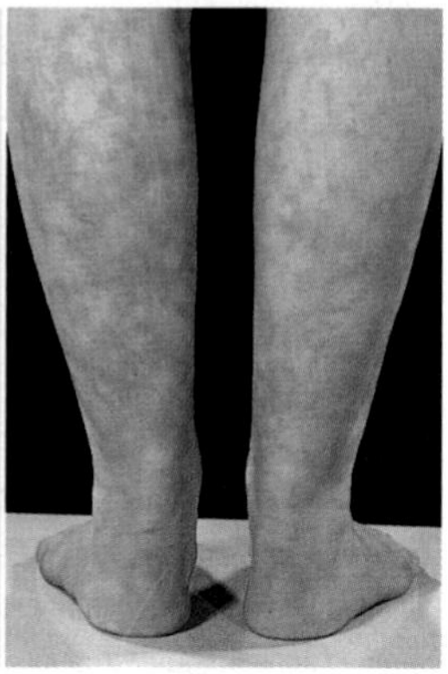

Figure 28.39.
Livido reticularis.

Figure 28.40.
Legs of a patient with erythralgia.

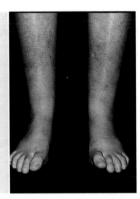

Figure 28.41.
Acute ischaemia of the left hand. This followed an untreated brachial artery embolus.

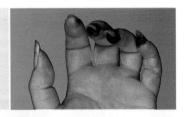

Figure 28.42.
Late demarcation of gangrenous fingertips. This followed an episode of acute distal ischaemia in a patient with rheumatoid arthritis.

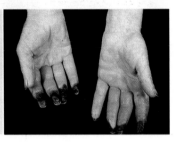

may be associated with gout or polycythaemia, or it may follow frostbite or previous injury. Vitamins are sometimes prescribed but there is no evidence of vitamin deficiency.

Sweating is under sympathetic control and is increased in emotional states and high temperatures. **Hyperhidrosis** gives rise to disturbing social problems, e.g. palmar sweating making the individual avoid contact, and soiling writing paper. Axillary sweating can spoil or ruin clothing and feet sweating can rot socks and shoes, as well as increasing the incidence of fungal infections. Autonomic denervation of affected limbs can increase sweating over the trunk. **Frey's syndrome** is increased sweating of the face, which can follow trauma or surgical incision due to cross-innervation between the facial and autonomic nerves of the face.

Vasculitic disorders

Pathological changes of small vessels occur in a wide variety of diseases, including a number of primary skin disorders. Common changes comprise a periarticular cuff of inflammatory cells with fibrinoid degeneration within a thickened arterial wall. This gives rise to narrowing and occlusion of the vessel with consequent distal ischaemia. The organ involved in the process dictates the clinical picture, as evidenced by the different presentations of collagen diseases, those of surgical importance being related to cutaneous manifestations of scleroderma and temporal arteritis.

The term vasculitis is also applied to occlusive disease of medium and larger vessels, and the pattern of these diseases ranges world-wide, examples of such syndromes have already been referred to – thromboangiitis obliterans; Takayasu's disease; moya moya – all of which are rare in the UK.

Proximal arterial disease may also give rise to distal vascular problems such as embolism (*Figure 28.41*), thoracic outlet syndrome (p. 366) and compartment syndromes (see below), the latter giving rise to symptoms from vascular compression.

Acute digital thrombosis can occur in collagen diseases such as rheumatoid arthritis (*Figure 28.42*) and scleroderma, and is occasionally seen associated with malignancy, giving rise to gangrene of one or more fingers.

Scleroderma (systemic sclerosis)

Collagen diseases are subject to inflammatory changes, thickened walls and narrowing of small arteries, with round cell infiltration and fibrinoid necrosis. Cutaneous involvement is most marked in scleroderma. The patients present with Raynaud's phenomenon, and this may be, for many years or long term, the only symptom. As subjects are usually female, in their twenties and thirties, the differential diagnosis from Raynaud's disease can be difficult.

In a few patients the disease progresses, involving the skin, particularly of the fingers, where the established features are termed **sclerodactyle** (*Figure 28.43a, b*). The skin and subcutaneous tissues become oedematous, thick, pale and rigid. There is reduced mobility and contractures, particularly of the interphalangeal joints. The skin cracks and recurrent ulceration, necrosis and scarring produce pulp atrophy and finger tapering. The nails are brittle and ridged, and recurrent paronychia is common. Pain may be severe and is due to necrosis, infection and associated calcinosis, the latter being calcification of necrosed fat around the finger tips and over the dorsum of the fingers and hands.

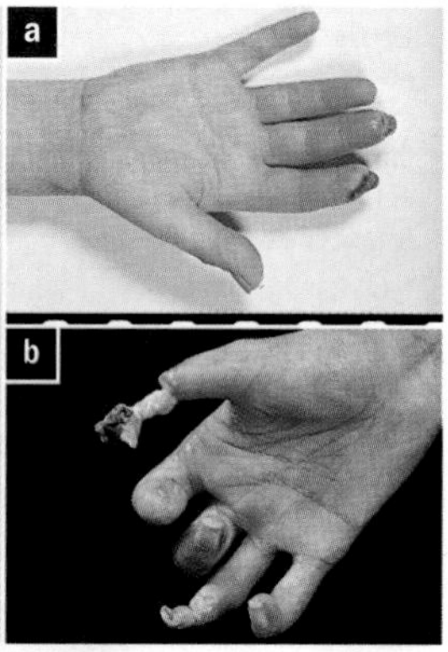

Figure 28.43.
Scleroderma. a. Distal ulceration. b. Severe sclero-dactyly with extensive tissue destruction.

Systemic involvement includes the small vessels of the heart, lungs and gastrointestinal tract. In the latter there may be reduced motility, ulceration, sclerosis, and stricture formation, producing dysphagia, constipation and abdominal colic. More rarely there may be haemorrhage or perforation. The **CREST syndrome** defines the advanced spectrum of the disease: calcinosis cutis, Raynaud's phenomenon, esophageal (*sic*) involvement, scleroderma and telangiectasia. The latter is common around the mouth, on the skin and mucosa, and the mouth is often small and contracted (microstoma; p. 146, *Figure 8.56*).

In **temporal arteritis** (p. 152; *Figure 9.7*) the inflammatory cell infiltrate includes giant cells. The patient complains of a severe headache and the temporal artery is palpable as a tender cord. The clinical importance of the condition is the associated disease of the ophthalmic artery, as occlusion of this vessel leads to blindness. Consequently the superficial temporal artery may need to be biopsied to confirm the diagnosis.

Compartment syndromes

Muscle groups are contained within fascial or fascio-osseous compartments. Increase in the muscle bulk within a compartment, for whatever reason, can compromise muscle blood flow. If this occurs it is termed a muscle compartment syndrome and it may be an acute or a chronic event.

A muscle's contraction temporarily inhibits its arterial inflow but it also empties its venous bed and this enhances inflow to the lowered resistant vessels during relaxation. Increase in compartment pressure can inhibit venous outflow, induce extracellular oedema and eventually inhibit muscle arterial supply.

Acute compartment syndrome usually follows injury. Bleeding may occur from muscle or other soft tissue damage and adjacent fractures. It may occur spontaneously in bleeding diatheses. Crushing and tearing of muscle produces oedema, which may be marked following reperfusion of a limb after arterial reconstruction, in trauma, or releasing a tourniquet or other external compression after some hours. Snake bites, prevalent in some countries, may give rise to severe local oedema within a muscle compartment. Late sequelae include Volkmann's ischaemic contracture (p. 421).

The symptoms are severe muscle pain and tense, tender muscle compartments. These symptoms may be difficult to differentiate from the underlying injury. Pressure measurements are liable to sudden change and are therefore difficult to obtain and interpret, while peripheral pulses may persist. Tense compartments should, therefore, be released whenever a compartment syndrome is considered as a possibility. In severe lower leg injury, and with major arterial reconstruction following a number of hours of ischaemia, all four vessel compartments should be released.

Chronic compartment syndrome occasionally complicates the overuse or overtraining of muscle groups. Characteristically they are commonest in the anterior compartment of the lower leg, though the other three compartments may also be involved. Such activity can increase muscle bulk by up to 20%. Pain accompanies exercise and usually subsides on cessation, but may persist as an ache for some time afterwards. The age group and physical fitness help to differentiate the condition from chronic arterial occlusive disease but popliteal entrapment syndrome and other musculoskeletal abnormalities have to be considered. Forearm compartment syndromes do occur in rowers, canoeists and wind surfers.

29 Venous and lymphatic diseases

Veins in the lower limb

The venous system consists of two parts: one of superficial veins, the other of deep veins, with communicating or perforating veins linking them. The superficial venous system (*Figure 29.1*) is made up of the long (great) and short (small) saphenous veins and their tributaries, they terminate at the saphenofemoral and saphenopopliteal junctions, respectively. The venous system in the lower limb (superficial, deep and perforating) contains a number of valves that only permit blood to flow in one direction, from the superficial to the deep veins. Valves are sited at any junction between the superficial and deep system (saphenofemoral and saphenopopliteal junctions), in the perforating veins, and along the course of

the deep and superficial veins. They have two main roles: to prevent retrograde blood flow from the deep to the superficial veins; and to reduce the venous pressure in the superficial and deep systems (due to gravity when standing).

Long saphenous system

This is the longest vein in the body and arises in front of the medial malleolus. It ascends superficially through the medial aspect of the calf, behind the medial femoral condyle, along the medial aspect of the thigh and terminates in the common femoral vein via the saphenous opening in the fascia at the groin. Along its course the long saphenous receives many tributaries of which the most important are:

- **The posterior arch – Leonardo's vein** starts behind the medial malleolus and runs upwards posterior to the long saphenous vein, joining it at knee level. This arch is important because it has three to four constant perforating veins – Cockett's perforators – at the posterior border of the tibia linking the superficial system with the posterior tibial veins (in the deep system). The arch has a tendency to become varicose and it is common for the long saphenous vein to be normal while the varicosities are related to the posterior arch vein.
- **The anterior superficial tibial vein** ascends along the shin and joins the long saphenous at the same level as the posterior arch vein.
- **The medial and lateral accessory saphenous veins** run posteromedially and anterolaterally along the thigh and join the long saphenous vein at variable levels near to the saphenofemoral junction.
- **The saphenofemoral junction tributaries** join the long saphenous vein just before it terminates in the common femoral vein at the groin. These tributaries are the superficial inferior epigastric, the superficial circumflex iliac and the superficial external pudendal vein.
- **Perforating veins** are commonly just above and below the knee and in the mid-thigh.

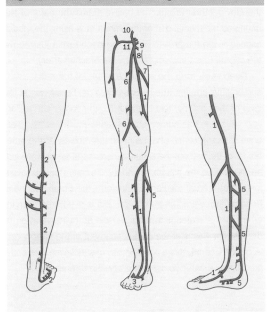

Figure 29.1. Anatomy of the superficial leg veins.

1. Long saphenous vein. 2. Short saphenous vein. 3. Dorsal venous arch. 4. Anterior superficial tibial vein. 5. Posterior arch vein. 6. Lateral accessory saphenous vein. 7. Medial accessory saphenous vein. 8. Medial superficial circumflex iliac vein. 9. Superficial external pudendal vein. 10. Superficial inferior epigastric vein. 11. Superficial circumflex iliac vein.

The short saphenous system

This vein starts laterally to the tendo Achilles, behind the lateral malleolus. It ascends superficially through the posterior aspect of the calf to terminate in the popliteal vein after piercing the deep fascia of the popliteal fossa. In about 50% of individuals the short saphenous terminates above the popliteal fossa. This may be in the muscular veins in the thigh or sometimes even higher, to the gluteal muscular veins.

Deep venous system

The deep veins below the knee are three pairs, each with its associated artery (anterior tibial, posterior tibial and peroneal). In the upper third of the calf, close to the popliteal fossa, they join to form the popliteal vein. Other calf veins include the gastrocnemial veins (a network of small veins draining the gastrocnemius muscle and eventually forming two veins, one for each muscular head, and draining to the popliteal vein at the same level as the short saphenous vein) and the soleal veins (which consist of sinusoids within the soleus muscle, are devoid of valves and drain to the posterior tibial, peroneal or distal popliteal veins).

The popliteal vein may be encircled by the origin of one head of the gastrocnemius muscle, causing popliteal vein entrapment syndrome. Proximally, the popliteal vein enters the adductor canal to become the superficial femoral. The deep femoral vein joins the superficial femoral vein 5–10 cm below the inguinal ligament to form the common femoral vein which then passes upwards underneath the inguinal ligament to become the external iliac vein.

The perforating veins

These veins link the superficial and deep veins by piercing the deep fascia. This linkage may be direct or indirect via a muscle sinusoid. Under normal circumstances the blood flow in the perforators is from the superficial to the deep venous system, retrograde flow being prevented by the presence of valves in the perforating veins. Perforating veins have been described in over 200 sites. In the case of the long saphenous vein, the main perforators are arranged in three sets, one in relation to the subsartorial canal at the medial aspect of the mid-thigh (Dodd's perforators), a second set in relation to the calf muscles just below knee level (Boyd's perforators) and a third set just above the ankle joint at the medial aspect (Cockett's perforators).

If the valves of the perforating veins become incompetent, contraction of the muscles pumps blood retrogradely, from the deep to the superficial veins, resulting in high pressure reflux and causing venous hypertension. Cockett has described this as a 'blow-out' syndrome. It is this high pressure reflux that gives rise to the flare sign (p. 388).

Perforating veins between the short saphenous vein and the deep veins include:

- Bassi's perforator is constantly encountered approximately 5 cm above the calcaneum and connects the short saphenous with the peroneal veins.
- The soleus point perforator connects the soleus veins with the short saphenous.
- The gastrocnemius point perforator connects the gastrocnemial veins with the short saphenous.

Veins in the upper limb

Superficial and deep veins exist in the upper limb; their valves only permit flow from the peripheral to the proximal veins. The two main superficial veins are the cephalic and the basilic veins; the cephalic drains the dorsal part of the hand and forearm and ascends along the lateral aspect of the forearm and upper arm, terminating in the axillary vein, after piercing the clavipectoral fascia. The basilic drains the palm of the hand and the medial part of the limb. It runs along the medial aspect of the forearm to pierce the deep fascia just above the cubital fossa and accompany the brachial artery.

Deep veins form the venae comitans of the radial, ulnar and brachial arteries. The latter receives the basilic vein at the level of the posterior fold of the axilla, to become the axillary vein. This vein has numerous tributaries which act as collaterals in the presence of axillary vein thrombosis. At the outer border of the first rib, the axillary becomes the subclavian vein, passing above the first rib behind the clavicle. The subclavian joins the internal jugular vein to form the brachiocephalic (innominate) vein. The subclavian vein is separated from its artery by the scalenus anterior muscle at its insertion on to the first rib. This is at the commencement of the narrow cervicoaxillary canal. It is a possible site of subclavian vein compression and can give rise to axillary vein thrombosis.

Physiology and haemodynamics of the venous system

Physiology

Limb veins have three principal functions: a pathway for blood return to the heart, blood storage and thermoregulation.

The venous system is a low resistance network, there being at least three times as many veins as arteries in the limbs. This venous network is fully interconnected, and thus blockage or removal of a single vein does not have the same consequences as in the arterial system. The deep system of the lower limb drains about two-thirds of its blood and is the main venous outflow tract.

About 70% of the body's blood is in the venous system at any one time. The capacitance of the venous system in the lower limb is very variable and depends on the venous tone. When the veins are dilated a large amount of blood is 'trapped' in the limbs while small changes in the calibre of the veins can markedly influence the cardiac output by increasing venous return.

Heat exchange is served by the dilatation of the superficial veins while heat conservation is by venoconstriction. Blood returning from the extremities is much cooler than that of the trunk and their mixing can maintain a stable core body temperature. This effective mechanism of thermoregulation is mainly controlled by sympathetic venoconstrictor nerves; it exists in normal superficial veins but is abolished in varicose veins.

Haemodynamics

The venous pressure at the calf level in a normal individual in the erect position is equal to the distance from the right atrium to the foot, if one takes the pressure in the right atrium as zero. This distance is equivalent to a pressure of 100–130 cm H_2O or 75–95 mmHg. On exercise, the muscles contract, producing a pressure of 100 mmHg, hence compressing the deep veins within the semirigid and rigid fascial and bony compartments propelling the blood to the heart, provided the venous valves are intact. This reduces the pressure in the deep system, generating a pressure gradient within the superficial system. As a result, blood flows from the superficial to the deep veins diminishing the pressure in the superficial veins to about 30–49 mmHg. If the valves are incompetent blood returns to the superficial and deep venous systems, resulting in failure to reduce the venous pressure in the limb, this venous insufficiency giving rise to venous hypertension.

Venous thrombosis

Formation of thrombus in the superficial veins (long or short saphenous systems) is called superficial thrombophlebitis, and in the deep veins, deep venous thrombosis.

Superficial thrombophlebitis affecting the superficial veins of the lower limb is not as serious as deep venous thrombosis, in terms of causing life-threatening pulmonary embolism (p. 244). However, when this thrombosis extends across the saphenofemoral or saphenopopliteal junctions, or through the perforating veins, a substantial risk of pulmonary embolism does exist. When the thrombosis affects the main long saphenous vein in the mid-thigh, the end of the thrombus probably reaches the saphenofemoral junction.

This form of thrombosis is not necessarily associated with infection but is always accompanied by a painful inflammatory response. Coexisting infection produces marked local symptoms but makes the thrombus adhere to the venous wall and thus unlikely to give rise to embolic complications. Sometimes superficial thrombophlebitis coexists with deep venous thrombosis. Direct injury, soft tissue infections, intravenous drips, varicose veins, long-term bedrest, surgery and autoimmune diseases – Behçet's syndrome – are common causes although the condition is often idiopathic.

Thrombophlebitis of a varicose vein (*Figure 29.2a, b*) becomes clinically evident by the presence of a firm palpable cord in the thrombosed portion of the varicose vein. Signs of inflammation are apparent – redness and stiffness in the overlying skin which is warm and tender along the thrombosed segment. Usually there is no apparent cause.

Two possible but uncommon complications may supervene: suppuration (a serious condition because it may give rise to septicaemia) and extension of the thrombus along a perforating vein or across the saphenofemoral or saphenopopliteal junctions to the deep veins with all the consequent dangers associated with deep venous thrombosis. It is advisable to mark the upper limit of the inflammation with a skin pen, so that progress can be monitored.

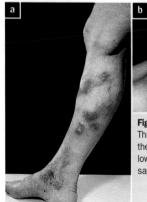
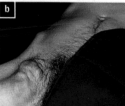

Figure 29.2.
Thromboses. a. Thrombosis of the long saphenous veins in the lower leg. b. Thrombosed right saphena varix of the right leg.

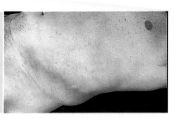

Figure 29.3.
Cutaneous staining of the left side of the abdomen on a superficial area of thrombophlebitis.

Phlebitis migrans (*Figure 29.3*) occurs in previously normal veins and often appears in patients who seem otherwise healthy. The phlebitis occurs spontaneously in almost any superficial vein and recurs at different sites, at intervals of days, weeks or months. The condition may be a sinister sign of underlying disease, in particular:

- Visceral carcinoma (Trousseau's sign), especially of the pancreas (p. 288) or the stomach (p. 282). A thorough examination of all the viscera is imperative.
- Thromboangiitis obliterans. Wandering superficial thrombophlebitis is one of the diagnostic features of this disease (p. 363).
- Autoimmune disease. The problem may occur in the course of Behçet's syndrome.

Mondor's disease (*phlébite-en-cordon*; string phlebitis, p. 231) is a self-limiting phlebitis of veins coursing over the upper chest wall towards the axilla. It is commoner in females, with a higher incidence in France than Britain. The subcutaneous cord or cords feel like those that occur in thrombosis of the dorsal vein of the penis (p. 352). In females, a vein overlying the breast may be affected and can be mistaken for carcinoma. This misdiagnosis has raised the condition from a curiosity to one of diagnostic importance.

Deep venous thrombosis (DVT) carries a risk of pulmonary embolism in the early stages and of post-thrombotic syndrome (secondary varicose veins, aching, swelling, skin changes and ulceration) later. The aetiology may be multifactorial but it is not unusual for it to be idiopathic. Venous stasis, coagulable states and endothelial injury – Virchow's triad – have all been implicated in the pathogenesis but thrombosis is not produced by one mechanism alone, requiring the combination of two or more factors.

The origin of thrombosis in the majority of the cases occurs at the calf veins (soleal and gastrocnemius) and the thrombi may remain locally or propagate to proximal veins. Carefully performed necropsies on patients who have been in bed for more than a week before death show a high incidence of thrombosis of the veins in these muscles. Sometimes thrombosis originates from the proximal veins (popliteal, superficial and common femoral, and iliac) and is due to direct venous injury, i.e. drug abuse, hip or knee replacement, pelvic fracture or pelvic surgery. Non-occlusive thrombi may be silent and only diagnosed when pulmonary embolism occurs. The more proximal the extension of the thrombosis the more evident is the symptomatology. Clinical diagnosis is rarely made in asymptomatic calf thrombi and only in about half of the patients with signs and symptoms suggestive of DVT. Certain risk factors are associated with a high incidence of postoperative DVT, these include female gender, age (>40), malignancy, previous DVT or pulmonary embolism (p. 244), type of surgery, immobility, varicose veins and obesity.

Low grade pyrexia, which fails to settle after surgery, occurrence of leg pain and swelling should raise suspicion. The patient experiences mild pain of gradual onset in the calf, with a sense of fullness, tightness or visible swelling. The extent of the thrombosis determines the severity of the symptoms. Thrombosis involving the popliteal vein may just produce ankle oedema, while iliofemoral thrombosis causes swelling of the whole limb; sometimes swelling is the only symptom.

Before commencing a routine examination in the patient with recent onset of symptoms, remember that dislodging the clot, although rare, can be produced by rough manipulation. The degree of pressure necessary to elicit tenderness is not great, therefore be gentle and do not hurry.

Have the bedclothes turned up (not down) to display the whole of both lower extremities, then carry out the following eight stages:

1. Observe the limbs for inequality of circumference, which is unlikely to be present in early cases. Pay particular attention to the relative prominence of the veins of the dorsum of the foot and look for visible, not varicose, veins coursing over the upper third of the tibia on the affected side (a useful sign of popliteal vein thrombosis). Note the skin colour, which may be purple in cases of extensive (iliofemoral) thrombosis in Caucasians.
2. Palpate the instep and follow this up by finger stroking around the groove beneath the medial malleolus and by examining the ankle for pitting oedema.
3. Pinch a small portion of skin in the ankle and calf. In very early oedema there is resistance that is not present on the normal side, owing to thickening of the dermis and subcutaneous tissues.

4. Dorsiflex the foot. This exerts slight traction on the posterior tibial veins and, if involved, causes pain in the calf: Homan's sign. In women accustomed to wearing high-heeled shoes, with therefore a short tendo Achilles, a false positive result is not unusual.

5. Examine the calves. Ask the patient to draw up the knee and lie quietly, keeping the leg in that position. Commencing near the tendo Achilles, grasp the calf and, while retracting it from the tibia, squeeze it gently. Proceed in this way in an upward direction until the main muscle belly is reached to ascertain whether the soleus is tender. Next alter the grip so as to be able to compress the main muscle belly forwards. Tenderness elicited in this way strongly suggests thrombosis of the posterior tibial vein. Comparative palpation of the bellies of both calf muscles is valuable.

6. Palpate the popliteal space for tenderness with the leg extended resting comfortably on the bed.

7. Seeking for tenderness in the thigh. Place the tip of the index finger over the saphenous opening (for surface marking, see *Figure 29.1*) and draw the finger downwards along the course of the femoral (not the long saphenous) vein.

8. Comparative measurement. Finally, make comparative circumferential measurements at identical points on the calf and thigh (*Figure 29.4*).

Phlegmasia alba dolens (white leg) results from iliofemoral DVT although not all iliofemoral thromboses produce this syndrome. It rarely occurs spontaneously but usually arises after immobilization in bed following an operation or childbirth. There is also an appreciable incidence among patients confined to bed with medical, as opposed to surgical, illnesses. Pregnancy-related cases occur in late pregnancy and the puerperium.

The process often commences in the commonest site, i.e. the veins of the soleus muscles, and the thrombosis propagates in an ascending fashion. However, clot formation commencing at a valve of the femoral vein or in the pelvic veins is not unusual.

In the sequence of events, the patient first experiences a vague, general malaise followed 24 hours later by an otherwise unexplained rise in temperature. Pain is felt in the groin and the medial aspect of the thigh. In a few instances the pain, which varies in severity, is located further down the leg. The femoral artery, which lies close to the vein, may go into spasm making it difficult to feel the femoral pulse. The leg becomes pale and the foot colder than its fellow. The differential diagnosis from acute ischaemia can be difficult at this stage but the difference later becomes apparent.

During the following 12 hours limb swelling occurs, commencing below the knee and spreading to the thigh (*Figure 29.5a, b*). Anteriorly, the swelling ceases abruptly at the inguinal fold; posteriorly, it involves a variable portion of the buttock. It is due to oedema and pits on pressure. There is tenderness along the course of the femoral vein and often deep tenderness in the corresponding iliac fossa. Enlargement of the lymph nodes of the groin is not unusual. The acute phase lasts 2–6 weeks if untreated. It may be followed by the chronic state, characterized by a swollen, oedematous limb requiring elastic stocking support, aching in the limb on walking (venous claudication) and skin changes or pigmentation and ulceration (p. 388).

Phlegmasia cerulea dolens (blue leg) is due to massive iliofemoral thrombosis. It may start as phlegmasia alba dolens but this is not necessarily so. Tingling and numbness of the extremity may be the first signs accompanied by severe painful cramp in the limb (calf or thigh). The limb soon becomes deeply cyanotic with marked swelling, especially below the knee. The pain continues, often being described as 'bursting'. The swollen portion of the limb feels tense, firm

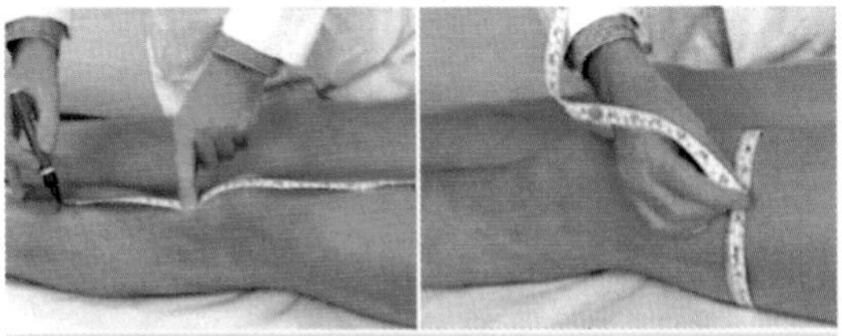

Figure 29.4. Measurement of circumference comparing the knees and thighs at fixed points, in this case 15cm and 20 cm below and above the tibial tubercle.

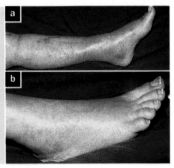

Figure 29.5. Phlegmasia alba dolens. a. Occurring in pregnancy. b. Occurring in a patient with an occult neoplasm of the bronchus.

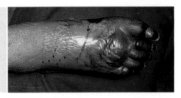

Figure 29.6.
Venous gangrene of the right foot.

yet rubbery, and there is relatively little pitting on pressure. Shock occurs soon after the iliofemoral occlusion due to the trapping of blood in the limb. The limb is initially warm but cools slowly to room temperature.

Gangrene appears to be extensive (*Figure 29.6*) but once the oedema has settled it is usually limited to the forefoot or toes. The condition can be misdiagnosed as arterial embolism due to the difficulty in feeling arterial pulsation in the tensely oedematous limb. However, absent pulses in a greatly swollen, warm and purple limb suggests that the main vein, not the main artery, is blocked.

Long-standing thrombosis of the superior or inferior vena cava, usually secondary to malignant disease, can give rise to varicosities across the abdominal wall (*Figure 29.7*). Superior vena caval obstruction can also give rise to oedema of the head and neck (*Figure 29.8*), plethora being accentuated by head dependency.

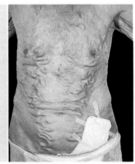

Figure 29.7.
Varicosities over the abdominal wall secondary to obstruction of the superior vena cava.

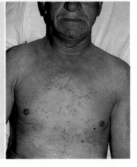

Figure 29.8.
Oedema and plethora of the head and neck due to obstruction of the superior vena cava.

Thrombosis of the axillary vein is commonly ascribed to trauma, although many patients have no history of an accident and first notice the abnormality on waking up in the morning. In a number of instances the swelling comes on after particularly strenuous use of the arm. Typically the patient is an active young or middle-aged individual, and in 80% of cases male. The temperature and pulse rate are normal. As a rule, the swelling involves the whole arm, from the shoulder girdle to the fingers; not infrequently there is also swelling of the lower part of the neck on the affected side. The superficial veins, especially those running to the superior thoracic inlet, are more prominent than usual. Although pain may be absent, a dull ache is often experienced in the arm and sometimes the axillary vein is palpable as a tender cord. The swollen arm (*Figure 29.9*) is firm but exhibits slight pitting on pressure. Fatal embolism has not been reported.

The crescent sign in calf haematoma: very often calf muscle haematoma – produced by minor tears of the soleus and gastrocnemius muscles – can simulate DVT, causing aching and swelling in the calf, while tenderness is elicited on calf palpation. The 'crescent sign' is an important diagnostic sign in patients with calf tenderness, and is produced because the blood in the calf tends to gravitate downwards and can be seen as an area of crescent-shaped bruising at the medial or lateral malleolus, or at both.

Differential diagnosis is critical because anticoagulation is contraindicated whereas it is absolutely indicated in DVT.

Rupture of the tendo Achilles can also be confused with DVT. The patient very often describes a history of sudden pain like receiving a kick on the back of the ankle followed by pain and restriction of walking.

With **rupture of Baker's cyst** (p. 481) the patient very often volunteers the presence of a long-lasting asymptomatic lump at the popliteal fossa. Sudden rupture may occur, with pain and swelling of the calf, while the lump may decrease in size or even disappear. A history of rheumatoid or chronic degenerative arthritis may co-exist.

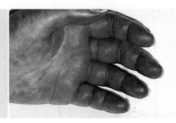

Figure 29.9.
Venous gangrene of the left hand.

Varicose veins

Varicose veins are by far the commonest of the peripheral vascular diseases. By definition, varicose veins are thin-walled, tortuous, dilated and lengthened, with incompetence of the contained valves. This excludes the normal, prominent and dilated veins on healthy muscular legs in non-obese people. Dilated venules ('spiders', 'rocket bursts') are related to the hormonal effects on soft skin and usually appear in females at certain periods such as the menarche, pregnancy, menopause and in other hormonal imbalances.

Primary varicose veins are those without any identifiable causative factor. Very often there is a familial predisposition and they appear in early teenage or the third decade; weakness of the venous wall is the most widely accepted theory for the pathogenesis of this situation.

Secondary varicose veins are usually the result of deep vein thrombosis. Other possible causes, though rare, are vascular malformations, arteriovenous (AV) fistulae and other congenital abnormalities, and post-traumatic effects secondary to gunshot injuries, stab wounds or surgery.

Varicosities usually involve either the long or short saphenous vein, or their tributaries (see *Figure 29.1*). The long saphenous vein (*Figure 29.10*) becomes varicose seven times more frequently; sometimes both systems are implicated.

Taking a history in patients with varicose veins can facilitate the diagnosis. The presence of varicose veins in teenage or early adolescence, no history of DVT, and positive family history suggest primary disease with a familial predisposition. Some patients have extremely severe varicose veins with mild or no symptoms, whereas other have severe symptoms with small varicosities. Aching, swelling, heaviness, cramps and itching are some of the most common symptoms. These are absent in the morning and become evident and aggravate while the day goes by. Symptoms very often become worse in warm weather (i.e. mostly in the summer) and the patient

finds relief with a cold shower or having the leg elevated; cosmesis is very often the only reason the patients are complaining. Pigmentation, skin changes and ulceration represent symptoms of severe disease which demands prompt diagnosis and treatment.

Examination of a patient suffering from varicose veins
Inspection

With the patient standing, the lower limbs are scrutinized from the umbilicus to the toes, remembering to view the backs of the legs as well as the front, to avoid overlooking varicosities of the short saphenous vein (*Figure 29.11*). A careful note is made of the anatomical distribution of the varices (*Figure 29.12a, b*) particularly of perforating veins, which produce a

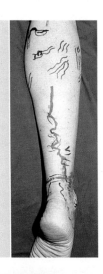

Figure 29.11.
Varicosities of the right short saphenous system marked preoperatively.

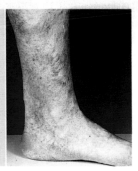

Figure 29.10.
Long saphenous varicose vein. This shows prominent skin bulges over the varicosities of the posterior arch vein, together with widespread venular dilatation and loss in ankle contour in a post-phlebitic leg.

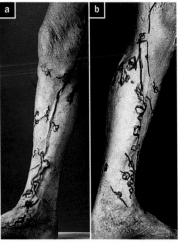

Figure 29.12a, b.
Lower leg varicosities of the long saphenous system, with preoperative marking of both legs.

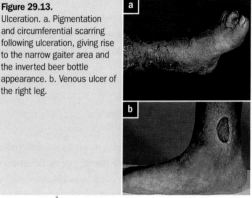

Figure 29.13.
Ulceration. a. Pigmentation and circumferential scarring following ulceration, giving rise to the narrow gaiter area and the inverted beer bottle appearance. b. Venous ulcer of the right leg.

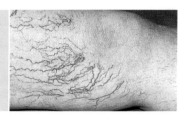

Figure 29.14.
Venous capillary deformities.

Venous stars (*Figure 29.14*) tend to occur in association with elevation of the venous pressure. They are common on the dorsum of the foot, as well as on the legs, especially above the knee on the medial aspect of the thigh of patients with varicose veins. They are particularly common in patients with obstruction to the vena cava and in pregnant women. Digital pressure easily squeezes blood from the star; upon sudden release, it fills from the centre.

discrete venous bulge, and of the presence of swelling, skin pigmentation, pre-ulcerative lesions, ulcers mainly just above the medial malleolus and any scars due to healed ulcers (*Figure 29.13a, b*).

Palpation

The limbs are palpated lightly, particularly over the courses of the short and long saphenous veins. In persons with fat limbs, superficial varicose veins are often palpable when they are not visible as soft subcutaneous gutters. This applies particularly to the areas immediately above an ulcer and to the proximal portions of both saphenous veins.

At this stage it is very important to make clear whether these varicose veins are primary or secondary, especially in cases of bilateral varicose veins or when some of the affected veins do not conform to the usual pattern, e.g. varicosities in the pubic area, lower abdominal or operation scars raising the possibility of a previous postoperative thrombosis. Apart from the postoperative DVT there are some other situations that cause the development of varicose veins and should be excluded:

The cough impulse test

When positive, this is a clear indication of the presence of incompetent valves in the long saphenous vein. The fingers are laid on the thigh over the saphenous opening, in such a way that the pulp of the middle finger rests upon the vein (*Figure 29.15*) or, when not clearly visible, where the vein should be. The patient is asked to cough. A fluid thrill is imparted to the finger if the valve at the saphenofemoral junction is incompetent.

The percussion or tap sign

With the patient still erect, place the fingers of the left hand just below the saphenous opening at the groin. Percuss the main bunch of varicosities once with the right middle finger. If a thrill is felt by the left hand at the groin one can conclude that the varicosities belong to the distribution of the long saphenous vein. Now percuss the long saphenous vein at the

- Pregnancy.
- An intrapelvic neoplasm (uterus, ovary or rectum) that can obstruct the venous return, resulting in venous hypertension of the lower limb and the development of varicose veins. Abdominal and rectal examination is necessary. Usually, however, the presence of such a tumour associated with varicosities is a coincidence.
- Superficial varicosities are often present with AV fistulae (p. 391).

Figure 29.15.
Right saphena varix. Note the bulge (arrowed) lateral to the groin crease. Palpation over this site demonstrated a cough impulse.

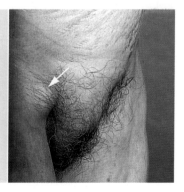

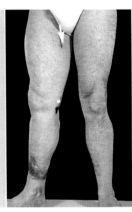

Figure 29.16.
Post-phlebitic limb with marked venous incompetence of the long saphenous system. When tapping over the saphenous vein in the groin (at the arrowed site), a transmitted impulse could be felt over the long saphenous vein where marked behind the knee.

groin with the right middle finger while the fingers of the left hand are placed on distal varicosities. When valves within the segment under review are incompetent there is no barrier to the downward wave of blood, and an impulse is felt by the fingers overlying the varicosities (*Figure 29.16*). In most instances anatomical charting of the distribution of veins together with the cough and tap signs are sufficient for the initial diagnosis.

The Brodie–Trendelenburg test

The patient lies down on a couch and the limb is raised to allow the blood to drain out of the veins. The saphenous vein at the upper third of the thigh is then compressed with a tourniquet and the patient is asked to stand up; the varices are observed for 30 seconds then the tourniquet is released. Normally the venous filling occurs from the periphery when the patient gets up and it takes more than 20 seconds. When the tourniquet is released the venous filling continues gradually from the periphery to the proximal sites. If the veins fill rapidly from below despite the applied tourniquet, this indicates incompetent perforating veins. Fast filling of the veins from above, after release of the tourniquet, indicates valvular incompetence of the saphenofemoral junction and the long saphenous vein. The test is positive when both or only one of the above findings are present. The exact site of any incompetent perforating veins can be further demonstrated by placing multiple tourniquets around the thigh and calf and observing which venous segment fills. The short saphenous vein can be assessed by the same manner, applying a tourniquet around the calf below the popliteal fossa, but the long saphenous vein should be occluded at the upper thigh as well for accurate interpretation.

Seeking the sites of perforators (Fegan's method)

Mark the varicosities with a skin pen while the patient stands; ask the patient to lay down and raise the affected limb, resting the heel against the examiner's upper chest. Palpate the line of the marked varicosities carefully for gaps in the deep fascia through which the perforating veins pass; they are felt as circular openings with sharp edges and are marked with an X. To confirm that the superficial varicosities fill from the perforators, the Brodie–Trendelenburg test can be applied or the examiner can digitally compress the marked sites during elevation and individually release them after dependency.

Test for patency of the deep veins (Perthes' test)

Deep veins that have been the site of thrombotic occlusion almost invariably recanalize with the passage of time. However, sometimes they remain occluded and so the venous outflow of the affected leg depends on the developed collateral circulation, which may not be adequate for compensation. If the patient complains of persistent 'bursting' pain in the lower leg on standing, the test for deep vein patency is carried out. While the patient stands, a rubber tourniquet is applied around the thigh, tight enough to occlude the long saphenous vein but not the deep veins. The patient then walks for 5 minutes. If the pain (of which the patient was complaining) is brought on, it is proof that the deep veins are still occluded. Additional evidence is that the superficial varicosities, if present, become more prominent as their exit (the long saphenous vein) is blocked by the tourniquet. Alternatively this test can be performed applying a tourniquet in the upper third of the calf with the patient in a standing position and making ten repeated tiptoe movements.

Congenital vascular defects

These defects may be either haemangiomas or vascular malformations, each having different pathogenetic origin and outcome.

Haemangiomas, although of vascular origin, result from cellular proliferation and differ from malformations which are embryonic, developmental abnormalities representing errors in vascular morphogenesis. *Table 29.1* illustrates the different characteristics of these two entities.

Haemangiomas usually become evident in the early neonatal period; approximately 80% of haemangiomas are single tumours and 20% occur in multiple sites. The tumour proliferates in the superficial dermis, the skin becomes raised, bosselated and a vivid crimson colour. If the haemangioma

Table 29.1. Characteristics distinguishing haemangiomas from malformations.

Haemangioma	Vascular malformation
Usually not present at birth	All present at birth but not necessarily apparent
Rapid postnatal growth; slow evolution	Commensurate growth; may expand
Female to male ratio 3 to 5:1	Female to male ratio 1:1
Endothelial hyperplasia	Flat endothelium
Increased mast cells	Normal mast cells
Multilaminated basement membrane	Thin unilaminated basement membrane
Primary platelet trapping (Kasabach–Merritt syndrome)	Primary venous stasis
	Local/disseminated intravascular coagulopathy
Infrequent pressure on adjacent bone	Defects with AV fistulae: hypertrophy
Rare overgrowth	Defects without AV fistulae; atrophy

lies in the deeper dermis or the subcutaneous tissue, the overlying skin is slightly elevated with a bluish hue.

The old terms 'cavernous' haemangioma to describe a deep lesion and 'capillary' for the superficial one are confusing and best avoided.

Palpation facilitates the differentiation of a haemangioma from a venous malformation. A haemangioma is a fibrofatty structure and its contained blood cannot be evacuated completely by compression (*Figure 29.17*). By contrast, a venous malformation is soft and easily evacuated by compression; it enlarges with dependency and disappears with elevation of the involved limb. The typical haemangioma grows rapidly over the first 6–8 months of life and reaches a plateau by 1 year. After this, signs of involution appear – the colour fades from vivid crimson to a dull purplish hue, the skin gradually pales, the tumour is less tense to palpation and its size slowly diminishes. Regression continues until the child reaches 5–10 years old.

Infants with limb haemangiomas are at a high risk of having visceral lesions, mainly multiple intrahepatic haemangiomas. These present with hepatomegaly, heart failure and anaemia. Platelet trapping – Kasabach–Merritt syndrome – is another complication of cutaneous haemangiomas. The involved skin becomes deep red-purple, tense and shiny with petechiae and ecchymoses often seen overlying and adjacent to the haemangioma. Severe thrombocytopenia carries a risk of haemorrhage, either gastrointestinal, peritoneal, pleuropneumonic or intracranial. Local bleeding and ulceration are two other complications. Bleeding, although frightening, can be controlled by 10 minutes' compression with a clean pad. Ulceration is rare and, when it occurs, may be complicated by infection. The site of the haemangioma may play an important role, for instance a small haemangioma in the eyelid can distort the growing cornea, producing astigmatism and amblyopia, and a subglottic haemangioma may be potentially life threatening, presenting insidiously as biphasic stridor at 6–8 weeks of life. Large, facial haemangiomas may grow to distort normal anatomic structures.

Congenital vascular malformations are clinical syndromes presenting with a variety of characteristics such as naevi (p. 146), port wine stain (*Figure 29.18*), varicosities, hypertrophy or atrophy of the extremities and oedema. The majority of these malformations are recognizable in childhood with an estimated prevalence of 1.2% of all 3-year-old children routinely examined in a hospital. They are the result of an interaction between genetic and environmental factors, and these factors are incorporated into the Hamburg classification (*Table 29.2*). This abandons less descriptive terms such as Klippel–Trenaunay and Parkes–Weber syndromes.

Although cutaneous vascular malformations are present at birth, not all are necessarily obvious. A **capillary malformation**, or port wine stain, is visible in a neonate and **lymphatic malformations** (*Figure 29.19*) are usually seen in the nursery or become evident within the first year of the life (a small

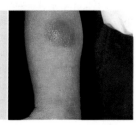

Figure 29.17.
Haemangioma of the right leg of an infant.

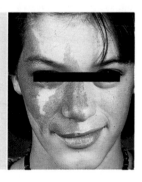

Figure 29.18.
Facial port wine staining.

Table 29.2. Hamburg classification of congenital vascular defects.

Type	Forms	
	Truncular	**Extratruncular**
Predominantly arterial defects	Aplasia or obstructive Dilation	Infiltrating or limited
Predominantly venous defects	Aplasia or obstructive Dilation	Infiltrating or limited
Predominantly lymphatic defects	Aplasia or obstructive	Infiltrating or limited
Predominantly AV shunting defects	Deep or superficial	Infiltrating or limited
Combined/mixed vascular defects	Arterial and venous, no AV shunt Haemolymphatic, with or without AV shunt	Infiltrating haemolymphatic or limited haemolymphatic

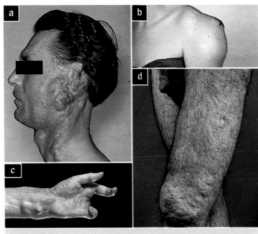

Figure 29.20.
Arteriovenous malformations. a. Left ear. b. Shoulder. c. Left hand; proximal shunting has caused distal ischaemia requiring amputation of the middle and ring fingers. d. Left leg.

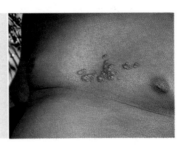

Figure 29.19.
Lymphatic vesicles from local lymphatic abnormality of the chest wall.

number appear in childhood). **Venous malformations** appear at birth, childhood or adolescence. **Arteriovenous fistulae** present signs during childhood or adolescence.

The lesions grow in parallel with the child but sometimes they may expand suddenly, as, for example, a lymphatic lesion when complicated with viral or bacterial infection. This also occurs when a venous lesion thromboses, or when venous and AV lesions are affected by hormonal changes. In general, the lesions are macular and sharply demarcated, with a colour ranging from pale pink to deep red. The overlying skin is normal in texture and varicosities, ectasias or localized spongy masses may be evident. In the early stages a pink stain and increased temperature of the surrounding skin are the only signs suggestive of an AV malformation. Gradually, distended veins occur, a thrill can be felt and an audible bruit appears (*Figure 29.20a–d*); eventually local pain and dystrophic skin changes manifest an ischaemic state. Limb hypertrophy or atrophy may occur. Malformations with AV fistulae are associated with hypertrophy whereas in those without AV fistulae atrophy is commonly seen.

Pathophysiologically, blood diverted from the arterial to the venous circulation through the fistulae results in distal hypoxia. Hypoxia and venostasis increase the precipitation of calcium phosphate, enhancing osteoblastic activity. Bone atrophy can be explained by both mechanical (increased vascular pressure on the bone metaphysis in childhood) and haemodynamic (reduction of the distal circulation due to arterial and/or venous hypoplasia) factors.

In a **congenital AV fistula** the lower extremity is the most common site but the upper extremity, the head or neck are involved in decreasing order of frequency. Presentation in youth is usual. Common signs include:

- Leg ulcer (p. 392) is frequently the presenting lesion and is sometimes known as a hot ulcer because the surrounding skin feels warmer than normal, due to the diversion of blood. It is often extremely painful.
- Varicose veins and port wine discoloration of the skin (*Figure 29.21*). This combination is always extremely suggestive of an AV fistula.
- Local gigantism. If, as is frequent, the AV connections are widespread and the patient is young, increased length and girth of the limb ensues (*Figure 29.22*). Care must be taken not to attribute inequality of limb lengths – and the scoliosis that follows – to shortness of the unaffected leg.

- Increased local warmth. The extremity is appreciably warmer and usually moister than that of the unaffected side.
- Collapsing arterial pulse (Corrigan pulse). This sign can be demonstrated on the foot pulses of the affected limb.
- Bradycardic reaction. Digital occlusion of the main artery to the limb is followed by a slowing of the pulse rate indicating that a considerable volume of blood is being short-circuited (Branham's sign).
- The machinery murmur. With a stethoscope applied over the fistula, a continuous high pitched bruit with systolic accentuation is pathognomonic.

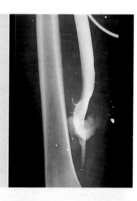

Figure 29.23.
Arteriogram of an acquired AV fistula of the right femoral artery and vein. Note the arterial dilatation, the early venous filling and the residual metal fragments from the original shrapnel injury.

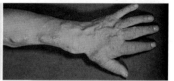

Figure 29.24.
Venous dilatation following a radial AV fistula fashioned for haemodialysis.

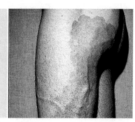

Figure 29.21.
Varicose veins and skin discoloration over the lateral aspect of the left leg.

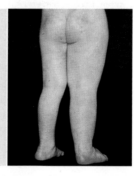

Figure 29.22.
Gigantism of the right leg due to a vascular malformation.

Leg ulcers

Ulceration is a common lower limb pathology, of diverse aetiology and very often causing considerable disability (*Figure 29.25a–x*). In general, the prevalence increases with age, from 0.5% in patients over 40 to 2% in those over 80, implying that an increase can be anticipated in western countries as the proportion of elderly people rises. Pain, offensive smell, time off work, loss of job and social isolation are only some of the problems encountered when dealing with these patients.

It is very important to take a detailed history as there is a large variety of causes of ulceration (*Table 29.3*). However, always bear in mind that 95% of ulcers are of vascular origin. Previous deep venous thrombosis and/or the presence of varicose veins suggest primary or secondary chronic venous insufficiency and cause ulcers in the gaiter area, immediately above the medial (and far less commonly the lateral) malleolus. The ulcer is associated with swelling, skin pigmentation and induration, all suggestive of venous hypertension. The surrounding skin is warm and moist.

A history of intermittent claudication or rest pain, with an absence of palpable arterial pulses, is suggestive of ischaemic arterial disease (p. 369). An ankle–brachial index of less than 0.9, as measured by the portable doppler device, confirms the presence of arterial disease. Loss of hair, dystrophic nails, pale and cold skin with poor capillary filling, are also present. However, a swollen leg with skin induration may also be present if the patient keeps the leg dependent for pain relief in

There are two varieties of congenital AV fistula – localized and diffuse. In the diffuse variety, which is relatively common, the AV communications are deep and clinically indiscernible, probably in the bone. In these, high flow signs are absent.

Acquired AV fistulae result from injuries, usually a stab wound or a through-and-through gunshot wound. Often the superficial situation of the involved vessels enables the clinician to palpate the resultant aneurysmal arterial dilatation (*Figure 29.23*). The signs of an aneurysm (p. 375) may be present. The other signs of AV fistula described above can be observed. The fistula may also have been surgically fashioned for access as, for example, in haemodialysis (*Figure 29.24*).

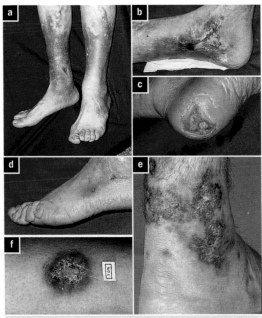

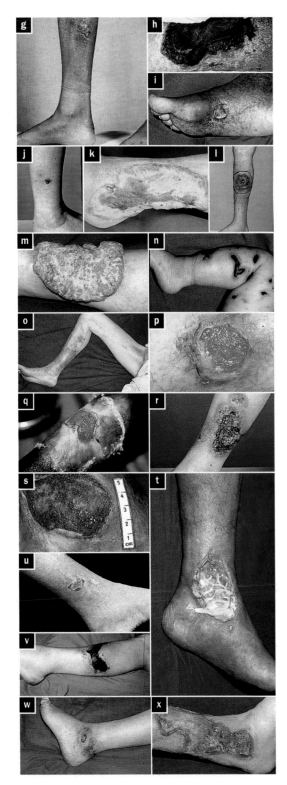

Figure 29.25.
Leg ulcers. a. Healing venous ulcer of the right medial shin. b. Mixed venous and arterial ulcer of the left malleolar region. c. Typical ischaemic ulcer of the heel. d. Vasculitic ulcer on the lateral aspect of the left foot. e. Allergic vasculitis. f. Necrobiosis lipoidica in a diabetic patient (see also p. 000). g. Healing ulcer in a patient with sickle cell disease. h. Leukaemic ulcer following chemo- and radiotherapy. i. Kaposi's sarcoma. j. Malignant melanoma. k. Malignant change in a chronic lower leg ulcer. l. Squamous cell carcinoma. m. Fungating malignant ulcer of the leg. n. Meningococcal septicaemic ulcers of an infant leg. o. Cellulitis with lymphangitis of the leg. p. Gumma of the right leg. q. Tropical ulcer. r. Leg ulcer in a patient with inflammatory bowel disease. s. Ulcer in a patient with rheumatoid arthritis. t. Ulcer in a patient with scleroderma. u. Healing ulcer following a cat bite. v. Eschar following trauma to the left shin. w. Ulcer in a patient following frostbite. x. Artefactual ulcer of the left leg.

profound ischaemia. Ischaemic ulcers tend to be dry, painful and deep, exposing tendons, fascia and bones. They develop more often in the foot but can also occur at any site in the leg, mainly in the anterior aspect where they can persist and enlarge following minor trauma. Mixed ulcers, with coexistent arterial and venous elements, make up 12% of all ulcers and add to the difficulty of diagnosis.

Diabetes mellitus can cause neuropathic or neuroischaemic ulcers (p. 371). Although it is difficult to exclude a neuropathic element in diabetic ulcers, there are differences between neuropathic and neuroischaemic lesions. A painless ulcer located over the metatarsal heads of the sole of the foot

Table 29.3. Causes of leg ulcers.

Vascular	Venous insufficiency (primary or secondary)
	Arterial obstructive disease
	AV malformations
	Vasculitis
Neuropathy	Diabetes mellitus
	Alcohol
	Syringomyelia
	Paralysis
Haematological	Sickle cell disease (p.30)
	Leukaemia
	Haemolytic jaundice
Malignancies	Kaposi's sarcoma
	Melanoma
	Basal cell cancer
	Epithelioma
Miscellaneous	Infection
	Syphilis
	Tropical (p.110)
	Pyoderma gangrenosum
	Skin diseases
	Rheumatoid arthritis
	Pressure sores (p.371)
	Trauma/burns
	Artefactual

with warm foot skin and palpable pedal pulses is more likely to be purely neuropathic in origin. Sensory impairment in the foot, mainly of pain and temperature changes, is very likely to be evident. Diabetic ulcers have a tendency to become infected. However, ischaemia should be suspected in ulcers showing no evidence of healing after 2 weeks of antibiotic therapy and local care.

Skin cancer may be the causative problem in long-standing ulcers without any tendency for healing, especially when they develop in the area of a previous burn or chronic ulceration (Marjolin's ulcer). Features that suggest this diagnosis are unusual or overabundant granulation and rolled irregular edges. Should any suspicion arise, biopsy of the ulcer must be undertaken.

Artefactual (factitious) ulcers are self-induced lesions from which the patient benefits, perhaps through increased attention or being the subject of litigation. They are usually produced on exposed sites by scratching with nails or implements, or by cigarette burns. They should be suspected when ulcers are of unusual or artefactual shapes, have delayed healing when a good healing edge and underlying granulation is present, or when unusual organisms are identified. Once suspected, an ulcer can be sealed and healing expected, provided continued trauma is not applied through or under the dressing.

Swollen leg

Oedema represents an increase of the tissue fluid which may affect any of the limbs or the whole body. When the oedema is generalized and symmetrical, the cause is a systemic abnormality whereas in localized swelling a local cause should be suspected.

In general, oedema represents an imbalance between capillary filtration and lymphatic drainage. A function of the lymphatic system is to compensate for any increase in capillary filtration; its role in the development of oedema is therefore substantial. However, this does not mean that all oedemas are lymphoedemas, as the latter only occur when the lymphatic system fails to drain the tissue fluid produced by normal capillary filtration. The pathophysiology of other forms of oedema is a redistribution of fluid from the arterial to venous end of the capillaries (Starling's law). Venous hypertension and cardiac failure increase the postcapillary venule pressure, resulting in back diffusion of fluid into the interstitial tissues. When the permeability of the capillaries increases, as for instance in an allergic reaction, there is exudation of protein-rich fluid into the tissue. Hyperproteinaemia reduces plasma osmolarity with an increase in capillary diffusion. The various causes of swelling are classified as:

- General. These are due to fluid retention and can cause either acute or chronic swelling. Examples are heart failure, renal failure and hypoproteinaemia (through liver failure or malnutrition).
- Local. These are due to venous or lymphatic insufficiency, inflammatory causes and a few uncommon conditions. **Acute conditions** are deep venous thrombosis, allergy, cellulitis, snake or insect bites, trauma and rheumatoid arthritis. **Chronic conditions** are venous insufficiency (primary or secondary), lymphoedema (primary or secondary), congenital vascular malformation, dependency of the limb and *oedem bleu*.

Clinical signs
Pattern and extent of the oedema
When oedema is widespread in the limbs and body, it is likely to be due to a systemic cause (heart or renal failure, or hypoproteinaemia). Swelling present in both lower limbs or in both upper limbs and the face indicates inferior or superior vena caval syndrome due to local disease in the abdomen or

the chest causing obstruction to the venous outflow. Unilateral swelling of a limb indicates local problems proximal to the upper limit of the swelling. If the feet are spared from the swelling it is more likely to be venous than lymphatic. Lipidemia, i.e. excess subcutaneous fat, also spares the feet.

Presence of skin changes

Varicose veins, lipodermatosclerosis, skin pigmentation and ulcers in the gaiter area are suggestive of venous insufficiency. Hyperkeratosis, thickened skin and enhanced skin creases resembling elephant hide, are characteristics of lymphoedema and thus the term 'elephantiasis'.

Pitting

Pitting oedema is usually systemic in origin. However, it is wrong to say that it cannot be lymphoedema because, in the early stages, lymphoedema does pit.

Kaposi–Stemmer sign

Failure to pick up or to pinch a fold of skin at the base of the second toe is characteristic of lymphoedema.

Lymphatics

Anatomy of the lymphatic system

The lymphatic system, like the venous system, is a pathway for the return of tissue fluid to the systemic circulation. The exchange of oxygen, nutrients and metabolites between the systemic circulation and tissues takes place at the capillaries. Lymphatic vessels start blindly from the tissues and contain valves that permit flow only in one direction. In the limbs they form superficial and deep plexuses in the dermis, and a subfascial plexus in the muscular compartments. Dermal lymphatics drain into the subcutaneous lymph vessels which follow the course of the superficial veins. In general the lymphatics drain into the lymph nodes which, in the limbs, are mainly placed in the axilla and the inguinal regions. Lymph flow in the limbs is facilitated by muscular activity and elevation. The lymph from the limbs and the body returns to the systemic circulation through the thoracic duct, which drains into the left subclavian vein. The large lymphatic vessels have some muscle cells in the wall allowing contractile activity of the lymphatics which propels the lymph centrally; retrograde flow is prevented by the presence of the valves.

Lymphatics are responsible for the resorption of 10–20% of tissue fluid and can transfer larger molecules (protein and protein debris) that cannot pass through the capillaries into

the venous system; 2–4 L of lymph with 70–200 g of protein pass daily into the systemic circulation from the lymphatic system. The lymph nodes are the sites where phagocytosis of particles and related matter occurs, and where foreign material is exposed to the immune system. Venous obstruction and inflammation increase the quantity of the lymphatic flow. Congenital anomalies of the lymph nodes or lymph vessels impair lymphatic drainage; the consequent increase in tissue fluid is termed lymphoedema.

Signs associated with lymphatic obstruction

Oedema of the extremities may be from venous or lymphatic obstruction though they may rarely coexist. Persistent swelling of a limb is seldom due to venous obstruction unless the inferior vena cava is occluded (bilateral swelling up to the groin) or a common iliac vein is obstructed (unilateral swelling). Proximal DVT must be excluded. For this reason signs and symptoms suggestive of thrombosis and developed collateral circulation should be sought. Most instances of long-continued limb oedema are due to lymphatic disease – lymphoedema – in which the oedema is firm or solid but pits to a variable extent, particularly in the early stages. Ulceration is rare.

Two varieties of lymphoedema can be distinguished, **secondary** which is by far the commonest and **primary** which is seen more often in vascular clinics. The former follows damage and obstruction of the lymphatic pathways by malignant disease involving lymph nodes (*Figure 29.26a, b*), by filariasis (*Figure 29.29*) and by surgical block dissections. Repeated attacks of inflammation – cellulitis – are common

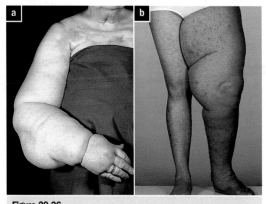

Figure 29.26.
Secondary lymphoedema following excision of regional lymph nodes and subsequent radiotherapy. a. Malignant disease of the right breast. b. Malignancy of the left ureter.

Figure 29.27. Congenital lymphoedema affecting the limbs and face.

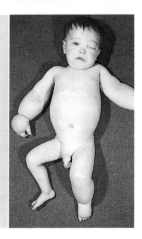

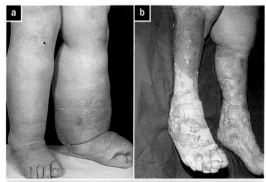

Figure 29.28.
Lymphoedema. a. Lymphoedema tarda. Progression of the lymphoedema is often at a different rate in the two legs. b. Late skin changes following a reduction operation around both lower legs. Note the extensive oedema of the feet and marked hyperkeratosis and skin changes.

Figure 29.29.
Elephantiasis of the scrotum.

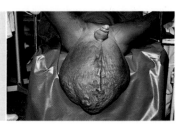

in both types and the swelling tends to increase with each attack, so that in time the limb can reach massive proportions: elephantiasis. The skin becomes hyperkeratotic and fissured so that the limb is pachydermatous in appearance as well as size.

Primary lymphoedema is due to congenital anomalies of the lymphatic system. The condition is classified by the type of the abnormality and the age of the onset of the disease; there is a 3:1 female preponderance. Milroy's disease is the term given to familial lymphoedema; it differs from the other forms in having an equal sex distribution.

Aplasia is rare. There are no subcutaneous lymph trunks and swelling is usually present from birth (lymphoedema congenitalia, *Figure 29.27*).

Hypoplasia is the commonest variety. The lymphatics are probably progressively obliterated together with an increase in fibrosis in the inguinal and pelvic lymph nodes. The oedema presents in the teens or twenties (lymphoedema praecox) but may be delayed until late life (lymphoedema tarda, *Figure 29.28a, b*). Attacks of cellulitis are common following trauma or an insect bite and may be the starting point for the presentation of the lymphoedema.

In **hyperplasia** the lymphatics are enlarged, increased in number and tortuous. This variety is thus analogous with varicose veins. Chyle often runs downwards past incompetent valves and appears on the skin surface as discharging vesicles of milky liquid. This is a unique sign.

Lymphoedema in the tropics. Although filariasis is the classical cause, in practice tuberculous lymphadenitis is commoner, with chronic sepsis in second place. The scrotum, which may become enormous (*Figure 29.29*), the labia and the lower limbs are notably affected. At first pitting on pressure can be demonstrated but with chronicity the swelling becomes solid.

Lymphangiosarcoma (p. 148) is a rare complication of long-standing lymphoedema. A localized increase in the swelling is noted which relentlessly increases in size. The condition is rapidly fatal unless an early extensive amputation – forequarter or hindquarter – is feasible.

30 The spine

History

A thorough and detailed history is an essential prerequisite to the examination and investigation of spinal disorders. This includes information on the age and maturity of the patient, the onset and nature of pain or deformity, its effects on the patient and his or her general health, and the family and social/occupational history. Note should be made of any pending industrial or legal complaints related to the patient's presentation as these invariably affect the ultimate prognosis.

The location, nature and radiation of pain are important, as are aggravating and relieving factors. The distinction between leg pain and back pain is particularly significant. Exacerbation by coughing or sneezing should be noted, as should its effects on everyday activities and sleep. Neurological symptoms, including bladder and bowel dysfunction, should be identified. Back pain in the skeletally immature should always be considered organic and fully investigated.

If the patient presents with spinal deformity, determine the time of onset, any precipitating factors, its progression and its effects on the physical and psychological health of the patient. In particular, secondary cardiorespiratory and neurological symptoms should be sought. Previous treatment and the level of compliance with this should be recorded. In children and adolescents spinal deformities are not usually accompanied by pain, and if this is present, more sinister causes must always be considered and excluded.

In all cases accurate recording of the history and examination, including the patient's mental state, will later prove invaluable.

Observation

The appearance and demeanour of the patient in the waiting area, their gait, their communication methods and the ease with which they undress all provide useful information. Adequate exposure is essential. The patient must be examined in a warm, relaxed and friendly environment and should undress to their underwear for assessment of their back.

The overall body habitus and facies of the patient can be used as a guide to congenital, endocrine or metabolic diseases. Sitting and standing heights, weight and arm span can be recorded.

An **antalgic gait** is seen when the patient spends less time weightbearing on a limb due to pain; this is suggestive of hip or knee pathology. A **shuffling gait** might suggest a neurological lesion and a **flexed gait** spinal stenosis.

Inspection from the side, while the patient is standing, allows assessment of their posture. An increase or decrease in the lumbar lordosis or thoracic kyphosis soon becomes evident.

Kyphosis (*Figure 30.1*) is the general term used to describe excessive convex posterior curvature of the back such as a round back or humpback deformity. In postural kyphosis the curve is mobile and regular and the flow of spinal movement is smooth. This can also be secondary to hip deformity or muscle weakness, both of which also lead to an increased lumbar lordosis. If the kyphosis is fixed, however, other causes such as senile kyphosis due to vertebral collapse, Scheuermann's disease and ankylosing spondylitis should be considered. A sharp angular kyphosis with a gibbus – exaggerated prominence of a spinous process – points to a vertebral fracture (either traumatic or pathological/malignant), to TB of the spine or to a congenital vertebral anomaly (*Figure 30.2a, b, c*).

Lordosis refers to convex anterior curvature of the spine. Flattening of the normal lumbar **lordosis** is commonly seen with prolapsed intervertebral discs, vertebral osteomyelitis,

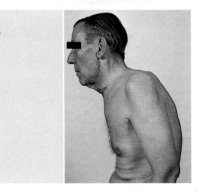

Figure 30.1.
Senile kyphosis.

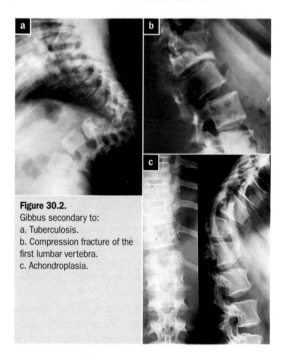

Figure 30.2.
Gibbus secondary to:
a. Tuberculosis.
b. Compression fracture of the first lumbar vertebra.
c. Achondroplasia.

ankylosing spondylitis and in the patient with a degenerative lumbar spine. The patient who presents with the spine, hips and knees flexed, the 'simian stance', should be assessed for spinal stenosis.

An increase in the lumbar curvature can be a normal racial variant which is more frequently seen in women, notably in pregnancy. It may also be secondary to spondylolisthesis or to a fixed deformity of the thoracic spine or hips, both of which should be examined (*Figure 30.3*).

Inspection from the back of the patient reveals a **scoliosis** (*Figure 30.4*), i.e. a lateral curvature of the spine. A curve is labelled according to the direction of its convex side. Further assessment of such a deformity is necessary to establish whether it is postural, compensatory, structural or related to pain and muscular spasm. One must first note whether there are one or more curves and whether they are mobile or fixed. In balanced deformities, the occiput lies above the midline; this can be confirmed with a plumb line. Any deviation can be measured in centimetres from the natal cleft and suggests an unbalanced curve. Shoulders, breasts and skin creases should also be asymmetrical and the extent of any difference should be recorded. A scoliometer or spirit level can be used to record the degree of asymmetry. Pelvic tilt must also be assessed.

A **postural curve** is usually a simple single curve that corrects in flexion. This is most often to the left side in adolescent girls and treatment consists mainly of reassurance.

A **compensatory scoliosis** can be secondary to previous thoracic surgery, to hip pathology or to leg length discrepancy. In the latter the curve corrects when the patient sits down.

A **sciatic scoliosis** or **list** is due to muscle spasm and its convexity is usually directed to the side of the intervertebral disc prolapse. It is associated with flattening of the lumbar lordosis and frequently with hip and knee flexion both at rest and on standing (*Figure 30.5*).

A **structural scoliosis** is fixed in comparison to the mobile curves above. It is always associated with rotation of the vertebral bodies towards the convexity of the curve. Secondary compensatory curves develop and can in time also become fixed curves. With thoracic curves in particular, vertebral rotation leads to a prominent rib hump deformity that can also be measured with special instruments.

Figure 30.3. Illustration of the lateral contour of the lumbar spine.
a. Normal. b. Spasm. c. Spondylolisthesis.

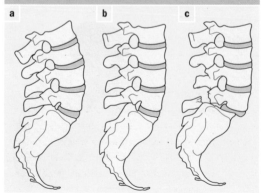

Figure 30.4.
Scoliosis, demonstrating the posterior aspect of a long neuromuscular curve. There is a dip in the left shoulder and pelvic obliquity. The plumb line indicates the displacement of the centre of gravity.

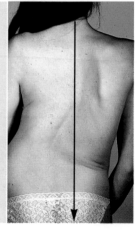

Figure 30.5.
Sciatic list. Secondary to prolapsed intervertebral disc. (Reproduced with permission from *Physical Examination in Orthopaedics*, by A. Graham Apley and Louis Solomon, Butterworth–Heinemann, 1997.)

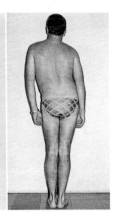

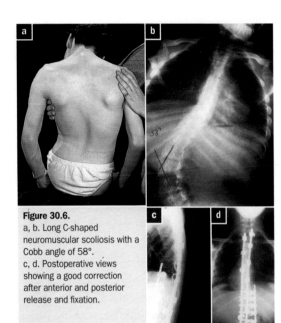

Figure 30.6.
a, b. Long C-shaped neuromuscular scoliosis with a Cobb angle of 58°.
c, d. Postoperative views showing a good correction after anterior and posterior release and fixation.

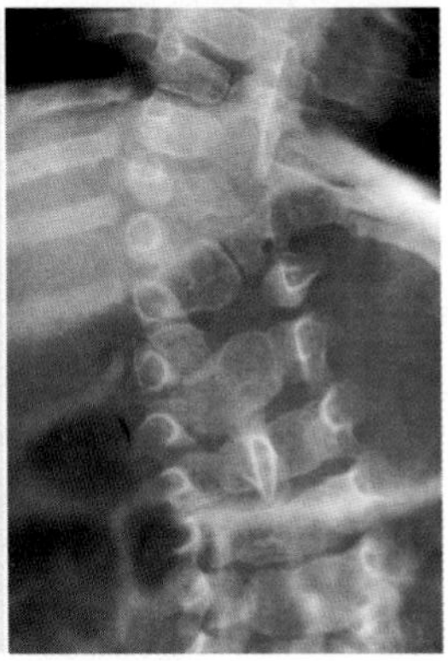

Of the structural curves, 80% are idiopathic. These are commonly seen in adolescent girls with most thoracic curves being right sided, and lumbar curves left sided. A high curve, where rib rotation exaggerates the deformity, is likely to present earlier than a well-balanced thoracolumbar curve.

Other causes include neuromuscular curves such as those seen in cerebral palsy or in the muscular dystrophies (*Figure 30.6a–d*). These are typically paralytic, long, C-shaped curves that are convex towards the weaker side. There is invariably significant cardiorespiratory compromise. Costopelvic impingement can lead to pain and seating progressively becomes more difficult as the curves deteriorate.

Osteogenic curves usually present at a very early stage and are associated with a host of congenital anomalies including cardiac and renal malformations (*Figure 30.7*).

Inspection of the patient also reveals the scars of previous surgery, sinuses from previous bony sepsis, pigmentation/*café au lait* spots in relation to neurofibromatosis, or hairy patches or fat pads suggestive of spinal dysraphism. This represents failure of fusion of the cartilaginous bars forming the vertebral arch resulting in a posterior vertebral defect which can have neurological consequences.

During this phase of the examination, the patient is asked to point to the site of greatest pain and to its radiation. Suspicion of emotional overlay should be aroused when the patient will not touch the back.

The patient can be asked to stand on tiptoe as a preliminary assessment of gastrocnemius power and hence a motor assessment of the S1 root.

When the patient lies prone, comparison of the gluteals reveals wasting or atrophy in L5, S1 or S2 lesions. This can also be noted by the observant examiner as a sag in the buttock crease of the standing patient.

Figure 30.7.
Vertebral defects.

Palpation

The whole spine should be palpated from top to bottom in a systematic way to exclude any sharp irregularities such as a gibbus or any steps as seen at the lumbosacral junction in spondylolisthesis. Percussion with the examiner's fist is then used in an attempt to elicit tenderness at every spinal/interspinous level and in the paravertebral areas (*Figure 30.8a, b*).

The sacroiliac joints should also be palpated and any tenderness elicited.

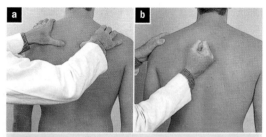

Figure 30.8.
a, b. Examination for spinal tenderness commences with digital pressure and, if no tenderness is elicited, this is followed by spinal percussion.

Movement

The patient is asked to touch their toes while keeping their knees extended (*Figure 30.9a–d*). This is a compound movement including thoracic, lumbar and hip flexion. The distance of the fingertips from the floor or from anatomical landmarks such as the tibial tuberosity or malleoli can then be recorded. Alternatively the spine is marked at predetermined points such as T1–L1 or L1–S1 and the increase in this distance noted with flexion (*Figure 30.10a, b*). Both parameters should increase by approximately 8 cm. Chest expansion can be similarly measured if rigidity suggests ankylosing spondylitis, with an expansion of less than 2.5 cm almost pathognomonic. If the patient constantly deviates to one side when bending forward, this is indicative of an irritative lesion such as a herniated disc, osteoid osteoma or spinal tumour, and should be investigated further. Reversal of the normal spinal rhythm on attempting to regain the erect posture is characteristic of disc degeneration with posterior facet pain.

A similar manoeuvre can be used to measure spinal extension with the reduction in the measured distance being recorded.

Lateral flexion is assessed by asking the patient to slide their hand down the side of each leg in turn (*Figure 30.9c*). The distance from the floor or from fixed anatomical landmarks can then be recorded.

Rotation is measured by folding the patient's arms across their chest in the seated position and asking them to twist to either side. This usually measures less than 40° and is almost entirely thoracic (*Figure 30.9d*).

Leg lengths with the patient supine, and range of movement of the hips, are measured to exclude their contribution to the patient's presentation. Whilst the patient is lying flat, compression and distraction of the pelvis can be attempted

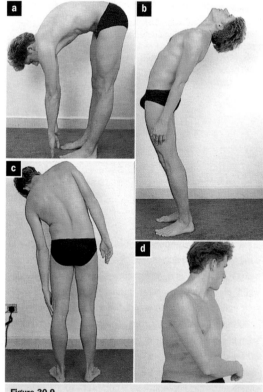

Figure 30.9.
a–d. Spinal movements.

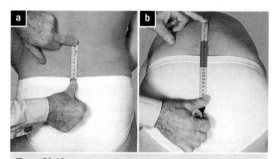

Figure 30.10.
a, b. Schober's test of spinal flexion. (Reproduced with permission from *Physical Examination in Orthopaedics*, by A. Graham Apley and Louis Solomon, Butterworth–Heinemann, 1997.)

by grasping the anterior superior iliac spines; reproduction of the patient's pain is suggestive of sacroiliac pathology. The sacroiliac joints can also be stressed by flexing the hip and knee and adducting the thigh – the pump handle test. This is a non-specific test but can suggest sacroiliac pathology including inflammatory and infectious arthropathies.

Examination of the back is incomplete without a full abdominal, rectal and vascular examination.

A series of tests have been developed to assess nerve root tension, namely the reproduction of extremity pain by stretching a peripheral nerve.

Straight leg raising (Lasègue's test):

This is a passive test with each leg being tested individually. With the patient supine, the hip medially rotated and the knee extended, the examiner gently and gradually flexes the hip until the patient complains of pain or tightness. The leg is then dropped back to a level which causes no symptoms and the ankle is dorsiflexed. If such a manoeuvre recreates pain radiating down the back of the leg, the test is considered positive and indicates stretching of the dura mater, primarily at the L5, S1 and S2 levels. Pain that does not increase with ankle dorsiflexion is suggestive of tight hamstrings or of a mechanical lumbosacral cause. The same test is then repeated on the other side for comparison (*Figure 30.11a, b*).

It cannot be overemphasized that it is leg/radicular pain and not merely back pain which signifies a positive test. This distinction between nerve root pain and mechanical back pain is significant both in terms of treatment and prognosis. The level at which the test is positive is recorded for future comparison.

If contralateral pain is felt during a straight leg raise – the cross over sign – this is highly indicative of a space-occupying lesion in the spinal canal such as a prolapsed intervertebral disc.

Bilateral simultaneous straight leg raising causes the pelvis to rotate and hyperextends the lumbar spine. In the presence of disc degeneration this leads to pain and is a indicator of painful segmental instability.

Bowstring test

This is carried out in a similar manner to a straight leg raise. Once the patient experiences symptoms, the knee is flexed by approximately 20°. This leads to pain relief in the patient with nerve root irritation. Thumb or finger pressure is then applied to the popliteal area. If this recreates the patient's radicular symptoms, it is indicative of nerve root tension (*Figure 30.12a, b*).

Femoral stretch test

With the patient either prone or in the lateral decubitus position, and the back not hyperextended, the knee is flexed whilst maintaining the hip in neutral rotation. The hip is then gradually extended. Limited knee flexion/hip extension with pain radiating down the anterior aspect of the thigh is due to stretching of the femoral nerve and is indicative of an L2, L3 or L4 lesion. As with the straight leg raising test, contralateral pain is of considerable significance (*Figure 30.13*).

Stoop test

This is done to confirm neurogenic spinal claudication. After exertion, the patient's buttock and leg pain is relieved by bending forward. Conversely, symptoms are exacerbated by extending the spine.

A focused neurological examination is vital. Muscle bulk/girth, tone, power, reflexes and sensation are sequentially assessed (*Table 30.1*).

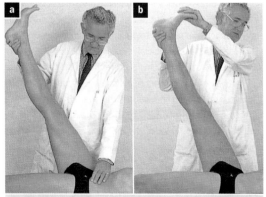

Figure 30.11.
a, b. Straight leg raising to elicit nerve root tension.

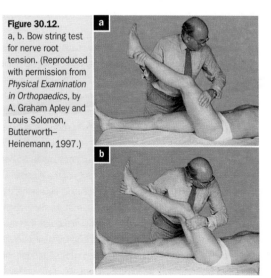

Figure 30.12.
a, b. Bow string test for nerve root tension. (Reproduced with permission from *Physical Examination in Orthopaedics*, by A. Graham Apley and Louis Solomon, Butterworth–Heinemann, 1997.)

Figure 30.13. Femoral nerve stretch test. This can be performed prone or on the patient's side.

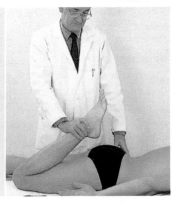

Table 30.1. Potential findings in nerve root dysfunction.

Level	Wasting	Motor weakness	Reflex depression	Sensory disturbance
L4	Thigh/ quadriceps	Knee extension	Knee jerk	Medial aspect of calf and ankle
L5	Calf	Extensor hallucis longus (ankle dorsiflexors)		Lateral aspect of calf and medial dorsum of foot
S1	Calf	Flexor hallucis longus (ankle plantarflexors)	Ankle jerk	Posterior aspect of calf; lateral border of foot and sole

Thigh/quadriceps girth should be compared to the contralateral side and may be decreased secondary to an L4 lesion or to disuse. With lesions of the fourth lumbar root, the quadriceps may be weak and tender to palpation. This is tested by asking the patient to extend the flexed knee against the examiner's resistance. The knee/patellar tendon jerk may be reduced or absent.

Lesions of the fifth lumbar root may cause weakness of the extensor hallucis longus prior to any demonstrable ankle dorsiflexor weakness. Alternatively, wasting of extensor digitorum brevis is another sensitive sign of an L5 lesion. Ankle dorsiflexion should be tested with the knees flexed, as resisting plantar flexion with the hip and knee extended may exacerbate sciatic pain.

With an S1 lesion, toe and subsequently ankle flexion become weak. In early lesions, fatiguability of the gastrocnemius should be compared to the other side by asking the patient to repeatedly rise on tiptoe. Ultimately, the patient may be unable to stand on tiptoe at all, although this may also be difficult in the presence of quadriceps weakness. With first sacral root irritation the calf muscles may be tender and the ankle jerk may also become deficient.

Figure 30.14. Dermatomal maps.

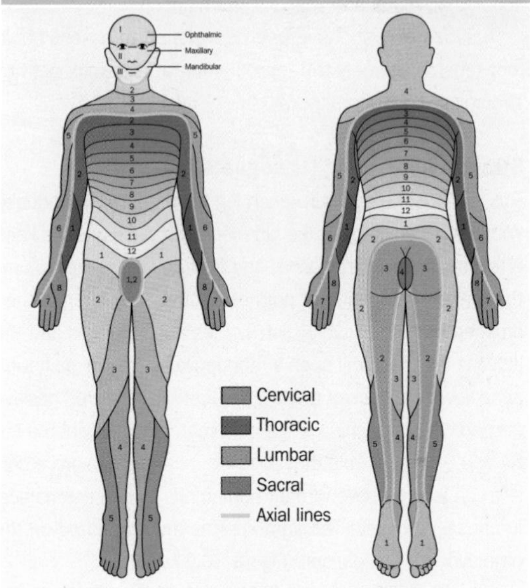

■	Cervical
■	Thoracic
■	Lumbar
■	Sacral
—	Axial lines

Sensory testing should be performed including light touch, pinprick and vibration sense in those under 50. It should be remembered that the distribution of the L4 dermatome comprises the anteromedial thigh and lower leg, the L5 dermatome the dorsum of the foot and anterior lower leg, and the S1 dermatome the sole of the foot and the outer border of the foot and lower leg. These territories are useful both in interpreting the radiation of the patient's pain and in assessing any root sensory deficit (*Figure 30.14*).

Difficulty with micturition, urinary retention, loss of anal sphincter tone or faecal incontinence, progressive motor loss and saddle anaesthesia are all suggestive of central cord compression and require urgent imaging and decompression.

Absence of the superficial abdominal reflex may be the only abnormality noted in the initial presentation of syringomyelia.

At the end of the neurological assessment, the history, general examination findings and motor and sensory findings should be collated to identify the anatomical level of any spinal pathology. This can then be confirmed by radiological investigation before any intervention is planned.

The neonate/congenital disorders

Spinal dysraphism represents failure of fusion of the cartilaginous bars forming the vertebral arch resulting in a posterior vertebral defect. Its incidence is decreasing due to improved

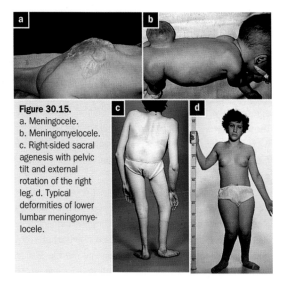

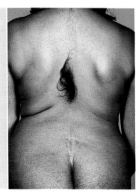

Figure 30.16.
Spinal bifida with faun tail and scar from previous surgery.

Figure 30.15.
a. Meningocele.
b. Meningomyelocele.
c. Right-sided sacral agenesis with pelvic tilt and external rotation of the right leg. d. Typical deformities of lower lumbar meningomyelocele.

prenatal diagnosis and prevention. However, there are still a variety of forms that can affect any level of the spinal column but are most frequently seen in the lumbosacral region (*Figure 30.15a–d*).

- **Myelocele** – Both the neural and vertebral arches fail to close. Clinical examination reveals an oval, raw, uncovered defect communicating with the central canal of the spinal cord. The infant is usually stillborn or dies soon after birth.
- **Syringomyelocele** – The bulging defect includes a dilated cyst of the spinal cord and is associated with dense neurological lesions.
- **Meningocele** – The protruding meningeal sac only contains cerebrospinal fluid and is covered with healthy skin (*Figure 30.15a*).
- **Meningomyelocele** – A normally developed spinal cord or cauda equina lies within the protruding sac which is covered by unepithelialized meninges rather than skin (*Figure 30.15b*).

A transmitted impulse can be detected from the swelling to the anterior fontanelle. Assessment of the degree of paralysis and anal tone reveals the level of neurological injury. General examination of these infants may reveal **hydrocephalus** in relation to the **Arnold–Chiari malformation** where cerebellar herniation obstructs cerebrospinal fluid outflow.

Spina bifida occulta – often associated with a local patch of hair, skin dimples, sinuses or lipomas – is found in nearly 15% of the population and is asymptomatic. It is frequently an incidental finding when radiographic investigation of the back is undertaken. It may be associated with an abnormal filum terminale or spinal cord tethering which becomes significant if later operative intervention is planned.

Infantile idiopathic scoliosis is predominantly seen in boys with left-sided, high thoracic curves. Most resolve spontaneously although the progressive ones can become very severe.

Congenital **osteogenic scolioses** present a more difficult management problem. Causes include failures of fusion and/or vertebral segmentation. Skin angiomas, dimples, hairy tufts, naevi and fat pads often give a clue to the associated **spina bifida**. (*Figure 30.16*) and spinal cord tethering must be excluded/documented by MRI prior to any surgical intervention.

Back pain in children

Back pain is uncommon in childhood and is most often caused by neoplastic or infectious diseases. Although it is often vague and poorly localized, it must be thoroughly investigated as psychosomatic back pain is a diagnosis of exclusion in children. The most likely causes of back pain in childhood are **infections** such as discitis or osteomyelitis, and spinal/paraspinal **tumours**. In adolescence, inflammatory disorders such as ankylosing spondylitis or juvenile chronic arthritis must be considered. Mechanical causes such as osteochondritis, Scheuermann's disease, herniated intervertebral discs, spondylolysis and spondylolisthesis must also be excluded. Painful scolioses should be carefully assessed as many have a sinister cause.

Back pain in children should never be dismissed as non-organic and should always be promptly investigated.

Scheuermann's kyphosis

Scheuermann's disease was described in 1921 as a **thoracic kyphotic deformity** affecting young males usually prior to puberty, characterized by vertebral wedging and a subsequent growth disturbance of the vertebral end plate. The aetiology of this condition is not known. The curve is usually rigid, particularly at its apex. There are two main forms of the disease, the more common being the thoracolumbar type with the apex between T10 and T11. Scheuermann's disease is radiographically characterized by **irregular vertebral endplates**, Schmorl's nodes and a reduction in disc height with **anterior vertebral wedging**. Patients normally present with either pain or cosmetic deformity without neurological symptoms or signs. The pain tends to decline following skeletal maturity.

Discitis

This is usually a childhood affliction although it can occur as a complication after disc space surgery. The aetiology is not thought to be infectious in all cases. The average age of presentation is 2–6 years with males and females equally affected. The child classically complains of back pain increasing in intensity over 2–4 weeks.

On examination the child shows some spinal rigidity and maintains the posture of fixed hyperlordosis. A low-grade pyrexia may be noted. Intra-abdominal infection or hip sepsis must be excluded by examination. Plain radiographs can be normal in the early stages and magnetic resonance imaging scans and bone scintigraphy allow an earlier diagnosis.

The treatment of discitis is bed rest and spinal immobilization with a brace or cast. Antibiotics can be used where there are signs of systemic sepsis. Surgery is almost never indicated as most cases undergo spontaneous interbody fusion. The mild deformity thus formed is usually non-progressive.

Differential diagnosis of back pain

This requires a general examination of the patient and an assessment of the abdomen, the pelvis, the lower limbs and the peripheral vascular system, to exclude conditions such as peptic ulcer disease, renal or perirenal infections, renal stone disease, gallstones, pancreatitis, intrapelvic tumours, gynaecological infection (pelvic inflammatory disease), arthritis of the hip, an abdominal aortic aneurysm or vascular claudication.

Spondylosis

This is a **defect in the pars interarticularis** (*Figure 30.17*) in the posterior column of the lumbar spine. This is the most common cause of back pain in childhood and adolescence although neurological defects are rare in children under the age of five. If there are bilateral pars defects, **spondylolisthesis** (*Figure 30.18a, b, c*) may result. This represents forward slippage of one vertebra on another and is classified into five major types: congenital; isthmic; traumatic; degenerative or pathological.

Acquired defects are known to follow repeated stress on the pars region. These are particularly common in gymnasts, footballers and cricketers. The most common manifestation is back pain. Examination reveals localized lumbar back pain, minimal tenderness and some paraspinal muscle spasm. There may be decreased forward flexion of the spine. Radiological evaluation is usually with plain films, including oblique radiographs. The latter confirm the pars defect as a fracture in the neck of the 'Scottie dog'. The severity is graded

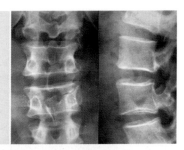

Figure 30.17.
Defect of the pars interarticularis.

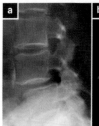
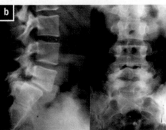
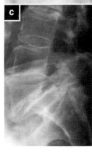

Figure 30.18.
Spondylolisthesis. a. L4–L5. b. L5–S1. c. L5–S1 with degenerative changes.

according to the percentage slip of one vertebra on the other, or the angle of rotation of the slip.

The management of spondylolisthesis remains controversial although most patients get better with non-operative measures.

Ankylosing spondylitis *(Figure 30.19a, b)*

This is a **sero-negative arthropathy** that progresses slowly to bony ankylosis of the joints of the spinal column and occasionally of the major limb joints. It affects 2 or 3 per 1000 with a **male preponderance**. Although it is related to HLA B27, the precise cause is not known.

The initial changes are seen in the **sacroiliac joints** and extend upwards to the **lumbar** and often the **thoracic spine**. The hips and shoulders can also be affected. The articular cartilage, synovium and ligaments all show chronic inflammatory changes and eventually become ossified. This condition should always be suspected when low back pain, which is worse in the morning and improves as the day progresses, is seen in young male patients.

The diagnosis is usually made on the basis of **reduced spinal movement** and **chest expansion** with possible sacroiliac or costochondral tenderness. Typical radiographic features include fuzziness of the sacroiliac joints and squaring/bridging of the lumbar vertebrae. In the early stages, a raised erythrocyte sedimentation rate and increased uptake at the sacroiliac joints on bone scan may be the only positive features.

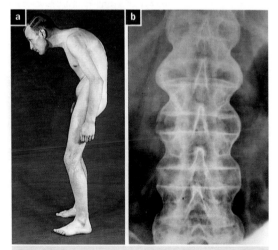

Figure 30.19.
Ankylosing spondylitis. a. Patient with a fixed thoracic kyphosis. b. Bamboo spine.

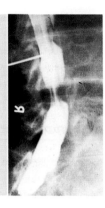

Figure 30.20.
Myelogram showing obstruction to passage of contrast medium due to spinal stenosis.

Spinal stenosis

This condition refers to a **narrowing of the spinal canal** (*Figure 30.20*) such as when the spinal cord and nerve roots are compromised. The patient presents with the insidious onset of back and leg pain. Symptoms are usually bilateral with leg pain being worse on standing and walking though sitting or flexing the spine forwards usually relieves the pain. The patient often experiences pain on walking a certain distance but can walk further leaning forwards (the 'simian stance'). This is because flexing the spine forwards increases the area of the spinal canal. Symptoms are often severe at night because the supine posture decreases the area in the spinal canal.

Spinal stenosis can be classified into **congenital** and **acquired**. The latter can be degenerative, secondary to a spondylolisthesis, iatrogenic, traumatic or in relation to miscellaneous disorders such as acromegaly, Paget's disease or ankylosing spondylitis. Moreover, combined causes can be noted in some cases, such as degenerative changes on the background of a congenitally narrow canal. The differential diagnosis of spinal stenosis includes **vascular claudication** and back pain and lumbar spondylosis without stenosis.

Coccydynia

This refers to any painful condition in the region of the coccyx. In practice these are often patients whose pain persists for weeks or months despite the absence of any demonstrable pathology. There is often a predisposing injury and the coccyx is very tender locally. Enquiry must be made as to whether the patient can pass their faeces normally, and a rectal examination should be performed.

The management of coccydynia entails the exclusion of organic disease and reassurance. Several treatment methods have been advocated, including physiotherapy, injections of local anaesthetic and steroid, and surgery (which remains particularly controversial).

Rheumatoid arthritis

Clinical manifestations from the thoracic and lumbar spine are relatively uncommon. This is unlike the cervical spine where rheumatoid disease can be extremely severe, can lead to myelopathy and must always be excluded prior to general anaesthesia.

Spinal infections

Vertebral osteomyelitis remains a common condition which requires a high index of clinical suspicion. The most common cause is **haematogenous spread** although infection can be from a contiguous focus or direct inoculation during a surgical procedure or a therapeutic injection. Most cases affect the lumbar spine. *Staphylococcus aureus* is the most commonly implicated organism, followed by streptococci and enterobacteriae. Patients with sickle cell anaemia have a known predisposition towards salmonella osteomyelitis and intravenous drug abusers have a high rate of infection with *Pseudomonas* sp.

The most common presentation is a deep, boring back pain that is not relieved by rest and is unaffected by changes in position. Patients occasionally complain of constitutional symptoms. Neurological deficits occur in 30% of patients. As well as careful examination, a full blood count, erythrocyte sedimentation rate and blood cultures should be taken. The diagnosis is often delayed as plain radiographic changes may not appear for 2–4 weeks. These include **loss of disc height** and **paravertebral soft tissue shadows**, followed ultimately by **endplate destruction**. The differential diagnosis includes renal osteodystrophy, non-pyogenic infection, ankylosing spondylitis and rheumatoid arthritis. In contrast, neoplastic vertebral destruction is more likely to be centred in the vertebral body and spare the disc space. An earlier diagnosis can be reached using MRI scanning or bone scintigraphy; CT scans are also more sensitive than plain radiography.

Tuberculosis

This remains the most common source of vertebral infection on a worldwide scale and it is particularly important at present with the advent of new strains of resistant mycobacteria; over 50% of cases are reported in the first decade of life. Infection can be acquired either directly from the lungs or by haematogenous spread. The infection begins at the anterior margin of the vertebral body near the intervertebral disc. The disc can be involved in an early stage. The extent of destruction varies – there is often complete destruction of one intervertebral disc with partial destruction of two adjacent vertebrae. The changes may extend over several spinal segments and anterior collapse of the infected vertebrae can lead to severe **angular kyphosis**, called a **gibbus** (*Figure 30.2a*).

Abscess formation is common and can form a paraspinal abscess (*Figure 30.21a*) or track down beneath the fascial sheath of the psoas muscle and burst into the compartment behind the iliacus fascia to form part of the abscess in the iliac fossa – the **psoas abscess** (*Figure 30.21b*). This abscess can also point posteriorly or into the groin. Neurological compromise may occur because of abscess formation within the spinal canal or secondary to a long-standing severe kyphosis.

Tuberculosis infection differs from pyogenic by its multisegment involvement, its spread along soft tissue planes and its propensity to lead to kyphosis and paravertebral abscess formation. Treatment consists of drug therapy or surgery where there is more than 5° of kyphosis or 50% vertebral body destruction and neurological compromise.

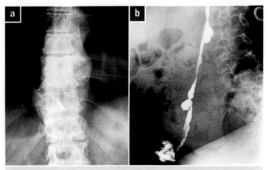

Figure 30.21.
Tuberculosis. a. Collapse of thoracic vertebrae and abscess formation. b. Sinogram of psoas abscess demonstrating the track from the thoracic vertebrae along the psoas sheath to the groin.

Osteoporosis

This is shown in *Figure 30.22a–c* and represents a **diminution of bone mass**. The composition of bone is normal but the amount per unit volume is decreased. With the advent of bone mineral density measurement using dual energy X-ray absorptiometry, osteoporosis is now defined as a reduction in bone mineral density more than 2.5 standard deviations from the young adult mean. It may be a primary disorder – as is most commonly seen in postmenopausal women – or secondary to nutritional disorders, a variety of hormonal diseases such as thyrotoxicosis, hyperparathyroidism, diabetes mellitus or Cushing's disease, or drug related, most notably with the use of corticosteroids.

Vertebral crush fractures (*Figure 30.22c*) represent one of the commonest sequelae of osteoporosis. The clinical presentation may only be of a progressive kyphosis – or dowager's hump – and the fractures often follow no trauma or the mildest stress to the spine. Successive fractures ultimately lead to **backache**, **kyphosis** and **loss of height**.

Plain radiographs of the spine reveal resorption of the horizontal trabeculae with biconcavity of the vertebral bodies. Compression fractures with anterior wedging most commonly occur around the **thoracolumbar junction**. Involvement of the pedicles suggests malignant pathology.

Spinal injuries *(Figure 30.23a–c)*

The vertebral column and spinal cord can be injured individually or together. Great care must therefore be taken in the primary assessment of all trauma victims. The spine must be immobilized during the resuscitation phase until a full clinical and neurological assessment is made and adequate radiographs are obtained.

The patient is therefore examined in a neutral position with the neck held with 'in-line' immobilization or stabilized with a collar and sandbags. The whole spine is initially held still, using a spine board when this is available. To assess the back of the spine the patient is log rolled – this requires *at the very least* one person to control the head, two to hold the pelvis and trunk, and one to examine the back.

Clinical examination should identify pain, tenderness, bruising, oedema or deformity. A full autonomic and neurological assessment is also undertaken. A conscious patient is able to locate the areas of greatest discomfort and to report any neurological disturbance. The abdomen, pelvis and extremities must be carefully examined as spinal cord injury may render serious pathology asymptomatic. In the unconscious patient, flaccid areflexia, diaphragmatic breathing, hypotension with bradycardia – **neurogenic shock** – and priapism are all suggestive of a spinal cord injury.

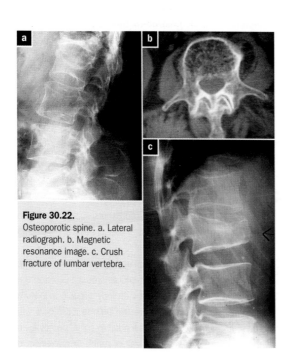

Figure 30.22.
Osteoporotic spine. a. Lateral radiograph. b. Magnetic resonance image. c. Crush fracture of lumbar vertebra.

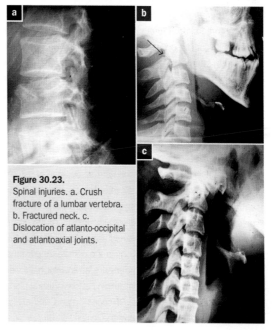

Figure 30.23.
Spinal injuries. a. Crush fracture of a lumbar vertebra. b. Fractured neck. c. Dislocation of atlanto-occipital and atlantoaxial joints.

Spinal shock refers to the flaccidity and areflexia seen immediately after spinal cord damage. It lasts up to 48 hours or until the return of the bulbocavernosus reflex. It is replaced in due course by spasticity, increased reflexes and upgoing plantar reflexes. Once this has occurred, the likely residual neurological deficit and prognosis can be determined. A motor and sensory level for spinal cord injury can then be defined and appropriate investigation, management and rehabilitation instituted.

Fractures (*Figure 30.23*) of the thoracolumbar spine can be divided into compression, burst, flexion–distraction injuries and fracture dislocations. The spine can be divided into anterior, middle and posterior columns. If more than one column is involved, the injury is likely to be unstable. The assessment of these injuries requires plain radiographs supplemented by CT and MRI. Advice from regional spinal injury units should be sought.

Tumours of the spine

Tumours in relation to the spinal column can be considered as those of the spinal column itself, those of the meninges and, rarely, those of the spinal cord. There are also neoplasms of the fibrous component of peripheral nerves and of adjacent soft tissues. The effects of these tumours can be divided into those of local destruction of the skeleton, compression of the spinal cord and interference with peripheral nerves. The degree of each of these determines the resulting symptomatology. Thorough clinical examination and imaging is necessary before any treatment can be considered.

Benign tumours (p. 427) usually affect patients in the second or third decade although sacral tumours occur in older age groups. The most common types are **giant cell tumours**, **osteoid osteomas**, **osteoblastomas**, **haemangiomas**, **osteochondromas** and **aneurysmal bone cysts**. The most common complaint is pain which may be local or radicular and which, particularly in children, must be thoroughly investigated. **Night pain** is a well recognized association of osteoid osteoma and osteoblastoma. **Scoliosis** may also be a presenting feature and is often seen without a compensatory curve. Most tumours have a characteristic radiographic appearance, e.g. osteoid osteomas and osteoblastomas frequently present as sclerotic lesions in the pedicle. Aneurysmal bone cysts and giant cell tumours are often expansile and lytic while eosinophilic granulomas can cause vertebral plana or a flat vertebra. Bone scans, CT scanning and MRI are all useful in delineating and defining the lesion.

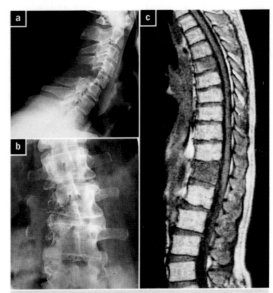

Figure 30.24.
Secondary deposits in the spine. a. C5. b. L3.
c. Multiple thoracic.

Malignant lesions (p. 429) within the vertebral column are predominantly **metastatic** (*Figure 30.24a–c*) as opposed to primary tumours arising in the spine itself. Common primary sites are the **breast, lung, prostate, kidney, thyroid, lymphoma** and the **gastrointestinal tract**. The pain associated with these lesions is classically relentlessly progressive, and unresponsive to rest and normal conservative measures. The patient often wakes up at night. There is scant radiographic evidence of the lesions as 50% vertebral body destruction is necessary before an abnormality can be detected on plain radiographs. Biopsy is frequently necessary to reach a diagnosis.

Non-organic back pain

Non-organic back/spinal pain represents such a significant clinical and medicolegal problem that it deserves particular attention.

Non-anatomical neurological symptoms and signs, particularly if these are inconsistent, should arouse suspicion that the patient's problems are not entirely organic in nature. Examples include cases where the pain is multifocal with some features that cannot be ascribed to spinal pathology, or when an entire extremity is weak or numb or gives way, or when the patient claims to be 'allergic' to all recommended treatments. The patient may complain of 'constant agony' but appear almost indifferent to it during the consultation. Diffuse weakness of all muscle groups, particularly the psoas, is highly suggestive of a functional or emotional deficit. This is also sometimes characterized by inconsistent jerky motor power.

These patients must be assessed particularly carefully, both to exclude unusual neurological disorders and to avoid unnecessary investigation which may reinforce the patient's illness behaviour. To this end a number of manoeuvres and distraction tests – which can easily be incorporated into the standard back examination – have been developed:

- Pain on gently touching or pinching the back, or refusal to touch their own back because it is too painful. Superficial stimulation does not usually reproduce spinal pain.
- The patient localizes the position of greatest pain to different points at the beginning and end of the consultation.
- Reproduction of symptoms by direct downward pressure on the patient's head.
- Reproduction of symptoms by trunk rotation with the patient's arms by their side, i.e. hip rotation.
- Pressure on the hamstrings during the bowstring test. This does not compromise the nerves and should therefore not recreate nerve root symptoms.
- The patient is unable to toe touch by flexing the spine in the standing position but can do so with legs straight when sitting on the examination couch (*Figure 30.25*).

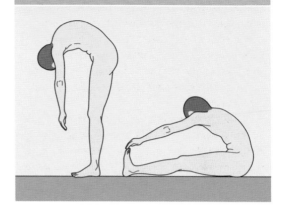

Figure 30.25.
Testing for functional back pain.

- The flip sign – The patient has a very positive straight leg raise but can sit up from a supine position without flexing the hips or knees. This is impossible in the presence of nerve root irritation as the tests are identical but merely have different starting points.
- Hoover test – The examiner places one hand behind the patient's heel while the patient attempts to straight leg raise on the contralateral side. The absence of downward pressure on the examiner's hand suggests that the patient is not making a significant effort to lift their leg.

31 Peripheral nerve injuries

Introduction

Peripheral nerve lesions present a difficult problem for the inexperienced observer as they do not necessarily provide a rational pathway to diagnosis. With the benefit of experience, however, recognizable classical diagnostic patterns emerge. The characteristic posture resulting from the nerve lesion is visible on inspection with the patient at rest, and abnormal movement may be detected during activity. The skin should be inspected and palpated for vasomotor changes, and motor and sensory testing should be carried out.

Posture

Certain nerve lesions produce characteristic postures:

- Winging of the scapula (p. 412) results from palsy of the accessory or long thoracic nerves.
- Horner's syndrome – drooping of the upper eyelid, enophthalmos, hemifacial absence of sweating; small pupillary diameter – is associated with avulsion or compression of the T1 spinal segment.
- The 'waiter's tip' (p. 413) results from rupture of the upper trunk of the brachial plexus – Erb's palsy.
- Wrist drop (p. 414) occurs as a result of paralysis of the radial nerve.
- The 'benediction sign' occurs in median nerve palsy (p. 414), while the claw-hand occurs as a result of combined median and ulnar nerve injury (p. 416) or injury to the lower trunk of the brachial plexus.

Classification of nerve injuries

The traditional classification is that of Sir Herbert Seddon. **Neurapraxia** is a nerve that does not function but is anatomically intact. **Axonotmesis** is a nerve where the fibres have been ruptured but the nerve sheath is intact. **Neurotmesis** is a completely divided nerve.

Current emphasis, however, is on **degenerative** and **non-degenerative** lesions. Injuries causing temporary or sublethal damage to nerve cells do not cause degeneration of the neurones while more significant injuries cause degeneration of the neurone distal to the site of injury. Key signs of degeneration are the loss of pseudomotor and vasomotor function – the skin is dry and red; these signs are evident 7–10 days after injury. In long-standing denervation in the limbs, the nails should be inspected for curvature, ridging, colour change and the absence of gloss. In general the treatment of degenerative lesions is surgical and non-degenerative lesions expectant.

Non-degenerative lesions

In these lesions there is blocked conduction but the nerve is in continuity, i.e. corresponding to Seddon's neurapraxia. Pseudomotor and vasomotor function are preserved, there being no cutaneous changes. Short-term conduction blocks can result from the application of a tourniquet or from excessive pressure over a nerve trunk in an unconscious patient. It usually resolves within an hour-and-a-half of removal of the cause.

Prolonged conduction blocks result from sustained compression on a nerve by tourniquet, callus, fibrosis and scarring or from surgical retraction. It is seen in some cases of obstetric brachial plexus injury and in sciatic and femoral nerve palsy after fractures, dislocations and hip replacement.

Degenerative lesions

These lesions are caused by the rupture of nerves in an intact sheath (axonotmesis) or complete division of the nerve (neurotmesis). It is characterized by loss of pseudomotor and vasomotor function, with redness and dryness of the denervated territory. Favourable lesions result from axonotmesis and are likely to recover spontaneously. Examples are from closed traction injuries, fractures, dislocations and ischaemia. As recovery takes place, the site of a positive Tinel's sign migrates distally along the course of the nerve. (In Tinel's test the nerve is tapped along its length and the patient experiences paraesthesia in the distribution of the damaged axon, when the end of the growing axon is tapped.) A nerve regenerates at approximately 1 mm a day from the site of injury until it reaches its end organ.

Unfavourable lesions result from neurotmesis and recovery is unlikely without surgical repair. These lesions are usually the result of open injuries; non-advancement of Tinel's sign signifies such a lesion. Recent penetrating injuries or visible scars of old injuries are unfavourable signs as they often signify nerve division. In clinical practice degenerative and non-degenerative injuries can be distinguished either by exploration or by repeated clinical examination.

Motor testing

The Medical Research Council grading system is widely accepted:

- 0 – No contraction.
- 1 – Flicker or trace of contraction.
- 2 – Active movement in a plane perpendicular to gravity.
- 3 – Active movement against gravity.
- 4 – Active movement against gravity and resistance.
- 5 – Normal power.

Grade 4 covers a wide range of activity, and more powerful non-normal activity can be graded as 4A.

The examiner should observe and palpate accessible muscles and tendons during contraction to confirm function. Be aware of the possibility of substitution ('trick') movements by alternative muscles to overcome a disability, and that some muscles, particularly in the hand, have dual innervation. Look for abnormal movements and muscle wasting, and examine relevant reflexes.

Sensory testing

Ask the patient to outline the appropriate area of abnormal sensation. Detailed examination of light touch is tested using a cotton wool ball, and pain using a sterile needle. The procedures are demonstrated to the patient and they are then asked to close their eyes during the examination.

Chronic denervation may also present with ulcers and burns over the denervated area.

The cervical plexus

The cervical plexus carries predominantly sensory fibres but it contributes motor fibres to the accessory nerve and some hyoid muscles. It is anatomically convenient to consider the cervical sympathetic chain at this point although its innervation is derived from thoracic nerves.

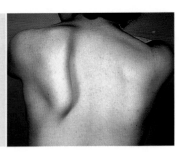

Figure 31.1.
Winging of the left scapula.

The **accessory (11th cranial) nerve** carries fibres from the third and fourth cervical nerve roots to supply the sternomastoid and trapezius muscles. It can be damaged by lesions of the posterior triangle of the neck or their surgical excision, such as biopsy of lymph nodes. The risk of damage is reduced by the use of a peroperative nerve stimulator.

When examining the patient look for scars behind the angle of the jaw and across the posterior triangle. The injury results in winging of the scapula (*Figure 31.1*) and, in long-standing cases, there is wasting of the trapezius with alteration in the contour of the lower neck and adjacent shoulder. The patient cannot shrug the shoulder on the affected side or turn their head away from the side of the injury against resistance. Palpate the sternomastoid for activity during the latter movement. There is no cutaneous sensory loss but there may be pain resulting from the injury.

The cervical sympathetic chain

Preganglionic nerve fibres passing to the head and neck are derived from the T1 spinal segment; damage to these fibres produces Horner's syndrome (*Figure 31.2*). This may accompany Klumpke's paralysis or complete brachial plexus injury (see below), penetrating neck wounds, apical lung tumours (p. 246) and surgical maneouvres such as cervical sympathectomy. The cervical sympathetic chain innervates part of the levator palpebrae superioris, and damage results in ipsilateral ptosis, also enophthalmos and a small pupil

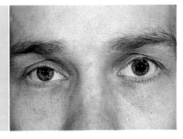

Figure 31.2.
Right Horner's syndrome following removal of a neoplasm from the right side of the neck.

(myosis), due to unopposed parasympathetic constriction. There is anhidrosis – absence of sweating – over the ipsilateral face and neck. In the case of cervical sympathectomy there is also loss of palmar sweating, as the aim of the procedure is usually to divide T2 sympathetic fibres in patients with hyperhidrosis.

The brachial plexus

The brachial plexus is deeply placed in the root of the neck but can be injured by penetrating injuries, such as in warfare, and can be avulsed, particularly in birth trauma and motorcycle accidents. Upper limb nerve injuries are more commonly of major branches of the brachial plexus, i.e. the radial, ulnar and median nerves.

Injuries of the nerve roots may result from complete avulsion of the brachial plexus or be confined to the upper (Erb's palsy) or lower (Klumpke's paralysis) roots. In complete brachial plexus paralysis the limb is flail and there is loss of sensation of the hand, forearm and lower arm. An associated Horner's syndrome indicates T1 damage. The latter, together with severe pain, and an avulsion rather than a compression injury, all carry a poor prognosis of recovery.

Erb's paralysis

This lesion is an injury of the fifth and sixth cervical nerve roots resulting from forced lateral flexion of the neck and depression of the shoulder, either in the fetus during labour or, in the adult, from motorcycle accidents. The characteristic posture is the waiter's tip position *(Figure 31.3)*. The patient cannot abduct the shoulder or flex the elbow, and wrist extension is weak. Hand movements are normal.

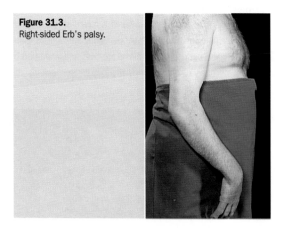

Figure 31.3.
Right-sided Erb's palsy.

Klumpke's paralysis

This is a lesion of the eighth cervical and first thoracic nerve roots, resulting from forced abduction and traction of the arm, such as during a difficult labour, or a violent upward pull, such as grabbing at a structure when falling from a height. The intrinsic muscles of the hand are paralysed but the shoulder and elbow motor function is relatively preserved. The ulnar border of the forearm and hand have reduced or absent sensation and are liable to trophic injury. If the T1 nerve has been avulsed from the spinal cord, there is an associated Horner's syndrome but this is absent if the root is damaged distal to the nerve root canal.

The **suprascapular nerve** is a branch of the C5 nerve root, supplying supraspinatus and infraspinatus muscles. The former initiates abduction and abducts and externally rotates the shoulder against resistance. The infraspinatus muscle is an external rotator of the shoulder. There is visible wasting in the supraspinatus and infraspinatus fossae, and reversal of the normal rhythm when the patient attempts to abduct the shoulder, i.e. shoulder abduction commences with rotation of the scapula. The supraspinatus fossa should be palpated while the patient abducts the arm against resistance, to detect the presence of any muscle contraction.

The **axillary nerve** can be torn or compressed in dislocation of the shoulder, in fracture of the neck of the humerus and, occasionally, in fracture of the scapula. The deltoid muscle is severely wasted and there is reduction of the power of abduction of the shoulder. Note, however, that if the suprascapular nerve is intact it is possible for a muscular individual to fully abduct the shoulder. To avoid 'trick' movements the arm must be held to the trunk when testing. In acute injuries, such as a recent dislocation, pain prevents motor testing, and sensory examination is of particular importance. The 'regimental patch' area over the attachment of the deltoid has reduced sensation.

The **musculocutaneous nerve** is at risk from lacerations of the arm, shoulder dislocation and at operation where the conjoint tendon is divided in the anterior approach to the shoulder joint. The biceps, coracobrachialis and brachialis muscles are paralysed and elbow flexion is reduced or eliminated. There is decreased sensation over the radial border of the forearm.

The **nerve to serratus anterior (long thoracic nerve of Bell)** is formed from the C5, C6 and C7 roots and may be damaged by heavy lifting or during radical mastectomy. The serratus anterior is the only muscle responsible for protracting the scapula. The muscle is observed and palpated when the patient pushes against a wall with outstretched hands. Normally the inferior pole of the scapula is drawn forwards by the serratus anterior but winging occurs when there is gross weakness. To differentiate between scapular winging from serratus anterior and trapezius weakness, ask the patient also to shrug their shoulders against resistance. This movement is absent with paralysis of the trapezius.

The **thoracodorsal nerve to latissimus dorsae** is sometimes damaged with radical mastectomy. There is usually surprisingly little abnormality, in view of the size of the muscle. The only movement to be lost is forced adduction of the shoulder joint. Grasp the muscle belly just below the inferior angle of the scapula and assess for muscle contraction when the patient is asked to cough.

The **radial nerve** is motor and sensory to the dorsal compartments of the arm and forearm. It divides at the elbow into the sensory superficial radial nerve and the motor posterior interosseous nerve. It is often injured in fractures of the shaft of the humerus and can be damaged at the axilla by an axillary crutch or by sleeping with the arm hanging over the back of a chair, usually when in an inebriated condition ('Saturday night palsy').

The characteristic posture is a wrist drop *(Figure 31.4)*. If the lesion is above the junction of the upper and middle third of the humerus, the power of the triceps is also lost. Ask the patient to extend the elbow against resistance; the bellies of the triceps are palpated to detect contraction.

If the lesion is in the midshaft of the humerus, the triceps and brachioradialis remain functional. The brachioradialis muscle is tested by asking the patient to flex the elbow against resistance with the arm in the pronated or midprone position; the brachioradialis can be palpated if it is innervated.

A lesion of the posterior interosseous nerve does not cause typical wrist drop because the radial wrist extensors are supplied by the radial nerve prior to the division into posterior interosseous and superficial radial. There is weakness, however, of finger and thumb extension and supination; wrist extension is accompanied by radial deviation.

The **median nerve** has no branches above the elbow. It supplies all the forearm flexor muscles except the flexor carpi ulnaris and part of the flexor digitorum profundus. In the hand the nerve supplies the thenar muscles and the first and second lumbricals. Its cutaneous supply is to the thumb and radial two-and-a-half fingers anteriorly and posteriorly as far proximally as the middle phalanx. The nerve is subject to injury through elbow dislocation, fractures and misplaced cubital injections, and at the wrist from carpal tunnel compression, lacerations and dislocations.

The median nerve controls coarse movements of the hand and the grip. In all injuries, regardless of level, the patient is unable to pick up a pin with thumb and index finger. This is partly due to sensory loss, and in part due to denervation of the flexor pollicis longus and the flexus digitorum profundis to the index finger if the lesion is above the mid forearm (anterior interosseous branch). A recent injury is easily missed on cursory inspection.

In lesions at or above the cubital fossa there is loss of flexion of the interphalangeal joints of the index finger. This can be demonstrated by Ochsner's clasping task, in which the patient clasps the hands firmly together – the affected index finger fails to flex due to denervation of the flexor digitorum sublimus.

Flexion of the terminal phalanx and abduction of the thumb are abolished but require specific testing to exclude movement by the adductor pollicis, interossei and extensor muscles. In long-standing lesions, the wasting of the muscles of the thenar eminence *(Figure 31.5)* and the unopposed action of extensor pollicis longus (supplied by the radial nerve) and the abductor pollicis (supplied by the ulnar nerve) turn the thumb, so its palmar surface lies in the same plane as the rest of the hand – the simian hand or ape-like thumb. Also, the outstretched index finger, together with flexion of the other fingers, produces a priest-like 'benediction attitude' *(Figure 31.6)* when the hand is held up with the palm facing forward.

Sensory loss is initially over the area of innervation although this can vary and later be reduced by cutaneous overlap. Elbow injuries of the nerve are also accompanied by trophic changes of the pulp of the digits, particularly the

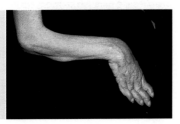

Figure 31.4.
Wrist drop from a radial nerve palsy.

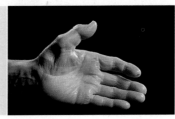

Figure 31.5.
Median nerve injury demonstrating wasting of the thenar muscles in a patient with a carpal tunnel syndrome.

Figure 31.6.
Median nerve injury demonstrating the 'benediction sign'.

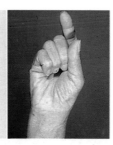

Figure 31.7.
Ulnar nerve palsy of the right hand demonstrating Froment's sign.

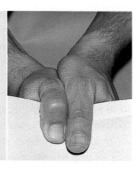

Figure 31.8.
Ulnar nerve palsy showing wasting of the hypothenar muscles of the left hand.

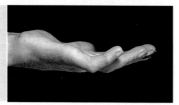

thumb and index finger. Median nerve injuries of the wrist produce thenar muscle weakness and hand sensory loss, as at the elbow, but the long flexor muscles are spared.

The **ulnar nerve** supplies the flexor carpi ulnaris and the flexor profunda digitorum in the forearm and the hypothenar, interossei, adductor pollicis and the third and fourth lumbrical muscles in the hand. Its sensory supply is to the anterior and posterior aspects of the medial one-and-a-half fingers. Ulnar nerve injuries, like those of the median nerve, can be considered to occur at the elbow and wrist since the muscle bulk of the upper arm and forearm protect the nerves in these areas.

At the level of the elbow joint the ulnar nerve lies behind the medial epicondyle and is subject to repeated trauma, as well as injury from fractures and their resultant callus. At this level the nerve is also subject to compression by aponeurotic bands and is stretched over the epicondyle in cubitus valgus deformities of the elbow joint. Lesions at or above this level present with pain along the medial aspect of the forearm and hand, weakness of the medial deep forearm flexor muscles and loss of fine movements of the hand. Paralysis of the flexor digitorum profundus allows unopposed hyperextension of the metacarpophalangeal joints of the little, ring and sometimes middle fingers. The tendon and adjacent muscle belly of the flexor carpi ulnaris is palpable just proximal to its attachment of the pisiform bone. Contraction can be assessed by flexing the fingers against resistance or resting the back of the forearm and hand on a table and asking the patient to flex and ulnar deviate the wrist.

Interossei weakness may be demonstrated by failure to grip paper between the fingers or pinch a sheet of paper between thumb and fingers. Froment's sign *(Figure 31.7)* assesses the adductor pollicis which is the only thenar muscle supplied by the ulnar nerve. The patient is asked to grip a sheet of paper with both thumbs placed alongside each other on top of the sheet. When this grip is increased, in ulnar nerve paresis there is flexion of the interphalangeal joint as tension in the flexor pollicis longus is increased to compensate for the weak adductor.

With ulnar nerve lesions at the level of the wrist joint, the long medial flexors are spared but paralysis of the small muscles of the hand is as described. The dorsal cutaneous nerve of the ulna arises 5 cm above the wrist and may be spared with lacerations of the wrist involving the main trunk. There is, therefore, preservation of sensation of the dorsal medial aspect of the hand to the level of the mid phalanx of the little and ring fingers.

In long-standing ulnar nerve lesions there is considerable wasting of the forearm and hand muscles *(Figure 31.8)* as evidenced by the flattening of the inner border of the forearm, loss of the bulk of the hypothenar eminence and, particularly, the loss of the bulk of the interossei. The latter is best seen on the back of the hand by the hollowing between the metacarpal bones. The little finger is held in abduction. This is more evident when the patient is asked to extend the finger, and is due to the unopposed action of the extensor muscles, which also abduct the little finger.

The **ulnar claw-hand** is considered with the claw-hand below.

Rapid methods for demonstrating injury of a major nerve of the upper limb

Key signs of major upper limb nerve injury are:

- Wrist drop in radial nerve damage.
- Ochsner's clasping test for median nerve injury.
- Froment's sign for ulnar nerve injury.

If fractures or other injuries prevent these tests being undertaken, examine for touch and/or pinprick sensation in the hand. This is for loss over the dorsal aspect of the metacarpal bone of the thumb (radial nerve), the thenar eminence (median nerve) or the medial aspect of the palm (ulnar nerve).

Claw hand (Main-en-griffe)

The term claw-hand describes the deformity produced by paralysis of all the small muscles of the hand. The long flexor and extensor muscles – acting unopposed by the lumbricals and interossei – hyperextend the metacarpophalangeal joints but extend the proximal and distal interphalangeal joints. The claw appearance is accentuated by interosseous muscle wasting.

Clawing of the little and ring fingers occurs with ulnar nerve injuries at the wrist – the ulnar claw-hand. The preservation of the first and second lumbricals – supplied by the median nerve – alters the tension of the flexor and extensor tendons along the index and middle fingers. In lesions of the ulnar nerve at the elbow joint and above, additional paralysis of the little and ring finger tendons of the flexor digitorum profundus prevents flexion at the interphalangeal joints and produces the **ulnar nerve paradox**: the higher the lesion, the less the deformity.

The diseases giving rise to the true claw-hand include:

- Lesions of both median and ulnar nerves (including leprosy).
- Lesions of the medial cord of the brachial plexus.
- Klumpke's paralysis.
- Anterior poliomyelitis.
- A number of neurological conditions, including syringomyelia (*Figure 31.9*), progressive muscular atrophy, polyneuritis and amyotrophic lateral sclerosis (a form of motor neuron disease).

Non-neurological causes of the condition include:

- Late and severe Volkmann's ischaemic contracture.
- The end result of a neglected suppurative tenosynovitis of the ulnar bursa.
- Advanced and untreated rheumatoid arthritis.

Nerves of the lower extremity

Femoral nerve injuries are uncommon but may be due to missile or knife wounds, or retraction during total hip replacement. The nerve can also be the site of a diabetic neuropathy and is temporarily but dramatically involved in the rare event of a spontaneous retroperitoneal haemorrhage, presenting as a mass in the loin, in patients with blood dyscrasias and those on anticoagulants. The resultant disability is marked since the denervated and wasted quadriceps is an essential extensor and stabilizer of the knee joint. The patient is unable to extend the knee when sitting over the edge of the examination couch.

There is some loss of hip flexion (iliopsoas; pectineus) and loss of sensation over the front and medial side of the thigh, leg and foot (anterior and medial femoral cutaneous, and saphenous nerves).

The **lateral cutaneous nerve of the thigh** may be compressed as it passes through the lateral aspect of the inguinal ligament or occasionally through the fascia lata. There is hyperaesthesia over the lateral upper thigh, and tingling pain in this region is worse on standing or walking but relieved by sitting. The condition is termed **meralgia paraesthetica**.

The sciatic nerve

Morphologically the sciatic nerve (*Figure 31.10*) is made up of two components, the tibial and common peroneal nerves,

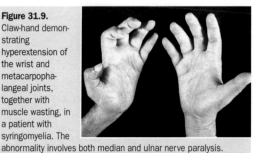

Figure 31.9.
Claw-hand demonstrating hyperextension of the wrist and metacarpophalangeal joints, together with muscle wasting, in a patient with syringomyelia. The abnormality involves both median and ulnar nerve paralysis.

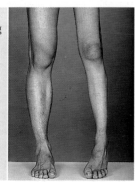

Figure 31.10.
Left sciatic nerve palsy showing wasting of the posterior thigh and all lower leg muscle groups. There is also disuse atrophy of the quadriceps and an equinus deformity of the foot.

respectively innervating the anterolateral and posterior muscle groups. The two components usually divide just above the popliteal fossa. This may be within the popliteal fossa or the components may remain separate throughout their course and be damaged independently in proximal lesions. The sciatic nerve may be damaged by missile and bullet wounds. It is also susceptible to trauma in posterior dislocation of the hip joint. Complete lesions cause paralysis of all muscles below the knee joint, and sensory loss over the lower leg and foot. A distal injury may spare the nerves supplying the hamstrings and allow some knee flexion.

The **tibial nerve** is the larger terminal division of the sciatic nerve. Division produces paralysis of the deep and superficial calf muscles and the intrinsic muscles of the sole of the foot. There is loss of plantar flexion of the ankle and toes and the patient cannot stand on tip toe. The foot is held in calcaneovalgus by the unopposed action of the extensors and everters. The disability is great and the patient has a pronounced limp due to the difficulty in 'taking off' from the affected foot. In time the disability in walking becomes less, owing to contracture of the calf muscle. The ankle jerk is absent.

An injury near the ankle denervates the small muscles of the sole, and the unopposed action of the long flexor and extensor muscles produces a highly arched foot. Sensory loss is over the sole of the foot and, if the injury is proximal to the origin of the sural nerve, there is also loss of sensation over the lateral side of the leg and foot.

The **common peroneal nerve** is the most frequently injured in the leg, often associated with fractures of the neck of the fibula or a badly fitting leg plaster. It is also subject to common peroneal nerve entrapment as the nerve winds round the neck of the fibula deep to the tendinus arch of origin of the peroneus longus. Division produces paralysis of the anterior and lateral compartments of the leg below the knee and the short extensors of the toes. The power of dorsiflexion (extensor muscles) and eversion (peroneal muscles) is lost, the foot drops and becomes inverted. There is a slapping gait and excess pressure on the outer side of the foot. The toe of the shoe is scuffed. There is sensory loss over the medial side of the dorsum of the foot.

The common peroneal nerve divides within the proximal part of the peroneus longus muscle into superficial and deep components. Injury to the **superficial peroneal (musculocutaneous) nerve** paralyses the peroneal muscles and the foot becomes inverted. There is sensory loss over the medial part of the dorsum of the foot. Injury to the **deep peroneal nerve** paralyses the tibialis anterior and other anterior compartment muscles, and the foot becomes inverted due to the unopposed action of the tibialis posterior. There is sensory loss between the first and second toes.

Diabetic neuropathy

Diabetic neuropathy *(Figure 31.11)* can affect every nerve in the body but it is of particular surgical importance in the feet. The motor neuropathy predominantly affects the small muscles of the foot, producing unopposed action of the long flexor and extensor tendons. This leads to a high medial arch of the foot and a 'cock up' deformity of the toes. The high arch increases the pressure on the heads of the first and second metatarsals, and this, together with the sensory neuropathy in the foot, leads to unfelt damage and perforating ulcers of the forefoot. The bent hammer toes are also subject to pressure necrosis in non-capacious footwear. Autonomic paralysis produces dry, vasodilated skin. This pinkness can give a false impression of a good blood supply, whereas these patients are, in fact, subject to arterial disease and also have an increased susceptibility to infection (p. 371).

Rapid methods for demonstrating injury of the major nerves of the lower limb

- Knee extension is lost in femoral nerve injury.
- Ankle flexion is lost in tibial nerve injury.
- Ankle extension is lost in common peroneal nerve injury.

Flexion and extension can also be assessed from movements of the big toe but first ensure that this is not the site of hallux rigidus. If fractures and pain from other injuries prevent motor testing, sensation is lost over the heel in tibial nerve injuries and over the dorsum of the foot with injuries of the common peroneal nerve.

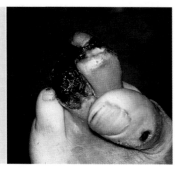

Figure 31.11.
Diabetic neuropathic foot. There is marked deformity and distal gangrene.

Entrapment and other specific injuries

Nerve entrapment denotes progressive, localized pressure on a nerve in an anatomical tunnel, usually near a joint. Ulnar nerve and common peroneal nerve entrapment and meralgia paraesthetica have already been referred to. Other common syndromes are carpal tunnel (p. 451), tarsal tunnel (p. 494), thoracic outlet (p. 366) and Morton's, i.e. Morton's metatarsalgia (p. 495).

Nerve damage may be caused by the inadvertent **injection** of drugs and noxious substances around nerves, this being particularly pertinent to the cubital fossa. **Radiation neuritis** is a late sequel of radiotherapy and is most commonly seen in the brachial plexus after treatment for breast neoplasia. The neuritis presents with severe pain rather than motor or sensory loss and can be very refractive to treatment. A **post-traumatic neuroma** presents with pain and there may be a palpable nodule. The neuroma is usually sited at the level of the injury, often with an overlying scar. The regenerating nerve ends have failed to enter the distal nerve sheath and produce a fibrous mass. A positive Tinel's sign may be present over the neuroma.

Certain nerve injuries are characterized by subsequent pain, often of a severe, intractable nature. Of particular note are avulsion injuries of the brachial plexus but severe pain may also accompany damage to sensory nerves, particularly the sural and superficial radial nerves.

Amputees may suffer **phantom limb** symptoms localized to the amputated part. The sensation varies from an awareness, to severe pain, localized to the missing limb. The pain may be a continuation of a pre-operative symptom but, more commonly, the symptom is seen in young individuals with traumatic amputation.

Causalgia was initially described as a sequel of severe nerve injuries incurred as war wounds, presenting with severe burning pain over the denervated area or beyond the usual distribution of the nerve. Subsequent studies in civilian prac-

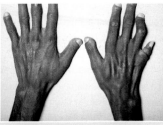

Figure 31.12. Tuberculoid leprosy. Motor neurone damage is present with extensive wasting of the small muscles of the right hand. The deformity of the hand, particularly noted in the ring and little fingers, is due to repeated trauma of the insensitive limb.

tice have shown that even minor nerve injuries may be associated with marked pain and sensitivity, and accompanying autonomic changes. The hypersensitivity is to light touch and particularly to pressure. The symptoms are accentuated by noise and surrounding hyperactivity. Pinprick and cold and hot stimuli, however, are well tolerated and do not precipitate the symptoms.

The vasomotor signs are a shiny, thin, red, dry skin with subcutaneous wasting and curved nails, which grow rapidly. **Reflex sympathetic dystrophy** is one of a number of names that have been applied to the syndrome, including algodystrophy, sympathetic neurovascular dystrophy and post-traumatic neurovascular pain. The terms **Sudeck's atrophy** or **Sudeck's syndrome** are used to describe the late onset of osteoporosis in denervated regions. This may be due to disuse or to autonomic neurovascular changes.

Allodynia is the perception of pain when a normal stimulus is applied.

Hyperpathia or **hyperalgesia** is the perception of disproportionately severe pain when a painful stimulus is applied. There may be associated components in causalgia or reflex sympathetic dystrophy.

For **neurofibromas** see p. 149, for leprosy (*Figure 31.12*) see p. 000 and for spinal injury see p. 110.

32 Bones and fractures

Introduction

Long bones in the body consist of an epiphysis at each end, a metaphyseal region next to the epiphysis and a diaphysis or shaft connecting the two ends. The outer portion of the bone is made of dense cortical bone, which is thickest in the diaphysis. The ends of the bone are composed of honeycombed cancellous bone, supported on the outside by a relatively thin cortex.

The examination of a bone in the extremities begins with **inspection** of the bone including exposure of the joint above and below. Any angular, rotational or size deformity is noted first. The soft tissues overlying the bone are inspected for the presence of scars (surgical or otherwise), signs of inflammation, swelling or colour change. **Palpation** of the bone begins with definition of the normal bone landmarks and any deformity of these. The skin temperature is compared to the opposite limb and the presence of oedema noted. Tenderness is elicited by digital pressure and percussion. The presence of **abnormal** movement and crepitus of the bone may suggest a fracture. The neurovascular status of the limb is assessed and finally the neighbouring joints are examined. This is summarized by remembering '**Look, Feel, Move.**' The final part of the examination is that of a radiograph but this must be preceded by a careful history and clinical examination.

Fractures

Fractures are caused when a force applied to the bone exceeds its ability to dissipate that force. This results in a discontinuity in the trabeculae in the bone, which is obvious if it is on the cortical aspect of the bone but may be more subtle if the fracture occurs in cancellous bone. Forces that greatly exceed normal physiological loads cause fractures. In pathological fractures, the strength of the bone is so weakened by disease that little or no violence causes fracture.

Displacement of the fracture refers to the abnormal orientation of the distal part in relation to the proximal. This may occur by translation medially, laterally, anteriorly or posteriorly, or by rotation, shortening, distraction and angulation.

Angulation of the fracture occurs when the distal fragment is tilted and is commonly referred to by the direction of tilting of the distal fragment, e.g. dorsally or medially. Traditionally, angulation was described by the direction of the point of the angulation but this is now used less commonly. The involved limb must be fully exposed by removal or cutting away clothing, and exposing the whole limb.

The early signs of a recent fracture
Inspection
The displaced long bone fracture is usually obvious to the patient and the clinician. Undisplaced fractures, fractures involving joints and carpal or tarsal fractures are more difficult to diagnose. The local physical signs on inspection include swelling, bruising, deformity and loss of function. Swelling and bruising are common in both soft tissue injuries and fractures and are not diagnostic of either; for example ankle sprains and ankle fractures present with pain, swelling and bruising. Deformity of the bone usually implies that there is displacement of the fracture and several typical patterns are seen in the hip with shortening and external rotation of the leg (p. 470) or the distal radius with dorsal and radial displacement (*Figure 32.1*). The presence of deformity should be confirmed by comparison with the uninvolved side. Loss of function is often one of the few signs of a fracture in the young child who has been noticed by the parents not to be using a limb after a fall. The patient resists any movement of the limb to avoid further pain from the fracture site.

A fracture is termed **compound** (p. 486; *Figure 39.5*) when there is an adjacent skin wound; this greatly increases the risk of subsequent infection and requires emergency treatment. Wounds are most commonly classified by the Gustilo and Andersson classification, which is best graded after operative exploration of the wound:

- Grade I – Less than 1 cm with minimal skin and soft tissue contusion.
- Grade II – Greater than 1 cm with skin and soft tissue contusion but without loss of muscle or bone. This grade should be applied when a wound occurs over a

deep muscle mass in association with a fracture, e.g. the femur.

- Grade III – A large and severe open wound with extensive skin and subcutaneous contusion, muscle crush and bone comminution. Subdivided into:
  IIIa – A comminuted fracture but the bone is covered by periosteum.
  IIIb – Loss of periosteal cover over the bone.
  IIIc – Fractures with major blood vessel injury.

Palpation

Palpation of the limb follows inspection. The skin and soft tissues may exhibit warmth from the fracture haematoma. Localized tenderness over the bone at one place is a very valuable sign; it may be the only sign of a crack fracture or greenstick fracture (see below). Palpation over a fracture may elicit **crepitus**, the grating of bone fragments against each other. Although this is diagnostic, as it is usually painful, local tenderness should avoid the need to demonstrate the sign. If the bone is subcutaneous, e.g. the tibia, then the entire length is palpated with the index finger and the patient's expression is observed for signs of pain. This may be the only positive finding in a child with an undisplaced fracture. If the bone is deeply placed, the bone is palpated by gently squeezing the affected part between finger and thumb; deformity of the bone may be palpated in this way. Finally, the extremity should be assessed for signs of vascular (p. 421) and neurological injury.

Move

If the fracture is painful the patient is usually unwilling to move the limb and this is noted as loss of function. In the case of the leg this may mean that the patient does not bear the full weight through the leg. In upper limb fractures the patient may support the arm with the other hand to prevent any painful movement at the fracture site. If the limb has an obvious fracture no attempt should be made to move the limb to assess crepitus and abnormal movement. Although these signs are characteristic of fractures they are painful for the patient and may cause further soft tissue injury. If there is no obvious fracture the limb can be gently moved to assess function and to examine the joints above and below the site of injury (see Chapter 29).

Fractures in special circumstances
Impacted fractures

These are fractures *(Figure 32.1)* where the distal fragment of bone is driven into the proximal fracture margin. These are common in the distal radius, proximal humerus and distal femur. The diagnostic pitfall is that the symptoms and signs are more compatible with a sprain than with a fracture. However, localized bone tenderness is present and this should be an appropriate indication for a radiograph. The fracture is termed **comminuted** *(Figure 32.2)* when the bone is fragmented.

Children's fractures

The **greenstick fracture** *(Figure 32.3)* is incomplete and involves one cortex, or both, but with the periosteum intact on one side of the bone. Cortical bone in children is more elastic than in adults and therefore able to tolerate bending without complete fracture. The bone may be angulated as a result of bending – **plastic deformation**. The absence of significant movement at the fracture site usually means that loss of function is less noticeable than with a complete fracture. Fractures involving the **epiphysis** occur in children and adolescents before closure of the growth plate. The bony physis may be displaced away from its anatomical position together with the distal part of the limb. A small bony fragment and the metaphysis

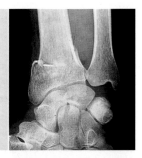

Figure 32.1.
Impacted fracture. The distal end of the radius has been driven into the shaft. Note that the radial and ulnar styloid processes are at a similar level. In the normal wrist the radial styloid should be 1 cm distal to that of the ulnar. (Cf. Figure 35.9.)

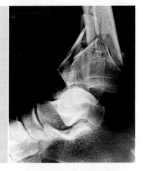

Figure 32.2.
Comminuted fracture of the lower end of the tibia and fibula.

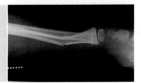

Figure 32.3.
Greenstick fracture of the left radius and ulna.

often accompany the displaced physis. The clinical appearance is identical to a bony fracture adjacent to the bone end.

Pathological fractures

These occur *(Figure 32.4)* when a bone breaks with little or no violence through a weakened area of bone. Most commonly this is as a result of a secondary bone tumour and the most common sources are the breast, bronchus, prostate, thyroid and kidney. Fractures occurring in osteoporotic or pagetic bone are also considered pathological.

Signs of complications of fractures

Fracture blisters

Untreated fractures or those associated with severe soft tissue injury may develop serous and blood-filled skin blisters *(Figure 32.5)* that usually appear 3–5 days after the injury. These are most commonly seen around the lower leg.

Arterial injury

Immediate arterial occlusion can occur from pressure or laceration from the bone fracture margin. It is associated with significant deformity and the distal pulse is usually absent together with impaired capillary circulation. If the limb is pulseless after initial reduction and splintage of the limb, arteriography may be needed to confirm the diagnosis. The complication is most often associated with high velocity injuries but should also be assessed carefully in supracondylar fractures of the humerus in children where the brachial artery is particularly at risk. Also see p. 449.

Bleeding

Substantial volumes of blood can be lost into fractures *(Figure 32.6)* – particularly the pelvis (3 L) and the femur (1.5 L) – leading to hypovolaemia and the signs of shock.

Compartment syndrome

Swelling within the confined fascial envelope around a bone may result in a rise in the compartment pressure above the capillary tissue perfusion pressure; this results in muscle ischaemia. Soft tissue injury followed by swelling and bleeding are the usual causes of a rise in compartment pressure. Swelling of a limb within a tightly constricting dressing or splint can also cause a rise in compartment pressure. The cardinal symptom is **increasing pain** despite reasonable splintage and analgesia. The most important sign is that of pain on passively stretching the involved ischaemic muscles – **stretch pain** – elicited by fully flexing and extending the joints distal to the injury. The diagnosis can be confirmed by measurement of intracompartmental pressures but must be presumed and treated on clinical grounds alone. The pulse is usually preserved unless the pressure within the compartment has reached very high levels. The long-term result of untreated muscle ischaemia is that of necrosis leading to repair by fibrosis and subsequent contracture – **Volkmann's ischaemic contracture** *(Figure 32.7)*. This presents in the forearm with wasting of the muscles and clawing of all of the fingers that are relieved by flexing the wrist. Also see pp. 368 and 380.

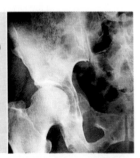

Figure 32.4.
Pathological fracture of the superior pubic ramus, through a metastatic deposit.

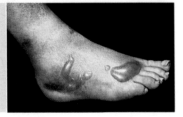

Figure 32.5.
Fracture blisters in a patient with a fracture of the right calcaneum.

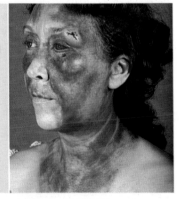

Figure 32.6.
Haematoma associated with a facial fracture. Blood loss can be one or more litres in a major fracture, and this may be concealed, as in fractures of the pelvis and thigh.

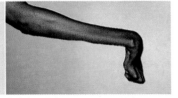

Figure 32.7.
Volkmann's ischaemic contracture of the right forearm and hand.

Nerve injuries

Nerves adjacent to the fracture are most likely to be stretched or compressed – neurapraxia or axonotmesis. Also see p. 411.

Adult respiratory distress syndrome

This syndrome (*Figure 32.8*) is a form of respiratory failure resulting from aspiration, sepsis, shock and particulate emboli.

Fat emboli

The aetiology of this disorder remains obscure but this is partly due the systemic release of bone marrow fat into the circulation. It is characterized by a disturbance of the mental state, tachycardia, tachypnoea, hypoxia, oliguria and upper trunk and conjunctival petechiae.

Delayed union and non-union

Union of the fracture is said to be delayed when there is still movement at the fracture site at the time one would normally expect the fracture to have united. Non-union is the absence of union after 12 months. A non-union may be hypertrophic, with abundant palpable callus, or atrophic. Persisting movement with tenderness at the fracture site is the sign of non-union. Although loss of function is usually present, a stable fibrous non-union can occur, which is functionally satisfactory, even though the bone has not united.

Malunion

Malunion (*Figure 32.9*) occurs when a fracture has not united in the anatomical position and gives rise to deformity. This may be as a result of delayed diagnosis, delayed treatment or from inadequate stabilization of the fracture.

Infection

Infection is a significant risk with any open fracture. The initial infection presents with swelling, redness of the adjacent skin and the presence of a purulent discharge. Chronic osteomyelitis may result.

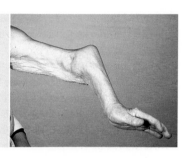

Figure 32.9.
Malunion of a left elbow fracture.

Deep vein thrombosis and pulmonary embolism

Deep vein thrombosis and pulmonary embolism (pp. 384 and 244) often result from prolonged recumbency or from fractures involving the pelvis, femur or tibia.

Reflex sympathetic dystrophy

Reflex sympathetic dystrophy follows bony injury adjacent to a joint. This often presents when mobilization of the joint is attempted at the end of plaster immobilization or internal fixation. There is initially pain, out of proportion to the injury, and stiffness in the joint. The pain is exacerbated by movement and this contributes to further stiffness. Subsequently there are changes of the skin with the presence of smooth, mottled skin. Radiographs may demonstrate widespread mottling and decalcification of the bone (*Figure 32.10*).

Myositis ossificans

Myositis ossificans is the formation of bone within muscle and is common after elbow and hip fractures and dislocations; there is pain and stiffness in the joint. Palpation of the musculature adjacent to the joint demonstrates firm masses that are opaque on radiographs.

Post-traumatic osteoarthritis

Post-traumatic osteoarthritis most commonly results from intra-articular fractures. Premature osteoarthritis develops as a result of direct injury to the articular surface.

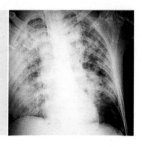

Figure 32.8.
Shock lung, following multiple injury and ventilation. There is widespread bilateral diffuse interstitial shadowing.

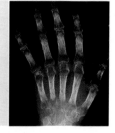

Figure 32.10.
Reflex sympathetic dystrophy (Sudeck's osteodystrophy). Rarefaction involves all joints of the left hand: the changes are particularly marked in the midcarpal region.

Infection

Infection in bone can occur by direct contamination in the case of an open fracture or by haematogenous spread. Bacterial, tubercular, spirochaetal, fungal and parasitic infections all occur though the bacterial and tubercular versions account for the majority.

Acute osteomyelitis

In children

Acute osteomyelitis occurs most frequently in childhood as a result of blood-borne spread. The source of infection may be introduced through a trivial lesion such as a skin abrasion or cutaneous abscess. The infection settles in bone at a region of rich blood supply, usually the metaphysis of a long bone. The most common region is the metaphysis adjacent to the knee. Less commonly in infants the infection settles in the epiphysis.

The patient may present with a pyrexia and malaise or may only be vaguely unwell. The child may be able to point to the involved area though in infants this is not usually the case. Local swelling may be seen but erythema is a late sign. The local area should be palpated for heat though metaphyseal tenderness is the most reliable sign. Palpable swelling is indicative of subperiosteal pus, and fluctuance suggests a subcutaneous abscess. There is often loss of function of the neighbouring joint, which may have a sympathetic effusion, but in neglected cases penetration of infection into the joint can cause a septic arthritis. Initial radiographs are normal.

In adults

Adult acute osteomyelitis usually results from open fractures. It is occasionally the result of haematogenous spread and effects the immunocompromised or IV drug abuser. The source of infection may be from arterial or venous medical monitoring lines, or from multiple venous puncture wounds; the midshaft of long bones is commonly involved. There are signs of generalized sepsis together with swelling, adjacent cutaneous erythema and a discharge at the site of injury. Localized bone tenderness and warmth are usually present.

Differential diagnosis of acute osteomyelitis

Acute septic arthritis

Although it is common to have a reactive synovitis in the presence of osteomyelitis adjacent to a joint, septic arthritis presents with considerable swelling, redness, heat and restriction of movement at the joint. Localized bony tenderness is absent.

Cellulitis

Any localized cellulitis overlying a metaphysis in a child may be from osteomyelitis and should be held to be thus until proven otherwise.

Malignant bone neoplasm

Malignant bone neoplasm can present in an identical fashion to an acute osteomyelitis and can only be confirmed by biopsy.

Fracture

The local signs of fractures in infants may be clinically very similar to acute osteomyelitis. The absence of systemic features and the radiological findings are usually conclusive.

Chronic osteomyelitis

This is shown in *Figures 32.11* and *32.12a, b*. It most frequently presents as a sequel to acute osteomyelitis associated with an open fracture. There is an area of bone that has been destroyed by the acute infection. These areas are surrounded by reactive dense sclerotic bone – **involucrum**. The incarcerated necrotic areas, the **sequestra**, act as irritants provoking a chronic discharge that escapes through **cloacae** in the involucrum and hence through a **sinus** in the soft tissues. The infection may remain dormant or asymptomatic for long periods followed by episodes of acute inflammation.

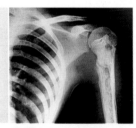

Figure 32.11.
Chronic osteomyelitis of the left humerus, showing patchy sclerotic central bone changes and subperiosteal new bone formation.

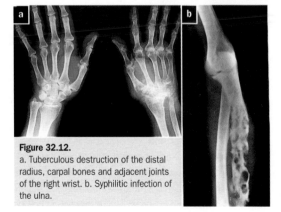

Figure 32.12.
a. Tuberculous destruction of the distal radius, carpal bones and adjacent joints of the right wrist. b. Syphilitic infection of the ulna.

Figure 32.13.
Brodie's abscess of the shaft of the fibula.

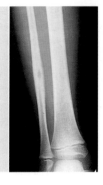

The patient presents with a history of open fracture or surgery. There is pain, redness and local tenderness. A deformity may be present from the old fracture, and a discharging sinus or healed sinuses may be apparent.

Brodie's abscess

This *(Figure 32.13)* is a localized, low-grade infection in adults presenting with intermittent episodes of pain, often worse at night, and swelling. The only sign may be deep tenderness at the site of the lesion but swelling and redness may be apparent. The most common sites are the upper and lower ends of the tibia, the distal femur and the proximal humerus. Plain radiographs demonstrate the architectural changes of the bone where the abscess is present.

Generalized bone disease

Osteoporosis

Osteoporosis (p. 407; *Figure 30.22a*) is a decrease in density of greater than 2.5 standard deviations below the mean of an age and sex matched normal population. Localized osteoporosis results from immobilization or disuse. Generalized osteoporosis occurs with advancing age. Skeletal mass decreases in both men and women from the third decade onwards and the hormonal changes after the menopause or oophorectomy lead to an increased rate of bone loss in women.

Individuals suffer loss of height and a stooped spine as a result of vertebral collapse. Osteoporotic fractures most commonly affect the vertebral bodies, hip and distal radius.

Paget's disease of bone

This is a chronic bone dystrophy and 90% of cases are multifocal. There is an association with viral infection but the aetiology has not been demonstrated with certainty. It occurs more often in men than in women and usually occurs beyond

the age of 40. The lumbar vertebrae and sacrum, skull and pelvis are most commonly affected though the limb bones *(Figure 32.14a–c)* may also be involved.

The majority of patients are asymptomatic. Patients may suffer bone pain and tenderness, bowing of the lower limbs and an increase in skull size which may become clinically apparent because of blindness or deafness resulting from nerve compression.

Pathological fracture can occur through the involved areas, particularly a transverse fracture through the upper end of the femur. Malignant change to osteosarcoma, fibrosarcoma or occasionally chondrosarcoma infrequently occurs; the prognosis in these circumstances is very poor. Osteoarthritis results in adjacent joints from abnormal stresses caused by bone deformity. High output cardiac failure is described as a result of the highly vascular nature of the bone although it is very uncommon.

In 10% of cases the disease is monostotic and it is usually the tibia or femur that is involved with bowing. The diagnosis is confirmed by radiographs demonstrating deformity, cystic changes and stress fractures. Also see p. 43.

Fibrous dysplasia

This is a benign fibro-osseous abnormality of bone of unknown aetiology. It normally affects a single bone but can be multifocal. Most often the ribs, jaw, femur or tibia are

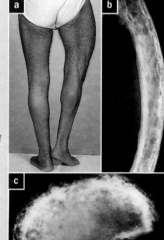

Figure 32.14.
a. Paget's deformity of the right femur, showing lateral bowing, most marked in the upper third. b. Paget's disease of the left femur, showing sclerotic changes and bowing. c. Paget's disease of the skull.

affected. In multifocal cases the femur and tibia are affected together with other bones.

Albright's syndrome is multifocal fibrous dysplasia together with associated precocious puberty and *café au lait* skin patches.

Osteomalacia

In osteomalacia *(Figure 32.15)* there is inadequate bone mineralization, and a large amount of unmineralized osteoid is present. It results from an inadequacy of vitamin D, from dietary deficiency, gastrointestinal disorders or renal osteodystrophy. In children it is known as rickets *(Figure 32.16)*. The abnormal bone is susceptible to pathological fracture which may be a microscopic stress fracture – Looser's zones – or a fracture of both cortices. Characteristic features are enlargement of the costochondral junction, bony deformities – predominantly bowing of the legs – and retarded growth. Radiographs demonstrate biconcave vertebral bodies – 'codfish vertebrae' – and abnormal cupped physes. Pathological fracture of the femoral neck occurs in adults with osteomalacia.

Scurvy

This results from a deficiency of vitamin C, i.e. ascorbic acid. There is abnormal collagen growth and repair. Patients present with fatigue, bleeding from the gums, bruising, joint effusions and iron deficiency; radiographs may show thin cortices and trabeculae.

Osteopetrosis (marble bone disease)

This disease *(Figure 32.17)* is characterized by decreased osteoclast function leading to failure of bone resorption. The bone becomes increasingly sclerotic and the medullary canal is obliterated. The most severe group is the so-called malignant form which is an autosomal recessive condition leading to dense sclerosis obliterating medullary canals on radiographs, hepatosplenomegaly and aplastic anaemia. The 'tarda' form is an autosomal dominant and demonstrates generalized osteosclerosis. Radiographs of the spine show the 'rugger jersey' appearance. Pathological fractures occur through the abnormal bone.

Hyperparathyroidism

Von Recklinghausen's disease of bone is a rare (5%) manifestation of hyperparathyroidism *(Figure 32.18a, b)*. The symptoms are those of hypercalcaemia with muscle weakness, gastrointestinal upsets and muscle pains. Cystic degeneration of bone is due to brown tumours of localized osteoclastic resorption and may be evident on radiographs. Also see p. 226.

Ochronosis

This is a congenital defect in tyrosine and phenylalanine metabolism that causes alkaptonuria. The urine turns dark on standing and pigment is deposited in the auricular cartilages, which look bluish. The sclera and the skin over bone prominences look slate blue. Arthritic change in the spine is common.

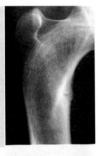

Figure 32.15.
Osteomalacia with a transverse stress fracture at the level of the lesser trochanter.

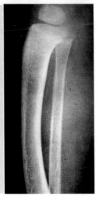

Figure 32.16.
Bowed tibia in a child with rickets.

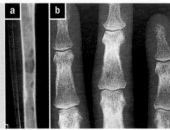

Figure 32.17.
Characteristic facial features of a patient with marble bone disease.

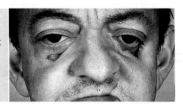

Figure 32.18.
Hyperparathyroidism. a. Cystic lesions within the tibia. b. Reabsorption of cortical bone in the phalanges.

Dwarfism

Short stature may be proportionate or disproportionate depending on whether the limbs are normal relative to the trunk size. Achondroplasia is the commonest example of short-limbed, disproportionate dwarfism. The rarer mucopolysaccharidoses give rise to proportionate dwarves. The problem is usually that of an intrinsic bone disturbance (dysplasia) or that caused by a metabolic or nutritional abnormality (dystrophy). Skeletal epiphyseal dysplasia can present in different forms of either short trunk or short limb varieties. Involvement of the spine, knees or hips should alert the examiner to the possibility of a dysplasia or dystrophy. Also see p. 43.

Achondroplasia

Achondroplasia *(Figure 32.19)* is inherited as an autosomal dominant but 80% are spontaneous mutations. The trunk is of normal length but the limbs are short. Achondroplasics have prominent foreheads and flat noses; there is often a thoracolumbar kyphosis with lumber hyperlordosis giving rise to prominent buttocks. Intelligence is normal. Adults may develop problems with spinal stenosis.

Spondyloepiphyseal dysplasia
Congenita

This is an autosomal dominant disorder characterized by a short trunk relative to the limbs with an association with cleft palate and increased lumbar lordosis. The vertebrae are flattened *(Figure 32.20)*.

Tarda

This is an X-linked recessive disorder characterized by scoliosis and abnormalities of the major joints, such as the hip, which are liable to early osteoarthritis.

Pseudoachondroplasic dysplasia

This is an autosomal dominant disorder characterized by normal facies but other features similar to achondroplasia. There is bowing of the tibia and craniocervical instability.

Multiple epiphyseal dysplasia

This is an autosomal dominant disorder characterized by short-limbed dwarfism. These may not become apparent until the early teenage years. It may present with a waddling gait because the proximal femur is often affected with bilateral irregularities of the femoral heads and concomitant abnormalities of the acetabula.

Mucopolysaccharidoses

These result from an accumulation of mucopolysaccharides resulting from an enzyme deficiency. Type 4 – Morquio's syndrome *(Figure 32.21)* – is the most common, in which there is short-limbed dwarfism together with a thickened skull, flat pelvis, coxa valga and abnormally shaped metacarpals. In particular there is instability at the atlantoaxial joint, and the child may present with progressive deterioration in walking as a result of spinal cord compression.

Osteogenesis imperfecta

This condition *(Figure 32.22a, b)* is a spectrum of the conditions where there is an abnormal cross-linking of collagen leading to decreased collagen secretion. The condition is transmitted as an autosomal dominant trait *(Figure 32.22a, b)*. The patient may suffer multiple fractures due to 'brittle' bones, short stature, scoliosis, hearing defects and ligamentous laxity. Blue sclera are seen in some of the forms. Severe forms are often fatal in infancy.

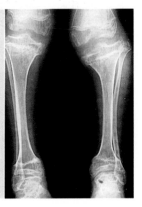

Figure 32.19.
Achondroplasia.

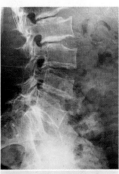

Figure 32.20.
Spondyloepiphyseal dysplasia.

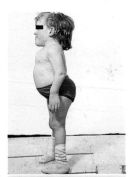

Figure 32.21.
Morquio's syndrome.
(Reproduced with permission of Mr. B. A. Taylor.)

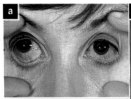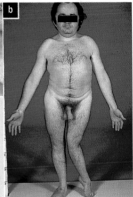

Figure 32.22.
Osteogenesis imperfecta.
a. Blue sclera. b. Limb
deformities in a patient with
brittle bone disease, showing
short stature with relative
sparing of the trunk.

Bone tumours

Palpation determines if the swelling on a bone is on one
aspect or around the whole circumference. The site of the
bone in relation to the epiphyses may help with the differential diagnosis because some tumours only arise at certain
sites, e.g. the giant cell tumour only arises in the epiphysis.
The following physical signs may help determine if the swelling
is benign or malignant (*Table 32.1*):

- **Benign** – Large; painless; normal temperature;
  slow growing.
- **Malignant** – Bone not greatly enlarged; often painful;
  warm; rapid recent growth.

Table 32.1. Tumours of bone and joints.

Origin	Benign	Malignant
Bone	Osteoid osteoma Osteoblastoma	Osteosarcoma
Bone marrow		Multiple myeloma Lymphoma
Cartilage	Osteochondroma (exostoses) Enchondroma (chondroma)	Chondrosarcoma
Fibrous tissue	Fibroma	Fibrosarcoma
Synovium	Synovioma	Malignant synovial sarcoma
Unknown aetiology	Giant cell tumour (osteoclastoma) Adamantinoma	Malignant giant cell tumour Ewing's tumour
Vascular	Haemangioma	
Other lesions	Aneurysmal bone cysts Bony dysplasias	

Benign neoplasms
Solitary (simple) bone cyst

This is a benign, non-neoplastic, unilocular, cystic lesion
(*Figure 32.23*) that occurs as a result of abnormal growth at
the epiphysis and is most commonly seen in the region of the
proximal humeral or femoral metaphyses in children and adolescents. The cyst is often seen as an incidental finding on a
radiograph. It can present with a pathological fracture occurring through the cyst. Occasionally it presents as a swelling
in the region of the metaphysis.

Osteochondroma

Osteochondroma (*Figure 32.24a*) is the most common
benign tumour. It is a bony excrescence occurring most commonly at the metaphyses of the long bones. The exostosis
(*Figure 32.24b*) may be solitary or multiple in which case it
may be associated with hereditary multiple exostoses – dia-
physeal aclasis. There is a 10% risk of sarcomatous change
in individuals with multiple lesions.

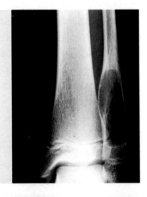

Figure 32.23.
Solitary bone cyst
of the lower end of the fibula.

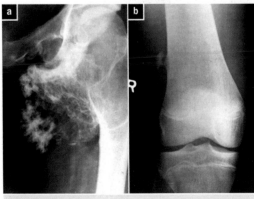

Figure 32.24.
Osteochondroma. a. A large exostosis arising from the neck of
the femur. b. Fractured exostosis of the lower end of the femur.

Enchondroma

Enchondroma *(Figure 32.25a, b)* is a benign cartilaginous lesion arising from the medullary surface, most commonly affecting the small bones of the hands and feet. The tumours may be solitary or multiple (Ollier's disease) or associated with multiple haemangiomas (Maffucci's syndrome). When phalanges are affected there is swelling and pain. Malignant transformation is rare in the solitary lesion but occurs in a small proportion of the multiple cases.

The term **chondroma** is applied to cartilaginous masses not restricted to the medulla. **Chondromyxoid fibromas** and **fibromas** are rare benign tumours made up of their defined tissue and usually presenting as incidental radiological findings. Fibromas differ from fibrous dysplasias in that there is no new bone within them.

Osteoid osteoma

Osteoid osteoma *(Figure 32.26)* is a benign lesion with a small osteoblastic centre with sclerosis, affecting the long bones or spine, and presenting with pain and tenderness in the region of the lesion. Characteristically pain is present at night and abolished by aspirin. **Osteoblastoma** *(Figure 32.27)* is a locally aggressive benign lesion of mature osteoid cells. Histological characteristics are similar to those of an osteoma but the lesion exceeds 1 cm across and may be of considerable size. Any bone can be affected but the spine and skull are common sites.

Aneurysmal bone cyst

Aneurysmal bone cyst *(Figure 32.28)* is a non-neoplastic condition affecting children and young adults, causing swelling of the long bones or vertebrae. The expanding osteolytic lesion contains a bloody fluid and may be the site of a pathological fracture.

Giant cell tumour (osteoclastoma)

This condition *(Figure 32.29a, b)* is a neoplasm of osteoclasts creating osteolytic tumours. It arises more often in the 20–40-year-old age group and occurs at the end of the long bones. The majority of tumours occur around the knee, with local swelling, heat and dilatation of superficial veins. Pathological fracture is common because of the osteolysis. Some tumours recur after excision and a small proportion are malignant from the outset.

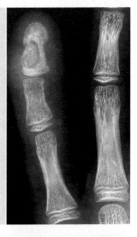

Figure 32.26.
Osteoid osteoma of the terminal phalanx of the right index finger, showing dense central bone with a lucent surround.

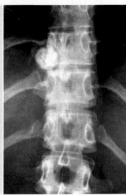

Figure 32.27.
Osteoblastoma.

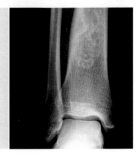

Figure 32.28.
Aneurysmal bone cyst of the lower end of the right tibia.

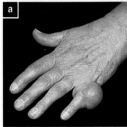
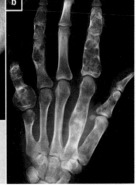

Figure 32.25.
a. Enchondroma of the left little finger. b. Multiple enchondromas (Ollier's disease).

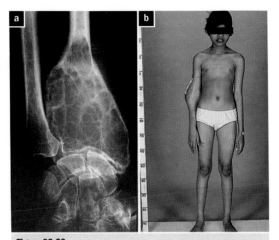

Figure 32.29.
a. Osteoclastoma of the distal radius. Note the characteristic 'soap bubble' appearance. b. Malignant change in an osteoclastoma of the right elbow region.

Malignant neoplasia

Multiple myeloma

This is the commonest primary malignant bone tumour (*Figure 32.30a, b*), which is a neoplastic proliferation of plasma cells or their precursors; it is rare before the age of 40. The common presentation of bony deposits is of pathological fractures affecting the ribs and vertebrae. The affected areas are osteolytic and the Bence Jones proteins are present. The diagnosis is confirmed on bone marrow biopsy.

Figure 32.30.
Multiple myeloma. a. Upper left femur. b. Extensive myeloma of the skull.

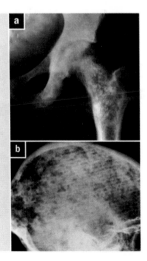

Osteosarcoma

Osteosarcoma (*Figure 32.31a, b*) is a malignant tumour in which osteoid is synthesized by sarcomatous cells. It occurs more commonly in males than females and 75% of patients are between the ages of 10 and 25; osteosarcoma in elderly patients often occurs as a complication of Paget's disease. Most sarcomas occur in the metaphyses of long bones. Many occur around the knee and the upper end of the femur and humerus. Patients present with increasing pain and swelling. Radiographs show characteristic abnormalities of the periosteum with a 'sunray' appearance of the bone and **Codman's triangle** of reactive bone at the junction with the periosteum. As with most sarcomas, spread of the tumour is usually by the bloodstream to the lungs.

Parosteal osteosarcoma

This is an uncommon malignant lesion (*Figure 32.32*) arising from the surface of the bone, often affecting the posterior surface of the distal femur, or upper tibia or humerus. There is a broad based swelling that grows and can encircle the shaft. Destruction of the cortex and medulla occurs late.

Figure 32.31.
a. Osteosarcoma of the left femur. b. Osteosarcoma commencing in the left lower humerus. Untreated tumours of this size are relatively rare in the UK.

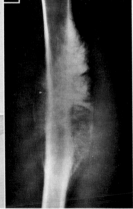

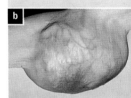

Figure 32.32.
Parosteal sarcoma of the right lower femur.

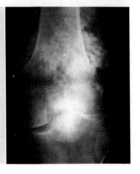

Chondrosarcoma

Chondrosarcoma *(Figure 32.33)* is a malignant neoplasia of cartilage. It occurs in an older age group than osteosarcoma, predominantly in the age range 40 to 70. About half of the lesions occur in the pelvic girdle and ribs, together with the proximal femur. The tumour may be situated within the bone or it may be on its periphery. The presentation is usually of an increasing size of a long-standing swelling in the axial skeleton. There is characteristic calcification on radiographs.

Fibrosarcoma

Fibrosarcomas *(Figure 32.34a)* are usually lytic lesions of the diaphysis or metaphysis and are of variable malignancy. **Synovial sarcomas** *(Figure 32.34b)* are usually associated with a major joint. They are highly malignant, invading locally and metastasizing to lymph nodes, as well as via the bloodstream. Both fibrosarcomas and synovial sarcomas may arise independently of bone, within muscle or subcutaneous tissues.

Giant cell tumour

This is a neoplasm of osteoclasts creating an osteolytic tumour. It arises most often in the 20–40-year-old age group and occurs at the ends of long bones. The majority of tumours occur around the knee and present with local swelling, heat and dilatation of superficial veins. Pathological fracture is also common because of the osteolysis.

Ewing's tumour

The histogenesis of this tumour *(Figure 32.35)* remains uncertain. It occurs most commonly between the ages of 5 and 20. The femur, tibia, humerus and fibula are most commonly involved but the pelvis and ribs can be affected. The tumour is usually osteolytic and penetration of the cortex, with raising of the periosteum, may give rise to a mass. The presentation is of pain and swelling of gradual onset. Fever and an elevated white cell count may simulate osteomyelitis.

Secondary neoplasia

These *(Figure 32.36a, b, c)* are the commonest bone tumours. The patient may present with a complication of the metastasis such as local pain or a pathological fracture. The most common causes are carcinoma of the breast, bronchus, kidney, thyroid and prostate.

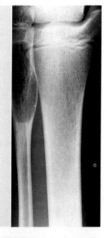

Figure 32.33.
Chondromyxosarcoma of the tibia.

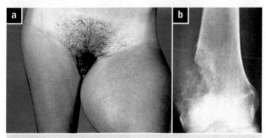

Figure 32.34.
a. Fibrosarcoma of the lower end of the left femur. b. Synovial sarcoma.

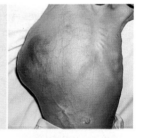

Figure 32.35.
Ewing's sarcoma arising in a rib.

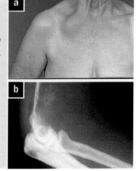

Figure 32.36.
a. Fracture through a metastasis in the right clavicle.
b. Lytic lesion due to secondary deposits from breast neoplasia.

33 Joints and muscles

Introduction

Orthopaedic nomenclature of joint movement differs slightly from descriptions in anatomical texts. The posterior surface of the forearm and hand are often referred to as the 'dorsal' surface. The anterior surface of the forearm is often referred to as the 'volar' surface and that of the palm as the 'palmar' surface. The weight-bearing surface of the foot is referred to as the 'plantar' surface and the non-weight-bearing as the 'dorsum'.

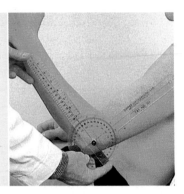

Figure 33.1.
Goniometer.

Movements

Measurement of movement of joints is recorded in degrees of motion in each direction; zero is the anatomical position. The movements should be measured using a goniometer (*Figure 33.1*). Normal movements at joints are:

- Flexion and extension at most joints are as described as movement in the sagittal plane towards or away from the ventral or dorsal surface of the limb. Movements at the ankle are referred to as plantarflexion and dorsiflexion.
- Abduction and adduction are movements in the coronal plane away from or towards the midline. These movements at the wrist are referred to as radial and ulnar deviation.
- Internal and external rotation take place around a longitudinal axis. There are joint specific rotatory movements, such as pronation and supination in the forearm, and opposition of the thumb.

Certain joints, most notably the hip, shoulder and those in the feet, have more complex descriptions of their movements. These are described in the relevant chapters.

Deformity

A **deformity** (*Figure 33.5*) of a joint occurs if the joint lies in abnormal alignment or if it lacks full movement. The deformity is usually referred to according to the position of the distal part with reference to the proximal part of the limb.

Abnormal alignment of a joint, such that if the distal part is deviated away from the midline, is referred to as a **valgus** deformity, and **varus** when the limb is deviated towards the midline at the joint. Lack of full extension at a joint is referred to as a **flexion deformity**. Kyphosis and **lordosis** (p. 397) refer to curves convex dorsally or ventrally in the spine. **Scoliosis** (p. 398) refers to abnormal curves of the spine in the coronal plane.

Dislocation (p. 450; *Figure 35.8*) of a joint is the complete loss of apposition of joint surfaces: known in former times as 'luxation'. Hence **subluxation** is the partial loss of apposition of joint surfaces.

Abnormal movement of a joint occurs when a joint can be moved in a plane in which little or no movement is normally expected. This may be due to a **ligament laxity**, which may be local or general, or due to loss of joint space in arthritis. Ligamentous laxity due to ligamentous injury is assessed by applying the appropriate stress to the joint concerned. The commonly accepted grading of ligamentous laxity is:

- 1+ denotes an increase in laxity as compared to the normal side.
- 2+ denotes an excessive amount of movement which is terminated by a firm endpoint, suggestive of partial rupture.
- 3+ denotes excessive movement with a soft or indistinct endpoint, suggestive of a complete rupture.

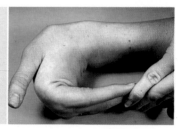

Figure 33.2.
Joint laxity.

Generalized joint laxity occurs in about 5% of the normal population. Hyperextension of the elbows, wrists, metacarpophalangeal joints and knees suggests this diagnosis. Abnormal joint laxity (*Figure 33.2*) is also associated with the rare connective tissue disorders of Marfan's and Ehlers–Danlos syndromes.

Routine examination of a joint

The elements of inspection, palpation, percussion and auscultation have been modified in orthopaedics into '**Look, Feel, Move**'. Examination of a joint should not be in isolation and should involve assessment of the whole individual and of the limb in general. The opposite joint should be examined first for comparison. The joint above and below the joint being examined need to be assessed because pain at one joint may be referred from the joint above, e.g. knee pain is often referred from the hip.

Look: If the joint to be examined is in the lower limb ask the patient to walk about so that you can observe the gait. Then observe the joint with the patient standing, looking for deformity. Look all around the joint for swelling, scars or sinuses and adjacent wasting of musculature, and look for evidence of vascular insufficiency. Measurement of leg length for hip examination, or of circumference of the upper arm or thigh for elbow or knee examination, usually take place at this time.

Feel: Ask the patient to point to any tender areas. Feel for excessive warmth of the skin. Examine for the presence of an effusion. Assess if any swelling is due to fluid, soft tissue or bone. Soft tissue swelling may be due to thickening of the synovium and capsule which can be palpated by rolling between or under the examining fingers. Define the normal bone landmarks and localize any tenderness. **Move**: Move the joint through the active range of movement followed by the maximum passive range. Feel for crepitus during this manoeuvre and document the range of movement. Examine for abnormal movement.

The arthritides

Osteoarthritis

Osteoarthritis of the knee is shown in *Figure 33.3*. Osteoarthritis is often known as osteoarthrosis because, strictly speaking, this is not primarily an inflammatory process. It is characterized by degeneration of the articular cartilage. This may be primary, resulting from a combination of age, hereditary and environmental factors, or secondary, resulting from trauma, infection or congenital disorders that increase the stresses upon the articular surfaces. It may affect one joint only or it may be widespread. There is degeneration of the articular bearing surface followed by the development of osteophytes. Subchondral sclerosis of the bone and the formation of cysts follow. Loose bodies may develop and can cause locking symptoms.

The patient complains of a painful and stiff joint. A deformity is often present due to capsule contracture or reduction in joint space. Osteophytes are often palpable and an effusion may be present. There is a decreased range of movement associated with crepitus, i.e. palpable grating.

Rheumatoid arthritis

This is the most common of the inflammatory arthritides (*Figure 33.4a, b*). The aetiology is unknown but it is likely to result from an autoimmune process. It is a polyarticular problem from the outset. Most commonly it is the hands and feet that are initially involved but the major joints of the upper and lower limb can also be affected. The primary pathological process is abnormal synovial proliferation known as pannus which is destructive to articular cartilage and bone. There are extra-articular effects of rheumatoid arthritis, such as pericarditis, and pulmonary abnormalities such as pleurisy, pulmonary nodules and fibrosis. Rheumatoid nodules may be palpable at the elbow. The disease is characterized by widespread deformity but is often most noticeable in the hands.

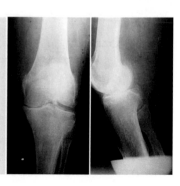

Figure 33.3.
Osteoarthritis of the knee.

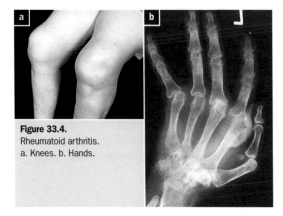

Figure 33.4.
Rheumatoid arthritis.
a. Knees. b. Hands.

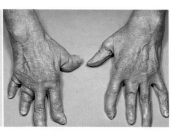

Figure 33.5.
Psoriatic arthropathy
of the hands.

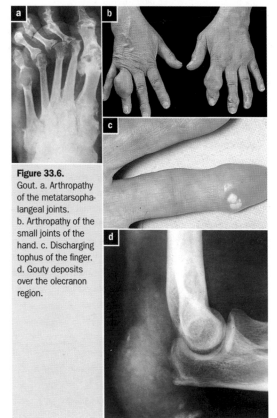

Figure 33.6.
Gout. a. Arthropathy
of the metatarsopha-
langeal joints.
b. Arthropathy of the
small joints of the
hand. c. Discharging
tophus of the finger.
d. Gouty deposits
over the olecranon
region.

Systemic lupus erythematosus

This is a chronic inflammatory arthropathy of unknown aetiology but likely to be an immunologically mediated disorder.
Women are predominantly affected. There is acute tender
swelling of the proximal interphalangeal joints, the metacarpophalangeal joints and the carpal joints of the hand; the
knee and other joints may also be involved. Extra-articular
manifestations include pyrexia, a butterfly rash of the face,
pancytopenia, pericarditis and nephritis.

Polymyalgia rheumatica

This is a disorder of elderly people and is characterized by
aching and stiffness in the shoulder and pelvic girdles. Malaise,
headache and anorexia are common. Few specific abnormalities can be found on examination but the disorder is characterized by a greatly increased erythrocyte sedimentation rate.

Ankylosing spondylitis

This is an inflammatory arthropathy involving the spine
(p. 405) and sacroiliac joints. It is often associated with anterior uveitis. There is progressive spinal pain and deformity
leading to kyphosis and spinal stiffness. Radiologically this
can result in a 'bamboo spine'. The HLA B27 is positive.

Psoriatic arthropathy

This occurs in a small proportion of patients with psoriasis.
The small joints of the hand (*Figure 33.5*) are predominantly
involved but any joint may be affected. HLA B27 is positive
in a large proportion of these patients.

Gout

Gout (*Figure 33.6a–d*) is a condition in which urate crystals
are deposited in joints due to a disorder of nucleic acid

metabolism. The synovium becomes greatly inflamed and the
joint becomes swollen and painful; it may mimic septic arthritis. It most commonly afflicts males in middle age – the great
toe metatarsophalangeal joint is the classic site. Crystals are
also deposited in gouty tophi in the helix of the ear, the eyelid
and around the elbow joint. The diagnosis is confirmed by the
presence of crystals in joint fluid. Pseudogout is similar to
gout but tends to affect the knee. Crystal analysis of joint
aspirate reveals pyrophosphate crystals, and radiographs
show evidence of calcification of the articular and semilunar
cartilages – chondrocalcinosis.

Reiter's syndrome

The condition is a sexually acquired reactive arthritis. It presents in young men with a triad of symptoms of urethritis, conjunctivitis (*Figure 33.7*) and arthritis. Usually only one joint is involved with a sudden onset of pain, heat and swelling. A large proportion of these patients are HLA B27 positive.

Septic arthritis

This occurs from either blood-borne spread, extension of juxta-articular osteomyelitis or a penetrating injury. In any joint that is hot, swollen, painful and restricted in its range of movement, septic arthritis must be presumed to be present until proved otherwise. Untreated, septic arthritis results in destruction of articular cartilage and long-term damage to the joint. The diagnosis can be confirmed by aspiration and microbiological examination of the joint fluid.

Tuberculous arthritis

This condition (*Figure 33.8*) should be suspected in otherwise unexplained monoarthropathy, especially in older patients and those from the tropics. There is marked wasting of the muscles with swelling of the joint due to synovial thickening. The tubercle bacillus can be cultured from the joint aspirate.

Haemophilia

An acute bleed into a joint causes a painful haemarthrosis (*Figure 33.9*) that presents as an acute arthritis. Recurrent attacks lead to progressive joint deformity.

Neuropathic arthropathy (Charcot's joint)

This (*Figure 33.10*) is osteoarthritis resulting from a lack of sensation in a joint. The most common cause is from diabetes mellitus causing neuropathy. Rarer causes include tabes dorsalis, syringomyelia, myelomeningocele, leprosy and congenital indifference to pain together with other neurological abnormalities. The joint is usually swollen, deformed, painless and unstable with the presence of abnormal movements. Radiographs often show advanced degenerative changes with gross destruction of the joint and multiple loose bodies.

Disorders of muscle

Muscles are subject to a large variety of disorders (*Table 33.1*). These may be subdivided into disorders of innervation, i.e. diseases of the peripheral and central nervous systems, and primary disorders of muscle, i.e. myopathies, and its attachments; myopathies may be due to primary pathology or secondary to biochemical or physiological abnormalities. The prime symptoms of muscular disorders are pain and weakness. Abnormal movements may be present and, on examination, there may be tenderness, wasting and deformity.

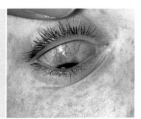
Figure 33.7. Conjunctivitis in Reiter's syndrome.

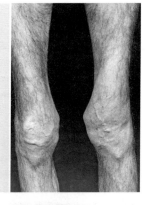
Figure 33.9. Knee joints of a patient with haemophilia showing the deformity produced by recurrent haemarthroses. Both knees are affected.

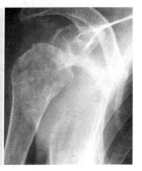
Figure 33.8. Tuberculosis of the right shoulder showing loss of normal joint contours.

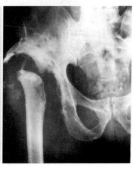
Figure 33.10. Charcot's joint of the right hip. Repeated trauma in an anaesthetic joint gives rise to gross bony and soft tissue deformity.

Table 33.1. Disorders of muscle.

Neurogenic myopathies	CNS
	  Cerebral palsy
	  Spina bifida (p. 403)
	  Poliomyelitis
	  Motor neurone disease
	  Multiple sclerosis

	Peripheral nerve injuries (p. 411)
	Disorders of neuromuscular transmission Myasthaenia gravis
Myositis	Infection Collagen disorders Idiopathic
Trauma	
Tumours	
Congenital absence of muscles	
Dystrophies	
Myotonia	
Arthrogryphoses	
Hormonal	
Metabolic	
Toxic	

Pain

Muscle pain is a common complaint and is often of unknown aetiology. It follows unaccustomed exercise, trauma, ischaemia, metabolic disorders, such as hypercalcaemia and glycogen disorders, and myositis. Muscle aches and pains also accompany many systemic diseases, particularly fevers. Painful **cramps** are known to most individuals, usually first noted in youth after excessive exercise. The incidence increases in pregnancy, uraemia and in old age, particularly at night.

Weakness

Weakness is present in most muscle disorders but varies in severity. In congenital disorders, weakness is often delayed in onset but is then progressive. In the muscular dystrophies, characteristic muscle groups are usually involved. In some metabolic disorders the weakness is periodic, whereas it is of sudden onset in inflammatory disease. There may be complete paralysis in a lower motor neurone lesion. **Fatigue** is characteristic of myasthaenia gravis and related disorders.

Wasting

Muscle wasting occurs with disuse and confinement to bed, or in any debilitating disease producing weight loss. It is most marked in lower motor neurone lesions such as a peripheral nerve injury, poliomyelitis, MS and motor neurone disease. Wasting is a characteristic feature of muscular dystrophies and is present in most myopathies. Ischaemia produces weakness and wasting, which is followed by fibrosis, with a resultant Volkmann's contracture (p. 421).

Deformity

Deformity may be due to muscular atrophy and contraction. There may also be spasm from upper motor neurone disease, swelling in myositis and abnormal posture to protect painful, or compensate for, weak muscle groups.

Abnormal movements

Abnormal movements are mostly related to diseases of the CNS. They include **tremor,** as seen in Parkinson's and cerebellar diseases, but also occur in toxic and metabolic myopathies, and after fatigue from extreme activities or cold exposure. **Athetoid movements** are characteristic of cerebral palsy while **choreiform movements** occur in Sydenham's and Huntington's choreas, and in vascular, toxic and metabolic cerebral disorders. **Myoclonic** and **tonic movements** occur in focal and generalized epilepsy, and hemiplegia, respectively.

Fasciculation

Muscle fasciculation – spontaneous muscle contraction – is usually a feature of disorders of the anterior horn cell, particularly motor neurone disease, but it can occur in thyrotoxicosis and polymyositis.

Fibrillation

Fibrillation – spontaneous contraction of small groups of muscle fibres – is an electrophysiological activity that follows muscle denervation; it cannot usually be seen through the skin but there may be a brief shimmering movement seen or felt.

As muscular disorders may be neurological as well as musculoskeletal in origin, examination must include the motor system. Initial impression is from the gait, posture, speech and a handshake. Motor assessment is of power, tone, co-ordination, reflexes, muscle wasting and abnormal movements, and the examination should include the whole body as well as the affected area. **Observe** the muscles for hypertrophy, atrophy, abnormal shape, such as tears and contractures, abnormality of surrounding tissues, such as inflammation or bruising, and abnormal movements.

Palpate individual muscles to assess their bulk, tone, texture, masses, such as haematomas, calcification and tumours, and tenderness; infiltration with fat affects tone, as does ischaemia and infarction. Tenderness may be due to inflammation, trauma or tears. **Tap** muscles to test for hyper-sensitivity, e.g. in motor neurone disease. Fasciculation may be felt as well as observed. Compare the two sides of the body visually and by measurement (p. 385; *Figure 29.4*) for muscle wasting. Palpate nerves for thickening and tap them to assess hypersensitivity and Tinel's sign (p. 411).

Active movement

Active movement of a muscle indicates its range and any painful limitation. Note the action of individual muscles, as well as muscle groups, and their agonists, checking for trick move-ments that are being made to overcome disability. Compare power on the two sides of the body and, if the history suggests, look for fatigue on repetitive movements. **Resisted** movement assesses power and discomfort while **passive** movement demonstrates abnormal mobility due to pain, joint stiffness, contractures, hypermobility, altered tone, e.g. rigidity, and spas-ticity, which may be classed like a cogwheel.

Co-ordination assesses smoothness of movement as well as direction and position sense. Inco-ordination can inter-fere with writing and eating, and produce intention tremors, loss of balance and ataxia. Abnormal movements are con-sidered above. Reflexes are reduced in lower motor nerve lesions and muscular dystrophies but may be brisk in myasthaenia and polymyositis.

Upper motor neurone lesions

These lesions are characterized by paralysis and hypotonia, giving rise to weakness, spasticity, hyper-reflexia and exten-sor plantar responses. **Extrapyramidal** lesions affect tone, co-ordination and balance, and there may be involuntary movements but usually no loss of power. **Cerebellar disor-ders** give rise to hypotonia and ataxia, while **lower motor neurone** damage produces weakness, wasting, hypotonia and areflexia.

Cerebral palsy

Cerebral palsy is usually related to a neonatal injury to the developing brain, common causes being anoxia, infection and haemorrhage. The condition has a higher incidence in pre-maturity. The motor damage results in spasticity, which involves the flexors more than the extensor muscles and leads to deformity of the limbs and spine. This may range from a minor equinus deformity of a foot to total body involvement and, correspondingly, the symptoms range from minor walk-ing difficulties to confinement to a wheelchair or a bedridden child. The lesions may be classified into spastic (usually a

monoplegia), athetoid (hemiplegia), ataxic (diplegia), atonic (quadriplegia) and rigid or mixed varieties.

Multiple sclerosis (MS)

Multiple sclerosis is a demyelinating disorder of unknown aeti-ology occurring in middle age and affecting motor and sen-sory neurones in any part of the nervous system. The lesions may be single or multiple, a common presentation being a monocular optic neuritis, producing blindness. This and other symptoms can be intermittent but there is usually slow pro-gression. Multiple sclerosis is the commonest cause of para-plegia in Europe and North America.

Motor neurone disease

This is a disease of spinal and cranial nerves and motor neu-rones. The disease has a world-wide distribution and usually occurs in middle age. The clinical picture is of weakness and wasting, commonly commencing in a single upper limb. Painful cramps are common, as well as fasciculation of affected muscles. The disease is progressive, giving rise to speech difficulties, dysarthria and respiratory distress. It is usually fatal in 2 to 4 years.

Poliomyelitis

Poliomyelitis – 'polio' – results from an infection by an enterovirus. Although rare in countries that practise routine vaccination, it is still common in the developing world and paralysis complicates 1–2% of infections. The paralysis occurs after destruction of more than 60% of the anterior horn cells, the cervical and, particularly, the lumbar enlarge-ments being susceptible. The pattern of paralysis deter-mines the subsequent joint deformity, limb contractures and spinal abnormality.

Myasthaenia gravis

Myasthaenia gravis (p. 41) is a disorder of neuromuscular innervation characterized by fatiguability. It is a congenital abnormality but is also associated with neoplastic syndromes, particularly anaplastic bronchial neoplasms. The latter, how-ever, differ from congenital myasthaenia in the loss of the long tendon reflexes.

Myositis

Inflammatory disorders of muscle comprise infective, colla-gen diseases and idiopathic types. There is pain and local-ized tenderness, which may be severe, together with the symptoms of the associated systemic disease. Acute viral infections, producing inflammatory changes in muscle,

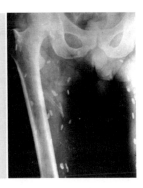

Figure 33.11. Cysticercosis. (See p. 74.) Widely distributed calcified cysts in the muscles and other soft tissues.

include influenza, Coxsackie, mumps, adenoviruses and dengue fever. Bacterial myositis usually follows trauma or ischaemia, e.g. clostridial (p. 70); acute suppurative (tropical) myositis is probably staphylococcal in origin. Other bacteria producing febrile myalgia include brucellosis, typhoid and leptospirosis.

A number of parasites migrate through human tissues, including smooth and striated muscle (*Figure 33.11*). Of note is the cysticercus stage of the pig tapeworm *Taenia solium*, toxoplasmosis and trichiniasis. Other organisms producing myositis include mycoplasma and malaria. Inflammatory disorders producing myositis include collagen diseases, particularly dermatomyositis, connective tissue disorders and sarcoid; idiopathic myositis is usually a diagnosis of exclusion. The condition may be focal or a polymyositis. There is rapid enlargement of the muscles, mimicking an abscess or a deep vein thrombosis, and accompanied by pain and weakness.

Trauma
Muscle tears

Muscle tears usually occur at the musculotendinous junction, the highest incidence being in the powerful limb muscles that cross two joints, such as the hamstrings, the rectus femoris and the gastrocnemius. They usually occur in explosive running, such as sprinting, and in soccer players, and are also seen in the pectoralis major muscle in weightlifters. They are more common with inadequate training, lack of warm-up, fatigue, previous injury and in occult nerve lesions such as a prolapsed intervertebral disc.

Intra- and intermuscular haemorrhage

A violent blow may produce intra- or intermuscular haemorrhage. Intramuscular haemorrhage is retained within the sheath, there is a tender swelling, and a local cyst may develop. Long-term disabilities include fibrosis and myositis

ossificans where there is persistent or new pain and swelling, stiffness and tenderness; ossification may be demonstrated radiologically. Movement is limited and, therefore, muscle wasting follows.

With intermuscular haemorrhage blood is dispersed and so bruising may be observed at distant sites tracking along tissue planes. Pain and long-term complications are usually less severe. Chronic symptoms usually follow acute cyst formation, occurring particularly in partial tears.

Acute traumatic tears

Acute traumatic tears are seen in the **tendons** of the long flexor and extensor digital muscles, tibialis anterior and posterior, and biceps brachiae. **Chronic** tears occurring in degenerate areas due to neovascularization, myxomatous degeneration, granulation and calcification (**tendonoses**) may be incomplete or complete. They occur in the supraspinatus, and the patellar and Achilles' tendons.

Tenosynovitis

Tenosynovitis due to inflammation of the paratenon gives rise to marked pain on movement and local tenderness. It occurs particularly around the wrist and ankle, a classic example being de Quervain's synovitis affecting the extensor tendons around the anatomical snuffbox of the wrist. **Suppurative tendinitis** occasionally follows infection of the tendon sheaths of the hand. Chronic sequelae of tendon inflammation include stenosing tenosynovitis, this resulting in trigger fingers and abnormalities of the peroneal and tibialis posterior tendons.

Repetitive strain injury (RSI)

This has become, particularly in recent years, a significant source of disability in the workplace. The increase in the disorder is due to advances in automation and mechanization, which have led to the need for rapid, repetitive movements, often involving the upper limbs or the hands and wrists alone. Although physical workloads may be lighter, the increased rate of work results in RSI and an associated overuse syndrome.

The repetitive strain syndrome can be defined as chronic pain affecting the neck/arm region due to the repetitive nature of the work. Psychological factors may contribute to the syndrome.

Clinical features include chronic pain in the neck, chest wall, arms and hands, with impairment of full work performance. There may be swelling of the hand, arm or forearm, as well as poor grip strength and taut proximal muscles.

Periarticular inflammation

Periarticular inflammation at a tendinous attachment to bone is termed **enthesopathy**. The diagnosis is often difficult as other periarticular pathologies may be simulated or coexist. Pain from an enthesopathy of the common extensor origin from the lateral epicondyle of the humerus – 'tennis elbow' – may be misdiagnosed as pain from a capsulitis or bursitis around the elbow, entrapment of the posterior interosseous nerve or pain from osteophytes of the radial head. Similarly, enthesopathic pain from the attachment of the common flexor origin to the medial epicondyle of the humerus – 'golfer's elbow' – may be confused with ulnar nerve compression symptoms. The differential diagnosis of symptoms from the attachment of the adductor longus – groin strain – include an incipient femoral hernia, that of the patellar tendon attachment, muscular tears and enthesopathic pain in the tendo Achillis, to bursitis and tendinitis (p. 486).

Inflammation of periarticular structures lined by synovial membrane include capsulitis of the shoulder joint – frozen shoulder – and congenital and acquired bursitis, particularly in congenital bursae around the elbow, knee and ankle, and acquired bursae around the foot. These conditions may be precipitated by trauma and are encountered in diabetes and rheumatoid arthritis. Fasciitis is characteristically seen in the plantar fascia and iliotibial tractitis can be precipitated in running long distances along a road camber.

Rhabdomyosarcoma

Rhabdomyosarcoma (*Figure 33.12*) is a tumour of striated muscle. It is a rare variety of soft tissue sarcoma, occurring mainly in infants, children and young adults. It particularly affects the lower limbs and trunk. The presentation is usually of a rapidly expanding, painless mass, and the lesion metastasizes early to the lungs. The benign form of striated muscle tumour is the **rhabdomyoma** while the smooth muscle equivalent is the **leiomyoma**. This lesion most commonly occurs in adolescence to middle age; it is slow-growing and often presents as a very large mass. The lesions can occur in limb

muscles, possibly arising from vascular smooth muscle, but are encountered in the gut mesentery and retroperitoneum. Postexcision recurrence is very rare.

Congenital muscular disorders

Congenital muscular disorders include the absence of muscles, the commonest example being that of the sternocostal head of pectoralis major (*Figure 33.13*).

Sprengel's deformity

Sprengel's deformity (*Figure 33.14*) is an abnormality of the scapula and its musculature, the bone being small, sited high on the chest wall and sometimes tethered to an abnormal spine.

Muscular dystrophy

Muscular dystrophies form a rare group of genetically determined abnormalities with a world-wide distribution. They usually commence in childhood, are more common in males and are characterized by progressive, symmetrical weakness, with reduced reflexes. There may be initial muscle hypertrophy but this is due to fatty infiltration, there being progressive atrophy of muscle fibres. Sensation is normal and there is no fasciculation. The disorder is remarkably selective in its pattern of distribution and is classified by the muscles involved. For example, facioscapulohumeral dystrophy is transmitted as an autosomal dominant and has equal distribution in the sexes.

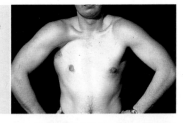

Figure 33.13. Congenital absence of the pectoral muscles.

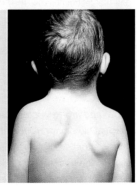

Figure 33.14. Sprengel's deformity.

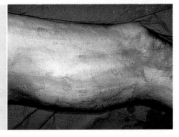

Figure 33.12. Rhabdomyosarcoma of the adductor muscles of the right thigh.

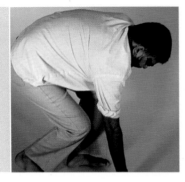

Figure 33.15. Gowers' sign in a patient with a proximal myopathy.

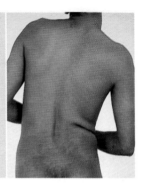

Figure 33.16. Abnormalities of posture and gait associated with a toxic myopathy, secondary to phenothiazine therapy.

Initially patients cannot whistle, pout their lips or close their eyes, but slow progression of the disease produces contractures and deformity with secondary disuse atrophy of muscles.

Patients with pelvic girdle disease can only walk slowly, cannot run, have difficulty climbing stairs and climb up their legs with their hands to stand – Gowers' sign (*Figure 33.15*). Patients with the Duchenne variety of muscular dystrophy are initially slow to walk, the diagnosis usually being made by 3 years old, the child being confined to a wheelchair by the age of 10.

Myotonia

Myotonia is persistent muscle contraction after voluntary cessation. Clinically it is recognized by slow, mechanical relaxation. The condition is transmitted as an autosomal dominant. There is initial enlargement of muscles, which are tender to percussion.

Myotonia congenitalia (Thomsen's disease)

This condition presents at birth, the symptoms being worse after rest or in the cold and being helped by exercise. A diffuse, generalized muscle hypertrophy may be present throughout life. Symptoms are most marked in infants, giving rise to feeding difficulties.

Dystrophica myotonia is a form of the disease presenting with a facial myopathy, distal muscle atrophy, frontal baldness, cataracts, cardiomyopathy, gonadal atrophy, mild endocrine abnormalities and, of later onset, dementia.

Arthrogryphoses

Arthrogryphoses are rare but extremely crippling disorders, characterized by joint fusion and muscle contractures. They are produced by retardation of joint development *in utero* and may be linked to a lack of normal intrauterine movement. Lesions do not usually progress after birth.

Metabolic myopathies

Metabolic myopathies occur in disorders of glycogen, pyruvate, xanthine and calcium metabolism, while **endocrine abnormalities** associated with myopathy include hyper- and hypothyroidism, Cushing's disease, Addison's disease, acromegaly and steroid therapy. **Toxic myopathy** has been reported with cimetidine, phenothiazine (*Figure 33.16*), vincristine, chloroquine, amphetamine, lithium and alcohol.

Gait

The observation of a patient's gait upon entering the consulting room can often reveal valuable information. Examination of any lower limb joint should be preceded by observation of the patient standing and walking. A limp is an abnormal gait.

The normal gait cycle has a heel strike, stance, toe off and a swing phase. Any abnormality can often be linked to the phase of the gait cycle, helping the diagnosis.

Heel strike

The foot makes contact with the ground through the heel initially before roll-over on to the rest of the foot. A patient with a painful heel avoids weight-bearing on the heel and therefore contacts the ground through the toes and metatarsal heads. A foot drop produces a characteristic slap as the whole foot contacts the ground. The heel strike is violent in tabes dorsalis.

Stance

As the body weight is swung through, the foot remains planted firmly on the ground. If the leg has a painful joint, the patient avoids prolonged weight bearing during this phase and therefore tends to rush to the next phase. The resulting **antalgic gait** is observed as hurrying off the involved leg.

A **short leg gait** is observed in this phase by vertical dipping of a shoulder. If the abductors are insufficiently strong to hold the pelvis upright in the stance phase, the body weight is thrown over the leg, resulting in a sideways dipping of the shoulder, the **Trendelenburg gait**. If this is bilateral it produces a characteristic waddle. A flexion deformity or ligament injury of the knee will often reveal itself in this phase.

Toe off

In this phase the body weight is transferred forward and the leg is raised from the ground. If there is a flexion deformity at the hip or knee, the heel rises too soon. If the body is thrown up as well as forward it suggests that the body is being moved to allow clearance of a stiff knee.

Swing

The leg is swung through. If there is a foot drop the leg must be lifted up to avoid the toe scuffing the ground. In tabes dorsalis both legs are elevated rather further than that of a drop foot. Stiffness of the hip causes a bold elevation of the side through the lumbar spine. Stiffness in the knee results in an abnormal swing phase with the leg being thrown out to the side for clearance. The **scissor gait** of spastic diplegia is most noticeable in the swing phase. The **hemiplegic gait** produces a similar picture on one side.

34 The shoulder joint and pectoral girdle

Introduction

The shoulder is a complex joint so any precise diagnosis of its disorders requires a methodical approach.

Inspection

The shoulder should be observed from in front and behind. Abnormal contours of the trapezius or deltoid muscles can result from denervation of the accessory or axillary nerves. There is a right angle appearance of the deltoid contour in the presence of an anterior dislocation. Wasting in the supraspinous fossa commonly results from a tear of the supraspinatus tendon and occasionally from a palsy of the suprascapular nerve.

Prominence of the sternoclavicular or acromioclavicular joints occurs as a result of subluxation or dislocation after degeneration or trauma. Swelling commencing in the interval between the tip of the acromion and the humeral head is associated with calcific tendinitis or subacromial bursitis. Winging of the scapula (p. 412) is present with a palsy of the nerve to serratus anterior or the accessory nerve, and there may be deformity due to congenital anomalies (p. 438; Figure 33.1).

Palpation

A convenient routine is to palpate the sternoclavicular joint, looking for abnormal movement and tenderness, which is suggestive of dislocation, then pass laterally along the subcutaneous border of the clavicle looking for tenderness in an acute fracture or tenderness and crepitus in a non-union, along to the acromioclavicular joint, which is tender in osteoarthritis. The coracoid process is palpable inferior to the clavicle in the deltopectoral groove (Figure 34.1).

Palpation in the area immediately lateral to the acromion reveals tenderness in supraspinatus tendinitis. Crepitus due to a supraspinatus tear can be palpated here although crepitus from osteoarthritis of the glenohumeral joint is also palpable. The joint is palpable, anteriorly and posteriorly, through

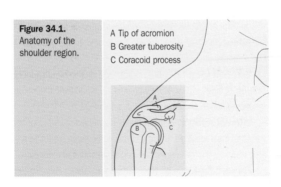

Figure 34.1.
Anatomy of the shoulder region.

A Tip of acromion
B Greater tuberosity
C Coracoid process

the deltoid, and the greater tuberosity laterally. The axillary artery and medial border of the neck and head of the humerus are palpable in the axilla, and this can also demonstrate osteophytes, especially in thin subjects.

Testing movement

This must be undertaken from behind in order to distinguish between scapulothoracic and glenohumeral movement.

Abduction normally occurs to 180°, the scapula contributing 90° of rotation. In order to discern pure glenohumeral movement the scapula must be fixed by the examiner, by placing a hand firmly on the superior border or holding the inferior angle of the scapula (Figure 34.2).

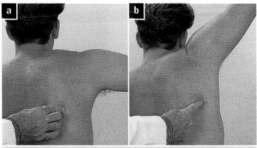

Figure 34.2.
Scapular involvement in shoulder abduction. a. Abduction to 90° with scapula restrained. b. Scapular rotation in full abduction.

Scapulohumeral rhythm

In normal **scapulohumeral rhythm**, the majority of movement from 0° to 90° occurs at the glenohumeral joint and subsequent **abduction** occurs mainly as a result of scapular rotation. Reverse glenohumeral rhythm, i.e. scapular rotation occurring early in abduction, is suggestive of a rotator cuff tear. Pain occurring in the midpart of the range of abduction, the painful arc, is suggestive of supraspinatus tendinitis.

Adduction normally allows the elbow to be brought to the midline.

External rotation is best compared by the simultaneous testing of both sides, thus allowing comparison; the range increases when the arm is abducted to 90°.

Internal rotation is traditionally described in terms of the vertebral level reached by the thumb but be aware that this test also requires the presence of a certain amount of extension.

Forward flexion is normally present to 160°. Forward and lateral elevation are functional terms and refer to forward flexion and abduction respectively, with the hand outstretched.

The rotator cuff

The majority of shoulder abnormalities arise in the rotator cuff. The aetiology of the lesions may be different but a common cycle of pathological processes occurs. Subacromial impingement or supraspinatus tendinitis can result in a tear of the tendon and, conversely, a tear can result in impingement or tendinitis. The spectrum of symptoms and signs resulting from the cycle makes a precise diagnosis difficult. Nevertheless, a systematic examination usually establishes the diagnosis (see below).

The supraspinatus muscle

Although the cuff includes the subscapularis, infraspinatus and teres minor, it is in the supraspinatus that most problems arise. The muscle arises in the supraspinous fossa, passes laterally below the acromion and forms a tendon, which inserts into the greater tuberosity of the humerus. The supraspinatus outlet is the space between the acromion and humerus through which the tendon passes. There is a region of the tendon proximal to the insertion that is a vascular watershed and is relatively hypovascular. This region is at risk of inflammation and tears.

Subacromial impingement

Impingement is pain resulting from pressure on the tendon as it passes through the outlet; this is made worse with for-

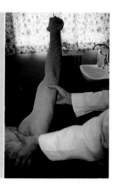

Figure 34.3.
Neer's impingement sign. The examiner's left hand is holding the scapula, while the right is flexing and adducting the humerus.

ward elevation when the tendon is pushed up against the acromion. The resultant inflammation of the tendon is known as supraspinatus tendinitis.

Primary or **outlet impingement** is due to a narrow subacromial outlet. This is a result of an abnormal shape or slope of the acromial process, prominence of the underside of the acromioclavicular joint or an anterior acromial spur.

Secondary or **non-outlet impingement** is due to traumatic or degenerative rupture of an abnormal supraspinatus tendon.

The clinical features of impingement/tendinitis include pain and a painful arc of movement; a number of manoeuvres produce pain and are useful in the diagnosis.

Neer's impingement sign *(Figure 34.3)* is an increase in pain when the humerus is pushed forward and elevated while the scapula is being controlled.

The **distraction test** is decrease of the painful arc with traction of the limb away from the axilla.

The **injection test** is temporary relief of pain when local anaesthetic is injected into the subacromial space.

Supraspinatus tear

The tendon is susceptible to rupture just proximal to its insertion because of the vascular watershed. A tear of the tendon results from degeneration with age, attrition from prolonged primary impingement or from trauma. There are two types of tear:

- An **incomplete tear** is on the deep or superficial surface, or is intratendinous, but there is no communication between the joint and the subacromial bursa. It causes inflammation and gives rise to the signs of secondary impingement.

- A **complete tear** is, in effect, a hole in the tendon, allowing communication between the joint and the subacromial space; it prevents the muscle from acting.

The **drop arm sign** is indicative of a complete tear; with the elbow flexed the arm is passively abducted to 90° and externally rotated. Ask the patient to keep the arm in this position and then let go. The arm drops a little when a tear is present.

There is atrophy of the supraspinatus muscle, and movement produces palpable crepitus in the supraspinous fossa; reverse glenohumeral rhythm is present.

Frozen shoulder (adhesive capsulitis)

This is a common diagnosis but should be one of exclusion. It is a syndrome characterized by a global restriction of glenohumeral movement, particularly external rotation, pain and muscle wasting. It is often preceded by minor trauma in the middle aged and elderly. As the immobility progresses the pain decreases. Spontaneous recovery occurs but may take up to 2 years.

Acute calcific tendinitis

This is a degenerative condition in which there is local deposition of calcium salts within the supraspinatus tendon *(Figure 34.4)* causing sudden severe pain and a limitation of movement. There is exquisite tenderness immediately lateral to the tip of the acromion. The diagnosis is confirmed by plain radiographs which show flecks of calcium.

Osteoarthritis

Osteoarthritis of the shoulder is less common than rheumatoid and is often secondary to humeral head and neck fractures. In osteoarthritis of the acromioclavicular joint there is tenderness and swelling of the joint and springiness to palpation.

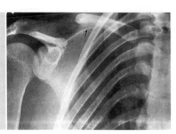

Figure 34.5.
Craniocleido-dysostosis. Incomplete clavicular development.

Rheumatoid arthritis

Rheumatoid arthritis gives rise to a painful erosive arthropathy with deformity and loss of movement. The sternoclavicular joint, i.e. the scapulothoracic union, is unaffected and some patients maintain useful shoulder function even when the glenohumeral joint is destroyed.

Congenital anomalies

Congenital anomalies of the shoulder girdle include the absence of muscle (p. 438; *Figure 33.13*), Sprengel's deformity (p. 438) and partial or complete absence of the clavicles (*Figure 34.5*). In the latter there may also be defection ossification of the skull, other bones and teeth – craniocleidodysostosis. The abnormal mobility of the pectoral girdle may enable the clavicles to meet in the midline.

Fractures of the shoulder girdle

Fractures of the **clavicle** (*Figure 34.6*) are common, particularly in children and young adults. They follow a fall on the outstretched hand. The fracture is usually in the midshaft and, in children, it may be of the greenstick variety. Although displacement can be considerable, non-union is very uncommon. Good remodelling occurs of malunion and of excess callus formation.

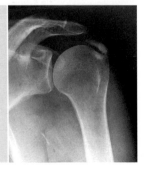

Figure 34.4.
Calcification of the supraspinatus tendon.

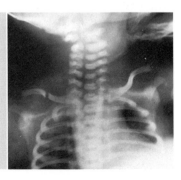

Figure 34.6.
Fracture of the right clavicle in a child.

Fractures of either end may be accompanied by a dislocation of the joint, with impaction of the fracture. The rare posterior dislocation of the head of the clavicle can impinge on to the great vessels and the trachea in the root of the neck. The patient may be in considerable distress from dyspnoea and cyanosis, and urgent reduction is necessary. Dislocation of the acromioclavicular joint *(Figure 34.7)* is accompanied by a tear of the coracoclavicular ligaments.

Fracture of the body of the **scapula** is due to a direct blow, which may also fracture the underlying ribs. A fracture of the neck of the scapula may follow a blow or a fall on the shoulder.

Fracture of the **neck of the humerus** *(Figure 34.8)* can occur with a fall on the outstretched hand, particularly in elderly women. There is often impaction without displacement. Pathological fractures are also common in the humerus, particularly through secondary deposits in the region of the neck. In younger individuals a fracture of the neck may be displaced and include dislocation of the shoulder and fracture of the greater tuberosity. The latter injury can also occur in isolation, due to a blow or as an avulsion injury when the action of supraspinatus is impeded, or as part of a dislocation of the shoulder. In children, fractures may occur through the upper humeral epiphysis, producing some angulation; dislocations are very uncommon in this age group.

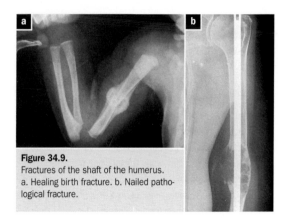

Figure 34.9.
Fractures of the shaft of the humerus.
a. Healing birth fracture. b. Nailed pathological fracture.

Fractures of the **shaft of the humerus** *(Figure 34.9a, b)* are produced when a fall on to the hand is accompanied by a twisting injury; the resulting fracture is of the spiral variety. There is usually angular deformity and the arm is rendered useless. The fracture may be further complicated by an injury to the radial nerve as it lies in contact with the bone, in the spiral groove, producing a wrist drop. Transverse and comminuted fractures are due to direct trauma. The shaft of the humerus is also the commonest fracture associated with a difficult delivery in a neonate.

Shoulder instability

This term includes acute and chronic dislocations, and subluxations, also patients with joint laxity or a fear of recurrent dislocation. In subluxation there is displacement of the articular surfaces but some contact remains.

Anterior instability
Acute anterior dislocation *(Figure 34.10)* constitutes the great majority of dislocations, usually resulting from forceful injury. The injured person holds the affected arm across the abdomen, supporting it with the good arm. The deltoid contour is lost and there is a virtual right angle at the tip of the acromion; local muscle spasm is present. The head of the humerus is palpable under the lateral aspect of the pectoralis major muscle. It is essential to test and record the function of the axillary nerve at the time of diagnosis. Pain prevents motor testing so it is necessary to test cutaneous sensation in the 'regimental patch' area, i.e. the area of skin over the attachment of the deltoid muscle. There is virtually no movement in acute dislocations although, in time, a surprising range of movement develops if the diagnosis is missed.

Figure 34.7.
Dislocation of the acromioclavicular joint.

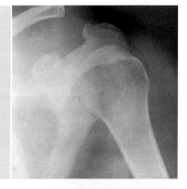

Figure 34.8.
Fracture of the neck of the humerus.

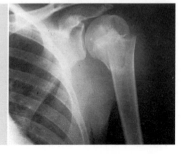

Figure 34.10.
Anterior dislocation of the shoulder joint.

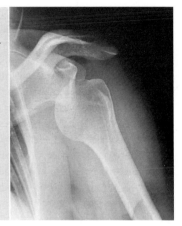

Figure 34.11.
Recurrent shoulder dislocation. Note the loss of contour of the deltoid muscle, due to displacement of the underlying head of the humerus, as compared to the opposite side.

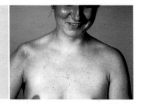

Figure 34.12.
Subluxation of the humeral head.

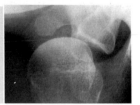

The complications of anterior dislocation are axillary nerve palsy, supraspinatus tear, and fracture of the surgical neck or greater tuberosity of the humerus.

Chronic anterior instability

This can be either an acute dislocation that has been neglected or a recurrent phenomenon. Recurrent instability can be traumatic or atraumatic. The pathological process in traumatic instability is a Bankart lesion, which is a rupture of the labrum and capsule from the anterior glenoid rim. In atraumatic instability the problem is laxity of the capsule.

Patients with **recurrent dislocation** *(Figure 34.11)* are usually asymptomatic until an incident provokes a painful dislocation. The degree of provocation required declines as the number of episodes increase, because the stabilizing mechanisms of the shoulder become more incompetent.

Patients with **recurrent subluxation** *(Figure 34.12)* have never suffered a dislocation but present either with pain on carrying out heavy or rapid overhead activities or with the 'dead arm syndrome'. This syndrome is characterized by pain, often of a sudden sharp paralysing nature, clicking, grinding and a heavy feeling. The patient may describe a feeling that the shoulder slips out of place.

Patients with **recurrent dislocation** and **subluxation** suffer symptoms of both occasional dislocation and subluxation.

Apprehension shoulder is a term applied to a group of patients with recurrent subluxation or dislocation but whose overriding symptom is a fear of dislocation in external rotation. They adopt activities and posture to avoid external rotation.

In **recurrent atraumatic anterior involuntary instability** the history differs from traumatic instability in that normal physical activities provoke the symptoms of instability. The physical signs are identical.

Posterior instability

Acute posterior dislocation is rare and initially the diagnosis can be easily missed. It can result from high energy trauma but also occurs after neurological seizures and, in the inebriated, with minor trauma. The shoulder is painful and there is muscle spasm. Characteristically there is significant loss of passive external rotation of the shoulder.

A missed posterior dislocation is subject to chronic dislocation. Recurrent instability tends to be subluxation rather than dislocation; there is pain on forward flexion, adduction and internal rotation.

Multidirectional instability

The principal pathology in these patients is a lax inferior axillary capsular pouch. Whilst the cause may have been traumatic and repetitive overuse, the recurrent problem is usually atraumatic. Patients present with shoulder pain, the feeling of the shoulder slipping down when carrying weight in addition to those symptoms described for anterior or posterior instability. The problem is often bilateral.

This group also includes patients with generalized laxity, such as Ehlers–Danlos syndrome. They also have the ability to bend the thumb back to touch the forearm and the ability to hyperextend the knees, elbows and fingers.

Assessment of instability
Apprehension testing

In the **crank test** the examiner stands behind the seated patient and stresses the arm into external rotation and abduction. Levering the head of the humerus anteriorly, while palpating anteriorly to prevent dislocation, provokes muscle contraction or an expression of apprehension from the patient. The fulcrum test is carried out with the shoulder on the edge of the examining couch and the arm externally rotated, abducted and extended. This similarly provokes an apprehension response. These tests are both positive in anterior instability. Occasionally internal rotation with the arm adducted and flexed forward elicits apprehension in posterior subluxation.

There are two grades of glenohumeral translation:

- Grade 1 – Translation of the humeral head up to the glenoid rim.
- Grade 2 – Translation of the humeral head over the glenoid rim, with spontaneous reduction.

In the **anterior drawer test** *(Figure 34.13)* the examiner stabilizes the scapula with one hand and the other hand grasps the humeral head from in front and behind. The humeral head is pushed anteriorly. The extent of translation is seen and felt. A modification of this test is the **load shift test**, which is carried out with the patient in both seated and supine positions. The scapula is fixed by the examiner and the humeral head is held from the lateral side and pushed medially into the glenoid ('load'). The head is then pushed anteriorly and posteriorly ('shift') and an assessment is made of the extent of translation, it is compared with the normal side. Grade 1 involves movement of the humeral head to the rim of the glenoid. Grade 2 involves movement of the head over the rim of the glenoid. The load and shift test is positive in anterior and posterior instability, and in multidirectional instability if this is associated with the sulcus sign. The **sulcus sign** *(Figure 34.14)* is present in multidirectional instability; it is elicited with the patient seated. Traction is applied to the arm and at the same time the examiner grasps the humerus and pushes it inferiorly. A visible skin sulcus beneath the acromion results when there is gross instability.

If an apprehension manoeuvre is positive, a **Jobe's relocation test** *(Figure 34.15)* may be added, the examiner applying a posterior force to the humeral head. Abolition of pain or apprehension, or an increased range of external rotation with this force, is indicative of anterior subluxation.

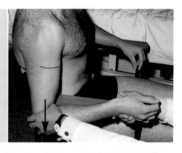

Figure 34.14.
Sulcus sign. The depression appears beneath the acromion.

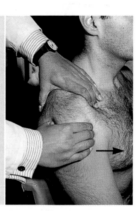

Figure 34.13.
Anterior drawer test. The examiner's left hand is fixing the scapula and the right hand is displacing the head of the humerus anteriorly.

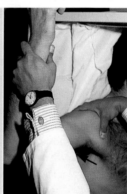

Figure 34.15.
Jobe's relocation test. The examiner's right hand is displacing the head of the humerus posteriorly.

35 The arm

The elbow joint

The important landmarks of this joint are easily palpable. The tip of the olecranon, and the medial and lateral epicondyles, form an equilateral triangle when the elbow is flexed. They are in line with the elbow extended. In traumatic cases this relationship is preserved in supracondylar fractures but it is lost in dislocations. Effusions are seen as a filling in of the concavity between the olecranon and the lateral epicondyle.

The 'carrying angle' is the physiological angulation of the forearm away from the midline when the arm is straight; it is 10° in males and 20° in females. An increased angulation is known as cubitus valgus, decreased angulation as cubitus varus (*Figure 35.1*). Flexion and extension occur at the elbow joint. Supination and pronation take place as the radial head rotates. The radial head, and its rotatory movement, is palpable 1 cm distal to the lateral epicondyle.

Tennis elbow (lateral epicondylitis)

This is a common overuse condition, often provoked by heavy repetitive physical activity involving rotation at the elbow. The site of the pain is the common extensor origin at the lateral epicondyle.

There is pain along the lateral border of the elbow, which radiates proximally and distally. The lateral epicondyle, or the common extensor tendon just distal to it, is tender (*Figure 35.2*).

In **Cozens' test** ask the patient to clench their fist, keep it clenched and then to extend the wrist. Grasp the lower forearm in the left hand and, while the patient continues to try to keep the wrist extended, flex the wrist firmly and steadily. This reproduces the characteristic pain.

In **Mills' manoeuvre**, with the elbow quite straight and the wrist flexed, pronation of the forearm brings on the pain.

Radial tunnel syndrome

This condition causes pain that mimics tennis elbow. The problem is produced by radial nerve compression as it passes through the radial tunnel. This point, 4–5 cm distal to the lateral epicondyle, is tender. The pain can be provoked by extension of the middle finger against resistance and by

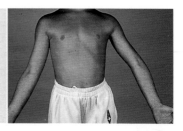

Figure 35.1. Left-sided cubitus varus.

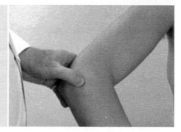

Figure 35.2. Palpation of the common extensor origin.

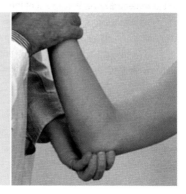

Figure 35.3. Palpation of the ulnar nerve behind the medial epicondyle of the humerus.

supination of the forearm against resistance. There is no motor or sensory loss.

Golfer's elbow (medial epicondylitis)

This is much less common than tennis elbow. There is pain, aggravated by throwing, and tenderness located at the medial epicondyle at the common flexor origin.

Cubital tunnel syndrome (ulnar nerve compression)

The ulnar nerve passes in the groove posterior to the medial epicondyle (*Figure 35.3*) with an overlying retinaculum forming the cubital tunnel. Proximal to this the nerve passes through the medial intermuscular septum. Distally it passes between the two heads of the flexor carpi ulnaris. Compression can occur at each site. Alternatively a marked cubitus valgus can lead to a traction neuritis.

There can be pain that passes from the medial epicondyle distally along the ulnar distribution. There is alteration of sensation and there may be wasting of the muscles of the hypothenar eminence, as well as the intrinsic muscles of the hand.

Palpation of the nerve in its groove causes pain and there is a positive Tinel's sign. There is decreased sensation in the ulnar nerve distribution.

Arthritis of the elbow joint
Osteoarthritis

Osteoarthritis is manifest by pain and a loss of range of motion. Occasionally there are loose bodies present in the joint, leading to the symptom of intermittent locking. Bony changes may be considerable in individuals moving the elbow for a repetitive throwing movement or when sensation to the joint is reduced (Clutton's joint), as in syphilis.

Rheumatoid arthritis

Rheumatoid arthritis is not uncommon in the elbow, with rheumatoid nodules occurring adjacent to the joint. The muscle wasting associated with **tuberculous infection** and joint swelling produces a fusiform configuration across the elbow joint.

Rupture of the biceps

The biceps is subject to rupture of its muscle belly and at both proximal and distal attachments. Rupture of the belly is usually painful and dramatic, and as a result of heavy lifting, producing two midarm bulges separated by a gap. Rupture of the long head of biceps occurs in the elderly and is due to attrition of the tendon as it passes through the bicipital groove. The rupture may be spontaneous or from minor

trauma, and the symptoms mild. The signs are more obvious, a bulge being present in the lower third of the arm, on flexion of the elbow against resistance (*Figure 35.4*). Rupture of the radial attachment of biceps follows forced flexion. There is marked pain and bruising of the cubital fossa.

Biceps and triceps tendinitis

Bicipital tendinitis causes pain in the anterior aspect of the upper arm and elbow as a result of overuse or strain. There is tenderness along the distal biceps tendon. **Yergason's sign** is positive when the elbow is flexed to 90° and the patient tries to supinate the forearm against resistance.

Tricipital tendinitis causes posterior elbow pain and tenderness at the triceps insertion. Extension of the elbow against resistance exacerbates the pain.

Valgus extension overload (pitcher's elbow)

This condition is caused by overuse of the elbow in recurrent throwing or overhead repetitive activities, such as pitching in baseball or javelin throwing. The syndrome has a number of components:

- **Ulnar collateral ligament injuries** – Valgus stresses can cause a partial or complete rupture. Laxity causes problems in the radiohumeral joint and in the posterior compartment of the posterior ulnar humeral joint. There is pain in the medial aspect of the elbow, just distal to the medial epicondyle. If a valgus stress is applied with the elbow in 30° of flexion there is increased laxity and provocation of pain.
- **Medial epicondylar apophysitis** – In young people with open epiphyses there can be pain during sporting activities with tenderness over the medial epicondyle.
- **Lateral compartment osteochondral defects** – The lax ulnar collateral ligament allows the transmission of excessive compressive forces into the radiohumeral joint, and results in damage to the articular surfaces of the radius and capitellum. Osteochondral loose bodies may be produced resulting in locking and crepitus. In young people osteochondritis dissecans occurs in this compartment and can also lead to loose bodies.
- **Posterior olecranon impingement** – Repetitive forceful extension with valgus stress results in impingement of the posteromedial aspect of the olecranon against the medial aspect of the olecranon fossa and an osteophyte or loose bodies may result.

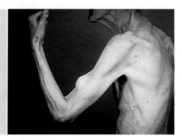

Figure 35.4.
Rupture of the long head of the biceps muscle.

There is posterior pain, tenderness over the olecranon, loss of extension, and pain when the elbow is passively extended with a valgus force by the examiner.

- **Olecranon bursitis** (*Figure 35.5*) – Inflammation of the olecranon bursa as a result of repeated trauma results in a painless swelling. Infection results in a painful olecranon bursitis; it is also referred to as student's or miner's elbow.

Acute injuries
Supracondylar fractures

Supracondylar fractures (*Figure 35.6*) are a common injury of children and adolescents, resulting from falling on the outstretched hand. The distal fragment of the humerus is displaced posteriorly and tilted dorsally. The relationship of the bony landmarks of the elbow is maintained. The presence of the radial pulse must be ascertained because the brachial artery is easily compromised at this site, with the risk of a Volkmann's contracture, if not corrected. Pain on passive straightening of the fingers is an important symptom of uncorrected acute ischaemia. Less commonly the median, radial or ulnar nerves are affected; usually they undergo spontaneous recovery. Malunion is common and may be a sideways, backwards or forwards tilt, or a rotational deformity.

Intercondylar T-shaped fractures

These fractures constitute the adult elbow fracture sustained through a fall on the elbow. The neurovascular structures are at risk, as in the child. The relationship of the bony landmarks of the elbow is preserved.

Fractures of the epicondyles

Fractures of the lateral epicondyle in adults and the epiphysis in children are produced by lateral angulatory forces applied to the fully extended elbow. The same forces can avulse the medial epicondylar epiphysis in children. The lateral epicondyle is subject to delayed or non-union, and healing of the medial epicondylar epiphysis is usually by a fibrous union. Ulnar neuritis is a common complication of both injuries, due respectively to stretching or compression and scarring.

In **fracture of the olecranon** there is swelling and tenderness of the olecranon. In a significant fracture the ability to extend the elbow against gravity, as a result of the action of triceps, is lost. There is a palpable and often visible gap across the fracture line.

Fracture of the radial head (*Figure 35.7*) follows a fall on the outstretched hand, particularly in children. An effusion is present, the elbow is painful in all movements and the radial head is tender to palpation. There may be associated damage to the capitellum and its overlying cartilage.

A **pulled elbow** is subluxation of the radial head through its annular ligament in a child, resulting from a sudden pull on the straight arm. The elbow is protected and palpation of the radial head causes pain. The injury is less common in the adult as the radial head conforms to the conical shape of the ligament.

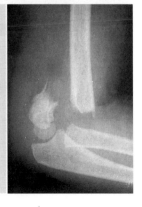

Figure 35.5.
Olecranon bursitis.

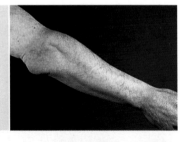

Figure 35.6.
Supracondylar fracture.

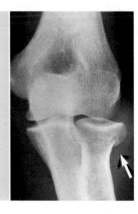

Figure 35.7.
Fracture (arrow) of the head of the radius.

Forearm fractures

These fractures interfere with pronation and supination. They are usually accompanied by deformity and are often palpable, the posterior border of the ulna lying subcutaneously. Combined fractures of both the radius and the ulna are common in direct trauma. When the fractures are complete there is usually angular and translation deformity but this is less so in the case of greenstick forearm fractures of children. It is important to remember that angular deformity in the fracture of a single bone cannot occur without an associated dislocation at one end or the other. A displaced ulnar fracture is accompanied by dislocation of the head of the radius – Monteggia fracture dislocation.

Isolated fractures of the **shaft of the radius** are less common than those of the ulna. Displacement is accompanied by dislocation of the distal radioulnar joint – Galeazzi fracture dislocation.

Dislocation

Dislocation (*Figure 35.8*) involves posterior displacement of the olecranon. The relationship of the bony landmarks of the elbow is lost. The injury may be accompanied by avulsion fractures of the medial epicondyle or coronoid process, and fracture of the head of the radius. Complications include nerve damage and myositis ossificans.

Myositis ossificans

This is an uncommon complication of fractures (p. 422) but is characteristically associated with elbow injuries.

The wrist

Anatomy of the wrist

In the anatomical position the radial and ulnar styloid processes are palpable on the sides of the wrist joint, the tip of the radial styloid being 1 cm distal to that of the ulna (*Figure 35.9a*). This relationship may change with fractures of the lower end of the radius. On pronation, the lower end of the radius rotates around the anterior surface of the head of the ulna, which becomes palpable (*Figure 35.9b*).

On flexion of the wrist against resistance, the flexor carpi radialis and ulnaris tendons stand out on either side of the anterior surface of the wrist. They are attached respectively to the scaphoid and pisiform bones. In the flexed position the palmaris longus tendon may stand out between the carpal flexors as it passes into the flexor retinaculum. If it is absent the median nerve becomes palpable.

Extension of the thumb demonstrates the tendons bordering the anatomical snuffbox. The abductor pollices longus and extensor pollices brevis lie anteriorly, and the extensor pollices longus posteriorly. Within the snuffbox the radial styloid and the scaphoid bone are palpable on either side of the wrist joint. The radial artery passes across the floor and the cephalic vein across the roof of the snuffbox. In the young adult the normal range of movement between full extension and full flexion is 150°. As age advances this range becomes slightly less. Although it is customary to attribute these movements to the wrist joint, they cannot be dissociated from movements in the midcarpal and intercarpal joints. These joints are also involved in radial and ulnar deviation, the sum of these movements being 60°.

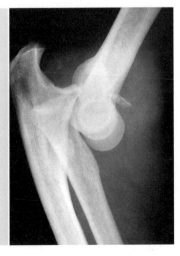

Figure 35.8.
Dislocation of the elbow joint.

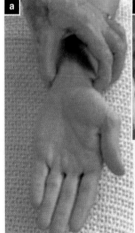
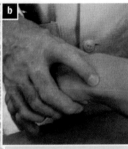

Figure 35.9.
a. Relative position of the radial and ulnar styloid processes.
b. Head of the ulna.

Soft tissue lesions of the wrist

Carpal tunnel syndrome (*Figure 35.10*) denotes a compression neuropathy of the median nerve as it passes beneath the flexor retinaculum. The majority of patients are women, many of them in the fifth or sixth decades. In more than 50% the symptoms are bilateral but more in evidence in the dominant hand. The complaint is of progressive weakness and clumsiness due to impairment of finer movements of the hand – e.g. picking up a pin, sewing, knitting – and associated with attacks of pain, tingling and numbness of the lateral three digits. Characteristically the attacks are nocturnal. Occasionally aching or pain radiates proximally even as far as the shoulder but sensory and motor changes are limited to the hand, the latter being the late onset of wasting of the thenar eminence (p. 414).

The **wrist flexion test** – Phalen's sign – for carpal tunnel syndrome is the exacerbation of paraesthesia when the patient is asked to maintain full wrist flexion for 60 seconds. The **tourniquet test**, when the cuff is pumped to systolic pressure for 60 seconds, has a similar effect. The diagnosis is supported by abnormal median nerve conduction studies.

De Quervain's disease – **stenosing tenosynovitis** – is a painful disabling condition affecting the common tendon sheath of the abductor pollicis longus and extensor pollicis brevis. It is due to inflammatory changes that may proceed to fibrosis and limitation of movement of the thumb. The condition only occurs in adults, usually female. There is always marked tenderness over the anterior border of the anatomical snuffbox. There may be associated swelling and fine crepitus. Pain is produced by passive adduction of the thumb across the palm with ulnar deviation of the wrist.

A **ganglion** (*Figure 35.11a, b*) is a myxomatous degeneration of connective tissue adjacent to a joint capsule. A cyst is formed, filled with crystal clear gelatinous fluid. The most common situation is on the dorsal aspect of the wrist over the scaphoid–lunate articulation. The swelling is rounded, sessile, it becomes tense and prominent when the wrist is flexed and may partially or wholly disappear on extension. The tensely filled cyst feels solid but occasionally fluctuation may be elicited and, if the swelling is large enough to be tested, it is translucent. Other common sites of ganglia are on the anterior aspect of the wrist, between the tendons of flexor carpi radialis and brachioradialis, along the finger (p. 456) and on the dorsum of the ankle and foot.

Arthritic changes around the wrist produce swelling, tenderness and limitation of movement. Osteoarthritis, following injury, and rheumatoid arthritis are both common findings, and the joint is often affected in **TB** in areas where the disease is prevalent. In the latter there is spindle-shaped enlargement across the joint, together with palmar flexion; abscess and sinus formation occur early, on account of the superficial nature of the joint surfaces.

Figure 35.10. Carpal tunnel, demonstrating the attachments of the flexor retinaculum and its relationship to the median and ulnar nerves.

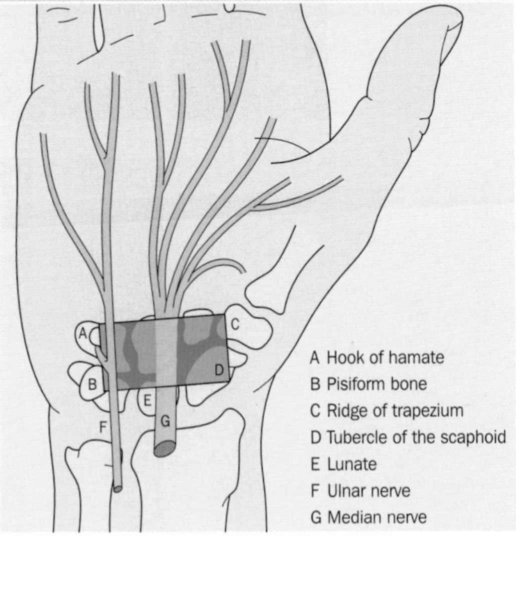

A Hook of hamate
B Pisiform bone
C Ridge of trapezium
D Tubercle of the scaphoid
E Lunate
F Ulnar nerve
G Median nerve

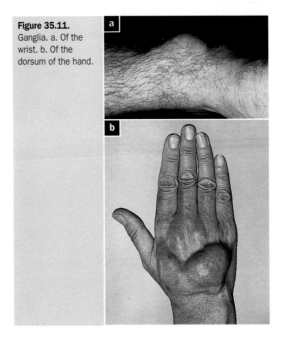

Figure 35.11. Ganglia. a. Of the wrist. b. Of the dorsum of the hand.

Ulnar tunnel syndrome

This is caused by compression of the ulnar nerve in Guyon's canal (a fascial compartment, anterior to the flexor retinaculum) and results in altered sensation in the ulnar digits or wasting of the hypothenar eminence.

Kienböck's disease

Kienböck's disease (*Figure 35.12*) is an avascular necrosis of the lunate bone usually diagnosed radiologically. It is often associated with a relatively long ulna. There is pain in the wrist and tenderness on the dorsum of the lunate, immediately distal to the hollow that is palpable on the dorsum of the wrist.

Fractures of the distal radius

A **Colles' fracture** (*Figure 35.13*) is produced by a fall on the outstretched hand and is a very common extra-articular fracture occurring within 2.5 cm of the articular surface of the radius. There is dorsal and radial displacement and tilting of the distal fragment together with shortening. Clinically there is a 'dinner fork' deformity with local bony tenderness.

Immediate complications include median nerve compression from direct pressure on the nerve. Late malunion, with dorsal tilting and shortening of the radius, may be asymptomatic or lead to pain from the radiocarpal or distal radioulnar joints.

Late attrition rupture of the extensor pollicis longus tendon may occur as it passes over the fracture site; active extension at the thumb interphalangeal joint is lost.

Smith's fracture (*Figure 35.14*) is caused by a fall on to a flexed wrist. The distal radius is tilted and displaced anteriorly and the fracture line may extend into the joint. Other wrist fractures include comminuted fracture of the distal radius (*Figure 35.15*) and displacement of the distal radial epiphysis in children (*Figure 35.16*). In the latter, the deformity is similar to that of the Colles' fracture.

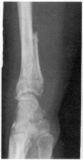

Figure 35.14. Smith's fracture.

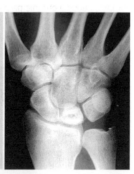

Figure 35.12. Kienböck's disease.

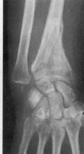

Figure 35.15. Distal comminuted fracture of the end of the radius, involving the wrist joint.

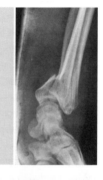

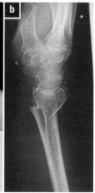

Figure 35.13. Colles' fracture. a. Typical 'dinner fork' deformity. b. Lateral view.

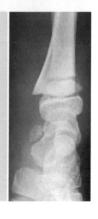

Figure 35.16. Fracture of the distal radial epiphysis.

Barton's fracture is an intra-articular fracture involving a dorsal or anterior rim of the distal margin of the radius.

A **radial styloid fracture** is caused by falling on to a wrist in radial deviation. There is tenderness in the anatomical snuffbox.

Scaphoid fracture

This common fracture is easily missed, resulting in serious consequences for the patient and the physician. It results from a fall on to the outstretched hand. The presentation may be immediate or delayed, with pain in the wrist and on gripping objects. Passive wrist movements may be painful. Palpation in the anatomical snuffbox (*Figure 35.17*) is more painful than in the unaffected side. Pain may be provoked by a tractive or compressive force applied to the thumb in its long axis and on direct pressure on the tubercle of the scaphoid.

The diagnosis can be confirmed radiologically with scaphoid views. In cases that present soon after injury the diagnosis should be made on clinical grounds even if radiographs do not demonstrate a fracture, and the scaphoid should be immobilized.

A chronic painful wrist may result as there is a relatively high rate of non-union and avascular necrosis of the proximal pole (*Figure 35.18*) due to the retrograde blood supply to the scaphoid.

Carpal dislocation

This also occurs through a fall on to the outstretched hand. There are two main categories:

- In **peridislocations** the entire carpus and hand are dorsally dislocated, with the exception of one or more of the proximal carpal row of bones. Most commonly it is the lunate which remains in the normal position – perilunate dislocation (*Figure 35.19*). On examination there is gross deformity of the wrist and minimal movement present. Radiographs are confirmatory.
- In **proximal row dislocation** the carpus and hand remain in alignment with the radius but one or more of the proximal carpal row of bones is dislocated, most commonly the lunate – lunate dislocation. The lunate is usually displaced anteriorly and there can be direct compression of the median nerve leading to pain and diminished sensation in its distribution. Radiographs are essential to establish the diagnosis.

Carpal instability

This is a group of conditions resulting from injury in which a loss of normal alignment of the carpal bones develops, early or late, causing chronic pain and weakness.

Figure 35.17.
Markings of the anatomical snuffbox.

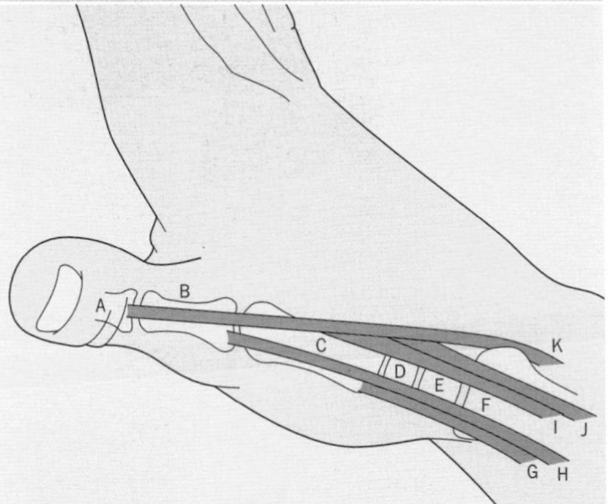

A Distal phalanx
B Proximal phalanx
C First metacarpal
D Trapezium
E Scaphoid
F Radius
G Abductor pollicis longus
H Extensor pollicis brevis
I Extensor carpi radialis longus
J Extensor carpi radialis brevis
K Extensor pollicis longus

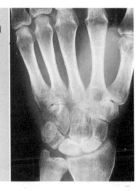

Figure 35.18.
Scaphoid fracture with proximal sclerosis from avascular necrosis.

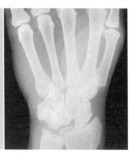

Figure 35.19.
Perilunate dislocation of the wrist.

The **pseudoinstability test** (*Figure 35.20*) is a non-specific indicator of carpal instability. The examiner firmly grasps the carpus with one hand and the distal forearm with the other, and applies an anteroposterior translation force. **Reduced translation** compared to the normal side is suggestive of instability. **Point tenderness** located over a carpal interosseous ligament is suggestive of its injury.

Dorsal intercalated segment instability results from a fall on to the outstretched hand on to the thenar eminence, with disruption of the scapholunate ligaments or associated with a scaphoid fracture. In the **Watson test** (*Figure 35.21a, b*), the examiner presses firmly on the tubercle of the scaphoid with the wrist in the ulnar deviation. The wrist is then rotated into radial deviation. There is a painful 'clunk' in scapholunate dissociation. A clenched fist posteroanterior radiograph confirms separation of the scaphoid and lunate. The lateral film shows an increased scapholunate angle.

Volar intercalated segment instability often follows a fall on to the hypothenar eminence, causing rupture of the radiocarpal ligaments of the ulnar side of the wrist. Intermittent traction across the wrist joint produces tapping of the mobile bones – lunotriquetral ballotement. The lateral radiograph shows a decreased scapholunate angle.

Instability of the distal radioulnar joint is characterized by pain over the ulnar aspect of the wrist and weakness in some movements. The piano key sign demonstrates pain or increased movement at the distal radioulnar joint (*Figure 35.22*).

Tears of the triangular fibrocartilage complex cause ulnar-sided wrist pain and is made worse with ulnar deviation of the wrist. There is tenderness in the sulcus distal to the ulnar styloid – the ulnar snuff box.

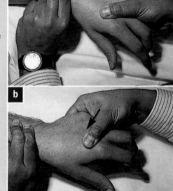

Figure 35.21.
Watson test.
a. The examiner's left thumb is applying pressure to the scaphoid.
b. Radial deviation of the wrist.

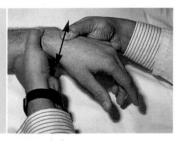

Figure 35.20.
Pseudostability test.

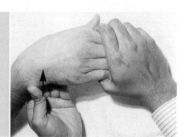

Figure 35.22.
Piano key sign.

36 The hand

Nomenclature

The anterior surface of the hand is referred to as the palmar surface, the posterior as the dorsal surface. The fingers should be referred to as index, middle, ring and little, in order to avoid confusion resulting from numerical descriptions. (Hand infections are considered on p. 75.)

Congenital hand abnormalities

Abnormalities of the digits

Syndactyly *(Figure 36.1)* is one of the most common congenital hand abnormalities. The fingers are joined, with the ring and middle fingers being most commonly affected. The abnormality can be simple, i.e. involving the skin only, or complex, i.e. involving fusion of phalanges. The lesion may be complete, involving the entire length of the finger, or incomplete. Syndactyly can be associated with other congenital abnormalities. Apert's syndrome causes syndactyly affecting all the digits and is associated with intellectual impairment, intra-abdominal abnormalities and abnormal facies.

Polydactyly *(Figure 36.2)* – duplicated fingers are a common hand abnormality. They most commonly affect the ulnar sided digits. The abnormality can vary from a simple case of extra soft tissue to duplication of bone, tendon and cartilage of the phalanges or even complete metacarpals.

Macrodactyly is the enlargement of a digit. This most commonly occurs in systemic disorders such as neurofibromatosis but may occur as an isolated lesion.

Clinodactyly is a deviation of the finger in the coronal plane and most commonly affects the little finger at a joint. There is often a trapezoid-shaped phalanx.

Camptodactyly is deviation of the finger in the sagittal plane. It most commonly affects the little finger at the proximal interphalangeal joint. The abnormality is often familial and presents in infancy or in later childhood.

Deltaphalanx is a triangular phalanx most commonly affecting the proximal phalanx of the thumb and little finger, and causing deviation in the coronal plane towards the middle finger.

Congenital trigger finger or thumb is caused by a stenosing tenosynovitis at the mouth of the A1 pulley. This may present primarily as flexion contractures and is often bilateral. Many present with classical triggering of the finger or thumb.

Constriction bands commonly affect the digits but can affect the limbs more proximally. *In utero* fibrous amniotic bands cause constriction of the extremities. They are associated with other intrauterine deformities such as syndactyly and club feet. Congenital amputation results either from the end stage of constriction bands or from developmental abnormalities.

Lobster claw hand and a thalidomide effect are shown in *Figures 36.3* and *36.4* respectively.

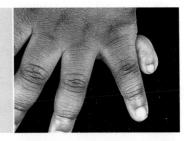

Figure 36.2.
Polydactyly.

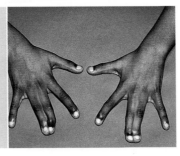

Figure 36.1.
Syndactyly.

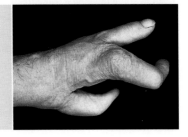

Figure 36.3.
Lobster claw hand.

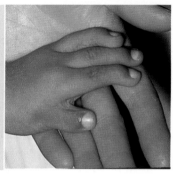

Figure 36.4.
Hand of a thalidomide-affected baby.

Abnormalities of the thumb

Hypoplasia of the thumb

Hypoplasia of the thumb is a spectrum of deformity. The following subgroups have been identified.

Thumb in palm deformity results from functional deficiency of the extensor pollicis brevis which is an X chromosome-linked recessive inheritance; it is often bilateral. The thumb cannot be extended and is held in the palm.

Congenital hypoplasia of the thumb is characterized by the presence of skeletal and vascular structures but the absence of the extensor pollicis longus and abductor pollicis longus.

The **floating thumb** is a structure attached by a somewhat thin pedicle to the radial border of the hand with a rudimentary skeletal and neurovascular structure but no intrinsic or extrinsic tendinous insertions.

Abnormalities of the forearm and hand

Radial clubhand is a spectrum of disorders of the development of the radius leading to shortness or absence of the scaphoid, stiff fingers and hypoplasia of the thumb. It is often associated with systemic congenital abnormalities.

Ulnar clubhand is uncommon. There is shortening or absence of the ulnar. This abnormality is usually associated with other musculoskeletal disorders but is not associated with systemic congenital abnormalities.

Congenital radioulnar synostosis is an abnormal union of the radius and ulnar causing limitation of pronation and supination of the forearm; it is often bilateral. The radius may be fused proximally, or along the substantial part of its length, with the ulnar. The forearm is usually stiff in pronation.

Madelung's deformity results from abnormal growth of the distal radial epiphysis with premature fusion of the ulnar half of the distal radial epiphysis. This causes ulnar and anterior angulation with a prominent distal ulnar.

Soft tissue swellings of the hand

An **implantation dermoid** (*Figure 36.5*) results from a penetrating injury to the finger, driving some epidermal tissue into the dermis. The original injury may be overlooked. As time passes the epidermal tissue proliferates and results in a cystic soft painless lesion, deep to the skin, but not adherent to it or the deep tissues.

A **ganglion of a digit** (*Figure 36.6*) can occur on the palmar or dorsal surface and is often referred to as a seed ganglion. There is a small tense swelling deep to the skin and adherent to the deep tissues. It is filled with viscous clear fluid (p. 451).

Pigmented villonodular synovitis (*Figure 36.7*) was formerly known as a giant cell tumour of a tendon sheath. It most commonly affects women between the ages of 30 and 50, and occurs on the fingers adjacent to tendons. The lesions are firm multilobular nodules deep to the skin and adherent to the deep tissues.

A **glomus tumour** (*Figure 36.8*) consists of a firm smooth nodule that is usually only a few millimetres in diameter. The lesion is derived from the glomus body which is a small AV anastomosis with a coiled arteriole and an abundant nerve supply. It can occur in the subcutaneous tissues of the finger or elsewhere in the body, but commonly in the nail bed, presenting as a focal tender red or violet subungual discoloration. Because of its abundant nerve endings, the lesion may be

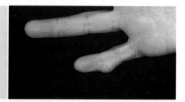

Figure 36.5.
Implantation dermoid.

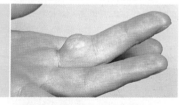

Figure 36.6.
Ganglion of digit

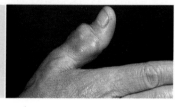

Figure 36.7.
Villonodular synovitis.

Figure 36.8.
Glomus tumour.

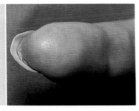

extremely sensitive to light touch or sometimes to temperature changes. The presentation is often with attacks of severe pain that should prompt a careful search for, and excision of, the offending lesion.

Dupuytren's contracture *(Figure 36.9a, b)* is a thickening and shortening of the palmar aponeurosis and its digital fascial extensions. It occurs predominantly in males and the disease is much more aggressive in young people than in the elderly. The disease may be familial and, for this reason, chromosomal transmission has been suggested. It is commoner in manual workers and is associated with anticonvulsant drugs, diabetes and cirrhosis, particularly alcoholic. There may be associated plantar fibromatosis and Peyronie's disease.

Initially, one or more nodules develop in the palm and the condition predominantly affects the ring and little fingers. As the disease develops there is a progressive contracture initially affecting the metacarpophalangeal joint and subsequently the proximal interphalangeal joint. The palpable bands radiating to the fingers from the palm are wholly separate from the flexor tendons. Prolonged presence of the disease results in flexion contractures of the affected joints. The Dupuytren's diatheses describes the generalized tendency in some individuals, particularly those affected early in life, to have widespread aggressive recurrent disease, which often affects both hands and feet.

Volkmann's ischaemic contracture (p. 421; *Figure 32.7*) results from a compartment syndrome in the anterior forearm compartment. The ischaemic damage may be secondary to a brachial artery injury or result from direct trauma giving rise to oedema and muscle compression. The injury may also be iatrogenic from a tight plaster or bandage. The vital early indicator of the problem is the presence of increasing pain in the affected area, despite splintage and analgesia. This is confirmed by provoking severe pain on passive extension of the fingers which causes stretch of the painful ischaemic muscle fibres.

Immediate fasciotomy, with or without arterial revascularization, must be undertaken. Awaiting further signs – such as the absence of major pulses, impaired microvascular circulation or sustained rise in compartment pressures – can lead to irreversible infarction of the forearm muscles. The late result is a contracture of the anterior compartment musculature, leading to a claw hand. Partial extension of the fingers occurs if the wrist is flexed. Although first described in the forearm in childhood injuries, the syndrome can follow ischaemia of other muscle compartments of the upper or lower limbs.

Tendon abnormalities

The retinacular pulley system

A fibrous retinacular sheath encloses the flexor tendon synovial sheath, from the neck of the metacarpal to the distal phalanx. Condensations of the sheath result in five heavy annular bands and three filmy cruciform ligaments. The pulleys prevent bowstringing of the flexor tendons. The A1 pulley extends from the neck of the metacarpal to the distal part of the base of the proximal phalanx. The A2 pulley commences 2 mm distal to the A1 pulley and runs for the length of the shaft of the proximal phalanx. The A3 pulley is a long, thick structure overlying the middle part of the middle phalanx. The A5 pulley is at the distal interphalangeal joint.

Trigger finger usually occurs in middle age and often follows a hand injury. There is a stenosing tenosynovitis of the mouth of the A1 flexor tendon pulley. As the nodular swelling in the tendon passes through the mouth of the pulley, there is a clicking sensation. As the problem progresses the patient is unable to extend the finger unless a passive force is applied with the other hand, at which time the finger extends with a sudden jolt. A long neglected lesion may result in a flexion contracture. When the thumb is affected, in **trigger thumb**, it is often as a congenital lesion presenting in infancy.

Figure 36.9. Dupuytren's contractures. a. Of the hand. b. Of the foot.

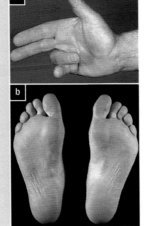

Mallet finger *(Figure 36.10a, b)* results from a direct blow to the tip of the finger, such as being struck by a ball while attempting to catch it. The distal interphalangeal joint is forcibly flexed by the injury and the terminal tendon of the extensor expansion is avulsed from its attachment to the base of the distal phalanx. The patient cannot extend the distal interphalangeal joint and the characteristic posture of the flexed distal interphalangeal joint is present.

Rupture of the intermediate part of the extensor digitoram tendon, which inserts into the base of the middle phalanx, results in weakness and inability to fully extend the proximal interphalangeal joint. The collateral slips of the extensor expansion can subsequently subluxate in the palmar direction and this results in the boutonnière deformity (see below).

Attrition rupture of the extensor pollicis longus results from abrasion in the region of Lister's tubercle as a result of a distal radial fracture or rheumatoid arthritis. The patient cannot extend the interphalangeal joint of the thumb.

Gamekeeper's thumb *(Figure 36.11)* is the rupture of the ulnar collateral ligament of the carpometacarpal joint of the thumb. It can be acute as a result of a direct injury or it can be a chronic lesion resulting from a repetitive strain. The thumb metacarpal is grasped by the examiner and a valgus stress is applied across the carpometacarpal joint. The ulnar side of the joint opens up when there is rupture of this ligament. Operative repair is often required.

Flexor digitorum profundus flexes the distal interphalangeal joint of the finger in a mass action with the other fingers. **Flexor digitorum superficialis** predominantly flexes the proximal interphalangeal joint and can act individually.

To test the flexor digitorum profundus tendon, the metacarpophalangeal and proximal interphalangeal joints of the finger concerned are held in extension by the examiner. The patient is then asked to flex the tip of the finger and this is palpated against resistance. To test the flexor digitorum superficialis to a finger, the remaining three fingers are held in full extension to eliminate the action of flexor digitorum profundus in the finger being observed. If flexor digitorum superficialis is intact, flexion is possible at the proximal interphalangeal joint.

In planning treatment, injuries to the flexor tendons are described in terms of the zone affected:

- Zone 1 is distal to the insertion of flexor digitorum superficialis. The flexor digitorum profundus may be avulsed or lacerated in this region.
- Zone 2 extends from the mouth of the A1 pulley, i.e. the fibro-osseous tunnel, which corresponds to the distal palmar crease, to the insertion of flexor digitorum superficialis. Any laceration in this region firstly divides the flexor digitorum superficialis and, if it is sufficiently deep, it divides the flexor digitorum profundus. Particular care is required in repair of flexor tendons in this region because of a high incidence of flexor sheath adhesion during healing.
- Zone 3 passes from the distal margin of the transverse carpal ligament to the mouth of the A1 pulley. The flexor digitorum superficialis and profundus are at risk in this region.
- Zone 4 constitutes the carpal tunnel.
- Zone 5 extends from the proximal margin of the carpal tunnel to the musculotendinous junctions in the forearm.

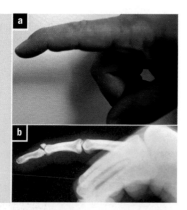

Figure 36.10.
a. Avulsed distal extensor tendon producing a mallet finger deformity.
b. Radiological appearance.

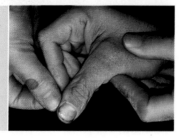

Figure 36.11.
Rupture of the ulnar collateral ligament of the carpometacarpal joint of the thumb.

The bones and joints of the hand

Heberden's nodes *(Figure 36.12)* result from osteoarthrosis. They occur on the dorsum of the distal interphalangeal joint and are small bony elevations on the terminal phalanges near the joint line. They result either from the primary osteoarthritis or from post-traumatic ossification of para-articular tissues.

Figure 36.12.
Heberden's nodes.

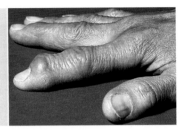

Figure 36.13.
Rheumatoid arthritis. a. Ulnar drift. b. Swan-neck deformity.
c. Rheumatoid knuckle pads. d. Rheumatoid nodule on the elbow.

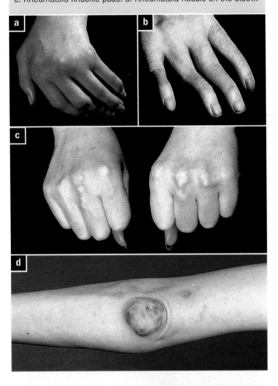

Osteoarthritis of the hand predominantly affects the distal interphalangeal joints. However, all joints can be affected and the carpometacarpal joint of the thumb is another common site.

The rheumatoid hand

The articular effect of rheumatoid arthritis is to cause an inflammatory synovitis. This results in erosion of cartilage and bone leading to swelling, pain and deformity of the joint. The periarticular tissues, such as tendons, are liable to attrition rupture. The common discrete deformities of the hand are as follows.

Ulnar drift *(Figure 36.13a)* occurs at the metacarpophalangeal joints as a result of stretching of the soft tissues, in particular the transverse bands of the base of the extensor hood. The extensor tendons bowstring to the ulnar and palmar side of the metacarpophalangeal joints. The result is the characteristic ulnar drift of the fingers, which are flexed and subluxed at the metacarpophalangeal joints.

The **boutonnière deformity** is an attrition rupture of the intermediate (central) slip of the extensor digitorum communis tendon. The lateral bands of the extensor hood sublux causing flexion of the proximal interphalangeal joint and extension of the distal interphalangeal joint.

Swan-neck deformity *(Figure 36.13b)* results from an imbalance in the tension of the structures of the extensor hood. This allows the transfer of the power of the extensor digitorum communis from its insertion into the distal phalanx to the insertion into the middle phalanx. This is precipitated by abnormalities at the metacarpophalangeal joint, weakness of the flexor digitorum superficialis, mallet deformity, laxity of the volar plate and abnormal joint surfaces *(Figure 36.13c, d)*. The characteristic deformity is hyperextension at the proximal interphalangeal joint and flexion at the distal interphalangeal joint.

Vaughn–Jackson syndrome is rupture of the extensor digitorum communis tendons to the ring and little fingers.

Mannerfelt syndrome is an attrition rupture of the flexor pollicis longus tendon. The patient is unable to flex the interphalangeal joint of the thumb.

Figure 36.14.
Bennett's fracture of the left thumb.

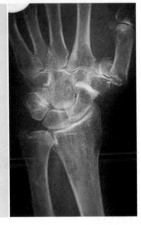

Bennett's fracture *(Figure 36.14)* is an intra-articular fracture of the base of the thumb metacarpal. All movements of the thumb are painful and there is considerable swelling over the thenar eminence and the dorsum of the thumb. The swelling can obscure the deformity and the subluxation at the carpometacarpal joint. The diagnosis is confirmed radiologically.

Figure 36.15.
Dislocated thumb.

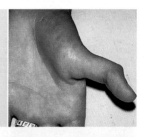

Figure 36.16. Metacarpal fractures.

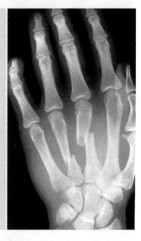

Figure 36.17.
Phalangeal fractures.

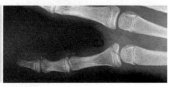

Digital fractures and dislocations

The bones of the fingers and thumb are largely subcutaneous so the deformity of fractures and dislocations is usually obvious. With undisplaced lesions local tenderness can be elicited by carefully palpating the full length of each bone. With the spiral fracture of a metacarpal bone, with shortening, there is loss of prominence of the relevant knuckle on making a fist. Tears in the joint capsule, due to angulation or dislocation, give rise to a spindle-shaped swelling of the digit, which persists for many months and, in severe cases, is permanent. Some fractures and dislocations are shown in *Figures 36.15–36.18.*

Figure 36.18. Dislocation of the proximal interphalangeal joint.

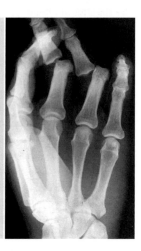

37 The pelvis, hip joint and thigh

Pelvic fractures

Anatomy

The pelvis is a ring structure composed of two innominate bones and the sacrum. The innominate bones are held together anteriorly by the ligaments of the symphysis pubis, and posteriorly by the strong posterior sacroiliac ligamentous complex. The latter consists of the strong interosseous ligaments, the anterior and posterior sacroiliac ligaments, the iliolumbar ligament, the sacrotuberous ligaments and the sacrospinous ligaments. Contained within the pelvic ring are the viscera and the iliac vessels. Passing through the pelvic outlet are the rectum, the urethra and, in the female, the vagina. All of these may be injured in pelvic fractures.

Injuries to the pelvis

Injuries to the pelvis are usually caused by falls or road traffic accidents. The mechanism of the injury determines the energy imparted to the pelvis and this is usually associated with the degree of the injury. Minor falls, particularly in the elderly, may produce isolated fractures of the pubic rami. Falls from a horse may cause severe ligamentous disruption or fracture in the pelvis, associated with visceral injuries. In road traffic accidents, force transmitted along the femurs or due to tightening of a lap seat-belt, can cause significant injury to the bony pelvis. Sporting activity in adolescence can cause avulsion fractures from the pelvis.

Fractures of the pelvis may be outside the pelvic ring and, therefore, not compromise the stability of the pelvic ring. Fractures or ligamentous disruption within the pelvic ring itself usually occur at two sites. The smaller fragment of the ring is unstable and may lead to displacement and later disability. Anterior ring lesions usually occur through the symphysis pubis or through the pubic rami. Posterior lesions usually occur through the sacroiliac joint or produce vertical fractures of the sacrum.

Fractures of the pelvis are thus classified into three types:

- **Type A** fractures or injuries outside the pelvic ring (Figure 37.1a). These lesions do not lead to instability of the pelvic ring itself or any long-term problems in weight bearing. Examples include fractures of the iliac wing, avulsion fractures or transverse fractures of the sacrum or coccyx.
- **Type B** injuries give rise to partial instability of the pelvic ring (Figure 37.1b). Typically, the injury causes rotational instability of half of the pelvis, which may be unstable to either external or internal rotation. Examples include separation of the symphysis pubis associated with a posterior lesion, such as partial separation of the sacroiliac joint retaining some ligamentous connection between the sacrum and the innominate bone. These remaining ligamentous connections prevent the half pelvis migrating superiorly. Wide separation of the symphysis pubis, or pubic rami fractures, are often associated with injury to the pelvic veins and can result in significant haemodynamic instability.
- **Type C** injuries also involve the pelvic ring in two places (Figure 37.1c). In contrast to Type B injuries, the posterior injury is complete, there being little or no ligamentous connection between the sacrum and the innominate bone. The fracture is thus unstable to rotation and vertical displacement. These injuries are often associated with visceral and vessel injury (p. 361).

Figure 37.1.
a. Isolated fracture of the left iliac bone. b. Fracture of left pubic ramus. c. Fracture of pubic ramus with disruption of the sacroiliac joint.

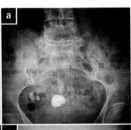
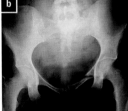
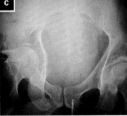

Presentation of pelvic fractures

The history of the mechanism of the accident often indicates whether the violence is of low or high energy. In high energy injuries, the patient may have multiple injuries and be in a state of shock. The assessment of such a patient includes resuscitation in accordance with the guidelines of the advanced trauma life support system (ATLS). Part of the initial evaluation of such a multiply injured patient includes an anteroposterior (AP) radiograph of the pelvis.

Examination of the pelvis in such a patient may reveal bruising or contusion around the pelvic area; evidence of such damage within the scrotum suggests a pelvic floor injury, and bleeding from the tip of the penis suggests a urethral injury. The attitude of the lower limbs may reveal rotational or length abnormality; if there is no long bone fracture in the leg the deformity is most likely to be due to a pelvic injury.

Assessment of stability of the pelvis needs to take place in both the rotational and vertical displacement planes. Rotational assessment is carried out by firmly gripping both iliac crests and attempting to squeeze them together and subsequently to push them apart *(Figure 37.2a, b)*. Abnormal mobility or crepitus suggests fracture or ligamentous disruption. Vertical stability assessment requires two people – one needs to hold both iliac crests to detect movement while the other applies longitudinal traction and compression through the leg to cause vertical displacement of the hemipelvis. This procedure needs to be undertaken with each leg in turn.

Any wounds in the pelvic area need to be carefully assessed, particularly those in the perineal area. Rectal and vaginal examination are mandatory to detect evidence of a rectal or vaginal tear. Tears indicate that the pelvic injury is open and very likely to be contaminated by vaginal or faecal organisms. Such open injuries carry a very much worse prognosis and require prompt surgical treatment. Rectal examination in the male may indicate that the prostate is high riding, implying a complete rupture of the urethra (p. 361).

Neurological examination of the lumbosacral plexus should be carried out and be complete, including assessment of the lower sacral nerves. In Type C injuries neurological abnormalities are seen in nearly 50% of cases. Early diagnosis of such an injury is important and should be documented in the medical notes.

The pelvis is subsequently assessed by examination of the pelvic radiographs, performed as part of the ATLS resuscitative protocol. Further evaluation is often carried out by pelvic inlet and outlet radiographs and by CT scan.

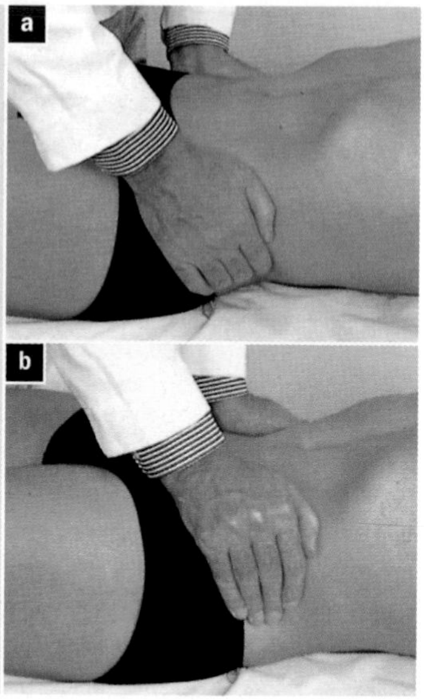

Figure 37.2. Assessing rotational stability of the pelvis. a. Side to side compression. b. Backward pressure at the iliac crests.

Acetabular fractures

Anatomy

The acetabulum is considered for the purposes of trauma to consist of anterior and posterior columns, extending from the ilium down to the pubis and the ischium respectively. Superiorly there is a weightbearing dome area and medially a quadrilateral plate of bone separating the acetabulum from the inside of the pelvis. Injuries to the acetabulum most commonly occur with severe violence, sustained in heavy falls or in road traffic accidents.

The direction of the force produces predictable patterns of injury, and fractures are often associated with dislocations of the hip. A fall on to the greater trochanter applies a force along the femoral neck, fracturing the quadrilateral plate, often in association with anterior and posterior column fractures, and forcing the head deeper into the pelvis.

A longitudinally applied force along the femoral shaft, often produced by a dashboard injury to the knee, results in a posteriorly directed force, leading to fracture of the posterior column. This injury is often associated with posterior dislocation of the hip.

Assessment of acetabular fracture

The history of the mechanism of the injury often alerts the examining doctor to the diagnosis *(Figure 37.3a, b)*. The patient may be shocked because of pelvic vessel injury but

Figure 37.3
a. Acetabular fracture of the left hip. b. CT reconstruction of the fracture shown in a. The orientation is reversed left to right.

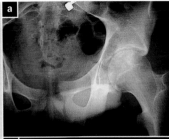

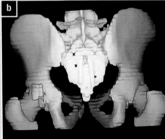

more commonly due to other injuries. Resuscitation and assessment should take place simultaneously. Contusion or bruising over the greater trochanter may suggest direct injury to that part. Evidence of injury to the front of the knee, femoral fracture or abnormal attitude of the leg may suggest a fracture dislocation of the hip. The leg may be shortened or abnormally rotated. Palpation in the groin often reveals tenderness, and any attempt at movement of the affected hip causes severe pain.

Assessment of stability of the pelvic ring should be carried out (see above) and palpation of the affected leg pulses and assessment of neurology must be undertaken. Sciatic nerve injury is not uncommon following posterior column fractures. Further assessment takes place with the AP radiograph and additional information is obtained from a 45° oblique radiograph of the affected hip and by CT scanning.

Gait

Examination of a hip joint must begin with observation of the gait, unless there is a suspected fracture. The **antalgic gait** results from pain in the joint and there is shortening of the period of the stance phase of the affected limb together with a more rapid swing phase of the contralateral limb. The **Trendelenburg gait** occurs as a result of weakness in the power of abduction in the affected hip joint and is characterized by a rapid movement of the shoulders towards the

affected side in order to maintain the centre of gravity while the affected leg is in the stance phase. If this is bilateral, the waddle of bilateral congenital dislocation of the hips should be suspected. The **short leg gait** occurs as a result of a leg length inequality, characterized by an excessive rise and fall of the ipsilateral shoulder with each full gait cycle.

Examination of the standing patient

Inspection

A painful condition of the hip joint leads the patient to stand with the affected side slightly flexed, to minimize the weight bearing. A patient with a short leg may stand with the contralateral longer leg flexed at the knee in order to be balanced. Identify the position of the anterior superior iliac spines and assess if there is a pelvic tilt. Look for wasting of the glutei, which is apparent where there has been chronic arthritis. Scars and sinuses indicate previous surgery or sepsis.

For the **Trendelenburg sign** *(Figure 37.4a, b)* the patient is observed from behind and is asked to lift up their bad leg by bending their knee behind and so keeping the hip extended. The iliac crest on the affected side is elevated as

Figure 37.4
a, b. Trendelenburg test. c. Diagram of failure of pelvic abduction on the side of the dislocated hip. (Reproduced with permission from *Physical Examination in Orthopaedics*, by A. Graham Apley and Louis Solomon, Butterworth–Heinemann, 1997.)

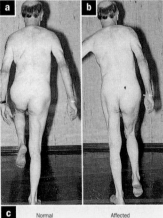

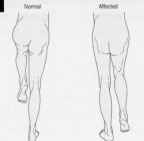

Normal   Affected

a result of the normal functioning of the abductor mechanism of the opposite hip. The patient is then asked to lift up the good leg while standing on the affected side. If the iliac crest on the unaffected side is seen to drop towards the floor due to weak abductor muscles, the patient may be forced to throw their shoulders towards the affected side in order to maintain their centre of gravity. A positive Trendelenburg sign may be due to weak abductor muscles, a shortened femoral neck reducing the lever arm for the muscles, lack of fulcrum in congenital dislocation of the hip or pain on movement of the abductors due to inflammation or injury.

Examination of the supine patient

Position

The patient should lie flat, preferably with only one pillow supporting the head. The anterior superior iliac spines should be palpated to ensure that the pelvis is square with the examining table. The legs are moved by the examiner so that they lie with the medial malleoli adjacent to the centre line of the examination table.

Inspection

A further inspection for scars and sinuses is performed and any deformity is noted. The state of the skin in the rest of the leg is assessed for signs of peripheral vascular disease or infection.

Feel

The normal bony landmarks of the hip are identified. The anterior superior iliac spines and the greater trochanters are palpated to identify their position and to feel for tenderness. The hip joint itself is palpated just below the inguinal ligament and lateral to the femoral artery pulsation. Absence of the femoral head may be obvious in congenital dislocation of the hip. The anterior superior iliac spines are palpated with the examiner's thumbs, which are hooked under the spines and the index fingers are placed over the greater trochanters (Figure 37.5a, b). A decrease in this anterior superior iliac spine to trochanter distance, as compared to the normal side, signifies shortening of the femoral neck or dislocation of the hip.

Measurement
Leg length

A tape measure must be used to measure from the anterior superior iliac spine to the medial malleolus. It is important to make the legs lie in the same attitude as any discrepancy constitutes a real shortening of the limb (Figure 37.6a, b). If short-

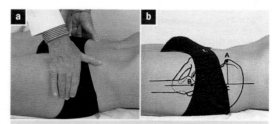

Figure 37.5.
a. Palpation of the anterior superior iliac spines and greater trochanters. b. A, Anterior superior iliac spine; B, Cranial limit of the greater trochanter; C, Bryant's triangle. The distance BC is shortened in fractures of the head of the femur, this being demonstrated by comparing the distance BC on the two sides.

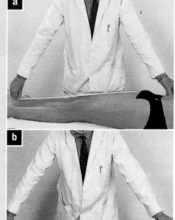

Figure 37.6.
Measurement of leg length. a. Looking for real shortening. b. Looking for apparent shortening.

ening is present the following method is used to localize the site. Both hips are flexed, the knees are flexed to 90° and the feet are placed together (Figure 37.7a, b, c). The knees are then observed from the side of the couch. Shortening in the tibia is demonstrated by a decrease in the level of the anterior surface of the distal femur of the affected side. Shortening in the femur is demonstrated by a relative depression of the proximal anterior surface of the tibia of the affected side.

Girth

Similar points are measured in both legs by marking a specific distance – in the thigh from the anterior superior iliac spine and in the shin from the tibial tuberosity. The circumference at these points indicates the wasting of muscles in the thigh or calf (Figure 29.4; p. 385).

Figure 37.7.
Leg shortening. a. Normal.
b. Shortening of the right thigh.
c. Shortening of the right lower leg.

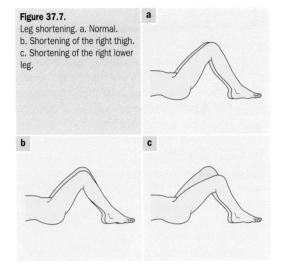

Thomas' test

This test *(Figure 37.8a–c)* is designed to demonstrate a fixed flexion deformity, or loss of the ability to extend, in the hip. The examiner passes one hand, palm upwards, underneath the lumbar spine of the patient. The examiner flexes the normal contralateral hip to its full extent and confirms that the lumbar lordosis is flattened. If there is a fixed flexion deformity, the affected limb becomes flexed at the hip and the knee rises from the couch. The degree of flexion of the hip when the lumbar lordosis is flattened constitutes the amount of the fixed flexion deformity.

Movements

Having confirmed that the pelvis is square to the examination table the following movements can be tested *(Figure 37.9a–g)*.

Figure 37.8.
Thomas' test. a. Patient flexing their own right knee and demonstrating how pelvic rotation takes place. The abnormality of the left hip does not allow extension to retain the leg on the couch. b. The left hand is placed behind the lumbar spine and demonstrates the moment at which the lumbar curve is flattened.

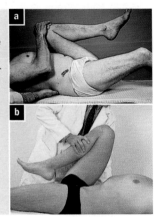

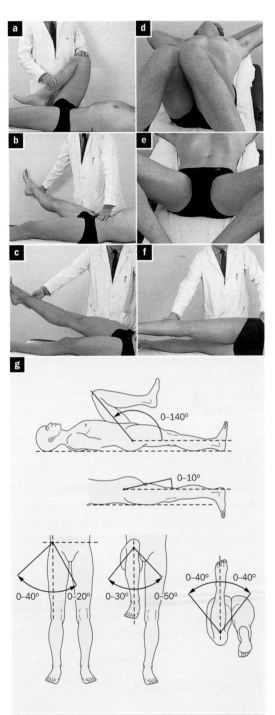

Figure 37.9.
Hip movements. a. Flexion. b. Abduction. c. Adduction. d. Internal rotation. e. External rotation. f. Extension. g. Normal ranges of movement at the hip.

Rotation

The examiner can stand at the end of the table and, holding both feet, can rotate the hip internally and externally. The patella should be observed as an indicator of the amount of rotation and any variation between the two sides can be observed. Rotation can also be measured when the hip and knee are flexed to 90°. Each side can be measured in turn and this is a useful method in the diagnosis of a slipped upper femoral epiphysis, in which a limitation of internal rotation in flexion is an early sign.

Adduction and abduction

The examiner firmly grasps the contralateral anterior superior iliac spine with one hand in order to detect any movement of the pelvis and the leg is deviated away from and towards the midline grasping the lower tibia or ankle with the other hand.

Flexion

Each hip is flexed as far as possible in turn.

Extension

The patient is asked to lie prone on one side and the hip is extended. This is normally only 10° and is limited early in any arthritic process. If Thomas' sign is positive there is no extension of the hip.

Paediatric hip conditions

Development dysplasia of the hip (DDH)

This is a common condition in children with an incidence of 1 in 1000 live births *(Figure 37.10)*. Females are affected four times more often than males and it is associated with

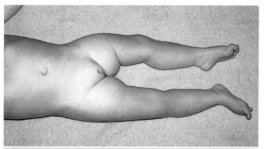

Figure 37.10.
Congenital dislocation of the left hip. There is shortening with extra skin creases on the affected side. The legs do not abduct and externally rotate equally, e.g. in nappy changing.

conditions such as torticollis and metatarsus adductus. There is often an associated family history of DDH and an increased incidence is seen in breach presentations and in oligohydramnios. There is a spectrum of disease ranging through dislocation, subluxation, instability and hip dysplasia. Despite the widespread screening of neonates there is a significant incidence of missed or late diagnosis of this condition. The clinical presentation depends on the age.

Neonate (0–6 months)

Most are diagnosed on routine screening in this age group. Correct diagnosis and treatment results in a 95% cure rate.

The key physical signs are:

- Limited abduction in flexion.
- Ortolani's test – This demonstrates a dislocated hip. The infant lies supine on a flat surface and the examiner places the knees and hips in a flexed position at 90°. The examiner pushes the greater trochanters anteriorly with the fingers, while abducting the hips. The examiner's thumbs are positioned over the femoral heads and a palpable jerk is felt as the femoral head reduces.
- Barlow's test – With the hips and knees flexed to 90° the examiner adducts the legs and applies a posteriorly directed force longitudinally through the femur. This causes a palpable jerk if the femoral head dislocates.

The examiner should be aware that in the case of an irreducible dislocation, neither Barlow's nor Ortolani's test is positive. These clinical tests should not be repeated unnecessarily because of the risk of a vascular necrosis of the head of the femur. In cases of doubt the definitive diagnosis is made by early ultrasound or plain radiographs taken at 3 months, when the upper femoral epiphysis is calcified and visible on radiographs.

Infant (6–18 months)

The infant is crawling or walking. The key signs are:

- Limited abduction.
- Shortening of the leg.
- Asymmetrical skin folds.

The hip is usually no longer reducible. Beware: the bilateral dislocation with symmetrical physical signs may make the diagnosis difficult.

Toddler (18 months to 3 years)

These children present with a delay in walking, limp, Trendelenburg gait and a hyperlordosis of the spine.

Adult life

Symptoms usually start in the early 30s with pain, weakness and limp. The leg is often short and a Trendelenburg gait or sign is present. Limited abduction and internal rotation is characteristic, due to the anteversion of the femoral neck and onset of degenerative arthritis.

Septic arthritis of the hip

This constitutes a surgical emergency because the infective process results in the destruction of articular cartilage. The common organisms are staphylococci, group B streptococci, *Haemophilus influenzae* and *Neisseria gonorrhoeae*. The symptoms are of pain in the hip and decreased range of movement. The generalized signs of sepsis may be present and infants may present with a pyrexia of unknown origin. Observation of the child often reveals that the leg is immobile – pseudoparalysis – due to pain. The hip may be held in the characteristic posture in infants – the 'frog position' – with the hip flexed, abducted and externally rotated. This position maximizes the intracapsular space and reduces the pain that results from excessive fluid pressure within the joint capsule. The hip is tender to palpation in the groin. Any movement of the hip is resisted and causes the child to scream in pain.

Transient synovitis of the hip

This is a common condition of the hip in childhood and should be a diagnosis of exclusion. There may be a history of trauma

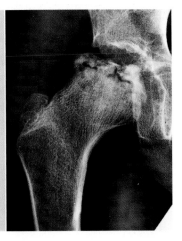

Figure 37.11.
Legg–Calvé–Perthes disease.

(< 5%) or an antecedent viral illness (30%). The child has a limp (85%), the pain is felt in the hip (80%) and may radiate to the knee (25%). All hip movements cause pain and the range of movement is limited but not so severely as in septic arthritis. **Gauvain's test** is often positive – passive sudden internal rotation of the leg is associated with reflex contraction of the abdominal muscles.

The pathological process is of a traumatic or immunologically mediated aseptic inflammation of the synovium, leading to an effusion within the hip joint. Infection should be excluded by observation for the symptoms and signs of sepsis and through haematological investigations. If real doubt exists the hip should be aspirated for microscopy and culture. If septic arthritis is excluded the child should be observed and rested. The application of skin traction can be of benefit in preventing the child from mobilizing. Transient synovitis normally improves within a few days of its commencement and a negative Gauvain's sign is a sign of resolution.

Tuberculous arthritis

Tuberculosis of the hip joint is now rarely seen in developed countries. It presents with a limp and pain, felt in the thigh or in the knee. Muscle wasting and a fixed flexion deformity – Thomas' sign – are characteristic. Neglected cases may develop an abscess or sinus.

Legg–Calvé–Perthes disease

There is necrosis of the head of the femur as a result of ischaemia, followed by revascularization and restoration of bony vasculature (*Figure 37.11*). It occurs most often in the age group between 4 and 8 years. Boys are affected more commonly than girls, with a ratio of 4:1, and 10% have bilateral problems. Associated factors with an increased incidence are seen in those patients with a positive family history, low birth weight and abnormal birth presentations. The pain is often felt in the knee rather than in the hip or thigh.

The child has a limp and a Trendelenburg gait is common. There is a decreased range of movement at the hip joint, particularly abduction and internal rotation. The diagnosis can be confirmed at the time of presentation by plain radiographs. The differential diagnosis can include juvenile rheumatoid arthritis, proximal femoral osteomyelitis and the irritable hip. Bilateral cases may mimic hypothyroidism and multiple epiphyseal dysplasia.

Revascularization and remodelling of the head of femur occur over a period of some years. A good outcome results from the restoration of the sphericity of the head at the time of healing.

Slipped upper femoral epiphysis

This is a common condition of adolescents and affects boys more frequently than girls, with a ratio of 3:2 *(Figure 37.12a, b, c)*. The classical description is of an obese child from hypogonadism but many cases are tall and thin. The patient presents with a limp and often complains only of pain in the knee. There may be a history of acute injury but the majority have had symptoms for weeks or months. On examination there is an antalgic or Trendelenburg gait. There may be an external rotation deformity. There is a painful limitation of internal rotation and of abduction of the hip.

The diagnosis is based on the radiographs. The usual direction of slippage of the epiphysis is posteriorly and medial to the femoral neck. The most sensitive investigation is the lateral plain radiograph; this demonstrates the posterior slippage before the medial slippage of the head becomes apparent on the AP film. The other hip is involved in 40% of cases but only 50% of these are symptomatic.

Figure 37.12.
Slipped upper femoral epiphysis. a. A line drawn along the superior margin of the neck of the femur on an anteroposterior radiograph intersects a small area of the supralateral part of the upper femoral epiphysis (shaded) in normal individuals. In a slipped upper femoral epiphysis a smaller area or no part of the epiphysis projects superior to this Trethowan's line. However, the lateral radiograph is a more sensitive guide to an early slip. b. Anteroposterior view of a slipped epiphysis of the left hip. c. Lateral views of a slipped epiphysis.

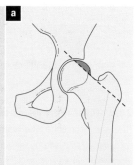

Trethowan's line

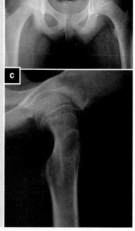

Adult conditions

Osteoarthrosis of the hip

This is a common condition of which the incidence increases with age *(Figure 37.13)*. The patient complains of pain which is often felt in the groin, radiating to the knee. Stiffness, particularly after a long period of rest, results in difficulty in putting on shoes and stockings. As the condition deteriorates, the walking distance is reduced and is associated with a limp. The patient goes on to suffer pain at night or at rest.

Examination of the hip demonstrates an antalgic or Trendelenburg gait. A small amount of shortening of the leg is often present. This may be due to **real shortening**, as the joint space is eroded, or from an adduction deformity of the hip, which gives an **apparent shorting** of the leg (p. 464). If the legs are placed in the same orientation and the length is measured from the anterior superior iliac spine to the medial malleolus; the only shortening that is measured is the real shortening due to loss of joint space. The apparent shortening is eliminated by placing both legs in the same orientation with respect to the pelvis. There is limitation of all hip movements and a fixed flexion deformity.

The majority of cases of osteoarthrosis of the hip constitute a primary condition. Premature osteoarthrosis of the hip can result as a secondary process from developmental dysplasia of the hip, Legg–Calvé–Perthes disease, slipped upper femoral epiphysis and osteonecrosis of the head of the femur.

Osteonecrosis of the femoral head

This condition results from an interruption of the blood supply to the head of femur. There is death of trabecular bone and bone marrow, which is followed by collapse of the bony architecture. In adults revascularization does not occur. The causes include the subcapital fracture of the neck of femur (see below) which leads to a traumatic interruption of the blood supply. Atraumatic causes of osteonecrosis are the use of corticosteroids, alcohol

Figure 37.13.
Osteoarthritis of the right hip.

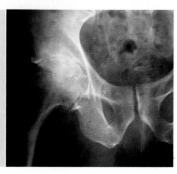

consumption, sickle cell anaemia, Gaucher's disease, myelo-proliferative disorders, chronic pancreatitis, Caisson disease – inadequate decompression after deep sea diving – and irradiation. Severe pain at night is the usual feature. In the early cases there may be only slight restriction of movement. In the later stages, after the femoral head bone has collapsed, there are similar signs to those of an arthritic hip. The diagnosis is confirmed in later cases by plain radiographs as these show collapse of the femoral head and narrowing of the joint space. Early cases are best detected by MRI.

Meralgia paraesthetica

This is a compression lesion of the lateral cutaneous nerve of the thigh as it passes through the inguinal ligament or occasionally through the fascia lata. There is an area of hyperaesthesia in the lateral aspect of the thigh and tingling in this area. This is worse on standing and walking but is relieved by sitting, where flexion of the hip shortens the course of the nerve. Percussion over the inguinal ligament may result in an exacerbation of the symptoms – Tinel's sign.

Psoas bursa

This condition is rare but should be considered in those patients who present with a swelling in the groin. The swelling is located in the femoral triangle but is too lateral to be a femoral hernia. It may not exhibit fluctuance due to it being tense and to the thick capsule around it. Palpation of the iliac fossa is often unrewarding because there is no palpable extension. The hip is often held flexed and externally rotated to relieve the tension in iliopsoas. Also see pp. 65 and 406 for psoas abscess.

The snapping hip

Patients occasionally present with a spectacular condition in which they can, with volition, bring about a distinct 'snap' with certain hip movements. It is sometimes associated with pain. The patient may be concerned that a form of dislocation or subluxation of the joint is occurring. This is a benign condition in which a tendon slips over a bony prominence, usually the iliotibial tract passing over the greater trochanter.

Complications of total hip replacement

This is now such a common orthopaedic procedure that there are many members of the population who have a total hip replacement *in situ*. Four complications are shown in (Figure 37.14a–d).

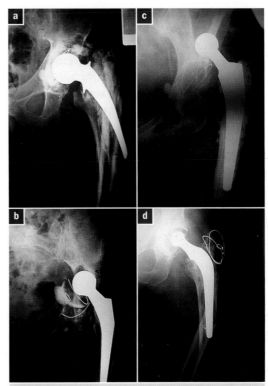

Figure 37.14.
Complications of total hip replacement. a. Aseptic loosening of the prosthesis. b. Loose cup. c. Dislocated prosthesis. d. Periprosthetic fracture.

Chronic low grade infection

The patient complains of a continuous ache in the groin or thigh, usually commencing some weeks or months after hip replacement. There is often a history of wound infection in the immediate postoperative period. Examination of the skin sometimes reveals an inflamed hip wound and possibly a sinus, and there is a noticeable limp with all hip movements possibly causing pain at the limit of exertion. Erythrocyte sedimentation rate and C-reactive protein level are elevated. The plain radiographs may show some signs of loosening and a bone scan is positive. The diagnosis is confirmed on hip aspiration.

Aseptic loosening of the hip

There may be a satisfactory outcome of the hip replacement for some years but then pain starts in the groin or the thigh. The pain may be exacerbated by getting up from rest in a chair. All hip movements cause pain at the limit of their excursion. Examine the hip by flexing it and the knee to 90° and apply axial compression or traction to the femur. This often produces pain as the femoral component of the prosthesis pistons within the femur. Rotation of the hip causes pain and may be associated with a 'clunking' sensation as the loose femoral component moves inside the femoral shaft. The plain radiograph shows demarcation between the bone and the prosthesis and, in advanced cases, migration of the prosthetic components.

Acute dislocation of the hip

The majority of successful total hip replacements use a prosthetic head of the femur that is of a much smaller diameter than the natural head. This affords particular advantages in allowing a good range of movement and reducing the frictional torque within the hip. However it allows an increased risk of dislocation. The direction of the dislocation is governed by the alignment of the acetabular and femoral components as well as the surgical approach used. The risk of dislocation is greatest when the hip is flexed and adducted. The patient complains of sudden severe pain in the hip and feels the hip popping out of the socket. In a posterior dislocation, the leg is short and internally rotated while in an anterior dislocation it is short and externally rotated.

Trochanteric bursitis

This is inflammation of the trochanteric bursa. Palpation over the greater trochanter causes pain. Asking the patient to abduct the leg against resistance by the examiner may cause pain. This condition can occur in patients who have not had hip surgery.

Heterotopic bone formation

This is when abnormal bone is formed in the soft tissues. In extensive cases there is progressive limitation of movement as bony islands can coalesce between the femur and pelvis.

Traumatic injuries of the hip

Fracture of the neck of the femur

Two types of fracture occur but the clinical picture is similar. The capsule of the hip joint extends down the neck of the femur as far as the top of the trochanters – fractures may occur inside or outside this capsule. The **intracapsular fracture** – or subcapital or cervical fracture *(Figure 37.15a, b)* – occurs through the femoral neck. At this point the blood supply to the head of the femur is often interrupted resulting in loss of blood supply to the head. Reduction of the fracture and internal fixation of the fracture may not always result in

satisfactory union of the fracture and a prosthetic replacement is often the treatment of choice in the elderly.

The **extracapsular fracture** *(Figure 37.15c)* occurs outside the hip capsule, usually at the base of the neck or between the trochanters, hence basicervical or intertrochanteric. The blood supply to the femoral head is not transgressed so reduction and internal fixation of the fracture usually leads to satisfactory union.

The majority of these fractures are through osteoporotic bone and occur in the elderly. They present having suffered a fall, often with little violence. There is pain in the hip and there may be bruising in the region of the greater trochanter. The leg is held in external rotation and there is usually shortening. If the leg is severely externally rotated (90°) and short, the fracture is probably extracapsular. Lesser degrees of external rotation and shortening are seen in intracapsular fractures due to the constraint of the hip capsule. Some intracapsular fractures are undisplaced, or the bone ends are impacted, giving rise to little or no deformity; the patient may even be able to raise their leg from the bed. The diagnosis of a fracture is confirmed by AP and lateral radiographs.

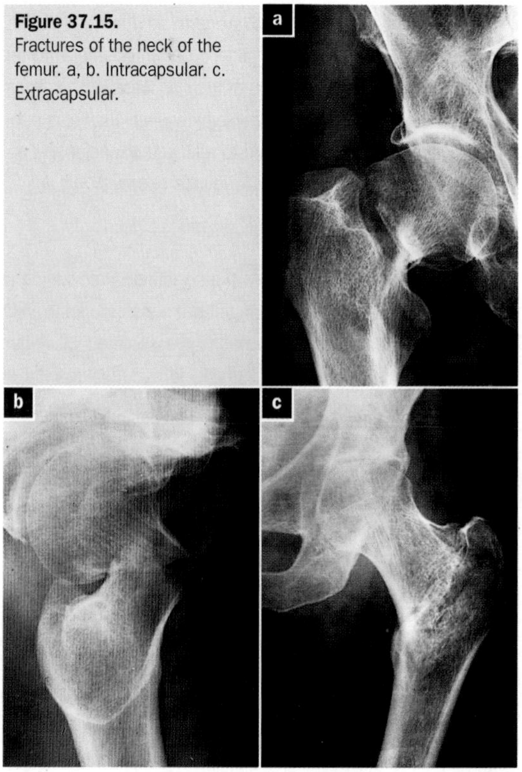

Figure 37.15.
Fractures of the neck of the femur. a, b. Intracapsular. c. Extracapsular.

Isolated trochanter fractures

A direct fall on to a hip can cause an isolated greater trochanter fracture. There is usually bruising and swelling around the trochanter with local tenderness. The hip movements are usually reasonably well preserved although painful; the diagnosis is confirmed radiologically. Avulsion of the lesser trochanter in isolation tends to occur in hurdling schoolchildren and is due to violent contraction of psoas. The patient is unable to actively flex the hip but other movements are intact – Ludloff's sign.

Fractures of the shaft of the femur result from extreme violence and range from simple transverse or spiral undisplaced fractures to severe, shattered, comminuted lesions, which are often compound and may be accompanied by vascular injury. The fractures occur in all ages but are commonest in young adults. In children, non-accidental injury must be considered. In the elderly, pathological fractures *(Figure 37.16)* occur in the upper third, these are usually through secondary deposits but may be in osteomalacia or osteoporotic bone, or in Paget's disease, where the brittle bone produces a characteristic transverse fracture.

Observing the patient in bed, the lower leg is laterally rotated and cannot be moved and there is true shortening of the limb.

Displacement is related to the direction and severity of the violence. In the upper third *(Figure 37.17)*, unopposed action of the iliopsoas and gluteal muscles flex, externally rotate and abduct the proximal fragment, while the quadriceps and hamstring muscles draw the distal fragment proximally. In mid and distal *(Figure 37.18)* third fractures, the distal fragment angulates posteriorly, together with the leg shortening.

A number of litres of blood may be discharged into the thigh but one litre may go unnoticed. The patient, therefore, may present in a state of hypovolaemic shock.

Traumatic dislocations of the hip

These are relatively rare and usually require considerable violence. The commonest form is the posterior dislocation, which usually results from a road traffic accident, when the victim's knee hits the dashboard and a longitudinal force is directed up the femur. The head of the femur is dislocated and often the posterior rim of the acetabulum is fractured *(Figure 37.19)*. There is severe pain in the groin. The leg lies internally rotated, shortened and is often slightly flexed at the hip. The greater trochanter appears unduly prominent. The sciatic nerve is injured in up to 10% of cases.

In central dislocation of the hip the head of the femur is driven through the floor of the acetabulum, which is fractured. There may be signs of a direct blow to the side of the hip and the leg tends to be abducted. Movements are painful.

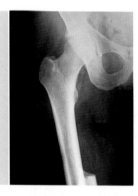

Figure 37.17.
Fracture of the upper third of the femur.

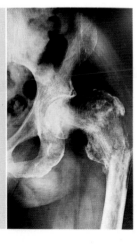

Figure 37.16.
Subtrochanteric pathological fracture of the femur.

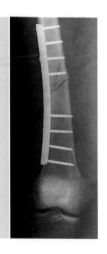

Figure 37.18.
Fracture of the lower third of the femur.

The anterior dislocation is very rare and usually occurs after falls from a height on to the feet. The leg is abducted, externally rotated and slightly flexed. The femoral head is palpable in the groin. There is usually no shortening because upward migration of the hip is prevented by the iliofemoral ligament.

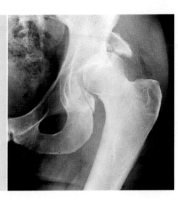

Figure 37.19. Dislocation of the hip with associated acetabular fracture.

38 The knee joint

General examination of the knee

Gait

An antalgic gait is present in conditions producing pain in the knee. The straight leg gait, where the patient circumducts the affected leg during its swing phase, results from fusion of the knee or from an advanced arthritic process, when there is little flexion. In long-standing weakness of the quadriceps muscle, hyperextension of the knee may be present in the stance phase.

Observation with the patient standing

Valgus or varus deformity at the knee joint becomes apparent on weightbearing. The normal physiological angulation between the shafts of the tibia and femur is 5–7° of valgus. An angulation in excess of this is genu valgum, i.e. knock knees *(Figure 38.1)*; angulation less than this constitutes genu varum, i.e. bow legs *(Figure 38.2)*. Childhood deformity may result from hereditary bone dysplasias or developmental growth plate abnormalities. In the adult it may result from previous trauma to the ligaments of the knee or from loss of articular cartilage in severe arthritis.

A flexion deformity, due to capsule contraction in arthritis or mechanical blockage due to a torn meniscus or loose body, may be obvious when the patient is standing. A recurvatum or hyperextension deformity may also be apparent in cases of hypermobility, ligamentous injury or long-standing quadriceps weakness. The presence of scars or sinuses should be noted.

Figure 38.1.
Knock knees.

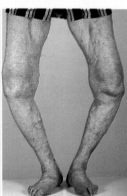

Figure 38.2.
Bow legs.

Examination with the patient supine

The back of the examination couch can be placed at 45° so that the patient is comfortable and the posterior structures of the lower limb can be relaxed when the knee is extended. The thigh should be observed for wasting of the quadriceps muscle. The circumference of the thigh can be measured at equivalent levels on both sides to give a numerical comparison of muscle wasting *(Figure 29.4; p. 385)*.

Observations should be made for generalized and local swelling around the knee. Generalized swelling, leading to obliteration of the medial and lateral parapatellar gutters, suggests that an effusion is present. A localized swelling with bruising on one or other side of the knee may indicate a recent ligament injury. Swelling at the joint line level may indicate osteophyte formation or a meniscal cyst. A swelling confined to the popliteal area is usually due to a fluid filled popliteal bursa – Baker's cyst. Redness of the skin and an increased temperature indicate an inflammatory process in the knee.

Palpation

Identification of the normal anatomical landmarks is difficult with the knee extended. With the knee flexed to 90° the medial and lateral joint lines, head of the fibula, tibial tuberosity and the femoral epicondyles can be palpated. Local tenderness is often a good clue to the site of the pathology *(Figure 38.3a, b)*. The superficial surface of the patella and the patellar ligament are palpated for tenderness.

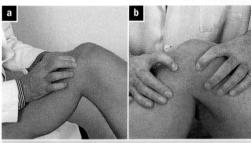

Figure 38.3.
Palpation of knee the joint. a. Palpation along the joint line.
b. Palpation of proximal and distal ends of the medial ligament.

With the knee extended, the medial and lateral borders of the articular surface of the patella are palpated; they are tender if an arthritic or inflammatory process is present. The knee should be flexed and extended passively by the examiner whilst one hand is placed symmetrically over the front of the knee, with thumb and fingers across the medial and lateral joint line. Crepitus *(Figure 38.4)* may be elicited from the movement of osteoarthritic articular surfaces over each other and the examiner can usually localize the compartment in which this occurs.

Testing for an effusion

A large effusion causes obliteration of the medial and lateral parapatellar gutters and there is fullness proximal to the patella in the suprapatellar pouch. In the **patellar tap test** *(Figure 38.5)* the suprapatellar pouch is emptied by pressing above the patella with one hand while the other examining

hand pushes the patella towards the examining couch. In normal circumstances there is no patellar movement. Where there is moderate effusion the examiner feels the patella move and then halt as it engages the trochlear groove.

The **stroke test** *(Figure 38.6)* is used to elicit a small effusion. The medial parapatellar gutter is stroked by one hand of the examiner to empty it of fluid. The lateral parapatellar gutter is then stroked from above downwards and the medial side is observed for movement as fluid passes from the lateral gutter into the medial gutter. If the test is negative it is repeated with one hand emptying the suprapatellar pouch from above and holding it closed. A small effusion can be demonstrated by this manoeuvre.

Movement

The patient is asked to dorsiflex the ankle and to press the knee into the examining couch, while tensing the quadriceps mechanism *(Figure 38.7a)*. An examining hand should be placed behind each knee simultaneously to determine if both knees are pushed back to the same degree. Inability to fully extend the knee – a fixed flexion deformity *(Figure 38.7b)* – may be due to capsule contracture in arthritis or a mechanical block to extension in the form of a meniscal tear or loose body.

The patient is then asked to lift the leg straight from the examining couch. In normal circumstances the knee extends to 0° or –10° during this manoeuvre. If the patient cannot fully extend the knee in this manner, but it can be extended further passively, the difference (measured in degrees) is known as the extensor lag. This indicates a failure of the normal func-

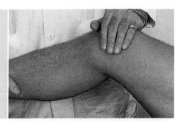

Figure 38.4.
Eliciting crepitus. The examiner's left hand is palpating the joint while the right is used to passively flex and extend the knee.

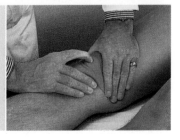

Figure 38.5.
Testing for a patellar tap.

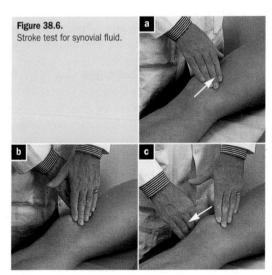

Figure 38.6.
Stroke test for synovial fluid.

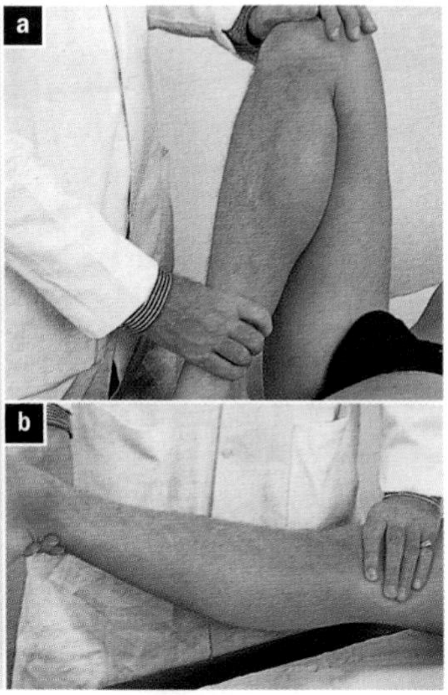

Figure 38.7.
Passive movements
of the knee.
a. Flexion.
b. Extension.

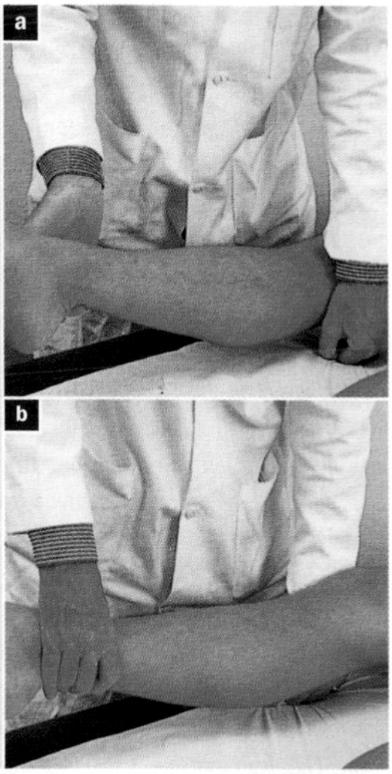

a

b

Figure 38.8.
a. Varus and b.
valgus stress test
(method 1).

a

b

tion of the quadriceps mechanism to extend the knee through the available range of passive motion. The patient is asked to flex the knee and this can normally occur until the soft tissues of the back of the leg and the thigh are in contact.

Tests for ligamentous laxity
Collateral ligaments

Varus and valgus stress tests are used to determine if there is injury to the medial or lateral collateral ligaments, and to assess if there is loss of joint space in arthritis. Two methods can be used.

A varus or valgus force can be applied by pressing the medial or lateral side of the knee respectively *(Figure 38.8a, b)*. The patient's ankle can be stabilized between the examiner's elbow and trunk *(Figure 38.9a, b)* allowing the examiner's hands to be placed either side of the knee. Movement in excess of the normal knee is noted.

The second method involves placing of one examining hand behind the knee with the fingers and the thumb on either side of the knee. The other hand grasps the ankle and applies a varus or valgus force while the femur is restrained by the hand behind the knee, applying an opposing force.

The test should be done in both full extension and slight flexion. Full extension of the knee causes tightening of the posterior capsule adding to stability of the knee. Abnormal movement in full extension indicates a major ligament rupture because the posterior capsule has been torn in addition to the collateral ligament. If the test is only positive in 20° of

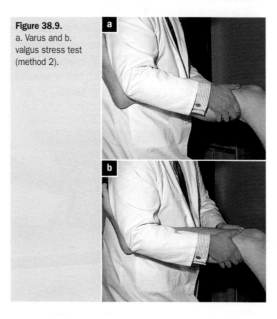

Figure 38.9.
a. Varus and b.
valgus stress test
(method 2).

a

b

flexion and not full extension, it implies a more limited injury to the collateral ligament. An arthritic knee may demonstrate abnormal collapsing of the knee into varus or valgus on stressing due to loss of the articular cartilage on either the medial or lateral side of the knee, respectively.

Anterior cruciate

In the **Lachman test** *(Figure 38.10)* the knee is flexed to 20° with the foot resting on the couch; the examiner grasps the thigh and lower leg with each hand. A forward translational force is applied to the tibia while the femur is pushed backwards at the same time. Both knees are compared and an increase in movement is suggestive of rupture of the anterior cruciate ligament.

To perform the **anterior drawer test** *(Figure 38.11)* the knees are flexed to 90°. The examiner steadies the feet by sitting lightly on the patient's toes and grasps the lower leg with both hands just below the tibial tubercle with the fingers palpating the hamstring tendons to confirm that they are relaxed. An anterior force is applied; excessive movement in the anterior direction is suggestive of a rupture of the anterior cruciate ligament.

The **pivot shift test** *(Figure 38.12a, b)* is used to confirm instability of the knee resulting from rupture of the anterior cruciate ligament. The patient lies supine with the hip in neutral rotation and slightly flexed. The knee is held extended initially. The examiner holds the foot internally rotated in one hand and applies a valgus stress to the knee with the other. This manoeuvre causes subluxation forward of the tibia on the femur when there is rupture of the anterior cruciate ligament. The knee is then flexed smoothly from full extension. There is a palpable clunk at about 20°–30° as the tibia reduces into its normal position if the pivot shift test is positive.

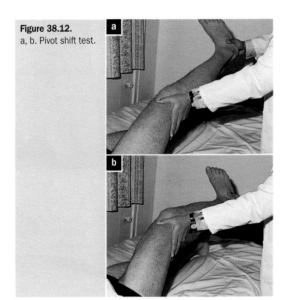

Figure 38.12.
a, b. Pivot shift test.

Posterior cruciate

In the **posterior drawer test** *(Figure 38.13)* both knees are flexed to 90° with both feet placed together. The knees are observed from the side and a posterior sag of the tibia on the femur indicates that there has been a rupture of the posterior cruciate ligament. A posteriorly directed force on the tibia may confirm this and an anterior force on the tibia should reduce the tibia to the normal position.

The arcuate ligament complex

The **arcuate ligament** is a thickening of the posterior capsule. It arises from the fibular head and diverges such that one limb is attached to the femoral condyle and popliteus tendon while the other limb curves over the popliteus and is attached to the back of the lateral meniscus. **Posterolateral**

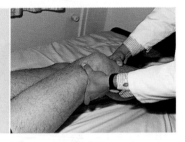

Figure 38.10.
Lachman test.

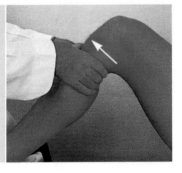

Figure 38.11.
Anterior drawer test.

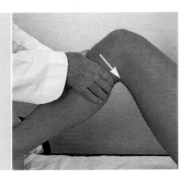

Figure 38.13.
Posterior drawer test.

rotatory instability of the knee results from disruption of the arcuate ligament complex which is made up of the arcuate ligament, the lateral collateral ligament, the tendoaponeurotic portion of the popliteus muscle and the lateral head of the gastrocnemius. The posterior cruciate ligament is also injured in the majority of cases. It usually occurs after sporting injury or a traffic accident.

The **external rotation recurvatum test** is positive in posterolateral rotatory instability. With the patient supine the legs are elevated from the examining table by grasping the great toes and lifting them. The test is positive if the knee falls into a varus angulation, with hyperextension and if the tibia rotates externally. In the **posterolateral drawer test** the knee is flexed to 90° and the examiner is seated gently on the toes. The tibia is pushed posteriorly and the test is positive when the lateral side of the tibial plateau is subluxed posteriorly in relation to the femoral condyle. The medial side of the tibial plateau remains stationary.

Signs of a meniscal injury

There may be **wasting** of the quadriceps muscle if the tear has been present for some weeks. There is often an effusion.

Tenderness can be elicited at the level of the joint line over the torn meniscus.

In the **McMurray test** *(Figure 38.14a, b)* the hip is flexed to 90° and the knee is flexed to over 90°. The examiner grasps the knee in one hand with his or her fingers over both joint lines and the foot in the other hand. The knee is taken from a position of abduction and external rotation to adduction and internal rotation by applying force to the foot. The test is repeated in varying degrees of flexion. The test is positive if there is a palpable click in the appropriate compartment of the knee as the torn meniscus becomes entrapped within the knee.

In **Apley's test** *(Figure 38.15a, b)* the patient lies prone with the knee flexed to 90°. The thigh is fixed by the examiner's knee and the foot is pulled upwards in order to distract the knee joint. At the same time a lateral rotation force is applied. If this causes pain it is suggestive of a lesion of the medial collateral ligament of the knee. If lateral rotation is repeated with compression applied through the knee the grinding test is positive, suggestive of a tear of the medial meniscus. To test the lateral compartment of the knee the test is repeated with the foot internally rotated.

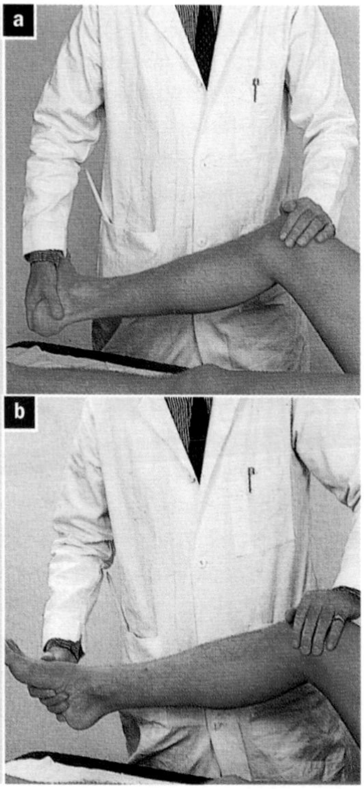

Figure 38.14.
a, b. McMurray test.

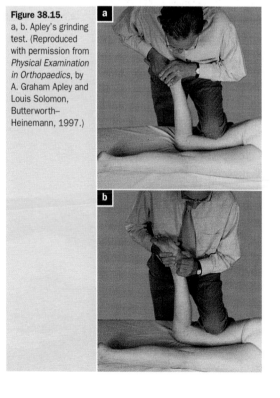

Figure 38.15.
a, b. Apley's grinding test. (Reproduced with permission from *Physical Examination in Orthopaedics*, by A. Graham Apley and Louis Solomon, Butterworth–Heinemann, 1997.)

Acute injuries of the knee

These are a common occurrence and involve either a direct blow to the knee or a twisting injury *(Figure 38.16)*. The patient presents with pain, swelling and limited movement in the knee. It is often difficult to make an accurate diagnosis on the initial assessment. Certain features should be sought. In the case of injury during a sporting event it is useful to know whether the patient was able to finish the event; if so it is less likely that there is a serious injury. If swelling occurs it is important to know the time period between the injury and the onset of swelling. Immediate swelling of the knee usually results from bleeding into the joint cavity – haemarthrosis – due to tearing of structures inside the knee. There is usually a tear of a ligament or meniscus but an intra-articular fracture may have occurred and therefore radiographs should be taken.

If a haemarthrosis is aspirated using an aseptic technique it is important to observe the fluid for globules of fat as this strongly suggests a fracture. An effusion that occurs some hours after the injury is suggestive of a traumatic synovitis, a usual occurrence after any knee injury. Muscle spasm and swelling make interpretation of limitation of movement difficult, while pain and apprehension limit testing of ligamentous laxity. In these circumstances it is important to re-examine the knee some days later when a more accurate assessment can be made.

The locked knee and meniscal injury

The menisci transmit a significant proportion of the body weight through the knee. These injuries occur most commonly in soccer players where there is a twisting injury when the leg is in the stance phase with sufficient violence to tear the meniscus. The locked knee is one of the few circumstances in which

a reasonable presumptive diagnosis can be made after an acute knee injury. The patient is **unable to fully extend the knee**. Passive knee extension by the examiner comes up against a firm resistance preventing full extension. This is strongly suggestive of a displaced bucket handle tear of the medial meniscus. The other causes of a locked knee are a loose body and a torn remnant of the anterior cruciate ligament.

The usual initial presentation is of an acute knee injury. However, in middle age the menisci undergo degenerate change and relatively minimal trauma can cause a tear. Subsequently the symptoms of the meniscal injury are as a result of the loose meniscal fragment interfering with the movement between the joint surfaces, particularly when the knee is flexed and twisted during normal activities. The patient complains of intermittent 'locking' of the knee. The patient's complaint of 'locking' should be carefully compared to the precise medical term locking which means an inability to fully extend the knee because of a mechanical obstruction to movement. **True locking** of the knee occurs as a result of a displaced bucket handle tear of the meniscus or a loose body obstructing the joint surfaces. The patient may be able to overcome the locking by shaking the limb or twisting the knee, resulting in a sudden freeing of knee movement. '**Pseudolocking**' often arises from patellofemoral joint disorders when the knee is painful to move from the flexed position; there is no true mechanical obstruction to joint movement.

Only 40% of all meniscal tears are displaced into the joint causing locking of the knee. Other symptoms include pain at the joint line especially on twisting or kneeling, repeated swelling and giving way of the knee. The other signs of a meniscal tear are quadriceps wasting, effusion, tenderness at the joint line and a positive McMurray or Apley's test.

Rupture of the ligaments

Ligamentous rupture requires a considerable degree of violence such as a traffic accident or a heavy tackle during a sport such as football. There is usually a haemarthrosis in the acute circumstance. Immediate diagnosis often cannot be made with certainty and therefore a little time must be allowed for these acute symptoms to settle.

Rupture of the **medial collateral ligament** results from vigorous ball games and skiing, in which a severe valgus force is applied to the knee. If the knee is examined a few days after the injury there may be visible swelling and bruising on the medial side of the knee. There is tenderness over the ligamentous attachments, the medial aspect of the knee and the joint line. When a valgus stress is applied to the knee there is

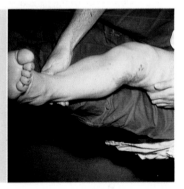

Figure 38.16.
Rupture of the medial and anterior cruciate ligaments.

excessive laxity and pain. Incomplete injuries are often more painful than complete ruptures on valgus stress, due to remaining injured but intact ligament fibres being stretched.

Rupture of the **lateral collateral ligament** of the knee occurs when severe varus forces are applied to the knee. The discrete cordlike ligament runs from the femoral condyle to the head of the fibula. When it is torn there may be swelling and bruising laterally, tenderness over the ligamentous attachments and lateral joint line, and excessive movement when a varus stress is applied to the knee. The injury can be associated with a palsy of the common peroneal nerve.

Rupture of the **anterior cruciate** ligament occurs in hyperextension injuries, when the ligament is tented over the intercondylar notch in the femur. It is also ruptured in severe valgus injuries of the knee when there is associated rupture of the medial collateral ligament of the knee and tearing of the medial meniscus – **O'Donohue's triad**. The physical signs of anterior cruciate ligament injury are of an effusion (often haemarthrosis), positive anterior draw test, positive Lachman's test and a positive pivot shift test.

Rupture of the **posterior cruciate ligament** results from a violent injury such as striking the dashboard of a car in an accident. In the acute injury there may be swelling and bruising in the popliteal fossa. The knee exhibits more hyperextension than the uninjured side when the legs are lifted off the couch by holding the heels. The posterior drawer test reveals a posterior sag of the tibia which can be increased by a posteriorly directed force and reduced to normal by an anterior force.

Injury to the **arcuate ligament complex** and the posterior cruciate ligament gives rise to **posterolateral rotatory instability** of the knee. It occurs after sporting injury or motor accident. The external rotation recurvatum and the posterolateral draw tests are positive.

Loose bodies

The patient often describes something moving in the joint and sometimes can even feel the body. There is often a history of the knee giving way or painful clicking. Very often there is no history of trauma. The physical findings are often non specific unless the joint is locked at the time of consultation. Radiographs are required to demonstrate the loose body.

Osteochondritis dissecans

This is a common cause of loose bodies in young people, predominantly males. The site of the lesion is usually the medial condyle of the femur, adjacent to the intercondylar notch. There is an area of necrosis and partial detachment of articular cartilage. The patient has symptoms of a loose body or joint line pain similar to that of a torn meniscus. If the patella is pressed against the femoral condyle and the knee is flexed and extended, this may exacerbate any discomfort over the lesion. This condition can also occur in the patella and give rise to anterior knee pain.

Anterior knee pain

Pain in the anterior aspect of the knee occurs in middle-aged and elderly patients as a result of patellofemoral osteoarthritis. However, this symptom is also common in adolescents and young adults in the conditions described below.

Malalignment

An altered quadriceps angle, weakness of the vastus medialis muscle and tight hamstring muscles can alter the mechanics of the patellofemoral joint leading to excessive forces across it and producing anterior knee pain.

Chondromalacia patellae

This is a self-limiting condition of young adults and adolescents. There is softening of the articular cartilage of the patella. On examination there may be wasting of the quadriceps muscle and an effusion. Patellofemoral crepitus is usual and direct pressure applied to the patellofemoral joint during flexion and extension may exacerbate the pain; the aetiology is unknown. However, it has been postulated that a direct blow to the kneecap, which may have been overlooked, initiates the abnormality in the articular cartilage. The natural history of this disorder is that it does improve although it may take many years.

Synovial shelf syndrome

The medial synovial shelf is a normal structure. Impingement of this synovial shelf on the femoral condyle can be a cause of anterior knee pain. It should be suspected when tenderness can be elicited along the patella retinaculum, adjacent to the medial aspect of the patella, during flexion and extension of the knee.

Excessive lateral pressure syndrome

Patellofemoral tenderness is exacerbated when the lateral facet of the patella is pushed laterally against the femur and is reduced when it is pushed medially by the examiner. The mobility of the patella is reduced in the medial direction, when the patient is relaxed, due to a tight lateral patellar retinaculum.

Patella tendonitis (jumper's knee)

The pain is localized to the centre of the patellar tendon near its insertion to the patella. A partial tear of the tendon has often been the initiating episode as a result of a severe strain.

Osgood–Schlatter's disease

This is a traction apophysitis of the tibial tubercle *(Figure 38.17)*. It occurs in adolescents during their growth spurt and is most common in athletic youngsters. The tibial tuberosity is tender and unusually prominent. The diagnosis is confirmed with radiographs.

Sindig–Larsen disease

This occurs predominantly in children under 10 years of age and is characterized by tenderness of the lower pole of the patella and the adjacent patellar tendon. The aetiology is similar to Osgood–Schlatter's disease.

Patellar instability

Under normal circumstances the patella engages the trochlear groove at 30°–40° of flexion. When the quadriceps muscle contracts with the knee in the extended position the patella should be pulled superiorly in a straight direction. Abnormalities of patella tracking can be shown by the fact that, at terminal extension, the patella may be seen to sublux laterally out of the trochlear groove. As the knee goes into flexion again the patella may be noted to jump back into the groove.

Sage's sign is indicative of a tight lateral retinaculum. The patient is supine and relaxed with the knee flexed to 20°. The examiner attempts to displace the patella medially – excursion of the patella of less than one quarter of its maximum width is considered positive, while 10 mm of displacement medially is considered normal and 5 mm or less is abnormal.

The **patellar apprehension test** is indicative of dynamic instability. The patient is supine with the knee flexed to 20°. The examiner displaces the patella laterally. Patients with instability find this particularly uncomfortable.

The quadriceps (Q) angle indicates the relative angle of insertion of the quadriceps mechanism. It is measured by drawing an imaginary line connecting the centre of the patella and the anterior superior iliac spine, marking the line of the pull of the quadriceps tendon. A reference line is drawn from the centre of the patella to the centre of the tibial tuberosity marking the pull of the patellar tendon. The angle of intersection of these lines is the Q angle. The average Q angle in males is 14°, in females 17°. A Q angle greater than 20° is considered abnormal and is associated with patellar instability.

Patellar dislocation

The acute dislocation is usually in the lateral direction and the patella is seen abnormally positioned over the lateral femoral condyle. When examined a few days after reduction of the patella there is usually bruising and swelling medial to the patella due to tearing on the medial capsule *(Figure 38.18)*. Radiographs should be examined carefully for evidence of a fracture of the patella or the lateral femoral condyle. Not infrequently an osteochondral fragment is sheared off during the dislocation and should be removed or fixed back into place. Examine the lateral radiograph for evidence of a lipohaemarthrosis, i.e. fat floating on top of the effusion seen in the suprapatellar bursa. If in doubt, aspirate the knee and look for fat globules floating on the haemarthrosis. A lipohaemarthrosis indicates that a fracture is present.

In cases of recurrent dislocation, the signs suggestive of patellar instability are Sage's sign and patellar apprehension. The diagnosis can be confirmed by examination under anaesthetic (EUA).

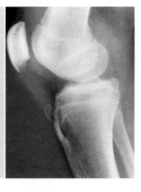

Figure 38.17.
Osgood–Schlatter's disease.

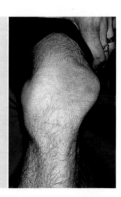

Figure 38.18.
Patellar dislocation.

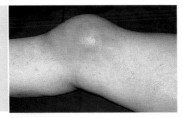

Figure 38.19.
Prepatellar bursitis.

Fat pad (Hoffa's) syndrome

There is a substantial fat pad lying deep to the patellar tendon. It may be injured by direct trauma to the knee. In the chronic condition there is pain when the knee is fully extended and tenderness with palpation of the fat pad which is adjacent to the patellar tendon medially and laterally.

Prepatellar bursitis (housemaid's knee)

This common condition is brought on by trauma to the anterior aspect of the knee, such as kneeling in carpet layers. Swelling in the prepatellar bursa ensues. Redness, swelling and tenderness anterior to the patella are the usual signs (Figure 38.19). If a penetrating injury has occurred, this bursa may be infected with pyogenic organisms and a surrounding cellulitis occurs. The range of movement in the knee should be well preserved, differentiating this condition from septic arthritis.

Infrapatellar bursitis (clergyman's knee)

There is a cystic subcutaneous swelling overlying the patellar tendon and tibial tuberosity caused by similar activities to that of prepatellar bursitis. The signs are similar but the swelling is more distal.

Cysts around the knee

Swellings at the front of the knee have been explained above.

The semimembranosus bursa

This lies between the medial head of the gastrocnemius and semimembranosus tendon and is found on the medial side of the popliteal fossa. It is tense when the knee is extended and flaccid when the joint is flexed. It does not communicate with the joint and cannot be emptied by compression.

Popliteal (Baker's) cyst

The swelling is more central and lower in the popliteal fossa than the semimembranosus bursa. The patient is likely to be in middle age or above. It is a diverticulum of the synovial

membrane through a hiatus in the capsule of the joint and is associated with rheumatoid arthritis or osteoarthritis. Although the cyst is in communication with the cavity of the knee joint, the channel may be very small and it may not be possible to express fluid from the cyst into the knee itself. The popliteal cyst is prone to spontaneous rupture, rupture after minor trauma (Figure 38.20) or strenuous exercise – which results in pain, swelling and tenderness in the calf – and a clinical picture that is similar to deep vein thrombosis.

The bursa anserina

This is placed between the tendons of the sartorius, gracilis and semitendinosus superficially and the medial collateral ligament of the knee deep to it. When distended and swollen it is apparent over the medial aspect of the knee. It is also referred to as breast-stroker's knee.

Meniscal cysts

This is a swelling on the medial or lateral aspect of the knee at the level of the joint line. The aetiology of the lesion is a degenerate tear within the meniscus which allows a synovial herniation that is filled with joint fluid. Depending on the nature of the opening between cyst and joint there may be intermittent or progressive enlargement. The '**disappearing sign**' is that the cyst is apparent when the knee is extended and less apparent or absent when the knee is flexed.

Lateral meniscal cyst

This is present on the lateral joint line around the posterior border of the lateral collateral ligament of the knee (Figure 38.21). The disappearing sign may be present as with the medial meniscal cyst.

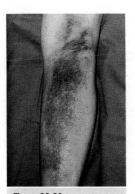

Figure 38.20.
Ruptured Baker's cyst.

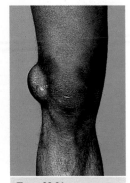

Figure 38.21.
Lateral meniscal cyst. This lesion is unusually large.

Arthritis of the knee

Septic arthritis of the knee

The knee is swollen and it is held in 20°–30° of flexion. The overlying skin is often red and hot. An effusion is present and the patient resists any movement at the joint. Any patient presenting in this manner must be presumed to have a septic arthritis until proved otherwise. The differential diagnosis includes osteomyelitis of the adjacent femur or tibia, an inflammatory arthropathy and crystal arthropathy – gout or pseudogout. Joint aspiration using a sterile technique is mandatory, followed by Gram stain and culture of the aspirate, to establish the diagnosis.

Osteoarthritis of the knee

This is a common condition in advancing age. Medial compartment disease is more common than lateral compartment. When there is genu varum the disease is in the medial compartment, similarly in genu valgum the lateral compartment of the knee is predominantly affected. Osteoarthritis of the patellofemoral joint can occur as a prominent feature, or it may be absent until the medial and lateral compartments are completely destroyed.

The patient walks with an antalgic gait. Examination of the patient standing reveals the varus or valgus deformity. Examination on the couch shows the knee to be held in fixed flexion due to capsular contraction; an effusion is often present. Osteophytes are palpable and there is joint line tenderness, crepitus and restriction of movement. The varus or valgus deformity can usually be corrected passively to neutral by doing a valgus or varus stress test *(Figure 38.22a, b)*.

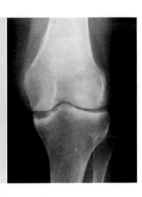

Figure 38.23.
Rheumatoid changes of the knee joint.

Rheumatoid arthritis

This inflammatory arthropathy causes widespread destruction in all three compartments of the knee *(Figure 38.23)*. Other joints are also involved – look at the hands of the patient – and the extra-articular manifestations of rheumatoid arthritis may be present (p. 432). Valgus deformity is much more common than in osteoarthritis and is usually associated with a fixed flexion deformity. Thickening of the synovium may be palpable in the suprapatellar bursa.

Tuberculosis

This condition is now rare in the western world but is still common in less developed countries. A patient, aged 10–30 years, presents with a painful swollen knee of several months' duration. A fixed flexion deformity and synovial thickening may be present. There is usually a good range of movement. Diagnosis is usually achieved by examination of an aspirate of the knee.

The popliteal fossa

Popliteal aneurysm

The popliteal pulse is usually difficult to palpate. When the pulse is very easily palpated, particularly in a middle-aged or elderly male, an aneurysm should be suspected (p. 373).

Tumour of the common peroneal nerve

The common peroneal nerve leaves the popliteal fossa and winds around the neck of the fibula. The rare tumour of the nerve is palpable in this area. It has the particular characteristic that it is mobile from side to side but not proximally and distally. Percussion over the nerve may elicit a Tinel's sign (p. 411) with radiating pain and paraesthesiae to the dorsum of the foot.

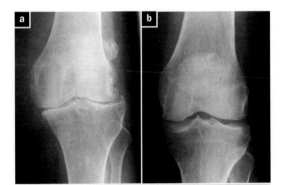

Figure 38.22.
Osteoarthritis of the knee. a. Typical changes. b. Destruction from wear and tear when the protective sensation of a joint is lost. (Charcot's joint.)

Injuries to the extensor mechanism

Rupture of the rectus femoris muscle occurs in the elderly or as a sports injury. There is pain around the patella and a characteristic hollow above the patella in the quadriceps tendon, where the fibres have been avulsed. If the patient cannot straight leg raise, operative repair should be considered.

Patellar fractures *(Figure 38.24a, b)* may be transverse or stellate. **Transverse fractures** are due to powerful contraction of the quadriceps and are avulsion fractures. A lipohaemarthrosis is present. Separation of the fragments occurs if the medial and lateral retinacular expansions of the quadriceps tendon are also torn. In these cases a gap is palpable in the patella and the patient is unable to straight leg raise. **Stellate fractures** are usually caused by a direct blow to the anterior aspect of the knee giving rise to local bruising. The retinacular expansions are rarely torn and marked separation of the fragments is less common than in transverse fractures; the straight leg raise is usually intact.

Ligamentum patellae ruptures occur in young adults due to sporting injuries or violent trauma. The injury can occur in the substance of the ligament or through an avulsion fracture of the tibial tuberosity in children, or the lower pole of the patella in adults. A puffy swelling develops over the ligament and the patella is riding high. The straight leg raise is absent.

Fractures about the knee

Patellar fractures have been mentioned above. Other fractures of the knee usually involve significant violence in children and young adults. In the elderly, osteoporosis significantly weakens the bone and fractures can occur with minimal trauma. As in all fractures, good quality radiographs are essential for accurate diagnosis.

A **supracondylar fracture of the femur** is usually clinically obvious as it is accompanied by pain, swelling, tenderness and an inability to move the leg. The gastrocnemial attachments to the distal fragment may produce posterior angulation at the fracture site. The foot pulses should always be assessed in view of the close relation of the fracture to the popliteal vessels. The comparable injury in children is the fracture separation of the lower femoral epiphysis.

A **fracture of a femoral condyle** *(Figure 38.25)* results in a lipohaemarthrosis. One or both condyles can be involved in a T or Y form, and may be displaced, such as after a direct blow when the patella is driven backwards, splitting the two femoral condyles.

Fractures of the tibial plateau (condyles) are relatively common and may be articular or non-articular. The lateral condyle is most frequently involved during falls or from side impact, typically from a car bumper – valgus force. A tear of the opposite collateral ligament is often present. The central portion of the condyle is often depressed making the knee unstable. This can only be assessed accurately by examination under anaesthetic by valgus or varus stress testing, depending on the condyle involved. A lipohaemarthrosis is present.

Figure 38.24.
Fractures of the patella. a. Transverse. b. Stellate.

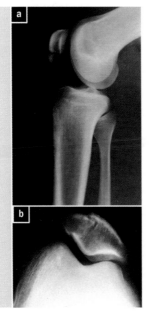

Figure 38.25.
Fracture of the medial femoral condyle.

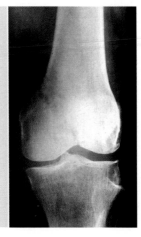

39 The leg and ankle joint

Soft tissue ruptures

The soft tissues of the leg are subject to a wide variety of ulcers (p. 393) and the leg and ankle are particularly vulnerable to trauma. The tibia and fibula are often injured in athletic pursuits or motorcycle accidents and constitute the commonest compound fractures in the body. The fibres of the powerful superficial calf muscles can be torn and occasionally the tendo Achillis is ruptured; the anterior muscles may be damaged in a compartment syndrome (p. 380). The ankle is subject to ligamentous and bone injuries in individuals from all walks of life, and the latter may be followed by premature arthritic problems. A swollen ankle is most commonly a post-traumatic problem but may also be part of systemic or lower limb disease (p. 394).

Rupture of the tendo Achillis most commonly occurs in middle-aged males, particularly while playing racket sports, but may follow even simply getting up from a seated position The rupture is usually complete but an incomplete lesion may rupture at a later date (see below). There is a sudden severe pain at the back of the lower leg, as though the patient had been kicked in the back of the ankle, and an individual cannot even limp without severe pain. The characteristic posture of the reclining foot is that it is held in a position less equinus than normal. The calf muscles are slightly contracted and drawn proximally and a defect can be felt in the tendo Achillis about 5 cm above its insertion.

Simmonds' test *(Figure 39.1)* is positive in complete rupture. In this test the patient lies prone with their feet hanging over the end of a couch and the calf is squeezed transversely. If the tendon is intact or incompletely ruptured the foot is seen to plantar flex. If the tendon is completely ruptured there is no movement of the foot.

Attrition rupture of the tendo Achillis occurs a few weeks after an incomplete rupture. The patient falls to the ground believing they have been tripped. There is surprisingly little pain compared with that of the primary event.

Tears of the soleus muscle are usually the sequelae of unaccustomed exercise. The condition used to be termed a ruptured plantaris tendon but it is now known to be due to tears of the soleus. The pain is sudden and severe, resembling

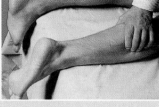

Figure 39.1.
Simmonds' test for a ruptured tendo Achillis. (Reproduced with permission from *Physical Examination in Orthopaedics*, by A. Graham Apley and Louis Solomon, Butterworth–Heinemann, 1997.)

that of a torn tendo Achillis but it is sited within the calf and the patient can usually still limp, albeit with marked discomfort. There is tenderness over the calf and, after a few days, bruising appears below the soleus muscle on the medial or lateral side of the tendon. If the patient remains ambulant the bruising descends to form a crescent above the malleolus. The **crescent sign** was originally thought to be indicative of calf vein thrombosis and this remains an important differential diagnosis when the problem is not clearly linked to exercise. Discomfort and a limp can take a number of weeks to resolve.

Shin pain occurring after unaccustomed exercise may also be produced by shin splints and an anterior compartment syndrome (p. 380). **Shin splints** are due to small muscle tears in the extensor muscles; there may be local tenderness but often there are no abnormal physical signs. The importance of the condition is the differential diagnosis of stress fractures of the tibia (see below) and compartment syndrome.

Painful heel

A painful heel may be due to lesions at the back of the foot or the back of the sole – the latter are considered on p. 497. Pain over the back of the foot is usually produced by tight narrow footwear and is common in young women and military recruits. The lesion produced is inflammation of an adventitious bursa, superficial or deep to the tendo Achillis, or over a calcaneal exostosis, which may exist just lateral to the tendon's attachment.

In **retrocalcaneal bursitis** the tenderness is deep to the tendo Achillis and the swelling is on either side of it. In **retro-**

Achillis bursitis *(Figure 39.2)* tenderness and swelling are superficial to the tendon. **Achillis tendonitis** is inflammation of the paratenon of the tendo Achillis. The pain, inflammation, degenerative changes *(Figure 39.3)* and tenderness are above the line of pressure from the heel of a shoe.

Osteochondritis of the calcaneum – Sever's disease *(Figure 39.4)* – occurs most often in boys 8–12 years old. As with Osgood–Schlatter's disease (p. 480) the condition is a traction injury of the epiphyseal cartilage. The first symptom is a limp, followed by dull pain in the back of the heel. There is tenderness and localized swelling over the posterior surface of the calcaneum below the attachment of the tendo Achillis.

Haglund's syndrome is a stress fracture of the calcaneal near the attachment of the tendo Achillis.

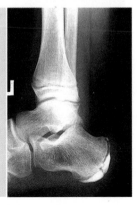

Figure 39.2.
Retro Achillis bursa.

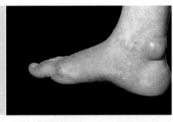

Figure 39.3.
Calcification of the tendo Achillis.

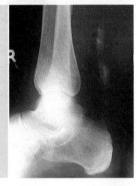

Figure 39.4. Osteochondritis of the calcaneum.

Fractures of the tibia and fibula

A **combined fracture of the tibia and fibula** *(Figure 39.5a–d)* is a common accident to men in the prime of life. This dual fracture is the commonest compound fracture, the overlying tissues being damaged either by direct injury or by a sharp end of one bone – usually the upper fragment of the tibia – transfixing the skin. The medial side of the great toe, the medial malleolus and medial side of the patella are usually in a straight line though this relationship is lost when both the tibia and fibula are fractured. Frequently the foot is rolled outwards and the deformity is obvious, in which case no attempt should be made to palpate or move the leg, thus avoiding further damage. Foot pulses, however, must always be checked to avoid missing distal ischaemia. As a rule the fibula is broken at a higher level than the tibia.

Isolated fractures of the shaft to the tibia may occur in a **young child** after a fall. There may be no pain or apparent abnormality when recumbent but the child refuses to bear weight and the cardinal sign is localized tenderness around the undisplaced spiral fracture. In the **adult** the fracture is usually due to a direct blow and is a transverse or slightly oblique fracture with overlying tissue damage, although when explored the injury may not be compound, i.e. the soft tissue injury may not extend down to the bone.

Isolated fractures of the shaft of the fibula are fractures of the adult, produced by direct trauma. The fracture is transverse and diagnosed clinically by local tenderness and, if in doubt, by **springing the fibula**. In the latter, place a knee

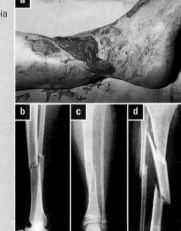

Figure 39.5.
Fractures of the tibia and fibula.
a. Compound fracture.
b. Transverse.
c. Spiral.
d. Segmented.

over the medial side of the middle of the leg and pull on the patient's knee and ankle. This opens up the fracture producing pain at the fracture site.

Stress fracture of the tibia is an incomplete fracture involving only the bone cortex. It is an overuse condition affecting athletes, professional dancers and soldiers in training. It causes a dull gnawing pain in the shin lasting for many hours. Deep palpation over the shin reveals an area of tenderness along the medial border of the subcutaneous tibia. Springing the tibia (see above re fibula) causes pain. The diagnosis is confirmed by plain radiographs although this may fail to demonstrate the fracture, in which case it can be seen on isotope bone scanning.

The ankle joint

The two malleoli are among the most obvious surface markings (Figure 39.6a, b) of the body. The lateral is a little less prominent and descends lower than the medial malleolus, the tip being 1 cm below and behind the corresponding landmark on the medial side. The line of the ankle joint lies on a plane 1 cm above the tip of the medial malleolus.

When the joint becomes distended with an effusion, the foot takes up a position of inversion and slight dorsiflexion. There is bulging beneath the extensor tendons as they cross the joint line and a fullness just anterior to the lateral and medial malleolar ligaments. A more extensive effusion causes bulging posteriorly filling up the hollow on either side of the tendo Achillis. To confirm the presence of fluid, place a finger on either side of the tendon (Figure 39.7); by digital compression some of the fluid can be displaced from one side to rebound against the watching finger on the other.

The neutral position of the ankle joint is with the foot at a right angle to the leg. Examine the ankle joint with the knee slightly flexed, to avoid tension in the tendo Achillis. On the left foot, grasp the heel with the left hand, and the forefoot with the right. In dorsiflexion the left hand pulls down and the right pushes up (Figure 39.8a, b). For plantar flexion the left is pushed up and the right pulled down. These movements occur principally at the ankle joint. Continue to hold the heel and, with the other hand, test inversion (turning the sole inwards) and eversion (turning the sole outwards) (Figure 39.9a, b). These movements occur principally at the subtalar joint. Rotation – valgus and varus – occurs at the midtarsal and plantar flexed ankle joint. The combination of rotation and inversion is termed supination, and rotation and eversion, pronation. In circumstances where there is laxity of the

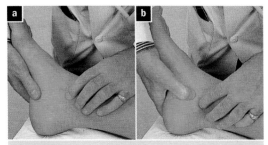

Figure 39.6.
Surface markings. a. Of the medial malleolus. b. Of the medial ligament.

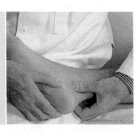

Figure 39.7.
Examining for the presence of fluid in the ankle joint.

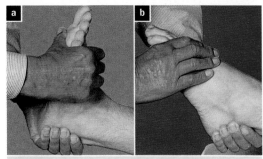

Figure 39.8.
a. Dorsiflexion and b. plantar flexion of the ankle. (Reproduced with permission from Physical Examination in Orthopaedics, by A. Graham Apley and Louis Solomon, Butterworth–Heinemann, 1997.)

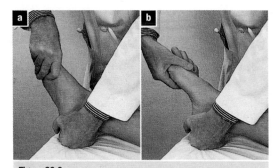

Figure 39.9.
a. Inversion and b. eversion of the foot.

medial or lateral ligament of the ankle joint there is an excessive valgus or varus movement. This is most often of the lateral ligament and is usually bilateral; such individuals are prone to recurrent inversion injuries.

As in other situations, **ligamentous injuries without fracture** may be incomplete or complete. The term 'sprain' is often used but should be reserved for *minor* ligamentous injuries and it is advisable to employ the terms incomplete or complete rupture for any substantial injury.

A sprained ankle is the result of a combined inversion and plantar flexion accident. Pain and tenderness are localized to the front of the ankle towards the fibula side. Directly after the accident, a haematoma appears at the site of the tear but it soon becomes obscured by generalized oedema.

In **rupture of the lateral ligament**, maximum tenderness is found below the tip of the malleolus, in contrast to a Pott's fracture dislocation (see below) where the tenderness is over the fibula itself. It is important to be able to distinguish a complete tear with avulsion of the ligament from an incomplete injury. Provided there is not marked discomfort, the ankle is slowly passively inverted – if the ligament is avulsed an obvious gap appears between the tip of the malleolus and talus on the anterolateral aspect of the joint. If pain prevents this manoeuvre it may be repeated after the injection of local anaesthetic. In doubtful cases the findings can be confirmed by a radiograph taken with the ankle held in full inversion and compared to the uninjured ankle.

As the medial ligament is much the strongest ligament of the ankle joint, **rupture of the medial ligament** is unusual without an associated fracture of the lateral malleolus and subluxation of the ankle joint.

In **fractures of the ankle** (Figure 39.10a–d) the patient usually makes the diagnosis of a displaced fracture themselves. In doubtful cases, or with an undisplaced fracture, there is swelling of the ankle, an inability to bear weight, a reduced range of movement and bony tenderness at the site of the fracture. Most commonly there is an isolated fracture of the lateral malleolus. With greater severity of injury there is a bimalleolar fracture, commonly of the lower end of the fibula, often 5 cm above the tip of the malleolus, associated with fracture of the tip of the medial malleolus. In almost every case there is some lateral or medial displacement of the talus. In many instances there is also an avulsion of the posterior malleolus of the ankle, this being the posterior aspect of articular surface of the tibia. Thus severe injuries are fracture subluxations although the displacement of the talus is usually insufficient to warrant the term dislocation. The term **Pott's fracture** – subluxation is often applied,

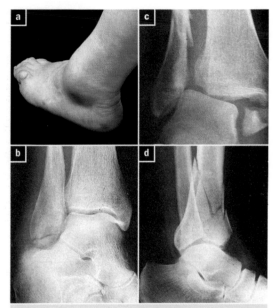

Figure 39.10.
Ankle fractures. a. Fracture of the lateral malleolus demonstrating marked local swelling. b. Fracture of the lateral malleolus. c. Fracture of medial malleolus with spiral fracture of the lower end of the fibula. d. Comminuted fracture of the lower end of the tibia.

named after the surgeon who carefully assessed his own equestrian injury.

In children and adolescents, severe ankle injuries involve displacement of the lower tibial epiphysis.

The **Maisonneuve fracture** is an important injury since it can be easily missed. There is a fibular fracture but this is above the syndesmosis and can be as high as the fibular neck. However, there is also rupture of the medial collateral ligament and tearing of the interosseous membrane, resulting in separation of the fibula and tibia, and diastasis of the ankle joint. The ankle is swollen and tender anteriorly and there is also tenderness over the fibular fracture. The diagnosis is confirmed radiologically.

Dupuytren's fracture is sustained by falling on to the feet from a height. The talus is driven upwards and the ligaments that support the inferior tibiofibular joint are torn, producing diastasis. The width of the ankle between the malleoli is increased and the distance from the malleoli to the sole shortened.

Fractures of the talus (Figure 39.11) are uncommon and, as with the calcaneum, the injury is usually due to a fall on to the feet from a height. The bone is usually fractured

Figure 39.11.
Fracture of the talus.

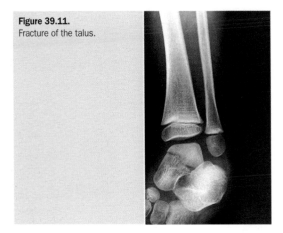

Figure 39.12.
Subtalar dislocation.

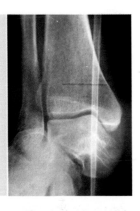

Figure 39.13.
Rheumatoid arthritis.

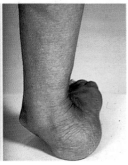

across the neck but comminuted fractures may enter the ankle joint. The absence of muscle attachments to the talus makes the bone subject to avascular necrosis, leading to non-union and subsequent arthritic change. The injury may also produce a subtalar dislocation *(Figure 39.12)*, this occurring with or without a talar fracture.

Osteoarthritis of the ankle joint occurs, often prematurely, as a result of ankle fractures or after repeated minor trauma, such as in football; swelling may be the presenting symptom. Osteophytes develop on the anterior and posterior lip of the anterior surface of the talus and may be palpable. In the case of the former, dorsiflexion of the ankle, and in the latter plantar flexion, cause pain upon impingement.

Rheumatoid arthritis is accompanied by loss of cartilage and osteoporosis that, in turn, produce joint destruction followed by bony collapse and deformity *(Figure 39.13)*.

In **TB of the ankle joint** the early signs are those of swelling and calf muscle wasting due to disuse atrophy. A limp is inevitable and there is pain in the joint, forcing the patient to walk on the forefoot to prevent full weightbearing. Untreated cases are subject to sinus formation.

Recurrent dislocation of the peroneal tendons from their groove is commonly an aftermath of an ankle injury,

there being laxity of their restraining ligaments; the displacement occurs on active extension with eversion and is sometimes very painful. The patient may be able to demonstrate the dislocation with an audible click or snap with this movement. The tendons are also subject to chronic **stenosing tenosynovitis** similar to that found around the wrist joint. There is tenderness and swelling along the course of these tendons, below and behind the lateral malleolus. Pain occurs only on inversion of the foot.

Patients who work or meditate in a cross-legged position occasionally develop an adventitious subcutaneous bursa over the lateral surface of the lateral malleolus. It is termed the tailor's bursa, from the occupational position that used to be common in this trade.

40 The foot

Introduction

The foot is subject to a wide variety of lesions in countries where footwear is not worn, and recurrent minor trauma and infection predominate. The latter, together with the problems of ingrowing toenails and plantar warts are considered in Chapter 4. The subsequent sections firstly consider the examination of the foot. This is followed by descriptions of the lesions affecting the whole of the foot, then those affecting the hindfoot (talus and calcaneum), the midfoot (remaining tarsal bones), and the forefoot and toes (metatarsals and phalanges). Finally lesions of the heel and sole and superficial tissues are discussed. The heel refers to both the posterior aspect of the foot and to the posterior aspect of the sole and is considered on pp. 485 and 497.

Examination of the foot

In view of the diversity of lesions, the system and extent of examination matches the presenting abnormality. This could involve the mechanism of the whole foot or be limited to a single toenail. Expose the foot and whole leg at least to thigh level – it is essential that both sides are exposed to allow for comparison.

The **gait** will have been observed if the patient has walked into the consultation. If not, and if the patient's age and disability permit, examine the gait for a limp and determine whether this is related to a disability of foot movement or foot discomfort. When the patient has removed their footwear examine their shoes, provided these have been regularly worn, since they may show evidence of abnormal wear or scuffing of an edge.

Examine the **stance** with the patient standing upright and in a balanced position, the feet being directed forward and slightly apart. To examine the feet in the standing position it is convenient to have the patient on a raised platform. In the normal stance an imaginary plumb line dropped from the middle of the patellar should bisect the space between the first and second metatarsals. Examine the arches of the foot as the medial longitudinal arch varies in its height amongst the normal population but look for flat feet or an abnormally high arch. Observe the heel from behind to check the normal alignment of the calcaneum with the tibia.

Examine the patient lying down on a couch. This examination follows the usual pattern of 'Look, Feel, Move' and, if appropriate, request radiographs. If a lesion is not obvious, ask the patient to point it out, together with the position of any associated pain. Inspection may reveal deformity of bones or joints, and abnormalities of subcutaneous tissues such as inflammation or pigmentation. Palpate the foot to confirm deformities and localize any tenderness. Active movement involves dorsal and plantar flexion and inversion and eversion, together with movement of the toes. During passive movement take into account any pain on active movement in order to avoid undue discomfort. Deformity, local tenderness, abnormal movements or undiagnosed pain may require radiological examination.

Deformities involving the whole foot

Clubfoot (talipes)
This is a congenital condition with a number of different morphological types. The abnormal postures of the foot are:

- Equinus (plantar flexion).
- Calcaneus (dorsiflexion).
- Varus (inversion).
- Valgus (eversion).

These various terms together with cavus – an undue hollowing of the instep – are used individually, or as a combination of any two, to describe any deformity.

Talipes equinovarus
This is the most common of the types of clubfoot *(Figure 40.1)*, the incidence is approximately 1 in 1000 live births, there is a strong familial tendency and boys are affected twice as often as girls. It is bilateral in one third of cases. In normal infants the foot can be passively dorsiflexed until the toes touch the anterior aspect of the leg by the examiner. In talipes equinovarus,

Figure 40.1.
Talipes equinovarus.

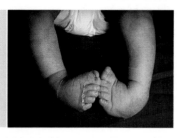

this movement is resisted and the foot may not even reach neutral or plantigrade. The flexures of the foot stand out with deep furrows and the tendo Achillis is short and prominent when dorsiflexion is attempted. The calf muscles can appear underdeveloped. This is an abnormality of uterine packaging and is associated with other abnormalities such as developmental dysplasia of the hip, femoral neck anteversion and tibial torsion. Other forms of club foot are rare.

Calcaneovarus is an extreme form of equinovarus. **Talipes calcaneovalgus** *(Figure 40.2)* occurs with a congenitally long tendo Achillis – a vertical talus is present and it can be classified as a form of this abnormality (p. 493).

Metatarsus varus – 'pigeon toes' – is a common congenital abnormality, the vast majority of cases correcting spontaneously by the age of four. The forefoot is medially deviated, the foot is plantigrade and the heel is normal.

An isolated **equinus deformity** *(Figure 40.3)* is an acquired disorder, usually due to paralysis of the extensor muscles of the foot or when shortening of a leg necessitates walking on tiptoe. It commonly occurs in patients with severe chronic venous ulceration where regular physiotherapy has not been undertaken. The deformity eventually becomes fixed but should be looked for with the knee fully extended since it can be obscured by a relaxed tendo Achillis. Callosities may be found beneath the head of the metatarsal bones.

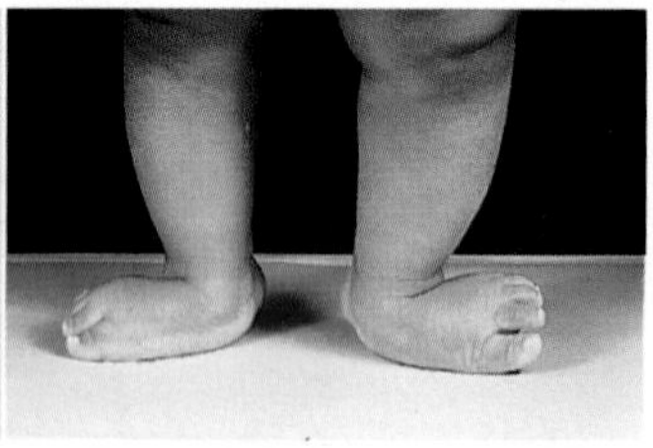

Calcaneus deformity occurs with any isolated paralysis of the gastrocnemius and soleus muscles. In acquired paralytic talipes, in both children and adults, the lesions are usually related to poliomyelitis. There is wasting of the affected muscle groups and the leg is usually cold and often discoloured. In the congenital lesions, always look for other congenital deformities, particularly spinal dysraphism.

Pes cavus

Pes cavus *(Figure 40.4)* is an exaggeration of the medial longitudinal arch. Most often it is idiopathic but several neurological and muscular disorders can produce the abnormality, in particular Charcot–Marie–Tooth disease, muscular dystrophy, Friedreich's ataxia and tibial nerve palsy. The toes are clawed and callosities form under the metatarsal heads.

A Volkmann's ischaemic contracture of the posterior compartment of the leg may result in a raised medial arch and claw toes. A Dupuytren's contracture can effect the plantar fascia resulting in contracture and an apparently elevated medial arch. The condition is usually unilateral and asymptomatic. It may be associated with hand involvement.

Pes planus (flatfoot)

Flatfoot *(Figure 40.5)* is one of the commonest foot abnormalities and is often referred to as a fallen arch. It is usually bilateral, most often an asymptomatic variation of normal, but may also be the result of other foot abnormalities. The longitudinal arches are most often affected but the transverse arch may also be affected, with splaying of the metatarsals. The condition is usually correctable by standing on tiptoe. Unilateral rigid, i.e. not correctable, flatfoot usually means there is an

Figure 40.2.
Talipes valgus

Figure 40.3.
Equinus deformity.

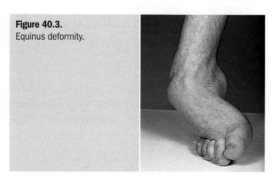

Figure 40.4.
Pes cavus following poliomyelitis.

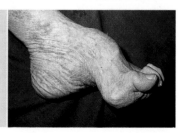

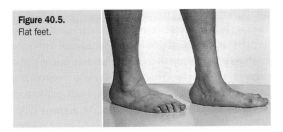

Figure 40.5.
Flat feet.

important and underlying pathology such as rupture of the tibialis posterior tendon or a hindfoot tarsal abnormality.

In the **pseudoflatfoot of infants** the medial fat pad is relatively large and obscures the appearance of the medial longitudinal arch. It normally disappears before the age of three.

In **congenital flatfoot due to talonavicular dislocation**, a congenital vertical talus is usually unilateral and the bony prominence of the dislocated head of the talus can be felt in the central part of the sole.

Rotational disorders include femoral anteversion and genu valgum; these give the appearance of a flat foot.

Acquired flatfoot – In adolescents and adults it is necessary to decide whether the foot assumes an arch just when it is non-weightbearing, when standing on tiptoe or whether the flatfoot is constant – rigid flatfoot. Note the arch when examining the stance and later when resting on a couch. A **mobile flatfoot**, when the arch is retained, is the commonest acquired flatfoot. It follows unaccustomed standing or accompanies rapid weight gain. **Foot strain** is a variety of relaxed flatfoot and follows unusual exercise or mobilization after confinement to bed. There is pain, tenderness and sometimes oedema over the medial longitudinal arch of the foot. The condition often occurs in middle-aged women, when the cause is likely to be due to rupture of the tibialis posterior tendon. A **rigid flatfoot**, seen in adolescents, is mainly due to congenital or post-traumatic tarsal abnormalities.

The metatarsophalangeal joint of the first ray and the fifth ray carry the bulk of the weight of the foot, with relative sparing of the second and fourth rays in **transverse flatfoot** – 'splay foot'. Flattening of the transverse arch can occur with age but is predominant in patients with rheumatoid arthritis where there is also subluxation of the metatarsophalangeal joints, and there may be symptoms of metatarsalgia (p. 494). The condition may be associated with hallux valgus (p. 495). Severe neuropathy of the foot (pp. 371 and 417) or gross infection (p. 79) can destroy the architecture of the foot, replacing the concavity of the foot with a convexity.

The hindfoot

The hindfoot comprises the calcaneum and talus and their joints. Also in this section are considered disorders of the posterior aspect of the foot. The posterior and sole aspects of the heel are considered on pp. 485 and 497 respectively.

Injuries of the talus are considered with the ankle joint; severe fractures are likely to be followed by chronic arthritic changes. The talus is also dislocated is some congenital forms of flatfoot (p. 492).

Fracture of the calcaneum *(Figure 40.6a, b)* is a common injury in people who work using ladders. It is produced by falling on to the feet from a height and is often bilateral. The fracture is associated with fracture of the vertebral column, particularly the first lumbar vertebra, the tibial plateau and, less frequently, fractures of the neck of the femur and the base of the skull. A fractured calcaneum presents with broadening of the heel, pain, swelling and bruising. Maximum tenderness is over the side of the bone rather than the plantar aspect. Ankle movements are limited, and inversion and eversion produce marked pain due to involvement of the subtalar joint. The subtalar joint is often involved and is therefore subject to premature arthritis. Stress fractures are considered on p. 487.

Premature osteoarthritis, in this case **subtalar arthritis**, often occurs after calcaneal fractures; rheumatoid arthritis and idiopathic osteoarthritis can also affect the area. There is pain in the foot, particularly on walking on uneven ground. Subtalar movement is assessed by holding the heel in one hand, steadying the tibia in the other and applying valgus and varus stresses to it. Movement on the affected side is reduced, as compared to the normal, and the patient's pain is reproduced at extremes of movement.

The **sinus tarsi syndrome** is a disorder of unknown aetiology although a history of trauma may be elicited. There is pain on the lateral side of the foot, which is reproduced when pressure is applied over the sinus tarsi, and a feeling of instability when walking over rough ground.

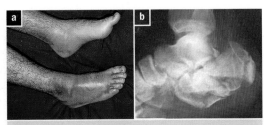

Figure 40.6.
Fracture of the calcaneum. a. Note the bruising and the bilateral injury. b. Calcaneal fracture.

The midfoot

Neuropathic arthropathy is a common cause of disruption and deformity of the midfoot. It occurs most frequently in diabetes mellitus (p. 371). Collapse of the midfoot can lead to early reversal of the longitudinal arches and produce the 'rocker bottom' foot. A sensory neuropathy, particularly with the loss of protective sensation, such as vibration pain and temperature, is present. The autonomic neuropathy leads to loss of sweating and temperature regulation, the skin becoming dry and inelastic. Plain radiographs show gross deformities in the midfoot joints.

Tarsal stress fractures occur in athletes and soldiers in training. The patients present with vague symptoms of pain in the midfoot. There is tenderness over the site of the fracture, which is usually the navicula or the cuboid. The diagnosis can occasionally be confirmed radiologically but this has a low sensitivity. Isotope bone scanning is the investigation of choice.

Tarsometatarsal (Lisfranc's) dislocation *(Figure 40.7)* is produced by a rotational injury and may be accompanied by metatarsal fractures. It is also accompanied by marked tissue swelling and, sometimes, distal ischaemic changes.

Köhler's disease *(Figure 40.8)* is an osteochondritis of the navicular bone. It normally commences in childhood and the patient suffers a limp and mild pain in the dorsum of the foot. There is tenderness over the navicular. The abnormality is confirmed on radiographs and it is usually self-limiting.

Tarsal tunnel syndrome is analogous to the carpal tunnel syndrome in the hand. The tibial nerve is compressed in the fibro-osseous tunnel deep to the flexor retinaculum, below and behind the medial malleolus. There is burning pain and tingling in the toes, and in the sole of the foot. Occlusion of the arterial blood supply with a sphygmomanometer for a minute reproduces the symptoms and electrophysiological studies establish the diagnosis.

The forefoot

The foot, like the hand (p. 455), is subject to a number of congenital bony abnormalities. These include syndactyly, polydactyly *(Figure 40.9)*, curly and over-riding toes and the absence of toes *(Figure 40.10)*. These deformities may also accompany various forms of talipes.

The forefoot comprises the metatarsal and phalangeal bones. The former are subject to pain and stress fractures, and with the proximal phalanx of the great toe, the deformity of hallux valgus. The toes may be deformed in congenital abnormalities such as talipes and are subject to trauma and infection.

Metatarsalgia is pain situated over the heads of the metatarsals. It results from abnormal loading of the metatarsal heads, such as in flattening of the transverse arch.

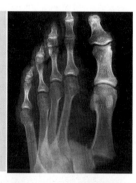

Figure 40.7.
Tarsometatarsal dislocation.

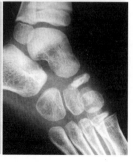

Figure 40.8.
Köhler's disease.

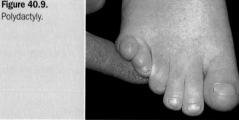

Figure 40.9.
Polydactyly.

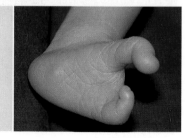

Figure 40.10.
Absent toes.

The term is also used to describe pain from other sources, such as hallux rigidus, corns and warts.

Morton's metatarsalgia results from a neuroma of the medial plantar nerve, most often affecting the third cleft, but occasionally affecting the second. There is severe pain that passes into the toes. Palpation between the metatarsal heads may elicit the pain, as may squeezing the forefoot; hyperaesthesia may be present over the nerve distribution.

A **stress fracture of a metatarsal** is traditionally an injury of recent military recruits and is termed a **march fracture** (*Figure 40.11*). It is a fatigue fracture occurring with repetitive stress, that is of an energy level well below that usually required to fracture the bone. There is pain and swelling over the dorsum of the forefoot, and tenderness to palpation of the appropriate metatarsal. As with many stress fractures, early radiographs may show no abnormality but the lesion is demonstrated on isotope bone scanning. After a few weeks the callus may be palpable as well as demonstrable radiologically.

Freiberg's disease (*Figure 40.12*) is avascular necrosis of a metatarsal head, most commonly the second. The condition is comparatively rare and most frequently affects young women. There is initially severe pain on pressure over the affected bone from the dorsal or plantar surface, and later joint stiffness. The abnormality is confirmed radiologically.

Hallux valgus (*Figure 40.13a–c*) is a common problem that is usually acquired, bilateral and found in women, largely as a result of pointed footwear. The valgus deformity of the proximal phalanx is accompanied by some pronation, so that the plantar surface faces laterally; an adventitious bursa (bunion) develops over the medial aspect of the metatarsophalangeal joint. The second toe is displaced dorsally as a hammer toe (see below). The hallux valgus may be symptomatic or asymptomatic and the symptoms may be due to bunion pain because of pressure or infection. Pressure symptoms may also result from compression or over-riding of the second toe. Widening of the forefoot may result in a loss of the transverse arch and there can be associated osteoarthritis over the metatarsophalangeal joint – **hallux rigidus**. Accompanying the valgus great toe is a varus deformity of the first metatarsal – **metatarsal primus varus**. This results in an increased separation between the head of the first and second metatarsals and consequent widening of the forefoot.

Hallux rigidus can result from trauma to the great toe or from a long-standing hallux valgus but is usually idiopathic. Flexion and particularly extension at the metatarsophalangeal joint is reduced and painful when the patient is asked to curl up the toes, and movement of the great toe only occurs at the interphalangeal joint. Osteophytes are prominent over the joint and radiographs confirm the loss of joint space.

A **bunionette** – tailor's bunion – is due to pressure from footwear on the head of the fifth metatarsal and results in

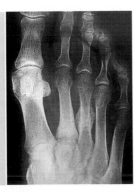

Figure 40.11.
March fracture of the third metatarsal. Repair has often commenced by the time of diagnosis: callus is seen on this radiograph.

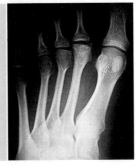

Figure 40.12.
Freiberg's disease. There is ischaemic osteosclerosis of the 1st and 2nd metatarsal bones.

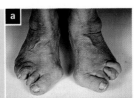

Figure 40.13.
a. Hallux valgus. b. Hallux valgus in a patient with rheumatoid arthritis.
c. Markings added to radiograph to demonstrate the angle of deformity.

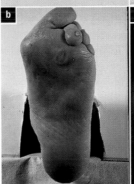

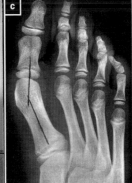

Figure 40.14.
Gouty deformity of the metatar-sophalangeal joints.

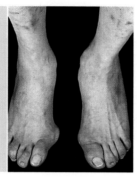

Figure 40.15.
Hammer toe. Displacement secondary to hallux valgus.

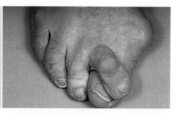

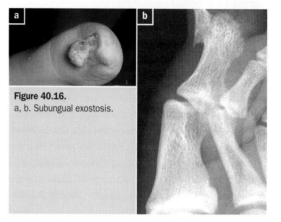

Figure 40.16.
a, b. Subungual exostosis.

inflammation of a bursa developed lateral to the metatar-sophalangeal joint. It is more common in those individuals with a broad forefoot.

Gout *(Figure 40.14)* is a systemic disorder of elevated uric acid levels and most commonly affects the first metatar-sophalangeal joint. There is exquisite tenderness in the joint which is dusky red and swollen; the patient resists any move-ment. The diagnosis is aided by the absence of a bunion, the male predominance and the presence of gouti tophi, usually on the helix of the ear, but also in olecranon bursae and the tendon sheaths of the hands and feet. Blood tests reveal the abnormally high uric acid levels. The intra-articular problem is caused by deposition of urate crystals.

Abnormalities of the sesamoid bones usually involve the medial sesamoid, which causes pain as a result of frac-ture, chondromalacia or osteoarthritis. There is local tender-ness over the involved bone.

Toes

The toes are subject to trauma and pressure effects from shoes. Phalangeal fractures are produced by forceful stub-bing of the toes or crushing with a heavy object; they are usu-ally closed injuries. They are painful and accompanied by bruising and oedema with local tenderness and limitation of movement. The great toe is particularly vulnerable to shoe deformity – hallux valgus, p. 495; infected ingrowing toenail, p. 495 – hallux rigidus and subungual abnormalities.

A **hammer toe** *(Figure 40.15)* usually affects the second toe and is often associated with hallux valgus. The toe is dis-placed dorsally, the metatarsophalangeal joint is hyperex-tended and the proximal interphalangeal joint is flexed. The distal interphalangeal joint may be flexed (claw toe) or extended (hammer toe). Excessive pressure gives rise to

corns and sometimes a bursa on the dorsum of the proximal interphalangeal joint and, with a flexed distal interphalangeal joint, on the tip of the toe. The condition is painful and dis-abling. An **overlapping fifth toe** is a common asymptomatic congenital abnormality; ainhum is considered on p. 109.

The commonest subungual lesion is a pigmented haematoma. The history and diagnosis are not usually in ques-tion, however other unusual conditions can give rise to diag-nostic problems, particularly malignant melanoma (see below). Bacterial infection usually involves the great toe nail (p. 79) but, in fungal discoloration, a number of nails are affected.

A **subungual exostosis** *(Figure 40.16a, b)* becomes apparent beneath the distal half of the nail, which is pushed upward and becomes discoloured. The exostosis can force its way through the nail by breaking or distorting it; it is cov-ered with granulation tissue. The exostosis is painless unless it is traumatized or becomes infected. In the early stages it can be difficult to distinguish from **onychomycosis**, a fungal infection that causes the nail to be discoloured, thickened, brittle and split longitudinally. It can also be mistaken for an ingrowing toenail. The diagnosis is established on a lateral radiograph of the toe.

A **subungual malignant melanoma** is usually misdiag-nosed and mistaken for a subungual haematoma or a fungal infection. There is usually deep pigmentation of the nail bed

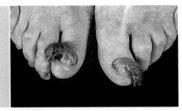

Figure 40.17.
Onychogryphosis.

but a third of lesions are amelanotic. Over the course of some months the proliferation of the lesion causes the nail to be lifted up and avulsed. The growth subsequently ulcerates and can become infected. A biopsy should be taken of all discoloured or undiagnosed lesions of the nail bed.

Junctional naevi may occur and complicate the diagnosis, as can a subungual pyogenic granuloma. A **subungual glomus tumour** is analogous to that occurring beneath the fingernail (p. 456) with similar severe bouts of pain, presenting difficulty in diagnosis. The smaller toenails are more commonly affected. Glomus tumours may also present elsewhere on the foot.

Onychogryphosis – 'ram's horn nail' *(Figure 40.17)* – is a deformed nail, usually of the great toe, following trauma to the nail bed. The nail separates from the underlying tissues and grows as a solid, curled, keratinized horn that causes pain in tight footwear or with secondary trauma or infection.

The heel, sole and superficial tissues

Some abnormalities of the sole have already been considered in flatfoot (p. 492) and pes cavus (p. 492), and the posterior heel has been described on p. 485. The plantar aspect of the heel is subject to disorders of the fat pad and of plantar fasciitis. The sole is susceptible to penetrating injuries and infection (p. 372); the neuropathic foot is at particular risk. Weight bearing and pressure areas develop callosities and corns.

Patients with fat pad atrophy complain of pain in the heel when walking. On examination the central weightbearing area of the heel is tender, and pressure reproduces the pain. The heel pads are soft and atrophic. **Inflammation of the fat pad** presents with pain in the heel on walking. It is often related to high impact activities, prolonged standing or direct trauma. There is tenderness in the central heel area without thinning of the fat pad.

Plantar fasciitis is an inflammatory process due to repetitive stress, predominantly in overweight men. It affects the insertion of the plantar fascia on the medial calcaneal

tuberosity. The patient has pain over the proximal insertion and distally along the plantar fascia; plantar flexion of the toes increases the pain. Note that heel spurs were previously implicated as a cause of this problem but it is now recognized that they are a coincidental finding.

A **callosity** is an area of hardened and thickened skin that occurs as a normal reaction when intermittent pressure is distributed over a reasonably large area. At the periphery, cornified skin ceases abruptly where it is continuous with normal skin. Callosities appear where the skin is normally thick, most frequently on the soles beneath the heads of one or more metatarsals, around the heel and on the inframedial side of the great toe. They are never present on the dorsum of the foot but may occur on the outer border of the foot in uncorrected talipes equinovarus.

A **hard corn** occurs when there is intermittent pressure over a very small area. There is a conical wedge of highly compressed keratotic epithelial cells and pressure on the corn is usually painful. There is a central core of white appearance composed of degenerate cells and cholesterol, encircled by a narrow area of keratotis that disappears gradually at the periphery. Palpation reveals the causative bony projection beneath the cutaneous lesion which occurs chiefly where the normal skin is thin; it is therefore found particularly on the fifth toe and over the dorsal projections of hammer toes.

A **soft corn** *(Figure 40.18)* occurs between the toes, where maceration of the skin takes place. It most commonly occurs between the fourth and fifth toes where opposing prominent bony projections of the bases of the proximal phalanges give rise to pressure and friction. Soft corns are particularly painful and are often mistaken for plantar warts (p. 80).

Neuropathic ulcers *(Figure 40.19)* most commonly occur over the metatarsal heads, particularly the first and the fifth. Diabetic neuropathy (p. 371), spinal disease or injury, and sciatic nerve palsies are potential causes. The foot has areas of anaesthesia and ulcers are associated with thick callosities. The distinction should be made between the ulcer and pregangrenous changes of toes due to vascular disease, where the pedal pulses are lost.

Figure 40.18.
Soft corn.

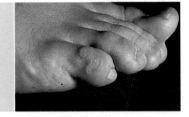

Figure 40.19.
Perforating ulcers in a neuropathic foot, secondary to diabetes.

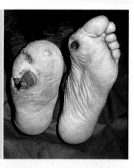

Figure 40.21.
Squamous cell carcinoma of the heel.

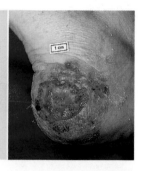

Figure 40.20.
Benign tumour of the foot.

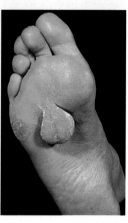

Figure 40.22.
Radionecrotic ulcer following treatment of a Kaposi's sarcoma of the sole.

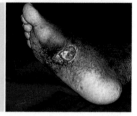

The superficial tissues of the foot are subject to the skin and subcutaneous lesions occurring elsewhere in the body (*Figure 40.20*) but of particular note are ganglia over the dorsum and cutaneous malignancies of the sole. Ganglia arise on the dorsum of the foot, particularly around the tarsus. They have the same clinical features as ganglia of the hand and wrist (p. 451) but are less common.

Malignant melanoma of the foot is uncommon but most often occurs on the instep. The lesions usually have pigmentation as a distinguishing feature but may go unnoticed until ulceration occurs. When suspected, the groin nodes and the liver must be examined. **Squamous cell carcinoma of the foot** (*Figure 40.21*) occurs over the weight-bearing areas of the foot and rapidly infiltrates the deep tissues. Other rare malignancies are occasionally encountered (*Figure 40.22*).

Index

Note: Figures and Tables are shown in *italics*. Where text occurs on the same page as the Figure and/or Table, the page number is given in roman; where reference is to the illustration alone, the page number is given in italic.